Cawson's Essentials of
Oral Pathology *and* Oral Medicine

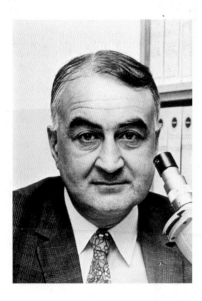

Professor Roderick A. Cawson

BDS, FDSRCS, LMSSA, MB BS, MD, FRCPath
1921–2007

For Elsevier
Commissioning Editor: *Alison Taylor*
Development Editor: *Veronika Watkins/Katie Golsby*
Project Manager: *Andrew Riley*
Designer: *Christian Bilbow*
Illustrator Manager: *Karen Giacomucci*

Ninth Edition

Cawson's Essentials of
Oral Pathology *and*
Oral Medicine

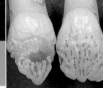

E.W. Odell

FDSRCS MSc PhD FRCPath

Professor of Oral Pathology and Medicine,
King's College London
Honorary Consultant in Oral Pathology,
Guy's and St Thomas' NHS
Foundation Trust, London

ELSEVIER

ELSEVIER

First edition 1962
Second edition 1968
Third edition 1978
Fourth edition 1984
Fifth edition 1991
Sixth edition 1998
Seventh edition 2002
Eighth edition 2008
Ninth edition 2017

ISBN 978-0-7020-4982-8
International Edition 9780702049811

Notices

Knowledge and best practice in this field are constantly changing. As new research and experience broaden our understanding, changes in research methods, professional practices, or medical treatment may become necessary.

Practitioners and researchers must always rely on their own experience and knowledge in evaluating and using any information, methods, compounds, or experiments described herein. In using such information or methods they should be mindful of their own safety and the safety of others, including parties for whom they have a professional responsibility.

With respect to any drug or pharmaceutical products identified, readers are advised to check the most current information provided (i) on procedures featured or (ii) by the manufacturer of each product to be administered, to verify the recommended dose or formula, the method and duration of administration, and contraindications. It is the responsibility of practitioners, relying on their own experience and knowledge of their patients, to make diagnoses, to determine dosages and the best treatment for each individual patient, and to take all appropriate safety precautions.

To the fullest extent of the law, neither the Publisher nor the authors, contributors, or editors, assume any liability for any injury and/or damage to persons or property as a matter of products liability, negligence or otherwise, or from any use or operation of any methods, products, instructions, or ideas contained in the material herein.

 ELSEVIER your source for books,
journals and multimedia
in the health sciences

www.elsevierhealth.com

  **Working together
to grow libraries in
developing countries**

www.elsevier.com • www.bookaid.org

The publisher's
policy is to use
**paper manufactured
from sustainable forests**

Printed in China

Contents

Preface   xv
References   xvii

1   **Principles of investigation, diagnosis and treatment**   1
   Taking a history   1
     Consent   5
   Clinical examination   6
   Medical examination   8
   Clinical differential diagnosis   8
   Investigations   9
     Imaging   9
     Histopathology   10
     Laboratory procedures   14
     Molecular biological tests   15
     Haematology, clinical chemistry and serology   18
     Microbiology   18
     Other clinical tests   20
     Interpreting investigations and making a diagnosis and treatment plan   20

SECTION 1: Hard tissue pathology   23

2   **Disorders of tooth development**   23
   Abnormalities in the number of teeth   23
     Anodontia and oligodontia   23
     Additional teeth: hyperdontia   24
     Syndromes associated with hyperdontia   25
   Defective enamel formation   25
     Defects of deciduous teeth   25
     Defects of permanent teeth   25
     Amelogenesis imperfecta   25
     Chronological hypoplasia   29
     Molar-incisor hypomineralisation   30
   Defective dentine formation   30
     Osteogenesis imperfecta with opalescent teeth   31
     Dentinogenesis imperfecta   31
     Dentinal dysplasia ('rootless' teeth)   32

   Defects of enamel and dentine   33
     Regional odontodysplasia (ghost teeth)   33
     Segmental odontomaxillary dysplasia   34
   Other systemic diseases affecting teeth   35
   Extrinsic agents affecting teeth   37
   Odontomes   41
   Disorders of eruption   42

3   **Disorders of development**   45
   Clefts of lip or palate   45
     Cleft lip and cleft palate   45
     Isolated cleft palate   48
     Syndromic cleft lip and palate   48
   Other facial clefts   48
   Stafne's idiopathic bone cavity   49
   Hereditary prognathism   49
   Ankyloglossia   49
   Cowden's syndrome   50
   Other craniofacial malformations   50

4   **Dental caries**   53
   Aetiology   53
   Bacterial plaque   53
   Microbiology   54
   Sucrose   57
   Susceptibility of teeth to caries   59
   Saliva and dental caries   60
   Pathology of enamel caries   61
   Pathology of dentine caries   65
   Clinical aspects of caries pathology   68
     Arrested caries and remineralisation   68
     Caries in deciduous teeth   69
     Hidden caries   70
     Root surface caries   70
     Clinical aspects of reactions to caries   70

5   **Pulpitis and apical periodontitis**   73
   Pulpitis   73
   Pulp calcifications   77
   Periapical periodontitis, abscess and granuloma   77
   Acute apical periodontitis   78
     Pathology and sequelae   78

Acute apical (dentoalveolar) abscess 79
Chronic apical periodontitis and periapical granuloma 81

6 Tooth wear, resorption, hypercementosis and osseointegration 85
Tooth wear 85
   Attrition 85
   Abrasion 85
   Erosion 86
   Abfraction 87
Bruxism 87
Resorption of teeth 88
Hypercementosis 91
Pathology of osseointegration 91

7 Gingival and periodontal diseases 95
The normal periodontal tissues 95
   Gingival and periodontal fibres 96
   Gingival crevicular fluid (exudate) 96
Classification of periodontal diseases 96
Chronic gingivitis 96
Chronic periodontitis 99
   Pathology 101
   Systemic predisposing factors 103
   General principles of management of chronic periodontitis 105
   Complications of chronic periodontitis 106
Gingival recession 107
Aggressive periodontitis 108
'Prepubertal' periodontitis 109
Periodontitis as a manifestation of systemic disease 109
   Down's syndrome 109
   Papillon–lefèvre syndrome 110
Periodontal (lateral) abscess 110
Acute pericoronitis 110
Acute necrotising ulcerative gingivitis 112
HIV-associated periodontitis 113
Gingival enlargement 113
   Hereditary gingival fibromatosis 113
   Drug-induced gingival overgrowth 114
Localised juvenile spongiotic gingivitis 115
Plasminogen deficiency gingivitis 115
Other inflammatory gingival swellings 115

8 Infections of the jaws 117
Normal healing of an extraction socket 117
Alveolar osteitis 117
Osteomyelitis of the jaws 120
Acute osteomyelitis 120
Chronic osteomyelitis 122
Diffuse sclerosing osteomyelitis 123
Chronic low-grade focal osteomyelitis and sclerosing osteitis 124
Osteoradionecrosis 124
Proliferative periostitis 125
Medication-related osteonecrosis of the jaws (MRONJ) 125
Traumatic sequestrum 127
Sclerotic bone islands 128

9 Major infections of the mouth and face 129
Periapical (dentoalveolar) abscess 129
Collateral oedema 129
'Fascial' or tissue space infections 129
Facial cellulitis 130
Facial abscess 132
Antibiotic abscess 133
Necrotising fasciitis 133
Cavernous sinus thrombosis 133
Noma (cancrum oris, necrotising stomatitis) 134
Actinomycosis 135
   Other 'actinomycoses' 136
The systemic mycoses 136
Systemic infections by oral bacteria 137

10 Cysts in and around the jaws 139
Classification of cysts 139
Common features of jaw cysts 140
Treatment of jaw cysts 141
Treatment of soft tissue cysts 142
Odontogenic cysts 142
   Radicular cyst 142
   Lateral radicular cyst 146
   Residual radicular cyst 146
   Inflammatory collateral cysts 146
   Dentigerous cysts 146
   Eruption cyst 148
   Odontogenic keratocyst 149
     Basal cell naevus syndrome 153
   Orthokeratinised odontogenic cyst 154

Lateral periodontal cysts 155
   Botryoid odontogenic cysts 155
Glandular odontogenic cyst 156
Calcifying odontogenic cyst 156
Carcinoma arising in odontogenic cysts 157
Gingival cyst of the newborn 157
Gingival cyst of adults 158
Non-odontogenic cysts 158
   Nasopalatine duct or incisive canal cyst 158
   Nasolabial cyst 160
   Sublingual dermoid cyst 160
   Thyroglossal duct cyst 161
   Branchial cyst 161
   Foregut cyst 162
Other cysts in other chapters 162

11 Odontogenic tumours and related jaw lesions **165**
Benign epithelial tumours 165
   Ameloblastomas 165
   Desmoplastic ameloblastoma 168
   Metastasising ameloblastoma 169
   Unicystic ameloblastoma 169
   Squamous odontogenic tumour 170
   Calcifying epithelial odontogenic tumour ... 170
   Adenomatoid odontogenic tumour 172
Benign epithelial and mesenchymal tumours ... 172
   Ameloblastic fibroma 172
   Ameloblastic fibrodentinoma and fibro-odontome 173
   Primordial odontogenic tumour 173
   Odontomes (odontomas*) 173
      Compound odontome 174
      Complex odontome 174
      Other types of odontome 175
Calcifying odontogenic cyst 176
Dentinogenic ghost cell tumour 176
Benign mesenchymal tumours 176
   Odontogenic fibroma 177
      Granular cell odontogenic tumour 177
   Odontogenic myxoma 177
      Normal dental follicle 178
   Cementoblastoma 178
      'Cementomas' 179

Fibroosseous odontogenic lesions 179
Cemento-ossifying fibromas 180
   Cemento-ossifying fibroma 180
   Juvenile ossifying fibroma 181
   Multiple and syndromic cemento-osseous fibromas 181
Cemento-osseous dysplasias 181
   Periapical cemental dysplasia 181
   Florid cemento-osseous dysplasia 182
   Focal cemento-osseous dysplasia 182
   Familial gigantiform cementoma 182
Malignant odontogenic tumours 183

12 Non-odontogenic tumours of the jaws ... **187**
Exostoses and tori 187
Osteochondroma 187
Central giant cell granuloma 188
   Noonan and other syndromes 190
Langerhans cell histiocytosis 190
Osteomas 192
   Gardner's syndrome 192
Ossifying fibromas 193
   Psammomatoid ossifying fibroma 193
Haemangioma of bone 194
Melanotic neuroectodermal tumour of infancy 195
Malignant neoplasms of bone 196
   Osteosarcoma 196
   Chondrosarcoma 197
   Ewing's sarcoma 198
   Myeloma 199
      Amyloidosis 200
   Solitary plasmacytoma 200
Lymphomas 200
Metastases to the jaws 200

13 Genetic, metabolic and other non-neoplastic bone diseases **205**
Genetic diseases of bone 205
   Osteogenesis imperfecta 205
   Gnathodiaphyseal dysplasia 207
   Osteopetrosis: marble bone disease 207
   Achondroplasia 207
   Cleidocranial dysplasia 208
   Cherubism 208
   Hypophosphatasia 209

Sickle cell anaemia and thalassaemia 210
Gigantism and acromegaly 211
Metabolic bone disease 211
Rickets 211
Vitamin D–resistant rickets 211
Hyperparathyroidism 211
Other bone diseases 213
Paget's disease of bone 213
Fibro-osseous lesions 216
Fibrous dysplasia 216
Monostotic fibrous dysplasia 216
Polyostotic fibrous dysplasia 218
Albright's syndrome 218
Osseous dysplasias 218
Bone 'cysts' 218
Solitary bone 'cyst' 218
Aneurysmal bone 'cyst' 220
Osteoporotic bone marrow defect 221

14 Disorders of the temporomandibular joints and trismus **223**
Temporary limitation of movement 223
Infection and inflammation 223
Injuries 223
Drugs 224
Persistent limitation of movement: extracapsular causes 224
Irradiation 224
Oral submucous fibrosis 224
Systemic sclerosis and scleroderma 224
CREST syndrome 225
Morphoea 225
Persistent limitation of movement: intracapsular causes 226
Arthritis 226
Rheumatoid arthritis 226
Osteoarthritis 227
Other types of arthritis 228
Condylar hyperplasia 228
Neoplasms 229
Synovial chondromatosis and loose bodies in the temporomandibular joints 229
Limitation of movement: muscle causes 229
TMJ pain dysfunction 'syndrome' 229

Giant cell arteritis (temporal arteritis) 231
Polymyalgia rheumatica 232
Tetanus and tetany 232
Pain referred to the joint 232
Dislocation 232
Ehlers–Danlos syndrome 233

SECTION 2: Soft tissue disease **235**

15 Diseases of the oral mucosa: mucosal infections **235**
Ulcers 235
Herpesvirus diseases 235
Primary herpetic stomatitis 235
Herpes labialis 238
Herpetic whitlow 239
Herpes zoster of the trigeminal nerve 239
Ramsay Hunt syndrome 240
Cytomegalovirus ulcers 240
Hand-foot-and-mouth disease 240
Herpangina 241
Measles 241
Chicken pox 241
Tuberculosis 242
Syphilis 242
Candidosis 244
Thrush 244
Angular cheilitis 246
Erythematous candidosis 246
Acute antibiotic stomatitis 246
Median rhomboid glossitis 247
Denture-induced stomatitis 248
Chronic hyperplastic candidosis 249
Chronic mucocutaneous candidosis syndromes 250

16 Diseases of the oral mucosa: non-infective stomatitis **255**
Ulcers 255
Traumatic ulcers 255
Eosinophilic ulcer (atypical or traumatic eosinophilic granuloma) 255
Factitious ulceration (self-inflicted oral ulcers) 255
Recurrent aphthous stomatitis 256

Behçet's disease 259
HIV-associated oral ulcers 261
Nicorandil-induced ulcers 261
Lichen planus and similar conditions 261
'Desquamative gingivitis' 262
Lichen planus 262
Vulvovaginal-gingival syndrome 267
Malignant change in lichen planus 267
Lichenoid reactions 268
Lichenoid drug reactions 268
Topical lichenoid reactions 268
Graft-versus-host disease 269
Lupus erythematosus 269
Chronic ulcerative stomatitis 270
Immunobullous disease 271
Pemphigus vulgaris 271
Paraneoplastic pemphigus 273
Mucous membrane pemphigoid 273
Erythema multiforme 275
Stevens Johnson syndrome 277
Toothpaste-induced epithelial peeling 277
Other mucosal allergic responses 277
Oral signs in reactive arthritis 277
Mucocutaneous lymph node syndrome
(Kawasaki's disease) 278
Miscellaneous mucosal ulcers 279
Wegener's granulomatosis 279
Oral reactions to drugs 279
Uncommon mucocutaneous diseases 279

17 **Tongue disorders** 283
Normal structures 283
Furred tongue 283
Foliate papillae 283
Lingual varicosities 283
Erythema migrans 283
Lingual papillitis 284
Hairy tongue and black hairy tongue 284
Glossitis 285
Anaemic glossitis 285
Glossodynia and the sore, physically
normal tongue 287
Macroglossia 287
Amyloidosis 287
Other diseases affecting the tongue 289

18 **Benign chronic white mucosal
lesions** 291
Fordyce spots 291
Leukoedema 292
Frictional keratosis 292
Cheek and tongue biting 293
Stomatitis nicotina 293
Oral hairy leukoplakia 294
White sponge naevus 295
Candidosis 296
Oral keratosis of renal failure 296
Skin grafts 296
Psoriasis 297
Other white lesions 297

19 **Potentially malignant disorders** 299
Terminology 299
Field change 299
Erythroplakia 300
Speckled leukoplakia 300
Leukoplakia 300
Proliferative verrucous leukoplakia 302
Smokeless tobacco-induced
keratoses 302
Chronic hyperplastic candidosis 304
Oral submucous fibrosis 304
Lichen planus 305
Lupus erythematosus 306
Dyskeratosis congenita 306
HPV-associated dysplasia 306
Syphilitic leukoplakia 306
Management of dysplastic lesions 307
Smoking cessation 312

20 **Oral cancer** 317
Epidemiology 317
Aetiology 318
'Early' and 'late' oral carcinoma 321
Oral cancer distribution 322
Pathology 322
Management 326
Role of the dentist 331
Oral cancer screening 332
Screening and detection aids 333
Verrucous carcinoma 333
Diagnostic catches 334

ix

21 Other mucosal and lip carcinomas 335
Lip carcinoma 335
Human papillomavirus–associated
oropharyngeal carcinomas 335
Nasopharyngeal carcinoma 339
Pseudocarcinomas and diagnostic catches 339

**22 Non-neoplastic diseases of salivary
glands** 341
Duct obstruction 341
Salivary calculi 341
Salivary duct strictures 342
Mucoceles and salivary cysts 342
Sialadenitis 344
Mumps 344
Bacterial parotitis 344
Chronic sialadenitis 345
Xerostomia 345
Sjögren's syndrome 346
Complications 349
HIV-associated salivary gland disease 350
IgG$_4$ sclerosing disease 350
Necrotising sialometaplasia 350
Sarcoidosis 350
Sialadenosis 350
Other salivary gland disorders 351
Hypersalivation (sialorrhoea or ptyalism) 352

23 Salivary gland neoplasms 355
Salivary gland neoplasms 355
Benign tumours 357
Pleomorphic adenoma 357
Warthin's tumour 358
Canalicular adenoma 359
Basal cell adenoma 359
Oncocytoma 359
Malignant salivary gland tumours 359
Mucoepidermoid carcinoma 360
Adenoid cystic carcinoma 361
Acinic cell carcinoma 362
Secretory carcinoma 362
Polymorphous adenocarcinoma 362
Salivary duct carcinoma 363
Epithelial-myoepithelial carcinoma 363
Undifferentiated carcinomas 363
Carcinoma ex pleomorphic adenoma 363

Adenocarcinoma not otherwise specified 363
Other epithelial lesions 363
Metastatic neoplasms 364
Non-epithelial tumours 364
Intraosseous salivary gland tumours 365
Tumour-like salivary gland swellings 365

24 Benign mucosal swellings 369
Fibroepithelial polyp, epulis and
denture-induced granuloma 369
Papillary hyperplasia of the palate 370
Pyogenic granuloma and pregnancy epulis 371
Giant-cell epulis 371
Papillomas 373
Squamous cell papilloma 374
Infective warts (verruca vulgaris) 374
Multifocal epithelial hyperplasia 374
Verruciform xanthoma 375
Calibre-persistent artery 375
Cosmetic implants 376

25 Soft tissue tumours 377
Benign tumours 377
Benign nerve sheath tumours 377
Lipoma and fibrolipoma 377
Granular cell tumour 378
Congenital (granular cell) epulis 378
Haemangiomas 379
Lymphangiomas 380
Malignant connective tissue tumours 380
Rhabdomyosarcoma 380
Sarcomas of fibroblasts 380
Kaposi's sarcoma 380

26 Oral pigmented lesions 383
Diffuse mucosal pigmentation 383
Localised melanin pigmentation 383
Physiological pigmentation 384
Melanotic macules 384
Oral melanotic macules associated with
HIV infection 384
Oral melanocytic naevi 384
Melanoacanthoma 385
Post-inflammatory pigmentation 385
Syndromes with oral pigmentation 385
Other localised pigmented lesions 386
Amalgam and other tattoos 386

Lead line and heavy metal poisoning 387
Soft tissue pigmentation 387
Melanoma 388

SECTION 3: Systemic disease in dentistry 391

27 Anaemias, leukaemias and lymphomas 391
Anaemia 391
Sickle cell disease and sickle cell trait 392
The thalassaemias 393
Leukaemia 393
   Acute leukaemia 393
   Chronic leukaemia 394
Lymphomas 394
   Hodgkin's lymphoma 395
   Non-Hodgkin lymphomas 395
   Burkitt's lymphoma 395
   MALT lymphoma 396
   Nasopharyngeal extranodal NK/T-cell lymphoma 396
   Other types of lymphoma 397
Leucopenia and agranulocytosis 397
   Aplastic anaemia 398
   Agranulocytosis 398
   Cyclic neutropenia 398

28 Haemorrhagic disorders 399
Preoperative investigation 399
Management of prolonged dental bleeding 399
Blood vessel abnormalities 399
   Hereditary haemorrhagic telangiectasia 399
   Angina bullosa haemorrhagica 400
Purpura and platelet disorders 401
Clotting disorders 402
   Haemophilia A 402
   Christmas disease (haemophilia B) 403
   Acquired clotting defects 403
Combined bleeding disorders 404
   Von Willebrand's disease 404
   Disseminated intravascular coagulation 404
Plasminogen deficiency 404

29 Immunodeficiency 407
Selective IgA deficiency 407
C1 esterase inhibitor deficiency 408

Leukopenia and agranulocytosis 408
Immunosuppressive treatment 408
   Bone marrow transplantation 408
   Graft-versus-host disease 408
Other organ transplants 408
HIV infection and AIDS 408
Oral lesions in HIV infection 411
   Candidosis 412
   Viral mucosal infections 413
   Bacterial infections 413
   Systemic mycoses 413
   Malignant neoplasms 413
   Lymphadenopathy 414
   Autoimmune disease 414
   Gingivitis and periodontitis 414
   Salivary gland disease 414
   Miscellaneous oral lesions 415
   Oral adverse effects of HAART 416
Risks of transmission of HIV infection 416

30 Allergy, autoimmune and autoinflammatory disease 419
Allergic or hypersensitivity reactions 419
   Atopy 419
   Contact dermatitis 419
   Latex allergy 420
   Allergy to local anaesthetic 421
   Asthma 422
   Other type 1 reactions 422
Mucosal allergic responses 422
   Oral allergy 'syndrome' 422
   Allergy to metals 422
Angio-oedema 423
Autoimmune diseases 423
   The connective tissue diseases 424
   Rheumatoid arthritis 424
   Sjögren's syndrome 424
   Systemic lupus erythematosus 424
   Systemic sclerosis (scleroderma) 425
Autoinflammatory diseases 425
   Sarcoidosis 425

31 Cervical lymphadenopathy 429
Tuberculous cervical lymphadenopathy 430
Atypical mycobacterial infection 431
Sarcoidosis 431

Syphilis	432
Cat-scratch disease	432
Lyme disease	432
Infectious mononucleosis	432
Acquired immune deficiency syndrome	433
Toxoplasmosis	433
Mucocutaneous lymph node syndrome	433
Langerhans cell histiocytosis	434
Sinus histiocytosis with massive lymphadenopathy	434
Castleman's disease	434
Drug-associated lymphadenopathy	435
Virchow's node	435
Delphian node	436

32 Cardiovascular disease — **437**
General aspects of management	437
Infective endocarditis	438
Prevention of endocarditis	439
Implanted cardiac devices	441

33 Respiratory tract disease — **443**
Acute sinusitis	443
Chronic sinusitis	443
Odontogenic sinusitis	444
Fungal sinusitis	444
Allergic fungal sinusitis	444
Invasive fungal sinusitis	445
Surgical damage to the maxillary antrum	445
Displacement of a root or tooth into the maxillary antrum	445
Oroantral communication	445
Aspiration of a tooth, root or instrument	446
Tuberculosis	446
Chronic obstructive airways disease	447
Asthma	447
Midfacial destructive lesions	447
Wegener's granulomatosis	447
Carcinoma of the antrum	448
Cystic fibrosis (mucoviscidosis)	449
Sleep apnoea syndrome	449
Bronchogenic carcinoma	449

34 Gastrointestinal and liver disease — **451**
Gastro-oesophageal reflux and gastric regurgitation	451

Coeliac disease	451
Crohn's disease	451
Orofacial granulomatosis	453
Malabsorption syndromes	453
Ulcerative colitis	453
Intestinal polyposis syndromes	454
Antibiotic-associated colitis	454
Liver disease	454
Viral hepatitis	455
Hepatitis A	455
Hepatitis E	455
Hepatitis B	455
Hepatitis D: the delta agent	457
Hepatitis C	457
Control of transmission of viral hepatitis	458

35 Nutritional deficiencies — **461**
Vitamin deficiencies	461
Vitamin A deficiency	461
Riboflavin (B_2) deficiency	461
Nicotinamide deficiency	461
Vitamin B_{12} deficiency	461
Folic acid deficiency	461
Vitamin C deficiency	461
Vitamin D deficiency	462

36 Endocrine disorders and pregnancy — **463**
Pituitary gigantism and acromegaly	463
Thyroid disease	464
Hyperthyroidism	464
Hypothyroidism	464
Lingual thyroid	464
Parathyroid disease	465
Hyperparathyroidism	465
Hypoparathyroidism	466
Pseudohypoparathyroidism	466
Adrenocortical diseases	466
Adrenocortical hypofunction or Addison's disease	466
Adrenocortical hyperfunction	467
Autoimmune polyendocrine syndromes	467
Diseases of the adrenal medulla	467
Phaeochromocytoma	467
Multiple endocrine neoplasia syndromes	468
Diabetes mellitus	468
Pregnancy	469

37 Renal disease	471
Chronic renal failure and dialysis	471
Renal transplantation	471

38 Pain and neurological disorders	473
Dental and periodontal pain	473
Pain in edentulous patients	474
Painful mucosal lesions	475
Pain in the jaws	475
Postsurgical pain and nerve damage	475
Pain induced by mastication	475
Pain from salivary glands	476
Neuralgia and neuropathy	476
Trigeminal neuralgia	476
Trigeminal neuralgia in multiple sclerosis	477
Trigeminal neuropathy	477
Glossopharyngeal neuralgia	477
Postherpetic neuralgia	478
Bell's palsy	478
Burning mouth 'syndrome'	478
Atypical facial pain	479
Atypical odontalgia	479
Paraesthesia of the lower lip	479
Facial palsy	480
Bell's palsy	480
Melkersson–Rosenthal syndrome	481
Other causes of facial palsy	482
Headache	482
Migraine	482
Migrainous neuralgia (cluster headache)	482
Intracranial tumours	483
Disturbances of taste and smell	483
Epilepsy	484

39 Physical and learning disability	487
UK discrimination legislation	488
Learning disability	488
Down's syndrome	489
Fragile X syndrome	490
Other chromosomal abnormalities	490
Behavioural disorders	491
Autism	491
Attention deficit hyperactivity disorder	491
Physical impairments	491
Cerebral palsy	491
Multiple sclerosis	492

Hydrocephalus	493
Spina bifida	493
The muscular dystrophies	493
Myasthenia gravis	493

40 Mental health disorders	495
Pain without medical cause	495
Anxiety disorders	496
Depression	496
Anorexia nervosa and bulimia nervosa	497
Psychoses and schizophrenia	497

41 Dentistry and elderly patients	499
Dementia	499
Other systemic diseases	500
Oral disease in the elderly	501

42 Complications of systemic drug treatment	503
Local analgesics with vasoconstrictors	505
Chemical dependence	505

43 Medical emergencies	507
Sudden loss of consciousness	507
Fainting	507
Acute hypoglycaemia	508
Anaphylactic reactions	508
Cardiac arrest	509
Strokes	510
Circulatory collapse in patients on corticosteroid treatment	510
Chest pain	511
Angina pectoris	511
Myocardial infarction	511
Respiratory difficulty	512
Severe asthma and status asthmaticus	512
Left ventricular failure	512
Convulsions	512
Epilepsy	512
Other emergencies	513
Haemorrhage	513
Violence	513

SECTION 4: Learning guide and self-assessment questions 515

44 Learning guide	515
Self-assessment questions	521
Index	529

Preface

It is interesting to see how this book has evolved over the last 50 years or more. The first edition was the first book to integrate oral medicine, pathology and surgery in a practical, student-orientated fashion. It was truly a book of essentials and was correspondingly small and concise. However, like all textbooks it has grown, fulfilling different functions from those originally envisaged.

The world into which this edition will be launched is very different from that of the last. The ready availability of information on the Internet, changing needs of students and innovative dental curricula have all had an impact. Though this edition contains more facts, its larger size is accounted for by considerably more explanation than previously included. This is intended to meet the higher-level understanding and application of knowledge required of students today.

The demise of the textbook has been long predicted, ever since the Internet was launched. My work on this edition reinforces my belief that the textbook accomplishes something the Internet is incapable of providing. In completely revising this text I have searched the Internet using the standard search engines and open access sources. I have been more than disappointed. Although a few sources provide accurate and up to date information, the majority of easily found Internet resources provide the opposite. Search engine results frequently offer websites with plagiarised and out of date information, fake and predatory open access journals with material that has not been properly peer reviewed, and images of misdiagnosed diseases. The textbook provides a repository of information that is subject to the author's professional scrutiny and comes with context and explanation. There is no comparison.

I hope students will like my attempt to provide more accessible sources to read up on the diseases that interest them. Lists of further reading have been dropped; I doubt they were much used, if at all. There are now PubMed ID references and websites provided where they are immediately relevant. Putting these numbers directly into a search engine will take the reader directly to a selected information source, from where further references can be trusted.

My thanks are due to Veronika Watkins, Alison Taylor, Clive Hewat, Christian Bilbow, and all the team at Elsevier for maintaining the excellent production standards of previous editions.

Producing a new edition such as this takes many hundreds of hours of intensive work, and I am grateful to my colleagues at work for their forbearance but most of all to my wonderful wife Wendy who has supported me unconditionally and maintained her sense of humour during the many months I spent in front of my computer.

E.W.O.
London 2017

References

References to further reading are now inserted throughout, immediately adjacent to the relevant text. To make searching for web URLs straightforward, links to the relevant websites can be found at http://sites.elsevier.com/cawsonsessentials. Various types of reference are provided, all designed to be immediately available through the internet. In the electronic version of this book they are direct links:

PubMed ID: These are shown with a few words of description and a number in the format PMID: 25556809. Entering the text PMID and number into an Internet search engine should take the reader direct to the reference. Alternatively, it can be entered direct into the PubMed website at http://www.ncbi.nlm.nih.gov/pubmed/ and this has the advantage of immediately showing the abstract and links to the full text of the article. References have been selected to be open access full text publications where possible, but it may be necessary to log in to publishers' websites or access through an institution library to obtain the full text. Use the references in these papers to direct onward reading.

PubMed Central ID: These are shown with a similar few words of description and a number in the format PMCID: PMC4334280. They can be resolved in the same way as above. If searching on the PubMed website itself, do not forget to select PMC in the window to the left of the search box.

ISBN numbers: These are ISBN13 codes to books in the format ISBN-13: 978-0723435938. The numbers can be entered either into a search engine, although a search in the website of an online bookseller or your university library will take you directly to the book title and a copy. Where possible, books available in electronic format have been selected.

Web Uniform Resource Locators URLs or web addresses. These may be entered directly into the address bar of a web browser. Some are long and complex and case sensitive. To avoid this, some are given just as the home page of an organisation with instructions on text words to enter into the search box. These should find the relevant resource directly.

DOI: Digital Object Indentifiers can be resolved at the DOI website https://www.doi.org/

Principles of investigation, diagnosis and treatment

The principles of patient investigation and diagnosis are summarised in Box 1.1.

TAKING A HISTORY

Taking a history and making a diagnosis are not completely generic skills that can be learned and then applied to any patient. Skills of gaining rapport, listening and questioning are always applicable, but to ask targeted incisive questions requires knowledge of disease. Effective history-taking and diagnosis of medical conditions are therefore founded in pathological knowledge.

Rapport is critical for eliciting useful information, and gaining rapport must take into account that almost all patients are nervous to a degree, some are inarticulate, and others are confused. History-taking needs to be tailored to the individual patient.

Initial questions should allow patients to speak at some length and to gain confidence. It is usually best to start with an 'open' question (Tables 1.1 and 1.2). Medical jargon should be avoided, because even regular hospital attenders who appear to understand medical terminology may use it wrongly and misunderstand. When a patient uses technical jargon, it is wise to check what they mean by it. Leading questions, which suggest a particular answer, should be avoided because patients may feel compelled to agree with the clinician.

It is sometimes difficult to avoid interrupting patients when trying to structure the history for the records. Structure can only be given after the patient has had time to give the information. Constant note-taking while patients are speaking is undesirable. Notes should be a summary of relevant information only.

Questioning technique is most critical when eliciting any relevant social or psychological history or dealing with embarrassing medical conditions. It may be appropriate to delay asking such questions until after rapport has been gained. Some patients do not consider medical questions to be the concern of the dentist, and it is important to give reasons for such questions when necessary.

During history-taking, the mental and emotional state of the patient should be assessed. This may have a bearing on some diseases and will also suggest what the patient expects to gain from the consultation and treatment. If the patient's expectations are unreasonable, it is important to try to modify them during the consultation, otherwise no reassurance or treatment may be satisfactory (Box 1.2).

Box 1.1 Principles of investigation and diagnosis

- A detailed medical and dental history
- Clinical examination
  - Extraoral
  - Intraoral
- Investigations selected for specific purposes
  - Testing vitality of teeth
  - Radiography or other imaging techniques
  - Biopsy for histopathology (including immunofluorescence, immunocytochemistry, molecular biological tests)
  - Specimens for microbial culture
  - Haematological or biochemical tests

Table 1.1 Types of questions

Type of question	Example
Open	Tell me about the pain.
Closed	What does the pain feel like?
Leading	Does the pain feel like an electric shock?

Table 1.2 Advantages and disadvantages of types of question

Types of question	Advantages	Disadvantages
Open	Allows patients to use their own words and summarise their view of the problem Allows patients partly to direct the history-taking, gives them confidence and quickly generates rapport	Clinicians must listen carefully and avoid interruptions to extract the relevant information Patients tend to decide what information is relevant
Closed	Elicits specific information quickly Useful to fill gaps in the information given in response to open questions Prevents vague patients from rambling away from the complaint	Patients may infer that the clinician is not really interested in their problem if only closed questions are asked Important information may be lost if not specifically requested Restricts the patient's opportunities to talk

Box 1.2 Essential principles of history-taking

- Introduce yourself and greet the patient by name
- Be culturally aware
- Act courteously and respectfully, maintain professional detachment
- Put patients at their ease, be empathic
- Start with an open question
- Mix open and closed questions
- Avoid leading questions
- Avoid medical and dental jargon and idiomatic expressions
- Listen 'actively'
- Explain the need for specific questions if asked
- Divide the consultation into manageable sections for the patient
- Summarise your findings back to the patient for confirmation of meaning
- Assess the patient's mental state
- Assess the patient's expectations from treatment

Box 1.3 History of the present complaint

- Record the description of the complaint *in the patient's own words*
- Elicit the exact meaning of those words
- Record the duration and the time course of any changes in symptoms or signs
- Include any relevant facts in the patient's medical history
- Note any temporal relationship between them and the present complaint
- Consider any previous treatments and their effectiveness
- Check previous investigations to avoid their unnecessary repetition

Table 1.3 Features required in a pain history

Characteristic	Informative features
Character	Ache, tenderness, dull pain, throbbing, stabbing, electric shock. These terms are of limited use, but information on the constancy of pain is useful
Severity	Mild – responds to mild analgesics (e.g. aspirin/paracetamol) Moderate – unresponsive to mild analgesics Severe – disturbs sleep
Duration	Time since onset. Duration of pain or attacks
Nature	Continuous, periodic or paroxysmal If not continuous, is pain present between attacks?
Initiating factors	Any potential initiating factors Association with dental treatment, or lack of it, is especially important in eliminating dental causes
Exacerbating and relieving factors	Record all and note especially hot and cold sensitivity or pain on eating as they suggest a dental cause
Localisation	The patient should map out the distribution of pain if possible. Is it well or poorly defined? Does it affect an area supplied by a particular nerve or artery? Is the distribution of the pain consistent with anatomy?
Referred pain	Try to determine whether the pain could be referred

Pain is completely subjective and, when physical signs are absent, special care must be taken to detail all its features (Table 1.3). Especially important are features suggesting a dental cause. A fractured tooth or cusp, dental hypersensitivity or pain on occlusion are easily misdiagnosed.

Factors triggering different causes of pain are discussed in detail in Chapter 38.

Demographic details

The age, gender, ethnic group and occupation of the patient should be noted routinely; even though apparently trivial, such information is occasionally critical. Increasing age predisposes to malignant neoplasms, autoimmune disease tends to have onset in middle-aged female patients and aphthous stomatitis is often diagnosed in the young. Identifying and recording a patient's racial or ethnic group can be misconstrued, but it cannot be avoided for fear of being considered racist. Many diseases have a restricted ethnic distribution that aids diagnosis., such as oral submucous fibrosis or florid cemento-osseous dysplasia.

History of the present complaint

Frequently, a complaint, such as toothache, suggests the diagnosis. In many cases, a detailed history (Box 1.3) is required and sometimes, as in aphthous ulceration, a provisional diagnosis can be made on the history alone.

If earlier treatment has been ineffective, the diagnosis should be reconsidered. Many patients' lives have been shortened by having malignant tumours treated with repeated courses of antibiotics.

Medical history

A medical history is important because it aids the diagnosis of oral manifestations of systemic disease. It also ensures that medical conditions and medications that affect dental or surgical treatment are identified.

To ensure that nothing significant is forgotten, a printed questionnaire for patients to complete is valuable and saves time. It also helps to avoid medicolegal problems by providing a written record that the patient's medical background has been considered. Some patients may find it easier to fill in a questionnaire than answer questions. However, a questionnaire alone does not constitute a medical history, and the information must be checked verbally, augmented as necessary and confirmed with the clinician's signature. It is important to assess whether the patient's reading ability and understanding are sufficient to provide valid answers to the questionnaire.

Medical history questionnaires vary widely in style and the questions asked. All dental surgeons should be able to take a history without the guidance of a questionnaire. The questionnaire itself is less important than understanding exactly why the questions are being asked and what follow-up questions are relevant (see Table 1.4). However,

Table 1.4 Questions to be included in a medical history and their relevance*

Question	Subsidiary or follow-up questions	Important features of relevance – not all can be included
Are you taking any medicines, medications or tablets at present?	Including over-the-counter drugs and complementary medicine such as herbal remedies	Potential interactions with treatment for oral conditions Potential oral adverse effects of drugs, of which there are many Steroid use and risk of steroid collapse, infections in immunosuppression Some herbal preparations interact with sedation drugs
	Include medication taken in the past	Patients may forget past courses of drugs with important effects such as bisphosphonates (risk of osteonecrosis), or gold injections (risk of lichenoid reaction) and others
Have you ever been in hospital for any illnesses or operations?	Any problems with the operation or the anaesthetic?	Hospitalisation usually indicates severe health problems; this general question should reveal information on malignant disease, chemotherapy, radiotherapy and immunosuppression
	… normal recovery, not readmitted, no allergies? How long were you in hospital?	Indicates previous reactions to anaesthetics and possibly bleeding problems or other medical complications
Do you carry any medication cards or MedicAlert, Medi-Tag, Mediband or similar devices?		Provide details of medications, doses and effect, usually anticoagulants, steroids, allergies and significant medical conditions Note that some of these alerts may carry patient-reported information as well as medically confirmed information.
Do you have, or have you had, any problems with your heart?	Elicit type, particularly valvular disease	Indicates risk of angina, myocardial infarct or other cardiac emergency in the dental surgery Potential anaesthetic problem Possible predisposition to infective endocarditis, depending on defect
Have you ever had rheumatic fever?	Do you have any heart damage as a result?	Possible predisposition to infective endocarditis
Do you have, or have you had, hepatitis or jaundice?	Known or likely type of hepatitis, if unknown clues may be in where and how it was contracted and the clinical course Questions to exclude non-infectious causes of jaundice such as haemolytic anaemias, gall stones, liver failure, alcohol, etc.	Infection control risk for hepatitis B and C Liver damage can cause coagulation defect, and the metabolic defect can contraindicate prescription of some drugs
Have you ever had epilepsy or other fits or faints?	Assess severity of epilepsy, type of seizure, frequency, duration and eliciting factors	Risk of epileptic attack or status epilepticus in the dental surgery Adverse effects of antiepileptic drugs such as phenytoin
	Degree of drug control and date and severity of last fit	Risk of vasovagal attack in dental surgery
	If other type of fits, what cause?	Fits of unknown cause may relate to head and neck neurological complaints and indicate a CNS cause
Do you have diabetes?	How is it managed? With insulin, other drugs or diet?	Risk of hypoglycaemic collapse in insulin dependent diabetics, and, less likely, hyperglycaemia
	How well controlled? Ever requiring hospital admission?	Diabetes predisposes to infection, particularly candidal but also bacterial and periodontal disease Dry mouth may result from dehydration
	How is blood glucose monitored? Normal levels and range	
Do you have high blood pressure?	Taking the blood pressure may be required and is a recommendation for dentists in some countries. Hypertension is often asymptomatic and dentists have a role in detecting and referring patients with poorly controlled or undetected hypertension.	May indicate risk of stroke, angina or myocardial infarction in the dental surgery Oral adverse reactions of antihypertensive drugs include dry mouth, gingival hyperplasia, lichenoid reactions, burning mouth and taste loss Risk of interaction with some vasoconstrictors in local anaesthetic Anaesthetic risk Patients may faint from hypotension after rising from a supine position for dental treatment
Have you ever been anaemic?	Do you know the reason?	Anaemia predisposes to numerous oral conditions including aphthous ulcers, candidosis, glossitis and burning mouth
	Do you or anyone in your family have thalassaemia?	Anaesthetic risk for sickle cell anaemia and thalassaemia Thalassaemia is now so geographically widespread that limiting questioning to those of Mediterranean heritage is too specific
	For patients of African heritage, do you or anyone in your family have sickle cell anaemia?	

Table 1.4   Questions to be included in a medical history and their relevance* (Continued)

Question	Subsidiary or follow-up questions	Important features of relevance – not all can be included
Do you have any allergies …	Ask specifically about penicillin and other drugs including local anaesthetic	Reveals atopic patients prone to allergy
… to medicines … to metals, foods, plasters, etc. … or asthma, hay fever, rashes, etc.?	Ask whether the patient has ever taken penicillin	Allergies to medication potentially prescribed by the dental surgeon, including related drugs Latex allergy and cross-reacting food allergies Identify potential triggers of attack relevant to dentistry Rashes may be cutaneous counterparts of oral disease Potential adverse effects of steroid inhalers used for asthma
Have you ever had any problems stopping bleeding after a cut or surgery?	Does anyone else in your family have problems with bleeding? Have problems followed tooth extraction? Have you ever taken Warfarin or any medicines to thin your blood?	Risk of haemorrhage following extraction, surgery or possibly local anaesthetic If familial, raises possibility of haemophilia and other inherited bleeding conditions Contraindicates prescription of drugs that prolong bleeding such as aspirin Anticoagulants interact with drugs prescribed for oral conditions and prolong bleeding after surgery
Have you ever come into contact with someone suffering human immunodeficiency virus (HIV) infection or acquired immunodeficiency syndrome (AIDS)? … or any other sexually transmitted infection?	An open question to allow patients to proffer relevant information in this sensitive area. Not usually followed up unless the patient offers that they are or may be HIV positive, in which case minimum information required is the name of the relevant physician and permission to contact them for details of the condition If positive ask about viral load, CD4 count and medication	Infection control risk following blood exposure Oral manifestations of immunosuppression Risk of significant medical complications that may present to the dental surgeon Oral adverse effects of anti-HIV medication and drug interactions Patients at risk should be encouraged to have an HIV test Gives an indication of degree of immunosuppression and infection risk
Do you smoke? Or use smokeless tobacco or betel quid …	Type and amount smoked, expressed in pack years (number of 20-cigarette packs per day multiplied by number of years of smoking). 25 g or 1 oz loose tobacco is equivalent to 50 cigarettes.	Predisposes to oral, nose and sinus and aerodigestive tract carcinoma Predisposes to atheroma, hypertension and cardiac disease Associated with oral red and white lesions and potentially malignant disorders Amenable to cessation advice in the dental setting
… or marijuana, cannabis or other drugs?		Cannabis carries additional health risks over smoking, possibly including oral carcinoma
Do you drink alcohol?	Units consumed per week and type of alcohol	Synergistic effect with smoking for oral potentially malignant disorders and oral cancer
For female patients, is there any chance you might be pregnant …	Stage of pregnancy	Risk from X-ray exposure Pregnancy modulates healing and is association with remission in aphthous stomatitis and predisposes to pyogenic granuloma and gingivitis
… or are trying to become pregnant?		Contraindicates prescription of many drugs
Are you otherwise generally fit and well?		An open question to allow patients to provide information that may not be covered by more specific questions
For parents of child patients – is your child receiving any other therapy or special support?	Type and reason Normal developmental milestones achieved? Any additional support at school?	A broad question to identify behavioural and developmental conditions that may affect provision of treatment
Do any diseases run in your family?		May reveal haemophilia and other bleeding disorders and a host of other genetic diseases and syndromes
Is there anything else about your health you would like to tell me?		May reveal general malaise, fevers, weight loss, psychiatric problems and reveal attitudes to health and disease not elicited by other questions
How is your mental health?		The stigma attached to mental health and learning difficulty problems requires a subtle approach if this is suspected but nothing has been elicited by previous questioning.

*There is deliberate 'redundancy' in medical history questioning, that is, a point of significance may be covered by questioning from more than one perspective to ensure nothing significant is missed. Thus, even if a patient claims that their heart is fine, rheumatic fever should be asked about specifically and jaundice and hepatitis both explored independently. Patients may well not recognise medical names and react to one question but not another.

This table groups conditions that are related, but some favour following a systems-based approach, a surgical sieve, various mnemonics or a medical history questionnaire. Clinicians should become adept at using whatever system they prefer and use the same system all the time to avoid inadvertent omissions.

generic terms such as 'benign neoplasm' or 'odontogenic tumour' to keep the list manageable.

When the list includes conditions with significant implications for the patient, such as a malignant neoplasm, it is traditional to put them at the top of the list even though their likelihood may be low. This ensures important diagnoses are not forgotten and that they are investigated and excluded first, before moving on to more likely, but less serious, conditions.

INVESTIGATIONS

Innumerable types of investigation are possible. It may be difficult to refrain from asking for every conceivable investigation so as not to miss something unsuspected and to avoid medicolegal complications. Although it may be tempting to explore every possibility, however remote, this approach may prove counterproductive in that it can produce a plethora of reports that confuse rather than inform. The more investigations performed, the more likely one will produce a spurious result.

The differential diagnosis forms the basis on which investigations are selected, and keeping focused on the list ensures that only appropriate investigations are requested. Every investigation must be selected to answer a specific question, and none should be regarded as 'routine tests'.

In all healthcare systems, investigations are expensive, some exceedingly so, and some can only be performed in specialised centres. It is the duty of every clinician to keep the cost-to-benefit ratio of investigations in mind and order only those that will confirm the differential diagnosis or exclude options from it. Often investigations that specifically exclude diseases are the most valuable.

A few diseases, such as mumps, may be diagnosed on the basis of a single test, but others, such as Sjögren's syndrome, may require many tests and some difficult interpretation to make the diagnosis.

Any test will occasionally produce an erroneous result. Sometimes this is the result of inappropriate samples or delay in specimen transport. However, for many blood tests, a result may be flagged as 'out of normal range' because the value is in the highest or lowest 5% of the population. This is not necessarily an abnormal result. Unexpected or inexplicable test results are often best repeated before accepting the result, provided the test is easily performed.

Screening and diagnostic tests

This book is primarily concerned with diagnosis, but the difference between screening and diagnostic tests must be appreciated.

To be useful in diagnosis, a test result, whether positive or negative, must indicate a specific disease or condition. This is measured by the parameters of the sensitivity, specificity, positive predictive value and negative predictive value of the test. The definitions of these parameters are shown in Table 1.9.

Sensitivity describes whether a test can correctly identify a condition, and the specificity determines whether it can correctly exclude a condition. However, no test is completely accurate, and there are always false-positive and false-negative (incorrect) results. You can also see from the definitions that the sensitivity and specificity are only measures that relate to a population in which the correct disease status is already known. That is not helpful when using the test in real life, and the value of the test is better described by the positive and negative predictive values. The ideal test

Table 1.9 Sensitivity, specificity, positive predictive value and negative predictive value

Parameter	Definition
Sensitivity	The proportion of patients known to have the disease who test positive
Specificity	The proportion of patients known to NOT have the disease who test NEGATIVE
Positive predictive value	The proportion of all positive results that are true positives (correct results)
Negative predictive value	The proportion of all negative results that are true negatives (correct results)

would have a high positive and a high negative predictive value.

A further complication is introduced by considering the value of tests when they are performed in different circumstances. Suppose a test is not very accurate, but the disease being tested for is very common. Under these circumstances, the test will perform well enough to be useful because a few false-positive results will be outweighed by the value in detecting the many patients with the disease. However, if the disease was very rare, the majority of the results would be false positive and the test would be useless.

The value of the test therefore depends on how it is used. If a clinician performs many tests on all patients, the positive predictive value will not be as high as if the test were used in a more focused manner. This explains why tests must be used to answer specific questions and not thrown randomly at difficult diagnostic dilemmas.

Diagnostic tests are required to have high predictive values, and the more significant the diagnosis, the higher the predictive value must be. Conversely, screening tests are used in population screening and are only intended to identify individuals who might have a disease. Screening tests need to be cheap and easily performed in great numbers, and a lower predictive value is acceptable. Patients who test positive for the screening test will then be referred for more accurate diagnostic tests.

Tests used for diagnosis in oral disease generally have high predictive values. Dentists need to be aware that many less-than-ethical companies sell tests to general dental practitioners for the diagnosis of diseases such as caries, periodontal disease, oral cancer and oral premalignant diseases. It is not always clear whether these are screening or diagnostic tests. In some countries these tests are marketed direct to patients. When evaluating whether using such a test is likely to be effective and its use ethical, it would be strongly advisable to find out what the predictive values of the test would be when used in your own patient population.

Imaging

The most informative imaging techniques in the head and neck are radiography and cone beam computerised tomography (CBCT), medical computerised tomography (CT), magnetic resonance imaging (MRI) and ultrasound. Their advantages and disadvantages are shown in Table 1.10.

Plain radiography is widely available, and simple additional techniques can add value (Box 1.6). Even simple manoeuvres, such as introducing a gutta percha point or probe into a sinus to trace its origins, may provide critical information. It is also advisable to request a formal radiologist's report on radiographic films whenever the radiographic

Table 1.10   Imaging techniques for lesions of the head and neck

Technique	Advantages	Limitations
Conventional radiography	Widely available and inexpensive Simple, many common lesions may be identified with a high degree of accuracy Panoramic radiographs can show unsuspected lesions	Small X-ray dose unavoidable Difficult to interpret in some areas of the jaws because of the complex anatomy Little information about soft tissue lesions
Computerised tomography (CT)	Good definition of soft tissue structures in any plane Useful for areas of complex anatomy such as maxilla or base of skull Definition further improved by use of contrast media	Expensive Available only in hospitals Frightening for patients. Scanner tunnel can provoke claustrophobia Shadows of dental restorations can obscure part of the image Larger X-ray dose than plain radiographs
Cone beam CT	Low-cost high-resolution CT ideal for the head and neck, oral surgery, implantology and endodontics	As CT but lower dose and higher resolution Has quickly become a routine radiological investigation for head and neck diagnosis Image density not directly proportional to bone density Relatively poor soft tissue resolution
Radiography or CT with contrast medium	Valuable for outlining extent of duct systems, hollow structures such as cysts or blood vessels (angiography), etc.	Requires more expertise than plain radiography
Magnetic resonance imaging (MRI)	Produces clear tomograms in any plane without superimposition Particularly good for soft tissue lesions, better than CT No X-ray dose Clear definition of bones and teeth	Expensive and limited availability Frighteningly noisy. May be refused by claustrophobic patient (as for CT) Slow, sometimes over 1 hour Possible risk to the fetus (unconfirmed)
Ultrasound	No X-ray dose Shows soft tissue masses and cysts well Useful for salivary gland cysts, Sjögren's syndrome, stones, and for thyroid and neck lesions May be combined with Doppler flow analysis to measure blood flow through a lesion	Requires expertise in interpretation A dynamic technique interpreted live and difficult to record effectively in pictures Overlying bone obscures soft tissue lesions
Scintigraphy	Uses a radioactive isotope to visualise particular types of cells With technetium 99^m provides an assessment of function in each salivary gland Can be used if sialography not possible Other isotopes are used for detection of bone metastases	Equipment not always available Small radiation dose but isotope rapidly cleared
Positron emission tomography (PET scanning)	Short-life radioactive isotope used to identify biochemical activity, usually glycolysis, to identify putative tumour size, location or metastasis Good for identifying unsuspected metastases Helps identify neoplasms when post-surgical artefact or inflammation obscure CT or MRI Also available as a combined PET-CT and PET-MRI scan, but with reduced CT or MRI resolution	Expensive Intake of radioactive substance

features appear unusual or beyond the experience of the clinician.

Imaging and diagnosis ISBN-13: 978-0702045998

Histopathology

Value and limitations

Removal of a biopsy specimen for histopathological examination is the mainstay of diagnosis for diseases of the mucosa, soft tissues and bone. In the few conditions in which a biopsy is not helpful, it may still be valuable to exclude other possible causes.

As with all other investigations, biopsy must address a specific question. For instance, recurrent minor aphthae lack specific microscopic features and biopsy is rarely justified. Conversely, a major aphtha may mimic a carcinoma that only microscopy will exclude.

Histological examination is not a 'test' in the same way as blood investigations. The pathologist will issue a report that describes the macroscopic and histological features seen in the specimen and provide an interpretation, usually specific, sometimes less so (Box 1.7). The interpretation will be based on the clinical information transmitted to the pathologist on the request form, and often this is critical to the reported diagnosis. Pathology reports, and not just the 'bottom line' diagnosis, need to be read and understood because they may contain important caveats about the confidence with which a diagnosis is made or suggestions for further investigations.

Box 1.6   Requirements for useful oral radiographic information

- Always take bitewings when dental pain is suspected. Small carious lesions may be missed in periapical films and poorly localised pain may originate in the opposing arch
- When imaging bony swellings with plain films, always take two views at right angles
- Panoramic tomograms often cannot provide high definition of bony lesions. Only a cross-section of the lesion is in the focal trough, and if the bone is greatly expanded, only a small portion will be in focus. To detect internal structure in bony lesions, plain films such as oblique lateral views of the mandible or oblique occlusal films are better. For better localisation where complex anatomical features are superimposed, cone beam computed tomography may be more useful
- Radiography of soft tissues is occasionally useful, for instance to detect a foreign body or calcification in lymph nodes

---

Box 1.7   Possible reasons for failures in histological diagnosis

- Specimen poorly fixed or damaged during removal (Figs 1.4 and 1.5)
- Specimen unrepresentative of the lesion or too small
- Plane of histological section does not include critical features
- The disease does not have diagnostic histological features, e.g. aphthous ulcers
- The histological features have several possible causes, e.g. granulomatous inflammation
- The histological features are difficult to interpret, e.g. malignant tumours may be so poorly differentiated that their type cannot be determined
- Inflammation may mask the correct diagnosis

Biopsy

Biopsy is the removal and examination of a part or the whole of a lesion.*

There are several different biopsy techniques (Box 1.8).

The most important technique is surgical biopsy. Leaving aside medical contraindications, the only important contraindications to biopsy are when the site of disease contains important structures, such as the facial nerve in the parotid gland, or when the biopsy risks seeding a tumour more widely in the tissues. The most common parotid neoplasm (pleomorphic adenoma) has an unusual tendency to spread and recur in the incision wound because of its gelatinous nature. In such instances, alternatives would be to perform a fine needle aspiration or excise the entire lesion with a margin of surrounding normal tissue and confirm the suspected diagnosis afterward.

---

*Biopsy is derived from the Greek words meaning 'to see in life'. Thus, a biopsy specimen is taken from a living patient. Its opposite is necropsy: 'to see in death'; a post-mortem or autopsy.

Box 1.8   Types of biopsy

- Surgical biopsy (incisional or excisional)
  - Fixed specimen for routine diagnosis
  - Frozen sections for rapid diagnosis
  - Fresh tissue for immunofluorescence, microbiological culture or molecular analysis
- Fine needle aspiration biopsy
- Wide needle/core biopsy

Selecting the biopsy site

If the wrong site is selected for biopsy, the chance of a definitive diagnosis is reduced. Choice of site is often a compromise between ease of access, chosen method and removing the ideal tissue.

Identifying the ideal tissue should take precedence and requires the clinician to understand the disease process at a tissue level so that the tissue most likely to show diagnostic features is selected. For large tumours, a central sample is often best, but it is critical to include the margin to assess the growth pattern and possible peripheral invasion. For mucosal disease, ulcers must be avoided because they are inflamed and have no epithelium. For potentially malignant diseases, red and speckled areas are the most important, followed by white areas. For immunobullous disease, the perilesional tissue is best because it is less friable and will not disintegrate on biopsy. However, samples for immunofluorescence should be taken away from the lesion, usually from clinically normal buccal mucosa, because they are used to identify bound autoantibody and not the histopathology of the disease.

It is often stated that a biopsy should include normal tissue at the margin. However, this is widely misunderstood. The pathologist does not require adjacent tissue for comparison; he or she will be very familiar with the normal histological variation in the mouth. However, there may be better reasons for choosing to include normal tissue in the sample. Cancers and some other lesions can be friable and disintegrate on biopsy so that having some normal tissue at one end helps support the sample and holds the suture more firmly. If a malignant process is suspected, the margin is where invasion of surrounding tissue will be seen. When performing an excision biopsy, a small collar of normal tissue may prevent recurrence of some lesions. However, always try to take the largest sample of lesional tissue and only include normal tissue for a specific reason.

Large lesions and those with areas that look or feel different may well require several biopsies to sample them adequately. Those in which the epithelial thickness is markedly increased, such as verrucous carcinoma, may need a sample several millimetres thick to include the underlying connective tissue needed to assess whether or not the carcinoma is invasive.

It can be seen that selecting the correct site can be a challenging intellectual exercise requiring a good differential diagnosis and knowledge of the basic histopathology of the likely disease – just one reason why dental students should know some basic histopathology.

Surgical biopsy methods

This is the surgical removal of tissue to determine the diagnosis before treatment and may be undertaken with a scalpel, biopsy punch, cutting laser, electrocautery or a wide cutting needle ('core biopsy'; Trucut biopsy). In general, a

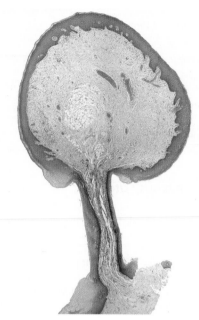

Fig. 1.4 An artefactual polyp produced by grasping normal mucosa with forceps to steady it during biopsy.

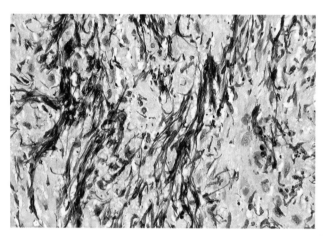

Fig. 1.5 Stringy artefact. This appearance is due to breakage of cells and their nuclei when the specimen is stretched or crushed. It is particularly common in lymphoma and some types of carcinoma.

scalpel biopsy is almost always preferred for intraoral sampling. The tissue is removed cleanly without damage, and the incision can be designed to heal by primary intention. Silk sutures are soft and comfortable in the mouth, and an appointment for removal a few days later provides an opportunity to review healing and discuss the diagnosis. Resorbable sutures may be used to avoid a second appointment but are less comfortable and often persist for many days in the mouth.

Removal of tissue with laser or electrocautery is useful to prevent bleeding, and the coagulated surface requires no sutures. These techniques are most useful to remove excess tissue or excise nodular lesions of the gingiva or mucosa. However, even when properly adjusted, the heat or electrical current will pass through the tissue and denature it, rendering a proportion of the sample unsuitable for diagnosis. Electrocautery is particularly prone to damage epithelium over a wide area and should never be used for a biopsy to assess dysplasia or other epithelial diseases.

Cutting needles or core biopsies are useful to remove a core of tissue, usually 1 mm or so in diameter, from deeper structures such as lymph nodes in the neck (Box 1.9).

A biopsy punch is a circular cutting blade designed to excise a circle of skin. These work well on skin because when the blade penetrates to the subcutaneous fat, a cylinder of skin is mobilised and can be lifted upwards and sliced off. However, punches are badly suited to oral biopsy. The circular blade will only cut taut tissue so that flexible mucosa has to be stretched before cutting. After cutting the sample springs back to its original size, and may then be too small, less than half the punch diameter. The round wound does not lend itself to healing by primary intention or easy closure with sutures. Punch biopsy is often recommended on firm tissue such as the palate and for salivary neoplasms on the palate. At these sites, it is easy to orientate the punch perpendicular to the tissue. Even here it can fail if the deep core of tissue remains fixed to the patient and only a disc of overlying mucosa comes away. Elsewhere a scalpel biopsy is almost always preferred. Despite this, punch biopsy has become popular with dentists because of its speed and simplicity. It is better to take a biopsy with a technique you are happy with than to avoid it, but biopsy punches must be used intelligently.

Surgical biopsy may be incisional or excisional. Incisional biopsy is the removal of part of the lesion for diagnosis only. In excisional biopsy, the whole lesion is removed. The latter is usually performed to confirm a confident clinical diagnosis or when a lesion is too small to require diagnosis and removal in separate steps.

Oral biopsy is a simple procedure that should be within the capability of any dentist. Avoiding or referring for a biopsy in the mistaken belief that the procedure is too unpleasant for general practice is unwarranted. Surveys show that patients rarely complain or suffer adverse consequences from mucosal biopsy, often take no analgesia afterward and much prefer to have their disease properly investigated. Occasionally, general anaesthesia is required for children or problem patients, and referral is necessary. For those that gag, a short-acting benzodiazepine is usually effective.

The pathology request form should contain all the clinical information used to reach the clinical diagnosis. The purpose is to ensure an accurate diagnosis and not (as some clinicians seem to think) to see whether the pathologist can guess it without the relevant information. If appropriate, give the vitality of teeth associated with the lesion.

> **Box 1.10   Essential biopsy principles**
>
> - Choose the most diagnostic or suspicious area, e.g. red area when potential malignancy is suspected
> - Avoid ulcers, sloughs or necrotic areas
> - Give regional or local anaesthetic – do not inject into the lesion
> - Include normal tissue margin if the lesion itself may be friable or malignancy is suspected
> - Specimen should preferably be at least 10 x 6 mm and 2 mm deep for mucosal disease, larger for large lesions, smaller on mucoperiosteum
> - For mucosal disease, specimen edges should be vertical, not bevelled
> - Design the sample shape and incision for easy primary closure
> - Before incising, pass a suture through the specimen to control it and prevent it being swallowed or aspirated by the suction
> - For large lesions, several areas may need to be sampled
> - Include every fragment removed for histological examination
> - Never open, incise or divide the specimen, always send it intact
> - Suture and control any post-operative bleeding
> - Label specimen bottle with patient's name and clinical details
> - Warn patient of possible soreness afterward. Give or recommend an analgesic
> - Check the histological diagnosis is consistent with the clinical diagnosis and investigations
> - Discuss with pathologist or repeat biopsy if diagnosis is unclear or not understood

> **Box 1.11   Advantages and limitations of frozen sections**
>
> - Can establish, at operation, whether or not a tumour is malignant and whether excision needs to be extended
> - Can confirm, at operation, that excision margins are free of tumour
> - Appearances differ from those in fixed material
> - Freezing artefacts due to poor technique can distort the cellular picture
> - Definitive diagnosis sometimes impossible
> - Only to be used when the result will alter the immediate surgical plan

> **Box 1.12   Principles and uses of fine needle aspiration biopsy**
>
> - A narrow (21-gauge) needle is inserted into the lesion and cells aspirated and smeared on a slide
> - Rapid and usually effective aid to diagnosis of swellings in lymph nodes and parotid tumours especially
> - Cells can be fixed, stained and examined within minutes
> - Valuable when surgical biopsy could spread tumour cells (e.g. pleomorphic adenomas)
> - For deep lesions, ultrasound or radiological guidance may be used to ensure that the needle enters the lesion
> - No significant complications
> - Small size of the needle avoids damage to vital structures in the head and neck
> - Cells may be pelleted and processed for sections to allow immunocytochemistry and other specialised stains
> - Some sample may be sent for microbiological culture
> - Small specimen may be unrepresentative; several 'needle passes' often taken
> - Definitive diagnosis not always possible (though a differential diagnosis may be very helpful to plan treatment)

The essential principles of biopsy are summarised in Box 1.10.

Patient view: PMID: 11235976

Frozen sections

Frozen section technique allows a stained slide to be examined within 10 minutes of taking the specimen (Box 1.11). The tissue is sent fresh to the laboratory to be frozen by immersion in liquid nitrogen (–196°C) or dry ice (–78°C), very cold to ensure freezing is near instantaneous and does not allow time for ice crystals to form in the tissue. A section is then cut on a refrigerated microtome and stained. The equipment for frozen sections is often in the theatre suite to speed the process even further.

Frozen sections can only be justified if the rapidity of the result will make an immediate difference to the operation in progress because the technique is less accurate than routine histopathology. This low risk of misdiagnosis means that frozen section is used more frequently to assess whether excision margins are free of a cancer than to make a primary diagnosis. If a rapid diagnosis is required in other circumstances, techniques such as fine needle aspiration biopsy or a routine specimen with special rapid laboratory processing are usually preferable.

Fine needle aspiration biopsy

Removing very small numbers of cells by aspiration using a fine needle, even if not completely conclusive, is often

sufficient to distinguish benign from malignant neoplasms, to initiate treatment or to indicate a need for further investigations. FNA should be used as an early step in the diagnosis of salivary neoplasms, lymph nodes in the neck, thyroid lumps and other deep tissues. Among the diagnoses that can be confidently made on FNA are many types of salivary neoplasm, tuberculosis and high-grade lymphomas (Box 1.12).

Brush biopsy and exfoliative cytology

This technique uses a round stiff-bristle brush to collect cells from the surface and subsurface layers of a lesion by vigorous abrasion and is discussed more fully in Chapter 20. It is an excellent method for taking small samples for experimental analysis but has not yet achieved an evidence base for oral diagnosis. The sample removed can be analysed in a variety of ways.

Exfoliative cytology is examination of cells scraped from the surface of a lesion but samples only surface cells and provides no information on deeper layers. It is no longer

Table 1.11   Examples of haematoxylin and eosin staining of various tissues

Eosin (acidic, red)	Haematoxylin (basic, blue)
Cytoplasm of most cells*	Nuclei (DNA and RNA)
Keratin	Mucopolysaccharide-rich ground substance
Muscle cytoplasm	Reversal lines in decalcified bone
Bone (decalcified only)	
Collagen	

*The cytoplasm of some cells (such as oncocytes in some salivary gland tumours) is intensely eosinophilic. In others such as plasma cells it is basophilic or intermediate (amphophilic).

Tissue processing

The fixed tissue is dehydrated by immersion in a series of solvents and impregnated with paraffin wax. The wax block is mounted on a slicing machine called a microtome and sections, usually 4 μm thick, are cut and mounted on glass microscope slides for staining. It takes 24–48 hours to fix, process, section and stain a specimen before the pathologist can report on it.

Some common stains used for microscopy

The combination of haematoxylin and eosin (H&E) is the most common routine histological stain. Haematoxylin is a blue-black basic dye; eosin is a red acid dye. Their typical staining patterns are shown in Table 1.11.

Periodic acid–Schiff (PAS) stain is probably the second most frequently used stain. It stains sugar residues in carbohydrates and glycosaminoglycans pink. This is useful to identify salivary and other mucins, glycogen and candidal hyphae in sections. Alcian blue is a turquoise stain for proteoglycans with negatively charged sugars, such as the sialic acid containing salivary mucins. Salivary mucins therefore stain with both PAS and Alcian blue, whereas ground substance in connective tissue stains only with Alcian blue.

Decalcified and ground (undecalcified) sections

Specimens containing bone and teeth need to be softened by decalcifying in acid to enable a thin section to be cut. This delays the diagnosis by days or weeks according to the size of the specimen and technique used.

Decalcification must be avoided if examination of dental enamel is required, for instance to aid diagnosis of amelogenesis imperfecta, because the heavily mineralised enamel is almost completely dissolved away. In such cases, a ground section is prepared by sawing and grinding using special saws and abrasives.

Immunofluorescent and immunohistochemical staining

Immunostaining methods make use of the highly specific binding between antibodies and antigens to stain specific molecules in the tissues.

Antibodies that recognise specific antigens of interest can be purchased. They are produced either by immunising animals with the purified target molecule and then purifying the resulting antibodies from serum, or generated in vitro (monoclonal antibodies). The staining process is shown in Figs 1.6–1.8. The antibody binds extremely specifically to the target molecule, and the combination is made visible, either by binding a fluorescent molecule that can be seen in an ultraviolet microscope or an enzyme such as peroxidase that can react with a soluble substrate to form a visible red

used in the mouth, brush biopsy (Box 1.13) having superseded it.

Laboratory procedures

Although a clinician does not need to understand the details of laboratory procedures, it is necessary to understand the principles to enable the optimal results to be obtained. Failure to prepare or send the specimen appropriately can prevent diagnosis and necessitate an additional biopsy.

Fixation

Fixation is a key process. The surgeon must immerse the specimen in ten times the specimen volume of 10% formal saline immediately on removal. Do not delay. In the absence of proper fixative, it is better to delay the biopsy and obtain the correct solution. Specimens placed in alcohols, saline or other materials commonly available in dental surgeries are frequently useless for diagnosis (Box 1.14). Do not confuse 10% formal saline (formol saline) with normal saline. Formal saline is formaldehyde dissolved in saline and kills and fixes tissue to prevent autolysis. Normal saline is isotonic saline infusion, not a fixative.

Special types of fixative are required for electron microscopy and for urgent specimens. Whenever microbiological culture is required, the specimen should be sent fresh to the laboratory or a separate specimen taken because fixation will kill any micro-organisms.

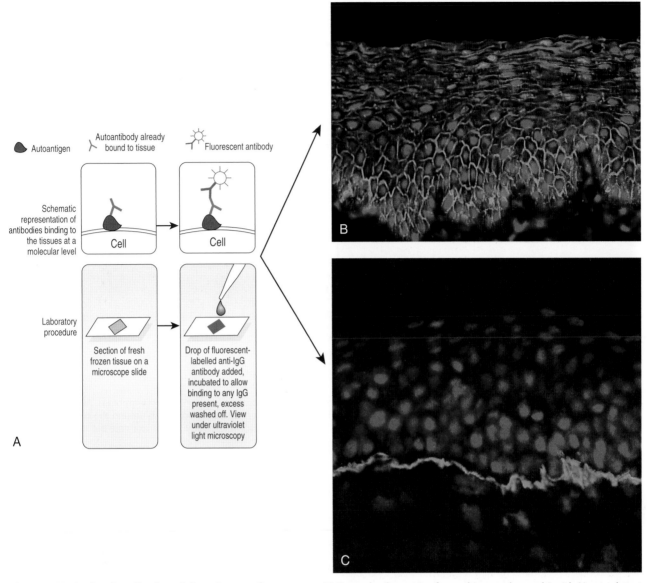

Fig. 1.6 Method and application of direct immunofluorescence. (A) Example: diagnosis of pemphigus and pemphigoid. Aim: to detect the site of the immunoglobulin (IgG) autoantibody already bound to the tissues in a biopsy. Green fluorescence indicates site of antibody binding; red fluorescence is a stain for cell nuclei to make the tissue structure more easily interpreted. (B) In pemphigus, green fluorescence reveals IgG autoantibody bound around the surface of the prickle cells in the epithelium (see Fig. 16.28). (C) In pemphigoid, green fluorescence reveals IgG autoantibody bound along the basement membrane (see Fig. 16.33). *(Images courtesy Dr Balbir Bhogal.)*

or brown deposit. Immunofluorescence is the more sensitive technique.

Immunostaining has revolutionised histological diagnosis. Antibodies are available for immunostaining many cell components and are widely used to identify epithelium (by staining cytokeratin molecules), lymphocyte subtypes (by staining T and B cell membrane antigens), viruses and cell proliferation (by staining molecules involved in the cell cycle). In most laboratories, immunostaining is a relatively cheap automated process.

It is important to know when immunostaining is required because fixation or decalcification may denature the antigens in the tissue and so prevent the antibody binding. Specimens for immunofluorescence must not be fixed in formalin but immediately be sent to the laboratory or sent in special transport medium.

The main circumstances in which diagnosis depends on immunostaining are shown in Table 1.12.

Molecular biological tests

Molecular diagnostic tests have revolutionised medical diagnosis, particularly in screening for and identifying genetic abnormalities and for rapid identification of bacteria and viruses. Techniques are evolving rapidly, and only principles will be illustrated. DNA sequencing and techniques for detecting messenger RNA expression are now rapid and inexpensive, and many medical tests based on single-sequence targets are being replaced by targeted sequencing of multiple specific genes or even whole-genome sequencing.

These methods are not yet widespread in dentistry, but are available in most large hospitals. When confronted with a difficult diagnosis, it is sensible to discuss the case with the pathologist or microbiologist before biopsy, to ensure that appropriate samples are available for these specialised tests.

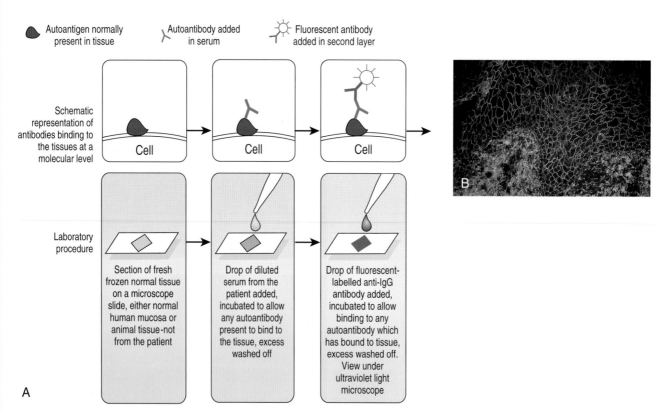

Fig. 1.7 Method and application of indirect immunofluorescence. (A) Example: control of treatment for pemphigus. Aim: to detect circulating autoantibody in the serum of patients with pemphigus. (B) If present, serum autoantibody binds around the surface of the prickle cells in the epithelium and is revealed by the binding to it of the green fluorescent antibody. In this example the nuclei are not counterstained red.

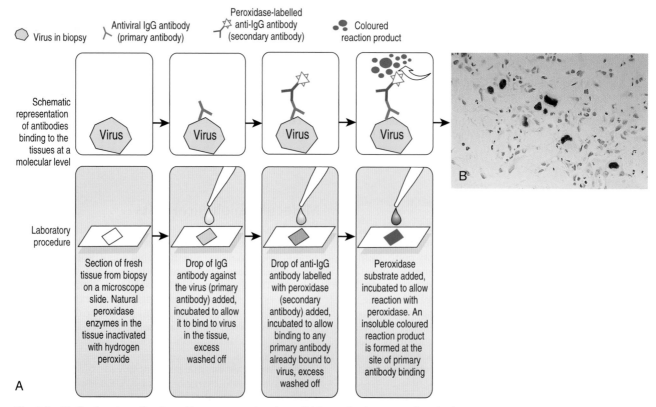

Fig. 1.8 Method and application of immunocytochemistry. (A) Example: diagnosis of viral infection. Aim: to detect viral antigens in infected cells. (B) In this example, brown reaction product identifies cells infected with cytomegalovirus.

Table 1.12 Important uses of immunostaining techniques

Disease	Molecule detected	Significance
Infections	Specific pathogens	Epstein Barr virus in epithelial cells in oral hairy leukoplakia, Treponema pallidum in ulcers indicates syphilis
Pemphigus	Autoantibody bound to epithelial desmosomes (desmoglein 3)	Indicates pemphigus
Pemphigoid	Autoantibody and/ or complement C3 bound to basement membrane	Indicates pemphigoid
Myeloma or B-cell lymphoma	Monoclonal production of kappa or lambda light chains of immunoglobulin	Monoclonal production (production of only one isotype of light chain) indicates a neoplastic process. Production of both types indicates a polyclonal infiltrate that is inflammatory in nature
Lymphomas	Cell surface markers specific for different types of T and B cells	Indicates whether a lymphoma is of B- or T-cell origin and its type
Undifferentiated tumours	Intermediate filaments (components of the cytoskeleton)	Presence of cytokeratins indicates an epithelial neoplasm, vimentin a mesenchymal neoplasm and desmin or myogenin a muscle neoplasm

NB Positive reactions, in themselves, are not necessarily diagnostic of disease and must be interpreted in the light of other histological and clinical findings.

Polymerase chain reaction and quantitative polymerase chain reaction analysis

When a known DNA or RNA sequence is associated with a specific disease, it can be detected by polymerase chain reaction (PCR). In this test, the clinical sample is solubilized, and the nucleic acids within it hybridised with probes complementary to the target sequence. If, and only if, the target sequence is present, PCR will copy the nucleic acid repeatedly until enough is synthesised to be detected, either in an electrophoresis gel (Fig. 1.9) or by another laboratory method. PCR is rapid and can be automated on robotic analysers.

Common applications of PCR are detecting pathogens or mutations in genes. Identification of mycobacteria is a good example of the value of this type of test. Previously, identification of mycobacterial infection required approximately 6 weeks to culture the sample. PCR can be performed in 48 hours, is more sensitive and differentiates different types of mycobacteria with a high degree of precision. PCR is also

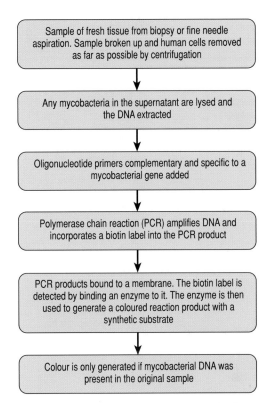

Fig. 1.9 Example application for the technique of polymerase chain reaction for identification of mycobacterial infection.

used to detect the causative mutation of fibrous dysplasia and to detect micrometastases in sentinel node biopsy.

PCR is extremely sensitive. It can detect a single copy of a sequence in a sample, but this high sensitivity makes it prone to false-positive results. Quantitative PCR (qPCR) is an automated process that detects the PCR product while the amplification is in progress and uses the rate of amplification to measure how many copies of the target sequence were originally present in the sample. This allows threshold values for a true positive result to be defined and adds a further level of confidence in the result.

In situ hybridisation and fluorescent in situ hybridisation analysis

Known DNA and RNA sequences can also be detected by in situ hybridisation (ISH) or fluorescent in situ hybridisation (FISH). As in PCR, the sequence of interest is detected by hybridising with a complementary probe, but the hybridisation is performed on tissue sections instead of on solubilised tissue. As in PCR, the probe will only bind if the target sequence is present. Once bound, the probe can be rendered visible by a fluorescent marker or enzyme reaction in the same way that antibodies are visualised in immunohistochemistry. In situ hybridisation is less sensitive than PCR but has the advantage that the location of the target sequence can be seen in the tissue, so that it can be confirmed it is in the expected place, in the correct tissue, and in the cell nucleus or cytoplasm. This adds an additional level of confidence that the test is detecting the correct target and makes it popular for tumour diagnosis. PCR, being performed on solubilised tissue, cannot demonstrate this.

In situ hybridisation is an automated staining process in many laboratories and often used to detect viruses in tissues. Epstein Barr virus and HPV type 16 genes integrated in

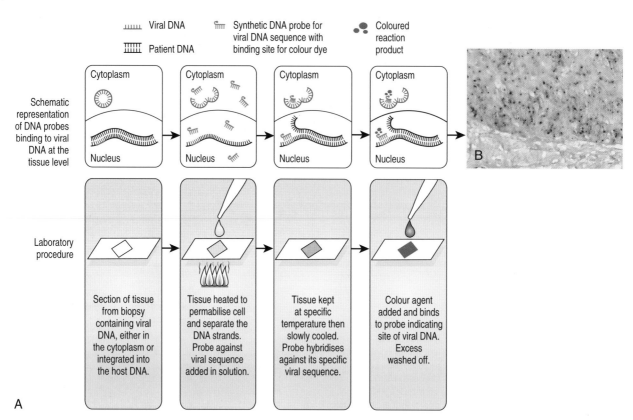

Viral DNA ⟋⟋⟋⟋⟋   Synthetic DNA probe for   Coloured
                     viral DNA sequence with   reaction
Patient DNA ⟍⟍⟍⟍   binding site for colour dye   product

Fig. 1.10 (A) Method and application of in situ hybridisation to detect viral DNA in tissues. (B) In this carcinoma, blue colour reaction product indicates the site of human papillomavirus DNA.

oropharyngeal carcinoma cells are common applications in dentistry.

It is also the method of choice to detect the fusion genes that result from chromosomal translocations, which are often specific to individual types of salivary neoplasms (Ch. 23). The break points in the chromosomes are known, and two probes labelled with different colour fluorescence markers are designed to bind on each side of the break point. In a normal cell the probes bind close together, one on each side of the potential break point, and can be seen down a microscope as four spots of colour in each nucleus (because there are two copies of each gene in a normal cell). Both colours are visible close together. If one of the gene copies is rearranged (the gene is broken), one pair of markers binding to the normal chromosome will show the normal pattern. The fluorescent markers on each side of the broken gene no longer bind close together and are seen as two widely separated spots of colour in the nucleus.

The application of in situ hybridisation is shown in Figs 1.10 and 1.11.

Haematology, clinical chemistry and serology

Blood investigations are clearly essential for the diagnosis of diseases such as leukaemias, myelomas or leukopenias which have oral manifestations, or for defects of haemostasis that can greatly affect management. Blood investigations are also helpful in the diagnosis of other conditions such as some infections and sore tongues or recurrent aphthae that are sometimes associated with anaemia.

As noted earlier, tests should address specific questions (Table 1.13). The request form should always be completed with sufficient clinical detail to allow the haematologist or clinical chemist to check that the appropriate tests have

been ordered and to allow the interpretation of the results. It is important to include details of any drug treatment on blood test request forms. Always put the blood into the appropriate tube because some anticoagulants are incompatible with certain tests. A haematologist will not be impressed by a request for assessment of clotting function on a specimen of coagulated blood.

Microbiology

Despite the fact that the most common oral diseases are infective, traditional microbiological culture of organisms is surprisingly rarely of practical diagnostic value in dentistry (Table 1.14, Box 1.15). Direct Gram-stained smears will quickly confirm the diagnosis of thrush or acute ulcerative gingivitis, and H&E-stained smears can show the distorted, virally infected epithelial cells in herpetic infections more easily than microbiological tests for the organisms themselves.

A key microbiological investigation is culture and sensitivity of pus organisms. Whenever pus is obtained from a soft tissue or bone infection, it should be sent for culture and determination of antibiotic sensitivity of the causative microbes. Those of osteomyelitis, cellulitis, acute parotitis or other severe infections need to be identified if appropriate antimicrobial treatment is to be given. However, such treatment has usually to be started empirically without this information; the sensitivity test may dictate a change of treatment.

Soft tissue infections of the head and neck are often treated without microbiological diagnosis. This is partly because the flora is complex and mixed with many anaerobes and organisms that are difficult to culture. The anaerobes do not survive ordinary sample-taking procedures. Culture results are usually a poor reflection of the actual

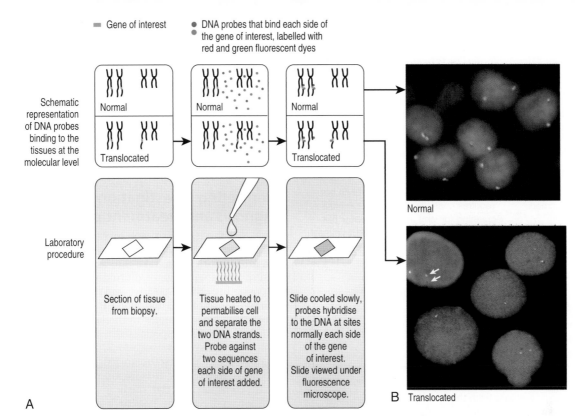

- Gene of interest
- DNA probes that bind each side of the gene of interest, labelled with red and green fluorescent dyes

Schematic representation of DNA probes binding to the tissues at the molecular level

Normal / Normal / Normal

Translocated / Translocated

Normal

Laboratory procedure

Section of tissue from biopsy.

Tissue heated to permabilise cell and separate the two DNA strands. Probe against two sequences each side of gene of interest added.

Slide cooled slowly, probes hybridise to the DNA at sites normally each side of the gene of interest. Slide viewed under fluorescence microscope.

B Translocated

A

Fig. 1.11 (A) Method and application of in situ hybridisation to detect a chromosomal translocation using 'break apart' probes. (B) In this salivary carcinoma, the *myb* gene is translocated to another chromosome. In the normal cell the red and green probes are seen to bind to the DNA close together, each side of the *myb* gene. In the cell with the translocation, one copy of the gene is normal, but the other shows 'break apart' of the red and green probes, indicating a translocation involving a break point between the binding sites of the two probes within or close to the gene of interest. For the *myb* gene, this indicates that the carcinoma is an adenoid cystic carcinoma. When the red and green fluorescent spots are very close, the red and green colours merge to produce yellow. The background blue is a DNA-binding dye to show the nuclei.

Table 1.13 Types of blood test useful in oral diagnosis (see also Appendix 1.1)

Test	Main uses
'Full blood picture' usually includes erythrocyte number, size and haemoglobin indices and differential white cell count	Anaemia and the effects of sideropaenia and vitamin B_{12} deficiency associated with several common oral disorders. Leukaemias
Blood film	Leukaemias, infectious mononucleosis, anaemias
Erythrocyte sedimentation rate	Raised in systemic inflammatory and autoimmune disorders Particularly important in giant cell arteritis and Wegener's granulomatosis
Serum iron and total iron-binding capacity	Iron deficiency associated with several common oral disorders
Serum ferritin	A more sensitive indicator of body stores of iron than serum iron and total iron-binding capacity but not available in all laboratories
Red cell folate level	Folic acid deficiency is sometimes associated with recurrent aphthous ulceration and recurrent candidosis
Vitamin B_{12} level	Vitamin B_{12} deficiency is sometimes associated with recurrent aphthous ulceration and recurrent candidosis
Autoantibodies (e.g. rheumatoid factor, antinuclear factor, DNA-binding antibodies, SS-A, SS-B)	Raised in autoimmune diseases. Specific autoantibody levels suggest certain diseases
Viral antibody titres (e.g. Herpes simplex, Varicella zoster, mumps virus)	A rising titre of specific antibody indicates active infection by the virus
Paul–Bunnell or monospot test	Infectious mononucleosis
Syphilis serology	Syphilis
Complement component levels	Occasionally useful in diagnosis of systemic lupus erythematosus or familial angio-oedema
Serum angiotensin-converting enzyme	Sarcoidosis
Serum calcium, phosphate and parathormone levels	Paget's disease and hyperparathyroidism
Human immunodeficiency virus (HIV) test	HIV infection
Skeletal serum alkaline phosphatase	Raised in conditions with increased bone turnover, e.g. Paget's disease and hyperparathyroidism Lowered in hypophosphatasia

Table 1.14 Microbiological tests useful in oral diagnosis

Test	Main uses
Culture and antibiotic sensitivity	Detect unusual pathogens, e.g. actinomyces in soft tissue infection Antibiotic sensitivity for all infections, particularly osteomyelitis and acute facial soft tissue infection
Smear for candida	Candidosis
Viral culture or antigen screen	Viral culture identifies many viruses but requires considerable time Screening for viral antigen is faster but detects a more limited range of viruses

Box 1.15 Reminders for microbiological investigation

- Always take a sample of pus for culture and antibiotic sensitivity from bone and soft tissue infections *before* giving an antibiotic
- Always take the temperature of any patient with a swollen face, enlarged lymph nodes, malaise or other symptom or sign which might indicate infection
- Culture of *Candida* from the mouth does not necessarily indicate infection because this is a commensal organism. Demonstration of hyphae in a scraping of epithelial cells indicates active infection.

flora unless specialised anaerobic sampling and culture are performed. When antibiotic treatment fails, advice should be sought from a microbiologist as to whether this type of sampling may help.

Viral identification is rarely required for oral diseases because many oral viral infections are clinically typical and indicate the causative virus. A smear alone may show the nuclear changes of herpetic infection in epithelial cells from the margins of mucosal ulcers. A more sensitive and almost as rapid result may be obtained by sending a swab for virus detection using ELISA (enzyme-linked immunosorbent assay) or electron microscopy.

Key reminders for microbiological investigations are in Box 1.15.

Other clinical tests

Urine tests are valuable for the diagnosis of diabetes (suggested by repeated candidal or periodontal infection), kidney damage which can have resulted from autoimmune disorders such as Wegener's granulomatosis and for the detection of Bence-Jones protein in myeloma.

Taking the patient's temperature is an easily forgotten investigation. The temperature should be noted whenever bone or soft tissue infections are suspected. It helps distinguish facial inflammatory oedema from cellulitis and indicates systemic effects of infections and the need for more aggressive therapy.

Interpreting investigations and making a diagnosis and treatment plan

Check that the results of each investigation are compatible with the preliminary diagnosis. If a result appears at odds with other information, take into account the normal variation, perhaps with age or diurnal variation, and consider the possibility of false-positive and false-negative results. A common cause of unusual blood test results is a delay in transporting blood samples to the laboratory.

Further advice and specialised tests may be appropriate, but more extensive investigations, those carrying risks or radiation dose, are best organised through other medical specialties. In referrals, it is important to state whether the dentist is requesting the medical specialist to exclude a condition and refer the patient back, or to take over the investigation. If the latter, it is essential that dental causes have been completely eliminated as the cause of the problem.

Finally, ensure that the patient's notes include a complete record of the consultation and investigation results. This must be correctly dated, legible, limited to relevant facts and include a clear complaint history, list of clinical findings, test results and plan of treatment organised in a suitable form for quick reappraisal. It must be signed by the clinician and, in addition, the name should be printed below if the signature is anything less than perfectly legible. It should be possible for another person to continue to investigate or treat the patient without difficulty on the basis of the clinical record.

Photography or computerised video imaging is a very valuable adjunct to the clinical record. Pictures are especially useful in monitoring lesions that vary in the course of a long follow-up, for instance, white patches. It is useful to include teeth or a scale in the frame to allow accurate assessment of small changes in size. Photographs may also be helpful in explaining to patients about their condition and to show the effects of treatment, but consent for the intended uses of the photographs must be obtained first, and digital image files must be stored securely in the same way as other patient-identifiable digital files.

Appendix 1.1

Normal haematological values

Red cells

Haemoglobin (adults)	Males 130–170 g/L	Females 115–165 g/L
Haematocrit (packed cell volume – PCV)	Males 0.40–0.54%	Females 0.36–0.47%
Mean cell volume (MCV)	80-100 fL	
Mean cell haemoglobin concentration (MCHC)	300–370 g/L	
Mean cell haemoglobin	27-32 pg	
Red cell count	Males 4.5–6.5 $\times10^{12}$/L	Females 3.8–5.8 $\times10^{12}$/L
Erythrocyte sedimentation rate (ESR)	Males 1-10 mm/h	Females 3-15 mm/h

White cells

Total count	3.6–11 $\times10^9$/L
Neutrophils	1.8–7.5 $\times10^9$/L
Lymphocytes	1–4 $\times10^9$/L
Monocytes	0.2–0.8 $\times10^9$/L
Eosinophils	0.1–0.4 $\times10^9$/L

Platelets   140–400 $\times10^9$/L

Note. These reference ranges are for adults and are calculated assuming a normal distribution of results and excluding the upper and lower 2.5% of the range as abnormal. Therefore, approximately 5% of normal persons have values outside the figures quoted above. These are average values and may vary slightly between laboratories, and you should always check normal values with the testing laboratory.

Principles of investigation, diagnosis and treatment

Disorders of tooth development

2

Development of an ideal dentition depends on many factors (Box 2.1).

Significant structural defects of teeth are much less common than irregularities of alignment of the teeth and abnormal relationship of the arches. The main groups of disorders affecting development of the dentition are summarised in Box 2.2 and Summary chart 2.1 and Summary chart 2.2.

ABNORMALITIES IN THE NUMBER OF TEETH

Anodontia

Total failure of development of a complete dentition (anodontia) is exceedingly rare. If the permanent dentition fails to form, the deciduous dentition is retained for many years. If the teeth survive caries, attrition will eventually destroy the crowns. Lack of alveolar bone growth may make implant placement difficult.

Isolated oligodontia

Oligodontia means few teeth. Failure of development of one or two teeth is relatively common and often hereditary. The

teeth most frequently missing are third molars, second premolars or maxillary second incisors (Fig. 2.1), the last teeth in each series. Absence of third molars can be a disadvantage if first or second molars, or both, have been lost; otherwise, orthodontic problems of alignment and space loss are the only effects.

Absence of lateral incisors can sometimes be conspicuous because the large, pointed canines erupt in the front of the mouth beside the central incisors. It is often impossible to prevent loss of space, even if the patient is seen early. It is also difficult and time consuming to make space by orthodontic means to replace the laterals, so combined procedures with prosthodontic replacement are often used. Disguising the shape of the canines is destructive of the tooth, usually unconvincing cosmetically and produces a poor contact.

Genetic causes PMID: 25910507

General review PMCID: PMC3844689

Oligodontia or anodontia with systemic defects

Anhidrotic (hereditary) ectodermal dysplasia

The main features are summarised in Box 2.3. In severe cases, no teeth form. More often, most of the deciduous teeth form, but there are few or no permanent teeth. The teeth are usually peg-shaped or conical (Fig. 2.2).

When there is anodontia, the alveolar process, without teeth to support, fails to develop and has too little bone to support standard implants without surgical bone augmentation. The profile then resembles that of an elderly person because of the gross loss of vertical dimension. The hair is fine and sparse (Fig. 2.3), particularly in the tonsural region. The skin is smooth, shiny and dry due to absence of sweat glands. Heat is therefore poorly tolerated. The finger nails are usually also defective. As a temporary measure, dentures or overdentures are usually well tolerated by children.

Box 2.1   Requirements for development of an ideal dentition

- Formation of a full complement of teeth
- Normal structural development of the dental tissues
- Eruption of each group of teeth at the appropriate time into an adequate space
- Normal development of jaw size and relationship
- Eruption of teeth into correct relationship to occlude with their opposite numbers
- Maintenance of tooth position by normal soft tissue size and pressure

---

Box 2.2   Disorders of development of teeth

- Abnormalities in number
  - Anodontia or oligodontia (hypodontia)
  - Additional teeth (hyperdontia)
- Disorders of eruption
- Defects of structure
  - Enamel defects
  - Dentine defects
  - Cementum defects
- Developmental anomalies of several dental tissues
- Developmental anomalies of dental tissues and adjacent bone
- Intrinsic pigmentation
- Odontomes

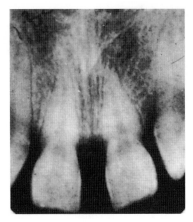

Fig. 2.1 Congenital absence of lateral incisors with spacing of the anterior teeth.

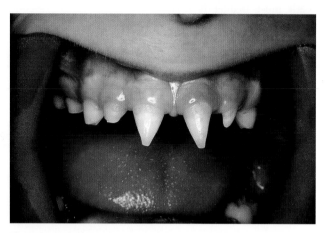

Fig. 2.2   Anhidrotic ectodermal dysplasia showing conical teeth.

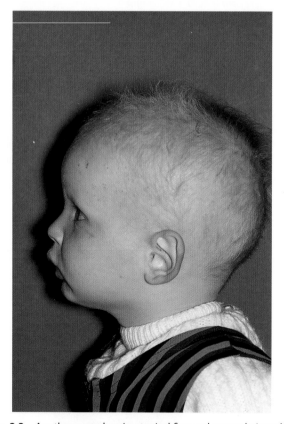

Fig. 2.3   Another case showing typical fine and scanty hair and loss of support for the facial soft tissues.

Implants cannot be placed in the maxilla during growth, but it may be possible to use mini implants or implants in the anterior mandible from a young age because, without teeth to erupt, alveolar growth is complete. Ultimately, a tooth-supported fixed partial denture or implant-supported overdenture is often a good solution.

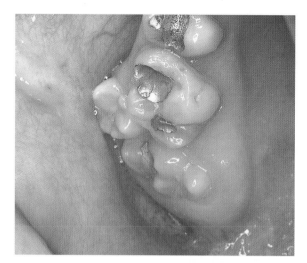

Fig. 2.4   A paramolar, a buccally placed supernumerary molar tooth.

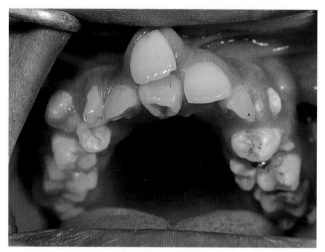

Fig. 2.5   Maleruption of a midline tuberculate supernumerary and two supplemental premolars.

Web URL 2.1 Ectodermal dysplasia URL: http://rarediseases.org/rare-diseases/hypohidrotic-ectodermal-dysplasia/

Other conditions associated with oligodontia

There are many rare syndromes in which oligodontia is a feature, but the only common one is Down's syndrome (Ch. 39). One or more third molars are absent in more than 90% of these patients, and absence of individual teeth is also common. Anodontia is rare.

Additional teeth: hyperdontia

Additional teeth are relatively common. They are usually of simple conical shape but less frequently resemble teeth of the normal series. These are the results of organised development and maturation under genetic control, not simple excessive growth of the dental lamina.

Supernumerary teeth This term is used for any additional tooth (Fig. 2.4). Conical or more seriously malformed additional teeth most frequently form in the incisor or molar region and, very occasionally, in the midline (mesiodens, Fig. 2.5).

Supplemental teeth These are supernumerary teeth with a normal morphology, and they are usually an extra tooth at the end of the incisor, premolar or molar series (also seen in Fig. 2.5).

Effects and treatment

Additional teeth usually erupt in abnormal positions, labial or buccal to the arch, creating stagnation areas and greater susceptibility to caries, gingivitis and periodontitis. Alternatively, a supernumerary tooth may prevent a normal tooth from erupting or cause crowding and malalignment. These additional teeth are usually best extracted.

Review PMCID: PMC3844689

Syndromes associated with hyperdontia

These syndromes are all rare, but probably the best known is cleidocranial dysplasia (Ch. 13), in which many additional teeth develop but fail to erupt.

DEFECTIVE ENAMEL FORMATION

Structural defects of the teeth, such as pitting, discoloration or more serious defects can only arise during development and are, therefore, markers of past disease. Hypoplasia of the teeth is not an important contributory cause of dental caries. Only normally formed enamel can become carious, and hypoplasia due to fluorosis is associated with enhanced resistance.

Defects of deciduous teeth

Calcification of deciduous teeth begins at approximately the fourth month of intrauterine life. Disturbances of metabolism or infections that affect the fetus at this early stage without causing abortion are rare. Defective structure of the deciduous teeth is therefore uncommon but, in a few places, such as parts of India, where the fluoride content of the water is excessively high, the deciduous teeth may be mottled.

The deciduous teeth may be discoloured by abnormal pigments circulating in the blood. Severe neonatal jaundice may cause the teeth to become yellow, or there may be bands of greenish discoloration. In congenital porphyria, a rare disorder of haemoglobin metabolism, the teeth are red or purple. Tetracycline given during dental development, contrary to guidelines, is now a rare cause of permanent discoloration.

Defects of permanent teeth

Single permanent teeth may be malformed as a result of local causes such as periapical infection of a predecessor (Turner teeth – Fig. 2.6), or trauma from intubation while a preterm neonate (Fig. 2.7). Multiple affected teeth usually indicate previous systemic disease as summarised in Box 2.4.

Amelogenesis imperfecta

→ Summary chart 2.1 p. 26

Amelogenesis imperfecta is a group of conditions caused by defects in the genes that encode enamel matrix proteins or other proteins or enzymes required to process or mineralise the matrix. Classification is complex and based on

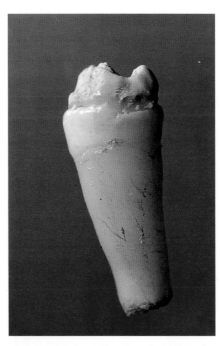

Fig. 2.6 Turner tooth, a hypoplastic tooth resulting from periapical infection, usually of a deciduous predecessor.

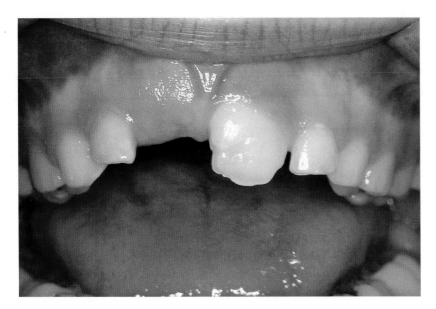

Fig. 2.7 **Localised dental disturbance caused by prolonged intubation during tooth development.** The upper left central incisor shows enamel pitting incisally, and the upper right central incisor is deformed and has failed to erupt.

Summary chart 2.1 Differential diagnosis of developmental defects of the teeth.

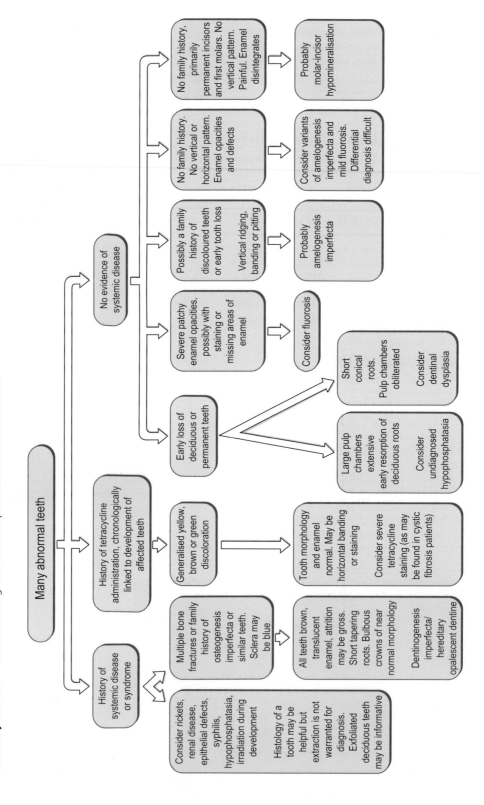

Summary chart 2.2 Differential diagnosis of developmental and acquired abnormalities of one or a group of teeth.

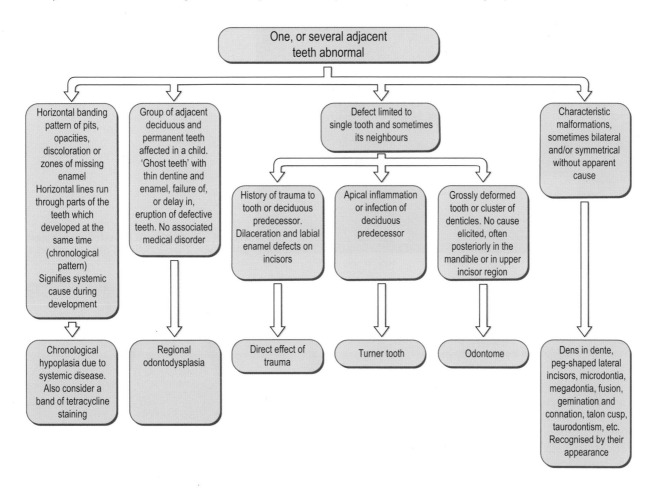

pattern of inheritance, type of defect (enamel hypoplasia, hypomineralisation or hypomaturation) and appearance (smooth, rough or pitted). At least 16 forms have been recognised on clinical grounds, but some are the same genetic condition with differing severity, and the classification is contentious.

Inheritance can be autosomal dominant, recessive or X-linked. However, the most common types have an autosomal inheritance and are thought to be caused by mutations in the genes for ameloblastin (C4), or genes for enamelin (C4) or tuftelin (C1). In the case of the autosomal dominant type of amelogenesis imperfecta, the defective gene is enamelin (C4).

The less common X-linked types are caused by a variety of defects in the AMELX genes encoding amelogenin, located on the X and Y chromosomes (the copy on the Y gene being inactive) and, confusingly, it seems the same mutation can sometimes cause hypoplasia, hypomineralisation or hypomaturation in different patients.

Genetic factors act throughout the whole duration of amelogenesis. Characteristically, therefore, all teeth are affected, and defects involve the whole enamel or randomly distributed patches of it. By contrast, exogenous factors affecting enamel formation (with the important exception of fluorosis) tend to act for a relatively brief period and produce defects related to that period of enamel formation (a chronological pattern).

Until there is a better understanding, dentists should at least be able to identify the three clinical types of hypoplasia,

hypocalcification and hypomaturation and take a family history, which may reveal an inheritance pattern.

Review types causes PMCID: PMC1847600

Hypoplastic amelogenesis imperfecta

The main defect in this type is deficient formation of matrix, so that the amount of enamel is reduced but normally mineralised. The enamel is randomly pitted, grooved or uniformly very thin, but hard and translucent (Fig. 2.8). The defects tend to become stained, but the teeth are not especially susceptible to caries unless the enamel is scanty and fractures to expose dentine.

The main patterns of inheritance are autosomal dominant and recessive, X-linked and (a genetic rarity) an X-linked dominant type. In the last type, there is almost complete failure of enamel formation in affected males, whereas in females the enamel is vertically ridged (Figs 2.9–2.12). Occasionally, cases are difficult to classify (Fig. 2.13).

Hypomaturation amelogenesis imperfecta

The enamel is normal in thickness on eruption but with opaque, white to brownish-yellow patches caused by failure of maturation, a process of matrix removal and increasing mineralisation that is partly developmental and partly posteruptive. The appearance can mimic fluorotic mottling if the spots are small (Figs 2.14 and 2.15). However, affected enamel is soft and vulnerable to attrition, though not as severely as the hypocalcified type.

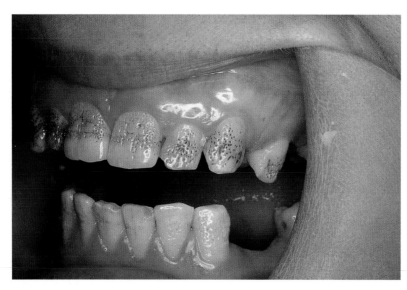

Fig. 2.8   Amelogenesis imperfecta, hypoplastic pitted type. Enamel between pits appears normal.

Box 2.4   Multiple malformed permanent teeth: important causes

Genetic
- Amelogenesis imperfecta
  - Hypoplastic
  - Hypomaturation
  - Hypocalcified
- Chronological hypoplasia
- Molar-incisor hypomineralisation
- Dentinogenesis imperfecta
  - Shell teeth
- Dentinal dysplasia
- Regional odontodysplasia
- Multisystem disorders with associated dental defects
- Hypophosphatasia

Infective
- Congenital syphilis

Metabolic
- Rickets
- Hypoparathyroidism

Drugs
- Tetracycline pigmentation
- Cytotoxic chemotherapy

Fluorosis

Other acquired developmental anomalies
- Fetal alcohol syndrome

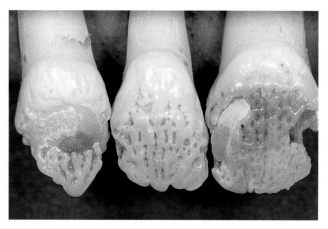

Fig. 2.9   Close-up of X-linked dominant hypoplastic type amelogenesis imperfecta. These teeth, from an affected female, show the typical vertical ridged pattern of normal and abnormal enamel as a result of Lyonisation.

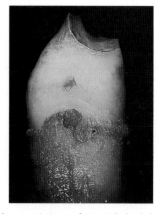

Fig. 2.10   Amelogenesis imperfecta X-linked dominant hypoplastic form in a male. This premolar has a cap of enamel so thin that the shape of the crown is virtually that of the dentine core.

There are several variants of hypomaturation defects such as a more severe, autosomal dominant type combined with hypoplasia and milder forms limited to only some tooth surfaces.

Hypocalcified amelogenesis imperfecta

Enamel matrix is formed in normal quantity but is poorly calcified. When newly erupted, the enamel is normal in thickness and form, but weak or chalky and opaque in appearance.

The teeth tend to become stained, and enamel is relatively rapidly worn away. The upper incisors may acquire a shoulder due to the chipping away of the thin, soft enamel of the incisal edge (Fig. 2.16). There are dominant and recessive patterns of inheritance.

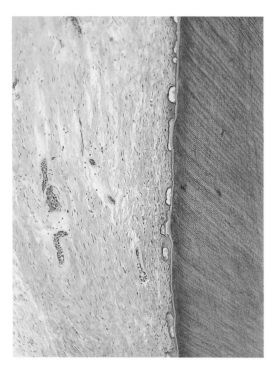

Fig. 2.11 Amelogenesis imperfecta X-linked dominant hypoplastic type in a male showing a thin translucent layer of defective enamel on the dentine surface.

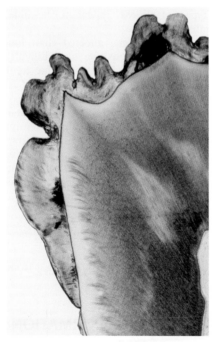

Fig. 2.12 Amelogenesis imperfecta, hypoplastic type. In this pitted hypoplastic type, the pits are seen to be focal areas of reduced enamel formation with incremental lines diverted around them. No enamel has been lost from the pit.

Chronological hypoplasia

➜ Summary chart 2.1 p. 26

Any severe disturbance of metabolism can halt enamel formation. Dentine formation is less sensitive to insult, so tooth formation will usually continue to produce a normally shaped tooth with only a band of enamel missing. The usual causes are the childhood fevers or severe infantile

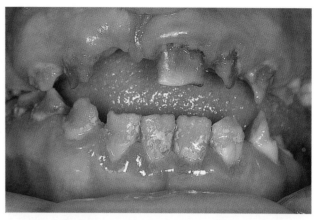

Fig. 2.13 Amelogenesis imperfecta, indeterminate type. Some cases, such as this, are difficult to classify but are clearly inherited, as shown by their long family history.

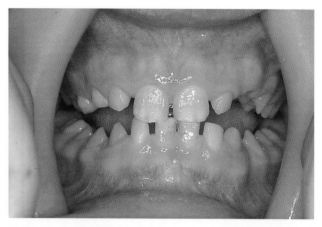

Fig. 2.14 Amelogenesis imperfecta, hypomaturation type. Tooth morphology is normal, but there are opaque white and discoloured patches.

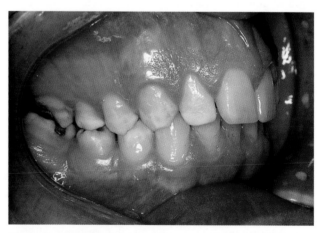

Fig. 2.15 Amelogenesis imperfecta, one of the several hypomaturation types. In this form there are opaque white flecks and patches affecting the occlusal half of the tooth surface.

gastroenteritis. Measles with severe secondary bacterial infection used to be the most common cause of this limited type of dental defect, but such defects have become uncommon since measles vaccination.

Unlike inherited forms of hypoplasia, only a restricted area of enamel is missing, corresponding to the sites of development at the time of the illness.

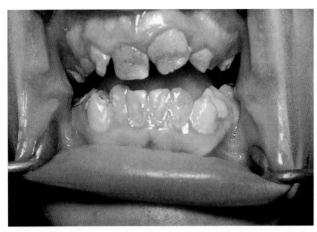

Fig. 2.16 **Amelogenesis imperfecta, hypocalcified type.** The soft chalky enamel was virtually of normal thickness and form but has chipped away during mastication leaving a characteristic shoulder, seen best on the upper left central incisor.

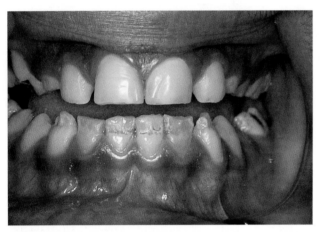

Fig. 2.17 **Chronological hypoplasia due to metabolic upset.** Unlike the hereditary types of amelogenesis imperfecta, defects are linear and thought to correspond to a short period of amelogenesis disturbed by a concurrent severe illness.

Clinically, the typical effect is one or more rows of horizontally disposed pits, grooves or a completely missing band of enamel horizontally across the crowns of the teeth. Defects are usually in the incisal third of incisors, suggesting that the disorder had its effect during the first year or two of life, when such infections cause the most severe systemic upset (Fig. 2.17). Metabolic disturbance *in utero* or around birth affects the primary teeth in addition (Fig. 2.18). The horizontal pattern is important in distinguishing chronological hypoplasia from genetic causes of hypoplasia and determining the timing of the systemic disease (Fig. 2.19).

Molar-incisor hypomineralisation

→ Summary chart 2.1 p. 26

Molar incisor hypomineralisation is an unexplained, apparently recently recognised and increasingly frequent condition defined by hypomineralisation of all first permanent molars and incisors (Fig. 2.20). The teeth erupt normally and have patchy opaque and yellow brown patches on the enamel of the occlusal third of the crowns.

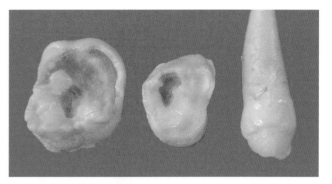

Fig. 2.18 Chronological hypoplasia with loss of primary molar occlusal enamel and a horizontal ridge on the upper canine.

The enamel surface is hard, but the underlying enamel is soft and breaks down, leaving a stained rough and soft surface that is prone to caries. The defects are sharply demarcated.

The cause is probably failure of enamel maturation, but the presentation and family history are distinct from amelogenesis imperfecta and chronological hypoplasia. It appears that many cases are similar to chronological hypoplasia in aetiology, but the systemic upset is milder and insufficient to cause the more severe defect of hypoplasia. A very wide range of types of illness appear to be able to cause hypomineralisation.

Molars are usually worse affected than incisors. The affected teeth are hypersensitive and difficult to anaesthetise. Restorations often fail, partly due to the adverse crown shape and partly because the enamel is not amenable to use of adhesive materials, even away from the clinically detectable defects. This makes treatment difficult, and after a period of preventive care to remineralise the molars and preserve them as space maintainers, extraction is often the best course of action. Otherwise full coverage restorations are required. Microabrasion is not sufficient to restore most affected incisors because the soft enamel extends deeply, and restorations or veneers are usually required.

Web URL 2.2 Review and treatment: http://www.aapd.org/assets/1/25/william2-28-3.pdf

Treatment PMID: 16805354, 26856002 and 23410530

Nature of enamel defect PMID: 23685033

DEFECTIVE DENTINE FORMATION

→ Summary chart 2.1 p. 26

The classification of hereditary dentine defects is unsatisfactory. As in amelogenesis imperfecta, the genetic findings do not correlate well with clinical presentation, and terminology is used inconsistently. The previous widely used classifications (of Witkop and of Shields) are now considered redundant, but no replacement is yet established.

The term *dentinogenesis imperfecta* (type I) was used when abnormal teeth were associated with bone defects, but this combination is now classified as *osteogenesis imperfecta*. The term dentinogenesis imperfecta is used when only the teeth are involved, replacing the term *hereditary opalescent dentine*.

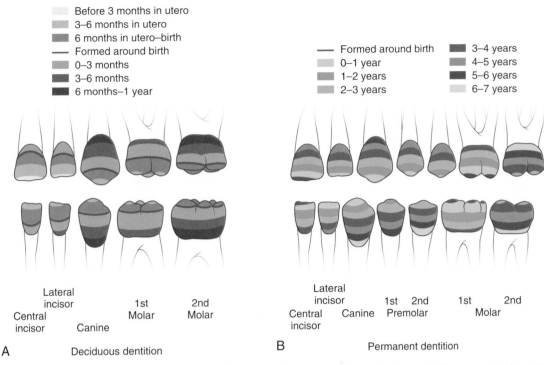

Before 3 months in utero
3–6 months in utero
6 months in utero–birth
Formed around birth
0–3 months
3–6 months
6 months–1 year

Formed around birth
0–1 year
1–2 years
2–3 years
3–4 years
4–5 years
5–6 years
6–7 years

Central incisor
Lateral incisor
Canine
1st Molar
2nd Molar

A   Deciduous dentition

Central incisor
Lateral incisor
Canine
1st Premolar
2nd Premolar
1st Molar
2nd Molar

B   Permanent dentition

Fig. 2.19   Charts to determine the chronology of enamel hypoplasia. Chronological hypoplasia should affect many teeth symmetrically consistent with the time of illness.

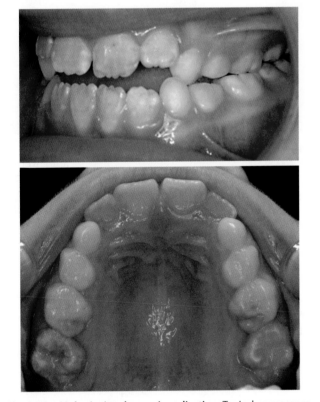

Fig. 2.20   Molar-incisor hypomineralisation. Typical appearance with discolouration and breakdown of enamel almost exclusively on permanent incisors and first molars.

Osteogenesis imperfecta with opalescent teeth → Summary chart 2.1 p. 26

This uncommon defect of collagen formation disturbs formation of both bone and dentine. Many forms are known, and the condition is described in Chapter 13. Types III and IV are those most frequently associated with dentine defects. Both are autosomal dominant traits with mutation in the genes COL1A1 and COL1A2 that prevent the procollagen alpha helix polymerising into normal type 1 collagen. The dentine is soft and has abnormally high water content.

In both these types, opalescent teeth are present in over 80% of patients in the primary dentition. Tooth discoloration and attrition is often most striking in the deciduous dentition. Class III malocclusion is associated in over 70% of patients. In type III disease, dental development is delayed in 20% but, in type IV disease, it is accelerated in over 20% of patients.

Dentinogenesis imperfecta

→ Summary chart 2.1 p. 26

This condition produces identical changes in appearance and structure of the teeth to those in osteogenesis imperfecta but is caused by mutations in dentine sialoprotein, a dentine matrix protein, rather than collagen genes. Previously there were thought to be two types (types II and III), but the condition of shell teeth is now thought to be just a more severe presentation of type II caused by defects in the same gene. Dentinogenesis imperfecta can be associated with developmental hearing loss.

Clinical features

The enamel appears normal but uniformly brownish or purplish and abnormally translucent (Fig. 2.21), giving an opal-like appearance that leads to the clinical description of 'hereditary opalescent dentine'. The appearance is caused by the dark dentine being visible through the enamel, which is usually normal but may have hypoplastic defects in a minority of patients. The shape and size of the crowns is essentially normal, but the roots are slender and stunted, giving the tooth a cervical constriction and bulbous outline radiographically (Fig. 2.22). Dentine formation progresses to obliterate the pulp chamber at an early age. There is a

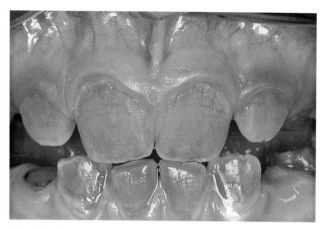

Fig. 2.21 **Dentinogenesis imperfecta.** Showing the grey-brown translucent appearance of the teeth which are of normal morphology.

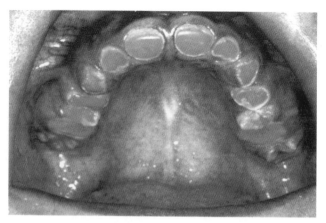

Fig. 2.23 **Dentinogenesis imperfecta.** In this 14-year-old, the teeth have worn down to gingival level, but the pulp chambers have become obliterated as part of the disease process. A rim of enamel remains around the necks of the posterior teeth.

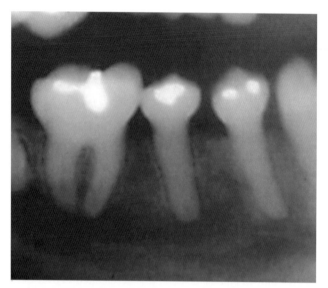

Fig. 2.22 **Dentinogenesis imperfecta.** Showing the slender roots and bulbous crowns of the 'tulip-shaped' teeth.

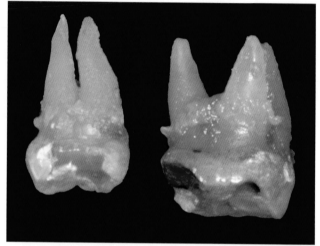

Fig. 2.24 **Dentinogenesis imperfecta.** Slender tapering roots and loss of enamel through fracturing.

weak zone in the dentine just below the amelodentine junction, and the lack of resilient dentine to support the enamel allows enamel to chip away, exposing the dentine, which is soft and rapidly wears away, eventually to the gingivae (Figs 2.23 and 2.24). In some patients, only a few teeth are severely affected, whereas the remainder appear normal.

Treatment aims to preserve vertical dimension, avoid extractions to prevent space loss and allow normal alveolar bone growth for implants later. Early application of occlusal composite onlays and preformed metal crowns on molars reduce wear. Worn roots may be used as temporary overdenture abutments but are too soft to survive long.

Severely affected patients may have shell teeth, with only a thin outer mantle layer of dentine tissue surrounding overlarge pulp chambers. Shell teeth are very difficult to manage conservatively.

Tooth structure

The earliest-formed dentine under the amelodentine junction usually appears normal. There is a sharp junction with the deeper defective dentine. This has few tubules, and they run in disorganised patterns. The uniform structure of dentine is absent; extensions of the pulp penetrate the dentine almost to the enamel (Fig. 2.25) and can be exposed by attrition to devitalise the teeth. Calcification is incomplete and the dentine soft.

The pulp chamber becomes obliterated early, and odontoblasts degenerate. Cellular inclusions in the dentine are common. In shell teeth, the dentine layer is very thin (Fig. 2.26).

Review PMCID: PMC2600777

Dentinal dysplasia ('rootless' teeth)

→ Summary chart 2.1 p. 26

Dentinal dysplasia (previously type 1 but now the only type)

In this rare disorder, the crowns are of normal shape and size, but the roots are either absent or very short and conical. The pulp chambers are obliterated by multiple nodules of poorly organised dentine containing tubules running in sheaves. A range of pulp shapes can result from differing severity, with almost complete obliteration producing crescent-shaped pulp at the level of the floor of the normal chamber. In the worst affected teeth, roots are absent. Teeth tend to be lost early in life (Fig. 2.27). There are pulpal extensions through dentine to the enamel, and vitality is

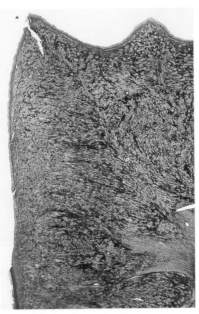

Fig. 2.25 Microscopic appearance of dentinogenesis imperfecta showing the grossly disorganised tubular structure with inclusions of pulp in the dentine and obliteration of the pulp cavity.

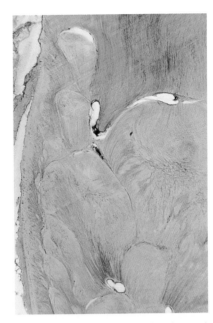

Fig. 2.28 **Dentinal dysplasia.** The pulp chamber in the short, broad root is obliterated by nodules of dentine with swirling patterns of tubules.

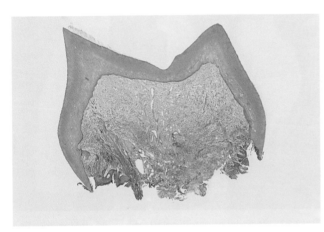

Fig. 2.26 **Shell tooth.** In this severe form of dentinogenesis imperfecta, only a thin mantle of dentine is formed, and no root develops.

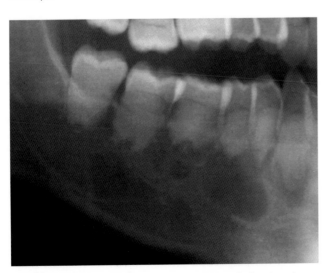

Fig. 2.27 **Dentinal dysplasia type 1.** Radiograph showing short roots, spontaneous pulp necrosis with apical areas, and obliterated crescent-shaped pulps.

lost quickly; otherwise the lack of roots predisposes to periodontitis.

The coronal dentine and enamel are normal or almost so, but dentinal tubule patterns in the root are abnormal (Fig. 2.28). Both dentitions are affected, the deciduous more severely.

Dentinal dysplasia 'type 2'

The defect in this rare disorder is in the dentine sialoprotein gene, so this disorder is better classified as a severely affected form of dentinogenesis imperfecta. The tooth crowns have the same opalescent appearance as dentinogenesis imperfecta in the deciduous dentition. The permanent dentition appears normal or nearly normal in colour, but the pulps are larger than normal. A tall, wide coronal pulp extends high into the crown (thistle pulp), sometimes with pulp stones, and more marked in the permanent dentition (Fig. 2.29).

Review PMCID: PMC2600777

DEFECTS OF ENAMEL AND DENTINE

→ Summary chart 2.1 p. 26

Regional odontodysplasia (ghost teeth)

→ Summary chart 2.2 p. 27

This localised disorder of development affects a group of teeth in which there are severe abnormalities of enamel, dentine and pulp. The disorder is not hereditary, and the aetiology is unknown. A few cases have been associated with facial vascular naevi or abnormalities such as hydrocephalus. There is no sex or racial predilection.

Clinically, regional odontodysplasia may be recognisable at the time of eruption of the deciduous teeth (2–4 years) or of the permanent teeth (7–11 years). The maxillary teeth are most frequently affected. Either or both dentitions, and one or, at most, two quadrants may be affected. The abnormal teeth frequently fail to erupt but, if they do, show yellowish deformed crowns with a rough surface.

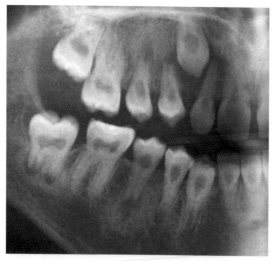

Fig. 2.29 Dentinogenesis imperfecta of dentinal dysplasia type 2 presentation. The pulp chambers are rounded, tall and wide in the developing dentition. The classical 'thistle-shaped' pulp appearance is seen in the lower canine and premolars.

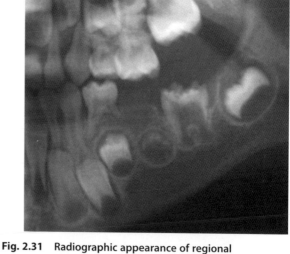

Fig. 2.31 Radiographic appearance of regional odontodysplasia. The lower left 5 and 6 are affected. Note their abnormal outline and radiodensity by comparison with the 4 and 7.

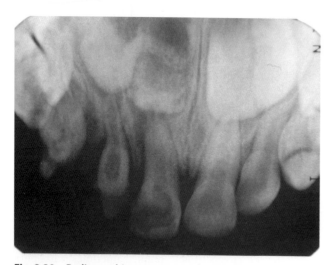

Fig. 2.30 Radiographic appearance of regional odontodysplasia. In the anterior regions the condition usually stops at the midline.

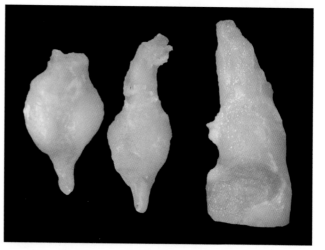

Fig. 2.32 Regional odontodysplasia. Distorted and hypoplastic teeth from the case shown in Fig. 2.30.

Review and cases PMID: 2549236

Cases PMID: 9524463

Natural history and treatment PMID: 17613259

Segmental odontomaxillary dysplasia

This rare disorder may be a mild form of the genetic condition hemimaxillofacial dysplasia; it can be mistaken for fibrous dysplasia or regional odontodysplasia.

Segmental odontomaxillary dysplasia causes unilateral expansion of the alveolar process of the maxilla in a child in the primary or mixed dentition. The premolar and molar regions are most frequently affected. Enlargement is due to both fibrous enlargement of the gingiva and swelling of the alveolar bone. The antrum is small, and the maxilla is distorted, although only rarely to the extent of causing facial asymmetry. Eruption of teeth in the affected area is delayed, and they are hypoplastic to varying degrees, with enlargement of the pulps, thin pitted enamel, an irregular pulp/dentine interface and many pseudoinclusions in poorly organised dentine, and pulp stones. Permanent successors, particularly the premolars, may be absent.

Affected teeth have very thin enamel and dentine surrounding a greatly enlarged pulp chamber. In radiographs, the teeth appear crumpled and abnormally radiolucent or hazy, due to the paucity of dental hard tissues, explaining the term 'ghost teeth' (Figs 2.30 and 2.31).

Histologically, the enamel thickness is highly irregular and lacks a well-defined prismatic structure. The dentine, which has a disorganised tubular structure, contains clefts and interglobular dentine mixed with amorphous mineralised tissue. The surrounding follicle soft tissue may contain small calcifications (Figs 2.33–2.34).

If they erupt, the teeth are susceptible to caries and fracture. If they can be preserved and restored, crown and root dentine continue to form, and the teeth may survive long enough to allow normal development of the alveolar ridge and occlusion. However, extractions are often required eventually. This should not be done until it is certain that eruption has completely failed or the defects are too severe to be treatable.

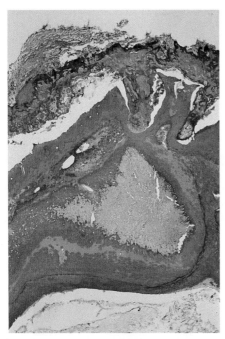

Fig. 2.33 Regional odontodysplasia. Both enamel and dentine are deformed, and there is calcification of the reduced enamel epithelium seen as a dark blue line at the top of the image.

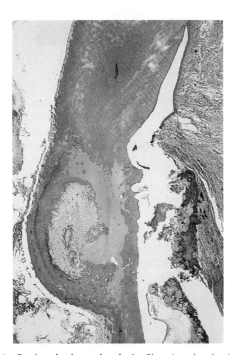

Fig. 2.34 Regional odontodysplasia. Showing dysplastic dentine with a disorganised tubule structure, an irregular enamel space and mineralised enamel epithelium.

Radiographically, there is a zone of bone sclerosis with a coarse trabecular pattern and loss of the cortex and missing and distorted teeth (Fig. 2.35). Histologically, the sclerotic zone consists of woven bone trabeculae in bland fibrous tissue and appears superficially similar to the regressing stage of fibrous dysplasia. Both radiographs and histology are therefore necessary for diagnosis.

Case series PMID: 21684782

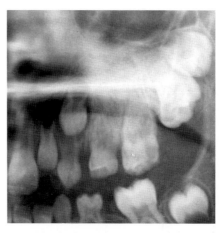

Fig. 2.35 Segmental odontomaxillary dysplasia. Showing abnormal upper primary molars that are indistinct against a background of even, coarsely trabecular bone. Permanent successors are absent.

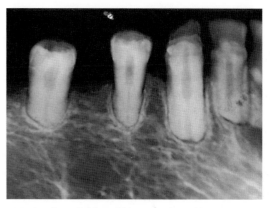

Fig. 2.36 Teeth in childhood hypoparathyroidism with short blunt roots, open apices and large pulp chambers.

OTHER SYSTEMIC DISEASES AFFECTING TEETH

Other metabolic disturbances

Rickets can cause hypocalcification of the teeth, but only if unusually severe (see Ch. 13).

Early-onset idiopathic hypoparathyroidism is rare. Ecto-dermal effects are associated. The teeth may therefore be hypoplastic with ridged enamel, short blunt roots and per-sistently open apices (Fig. 2.36). The nails may be defective, and there may be complete absence of hair. Patients with early-onset idiopathic hypoparathyroidism may later develop other endocrine deficiencies (polyendocrinopathy syn-drome), and chronic oral candidosis may be the first sign (Ch. 15).

Hypophosphatasia. This rare genetic disorder can have severe skeletal effects as a result of failure of development of mature bone. There may also be failure of cementum formation causing early loss of teeth (Fig. 2.37). In milder forms, premature loss of the deciduous incisors is charac-teristic and occasionally the only overt manifestation of the disease.

Hypophosphatasia dental effects PMID: 19232125

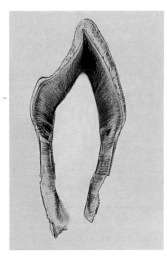

Fig. 2.37 Tooth in hypophosphatasia showing the enlarged pulp chamber and absence of cementum.

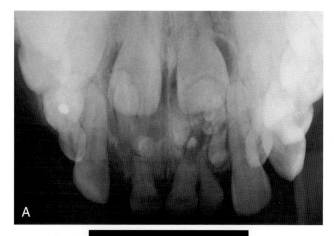

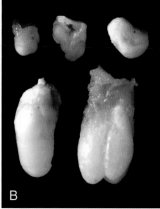

Fig. 2.39 Gardner's syndrome. Multiple unerupted abnormally formed supernumerary teeth. See also Fig. 12.16.

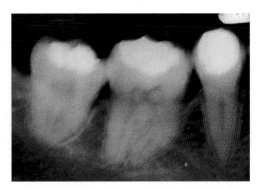

Fig. 2.38 Multiple pulp stones in a case of Ehlers–Danlos syndrome.

Ehlers–Danlos syndromes

This group of collagen disorders is characterised (to varying degrees) by hypermobile joints, loose hyperextensible skin, fragile oral mucosa and, in type VIII, early-onset periodontitis. There may also be temporomandibular joint symptoms such as recurrent dislocation (see main section in Ch.14).

The main dental abnormalities are small teeth with short roots and multiple pulp stones (Fig. 2.38).

Gardner's syndrome (familial adenomatous polyposis)

The Gardner variant of familial adenomatous polyposis (often referred to as Gardner's syndrome) is characterised by multiple osteomas, especially of the jaws, colonic polyps and skin tumours. The majority of patients have dental abnormalities. These include impacted teeth other than third molars, supernumerary or missing teeth and abnormal root formation (Fig. 2.39). This syndrome is discussed and illustrated further in Chapter 12.

Colon carcinoma develops in almost all patients by middle age, and the mortality is high. The dental abnormalities can be detected in childhood or adolescence, and recognition of this syndrome may be life saving.

Epidermolysis bullosa

Epidermolysis bullosa is a genetic blistering disease of skin and mucosae (Ch. 16). Dental abnormalities include fine or coarse pitting defects, or thin and uneven enamel, which may also lack prismatic structure. The amelodentinal junction may be smooth. Dental defects vary in the different subtypes of the disease but are most frequent in the autosomal recessive, scarring type of epidermolysis bullosa in which there may be delayed, or failure of, eruption. The defects result from poor adhesion between ameloblasts during development.

Congenital syphilis → Summary chart 2.1 p. 26

Prenatal syphilis, the result of maternal infection, can cause a characteristic dental deformity, described by Hutchinson in 1858.

If the fetus becomes infected at a very early stage, abortion follows. Infants born with stigmata of congenital syphilis result from later fetal infection, and only the permanent teeth are affected. The characteristic defects are usually seen in the upper central incisors.

The incisors (Hutchinson's incisors) are small, barrel-shaped and taper toward the tip (Fig. 2.40). The incisal edge sometimes shows a crescentic notch or deep fissure which forms before eruption and can be seen radiographically. An anterior open bite is also characteristic. The first molars may be dome shaped (Moon's molars) or may have a rough pitted occlusal surface with compressed nodules instead of cusps (mulberry molars) (Fig. 2.41). These defects are often thought largely of historical interest, but congenital syphilis has reappeared in developed countries including the UK. Several hundred cases of congenital syphilis occur every year in the United States, and worldwide half a million infants die from it every year.

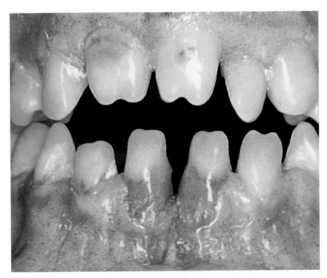

Fig. 2.40 Congenital syphilis: Hutchinson's teeth. The characteristics are the notched incisal edge and the peg shape tapering from neck to tip. *(From Cawson RA et al, 2001. Oral disease. 3rd ed. St Louis: Mosby.)*

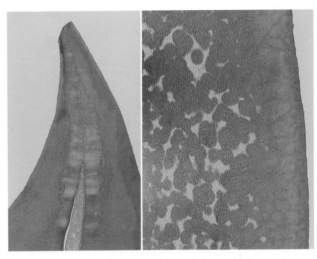

Fig. 2.42 Vitamin D-resistant rickets. A fine pulpal extension into the incisal dentine is just visible on the left. Right, at higher power, there is prominent globular mineralisation of dentine.

Vitamin D-resistant rickets

This term is given to familial hypophosphataemia, a rare X-linked dominant disease causing phosphate loss in the kidneys, and consequent rickets that does not respond to vitamin D. Patients have short legs, wide skull sutures and kyphosis develops during adulthood.

The teeth have abnormally large pulp chambers with fine extensions of the pulp horns to the tips of the cuspal dentine (Fig. 2.42). These are prone to exposure by attrition or fracture and are often invisible radiographically. A periapical granuloma on an apparently normal tooth is a common presentation.

Calcification of dentine is defective. The typical interglobular mineralisation of rickets is seen throughout the dentine.

EXTRINSIC AGENTS AFFECTING TEETH

→ Summary chart 2.1 p. 26

Drugs

Tetracycline pigmentation

Tetracycline is taken up by calcifying tissues, and the band of tetracycline-stained bone or tooth substance fluoresces bright yellow under ultraviolet light.

The teeth become stained only when tetracycline is given during their development, and it can cross the placenta to stain the developing teeth of the fetus. More frequently, permanent teeth are stained by tetracycline given during infancy. Tetracycline is deposited along the incremental lines of the dentine and, to a lesser extent, of the enamel.

The more prolonged the course of treatment, the broader the band of stain and the deeper the discoloration. The teeth are at first bright yellow but become a dirty brown or grey (Figs 2.43 and 2.44). The stain is permanent, and when the permanent incisors are affected, the dark appearance can only be disguised. When the history is vague, the brownish colour of tetracycline-stained teeth must be distinguished from dentinogenesis imperfecta. In dentinogenesis imperfecta, the teeth are obviously more translucent than normal and, in many cases, chipping of the enamel from the dentine can be seen. In tetracycline-induced defects, the enamel is not abnormally translucent and is firmly attached to

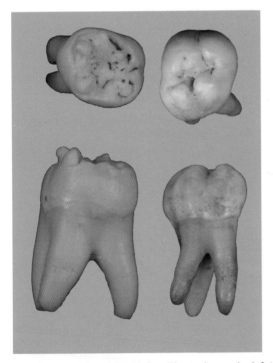

Fig. 2.41 Congenital syphilis: Molars. The molar on the left is a mulberry or Fournier molar with cusps surrounded by a hypoplastic groove producing a knobbly surface. That on the right is a Moon's molar, with a smooth rounded crown that tapers toward the occlusal surface. *(Copyright Museums at the Royal College of Surgeons.)*

The effects are due to infection of the dental follicle by *Treponema pallidum*. The postulated consequences are chronic inflammation, fibrosis of the tooth sac, compression of the developing tooth and distortion of the ameloblast layer. *T. pallidum* and inflammation are thought to cause proliferation of the odontogenic epithelium, which bulges and kinks into the dentine papilla, causing the characteristic central notch.

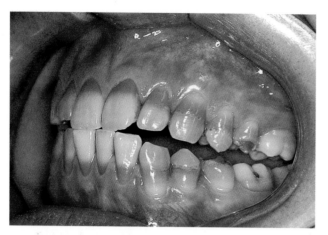

Fig. 2.43 **Tetracycline staining.** Note the chronological distribution of the dark-brown intrinsic stain.

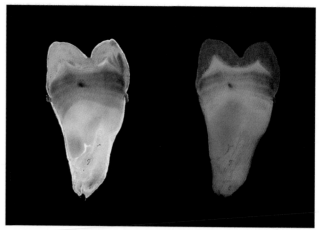

Fig. 2.45 **Tetracycline pigmentation.** Ground (undecalcified) section (*left*) shows the broad bands of tetracycline deposited along the incremental lines of the dentine; (*right*) same section viewed under ultraviolet light shows fluorescence of the bands of tetracycline.

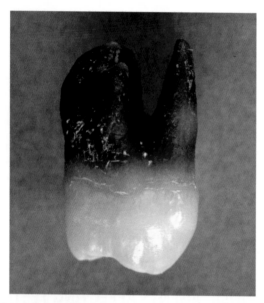

Fig. 2.44 **Tetracycline staining.** Now one of the commoner forms of staining, limited to third molar roots from use of minocycline during adolescence.

> **Box 2.5** **Dental fluorosis: distinctive features**
> - Limited to geographical areas where water-borne fluorides exceed approximately 2 parts per million
> - Only those who have lived in a high-fluoride area during dental development show mottling
> - The defect is not acquired by older visitors to the area
> - Permanent teeth are affected; mottling of deciduous teeth is rare
> - Mottled teeth are less susceptible to caries than normal teeth from low-fluoride areas
> - A typical effect is spotty paper-white enamel opacities
> - Brown extrinsic staining of these patches may be acquired after eruption

dentine. In very severe cases, intact teeth may fluoresce under ultraviolet light. Otherwise, the diagnosis can only be confirmed after a tooth has been extracted. In an undecalcified section, the yellow fluorescence of the tetracycline deposited along the incremental lines can be easily seen (Fig. 2.45).

It is no longer necessary to give tetracycline during dental development. There are equally effective alternatives, and it should be avoided from approximately the fourth month to at least the 12th year of childhood, ideally the 16th year. Nevertheless, tetracycline staining is still seen.

Minocycline stain PMID: 23887527

Cytotoxic chemotherapy

Increasing numbers of children are surviving malignant disease, particularly acute leukaemia, as a result of cytotoxic chemotherapy.

Among survivors, teeth that develop during treatment may have short roots, hypoplasia of the crowns and enamel defects. Microscopically, incremental lines may be more prominent, corresponding to growth arrest or delay during the period of chemotherapy. In extreme cases, tooth formation may be aborted so that oligodontia results.

Fluorosis → Summary chart 2.1 p. 26

Mottled enamel is the most frequently seen and most reliable sign of excess fluoride in the drinking water. It has distinctive features (Box 2.5). The highest fluoride levels completely disrupt amelogenesis, producing hypoplastic patches. Lower levels inhibit mineralisation and prevent enamel maturation.

Clinical features

Mottling ranges from paper-white matte patches to opaque, brown, pitted and brittle enamel. Clinically, it may be difficult to distinguish fluorotic defects from amelogenesis imperfecta when the degree of exposure to fluoride is unknown (Figs 2.46–2.48).

There is considerable individual variation in the effects of fluorides. A few patients acquire mottling after exposure to relatively low concentrations (Fig. 2.49), while others exposed to higher concentrations appear unaffected. Being a systemic effect, fluorosis is bilateral and usually affects all teeth, though a chronological pattern could result from a limited period of exposure. The perikymata are enhanced and visible clinically in severe cases, producing what appear

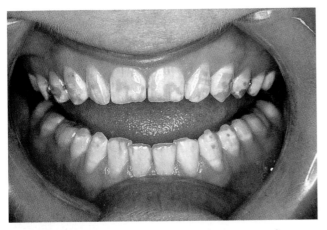

Fig. 2.46 Fluoride mottling. In this case, from an area of endemic fluorosis, there is generalised opaque white mottling with patchy enamel hypoplasia. Note the resemblance to the hypomaturation type of amelogenesis imperfecta.

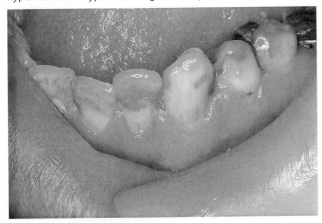

Fig. 2.47 Fluorosis. Moderate effects from an area of endemic fluorosis. Irregular patchy discoloration.

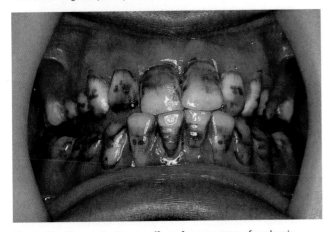

Fig. 2.48 Fluorosis. Severe effects from an area of endemic fluorosis. Closer view showing irregular depressions caused by hypoplasia and white opaque flecks and patches.

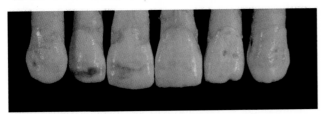

Fig. 2.49 Fluorosis from an area of endemic natural fluorosis in Gloucestershire.

Box 2.6   Grading of mottled enamel

- Very mild. Small paper-white areas involve less than 25% of surface
- Mild. Opaque areas involve as much as 50% of surface
- Moderate. The whole of the enamel surface may be affected with paper-white or brownish areas or both (Fig. 2.47)
- Severe. The enamel is grossly defective, opaque, pitted, stained brown and brittle (Fig. 2.48)

Table 2.1   Effects on enamel of raised fluoride levels

Fluoride concentration	Effects	Clinical appearance
Less than 0.5 ppm	Very mild or mild defects in as many as 6% of patients	Inconspicuous
0.5 to 1.5 ppm	At the upper limit, 22% show very mild defects	
2.5 ppm	Very mild or mild defects in more than 50% Moderate or severe defects in nearly 10%	Noticeable
4.5 ppm	Nearly all patients affected to some degree; 46% have 'moderate' and 18% 'severe' defects	Disfiguring
6.0 ppm and more	All patients affected; 50% severely disfiguring	

to be horizontal lines, which misleadingly suggests chronological hypoplasia.

Changes due to mottling are graded as shown in Box 2.6.

Pathology

Fluoride exerts its effects through inhibition of ameloblasts. At intermediate levels (2–6 ppm), the enamel matrix is normal in structure and quantity. The form of the tooth is unaffected, but there are patches of incomplete calcification beneath the surface layer. These appear as opacities because of high organic and water content that cause light reflection. Where there are high concentrations of fluorides (higher than 6 ppm), the enamel is pitted and brittle, with severe and widespread staining. Deciduous teeth are rarely mottled because excess fluoride is taken up by the maternal skeleton. However, when fluoride levels are excessively high (higher than 8 ppm), as in parts of India, mottling of deciduous teeth may be seen.

With severe mottling of the enamel, other effects of excessive fluoride intake, especially sclerosis of the skeleton, may develop. Radiographically, increased density of the skeleton may be seen in areas where the fluoride content of the water exceeds 8 ppm.

The severity of defects in relation to fluoride concentrations is shown in Table 2.1, and its relationship to caries prevalence in Fig. 2.50.

Mild dental fluorosis is not readily distinguishable from non-fluoride defects, and non-specific defects are more common in areas where the water contains less than 1 ppm of fluoride. Minimal mottling is associated with levels of 1 ppm fluoride in temperate climates and 0.7 ppm in hotter countries.

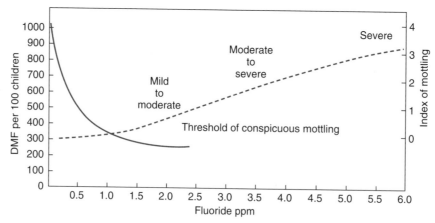

Fig. 2.50 Caries prevalence and mottling. The general relationship between the prevalence of caries (*continuous line*) and the severity of mottling (*broken line*) in persons continuously exposed to various levels of fluoride in the water during dental development. The optimum level of fluoride can be seen to be approximately 1 part per million. Higher concentrations of fluoride cause increasing incidence and severity of mottling without a comparable improvement in resistance to caries. The index of mottling is obtained by giving an arbitrary value for each degree of mottling and relating the numbers of patients with each grade to the total number examined.

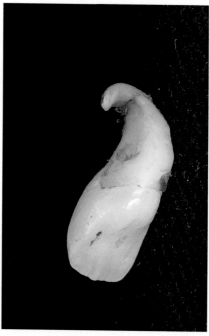

Fig. 2.51 A dilacerated upper central incisor. There has been an abrupt change in the direction of root growth after approximately one-third of the root was formed.

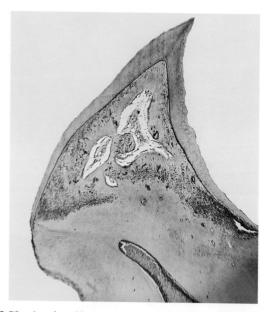

Fig. 2.52 Another dilacerated tooth showing, in addition to the deflected root, a change in enamel contour and disorganised coronal dentine formed after the causative trauma. The junction between dentine formed before and after trauma is clearly seen.

Mild enamel mottling has many causes that cannot usually be distinguished, even by analysis of an extracted or exfoliated tooth.

Treatment of opacities PMID: 26856002

Other acquired developmental anomalies
Dilaceration

Trauma to a developing tooth can cause the root to form at an angle to the normal axis of the tooth – a deformity known as *dilaceration*. The sudden disturbance to odontogenesis may cause the formation of highly irregular dentine at the bend, but the angulated root that develops after trauma is often of normal tubular dentine. The hook-shaped tooth is likely to be difficult to extract (Figs 2.51 and 2.52).

Fetal alcohol syndrome

Maternal alcoholism may cause developmental defects in the fetus. The eyes typically slant laterally, the lower half of the face is elongated and there is learning disability. Dental development may be delayed, and there may be enamel defects, such as mottled opacities in the enamel near the incisal margins, but elsewhere abnormal enamel translucency.

Rhesus incompatibility

Maternal-fetal rhesus blood group incompatibility causes haemolytic disease of the newborn, in which maternal antirhesus antibodies cross the placenta and cause haemolytic anaemia in a fetus with a rhesus-positive blood group. If jaundice is severe, bilirubin can bind to the developing teeth, causing green or grey-yellow discolouration (Fig. 2.53).

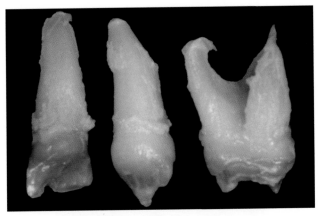

Fig. 2.53 **Rhesus incompatibility.** Deciduous teeth from a patient who suffered haemolytic anaemia from rhesus incompatibility. There is greenish discolouration of the dentine and enamel formed before birth.

ODONTOMES

Odontomes result from aberrant development of the dental lamina. The most minor examples, although they are not usually called odontomes, are slight malformations, such as an exaggerated cingulum or extra roots or cusps on otherwise normal teeth. All gradations exist between these anomalies and composite odontomes where the dental tissues have developed in a completely irregular and haphazard manner bearing no resemblance to a tooth and occasionally forming a large mass (Ch. 11).

Dens invaginatus is an exaggeration of the process of formation of a cingulum pit. Dentine and enamel-forming tissue invaginate into the pulp to appear radiographically as a tooth-within-a-tooth (*dens in dente*, Fig. 2.54). In the full dens invaginatus, also known as an invaginated or dilated odontome, the invagination extends the whole length of a tooth and sometimes through a widely dilated apex (Fig. 2.55). Often the invagination has incomplete walls allowing the exterior to communicate with the pulp and devitalising it. Alternatively, food debris lodges in the cavity to cause caries which rapidly penetrates the superficially located pulp chamber.

Dens evaginatus is the opposite, an enamel- and dentine-covered spur extending outward from the occlusal surface of a premolar or molar (Fig. 2.56). Fracture exposes the internal pulp horn.

Geminated teeth, meaning double or twinned teeth, are most common in the maxillary incisor region. The pulp chambers may be entirely separate, joined in the middle of the tooth or branched, with the pulp chambers of separated crowns sharing a common root canal. The crowns may be entirely separate or divided only by a shallow groove. The roots may be single or double. These defects are commoner in the deciduous dentition. In the past, effort has been expended trying to decide whether such teeth arise by fusion of two tooth germs or partial splitting of a single germ. This distinction is pointless, and it seems likely that the condition is genetic; it is often bilateral and is rarely seen in excessive crowding.

These malformed teeth usually need to be removed before they obstruct the eruption of other teeth or become infected, or for cosmetic reasons.

Enamel pearls are uncommon, minor abnormalities that are formed on otherwise normal teeth by ameloblasts that differentiate below the amelocemental junction. The pearls are usually round, a few millimetres in diameter and often

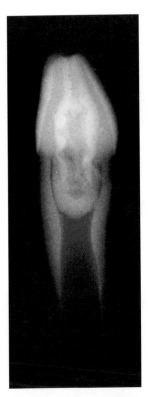

Fig. 2.54 **Dens in dente or mild invaginated odontome.** In this radiograph, the enamel-lined invagination and its communication with the exterior at the incisal tip are clearly seen. The pulp is compressed to the periphery.

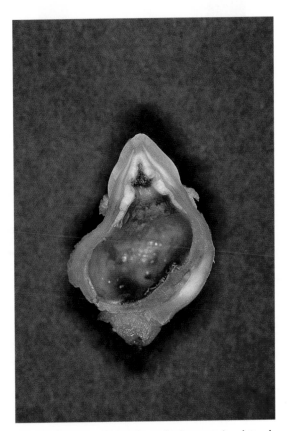

Fig. 2.55 **A dilated and invaginated odontome in a lateral incisor, sectioned vertically.** The central cavity communicates with the exterior through an invagination in the cusp tip.

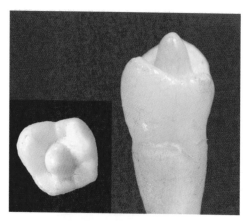

Fig. 2.56 Dens evaginatus from a lower premolar, occlusal surface inset.

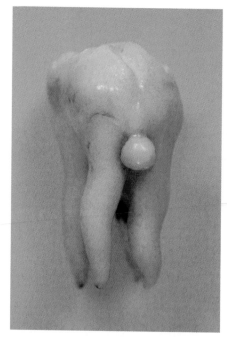

Fig. 2.58 Enamel pearl associated with a spur of enamel joining the crown to the pearl.

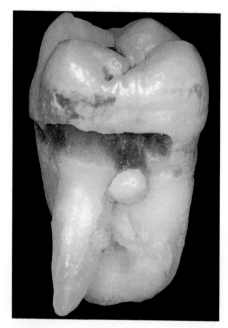

Fig. 2.57 **Enamel pearl.** There is a small mass of enamel at the root bifurcation.

> **Box 2.7   Normal teething**
>
> One-third of infants have no signs or symptoms. Many only have a few.
>
> - Effects are limited to a few days each side of the day of eruption
> - Increased biting and rubbing the gingiva
> - Reflex salivation and drooling
> - Irritability and sleep disturbance
> - Rubbing of face and ears
> - Facial reddening of the cheek
> - Decreased appetite
> - Mild temperature increase

form at the bifurcation of upper permanent molars (Figs 2.57 and 2.58).

Enamel pearls may consist of only a nodule of enamel attached to the dentine, or may have a core of dentine containing a horn of the pulp. They may cause a stagnation area at the gingival margin but, if they contain pulp, this will be exposed when the pearl is removed. The enamel and dentine are normal histologically.

DISORDERS OF ERUPTION

Normal eruption

Eighteenth-century parish registers are replete with the names of infants who died as a result of teething. Although this is now considered impossible, other myths about tooth eruption abound.

Teething coincides with a period of naturally low resistance to infection and declining maternal passive immunity during which viral infections are common. Eruption is associated with a very slight rise in temperature (not a fever), mild discomfort locally, reflex salivation causing drooling and, sometimes, reddening of cheeks. Systemic symptoms during teething should therefore be investigated because, if significant, they are more likely to be caused by primary herpetic gingivostomatitis or other treatable infection. In many infants teething passes unnoticed (Box 2.7). The signs and symptoms are not specific and are also seen in those not teething, in whom they pass unremarked.

Fusion of the enamel epithelium with the oral epithelium allows eruption without bleeding, but the urge to chew during teething is strong, and trauma to the mucosa may cause haemorrhage over an erupting tooth before it reaches the surface ('eruption haematoma', Fig. 10.23).

Very occasionally eruption of permanent molars is associated with painless loss of a small sequestrum. Bone lying in the concavity of the crown can be resorbed around the periphery while the cusps erupt, cutting off its blood supply from adjacent tissues ('eruption sequestrum'). Lower first permanent molars are the most frequently affected teeth.

Symptoms of teething PMID 10742315

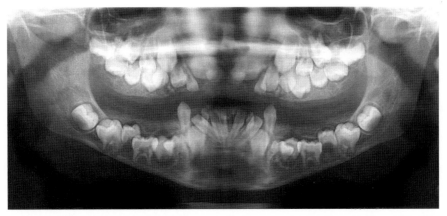

Fig. 2.59 **Primary failure of eruption.** A few teeth have erupted anteriorly, but after the last erupted tooth standing, none have erupted.

Natal teeth

Teeth present at birth or shortly afterward are called *natal teeth*. Almost always these are normal deciduous lower incisors that erupt prematurely. Occasionally they may be supernumerary teeth, though deciding this can be difficult as radiographs are difficult to take at such a young age. Removal may be required to aid feeding or when inadequate root development risks their displacement and inhalation, but they are best retained.

Bohn's nodules may be mistaken for erupting teeth in neonates.

Natal teeth are seen in a number of rare developmental disorders, pachyonychia congenita, Ellis-van Creveld and Hallermann-Streiff syndromes.

Delayed eruption

Eruption of deciduous teeth starts at approximately 6 months, usually with the appearance of the lower incisors, and is complete by approximately 2 years, earlier in females and with considerable individual variation in timing. Mass failure of eruption is very rare despite the biological complexity of the process. More often eruption delay has local causes and affects one or a few teeth.

Failure of a single tooth or adjacent teeth to appear in the mouth within a few months of the contralateral equivalent should trigger radiographic assessment to check for its presence and location. However, delayed appearance of the deciduous dentition in the absence of a cause does not warrant concern until it is delayed for 1 year provided no mechanical cause is evident, as eruption times are so variable.

In generalised delay caused by systemic illness, for instance in preterm infants, recovery normally allows eruption to proceed and after a few years eruption catches up with the normal timetable. Systemic diseases that cause delayed eruption are all rare. Eruption is complex, and many diseases can interfere with it. Both chemotherapy and radiotherapy arrest or interrupt eruption as well as tooth formation.

Single tooth failure of eruption is almost always due to a mechanical obstruction or ankylosis.

Primary eruption failure is a rare condition. Usually some teeth erupt, but then all teeth distally in the quadrant, sometimes all, remain unerupted and may eventually ankylose (Fig. 2.59). Half of cases are familial, and some are associated with mutation of the parathyroid hormone receptor gene. A common mild presentation is failure of eruption of only permanent molars, and the first permanent molars are almost always involved. There may be bilateral involvement, a Class 3 skeletal pattern and oligodontia associated. This condition does not cause delayed eruption of single teeth. Teeth in primary eruption failure do not respond to orthodontic traction, and treatment usually requires extraction. Restoration is then difficult due to lack of alveolar bone growth.

Causes of delayed eruption are shown in Box 2.8.

Primary eruption failure PMID: 17482073

Changes affecting buried teeth

Teeth may occasionally remain unerupted in the jaws for many years without complications, or may undergo varying degrees of hypercementosis or resorption (Ch. 6). Alternatively, dentigerous cysts may develop (see Ch. 10), as often happens in cleidocranial dysplasia.

Box 2.8   Causes of delayed eruption of permanent teeth

Localised

- Impaction, usually last teeth in any series
- Insufficient space in the arch, crowding, supernumerary teeth
- Retention of a deciduous predecessor, ankylosis
- Premature loss of a deciduous predecessor, before half of the successor root is formed
- Malposition
- Local pathological process
  - Odontogenic cysts and tumours
  - Cherubism
- Defects of the teeth
  - Dilaceration
  - Connate teeth
  - Turner teeth
  - Regional odontodysplasia
  - Segmental odontomaxillary dysplasia

Generalised

- Delayed development
  - Malnutrition
  - Down's syndrome (Ch. 39)
  - Hypothyroidism (cretinism) (Ch. 36)
  - Hypoparathyroidism and pseudohypoparathyroidism
  - Hypopituitarism

- Metabolic disease with delayed growth
  - Rickets (Ch. 13)
  - Infants with premature birth
  - Human immunodeficiency virus infection in infancy (Ch. 29)
- Increased resistance of overlying mucosa
  - Scarring
  - Hereditary gingival fibromatosis (Ch. 7)
  - Drug-induced gingival overgrowth (Ch. 7)
- Iatrogenic
  - Chemotherapy for malignant neoplasms
  - Radiotherapy to the jaws
- Increased resistance of bone or reduced bone turnover
  - Osteopetrosis
  - Gaucher's disease
- Complete or near complete failure of eruption
  - Cleidocranial dysplasia (Ch. 13)
  - Idiopathic or primary eruption failure

Disorders of development

3

Important developmental defects of the jaws are summarised in Box 3.1, and some are discussed more fully in other chapters.

CLEFTS OF LIP OR PALATE

Clefts of the palate alone and those of the lip, with or without cleft palate, are genetically distinct conditions. The embryology of the lower face and mechanisms of closure of the palatal shelves and fusion of the soft tissue processes to form the upper lip are very complex. Until around 6 weeks of development, the mouth and future nasal cavity are one. Then fusion of the median nasal process and maxillary processes of the first branchial arch forms the midline alveolar ridge and anterior palate, or primary palate. By the end of week 9, the secondary palate has formed by growth of the palatal shelves, their rotation and fusion. Formation of a complete palate therefore requires growth and migration of tissues, breakdown of epithelium to allow fusion and growth of the mandible to allow the tongue to drop out of the way. The process takes slightly longer in females, and the longer period of development makes them more prone to palatal clefts than males. Many genes are involved, and there is a relatively long period during which an environmental insult could interfere with the process. Approximately one in 700 babies have clefts of lip and/or palate. Mechanisms are summarised in Figs 3.1 and 3.2.

The sites of clefts vary because the lip and anterior palate (the primary palate) develop independently and before the hard and soft palates (the secondary palate). Isolated cleft lip is therefore the result of an early developmental disorder, whereas isolated cleft palate results from influences acting later, after the primary palate has closed. By contrast, a prolonged disorder of development can prevent both primary and secondary palates from closing and leaves a severe combined defect (Figs 3.3 and 3.4).

Clefts of lip and palate form because of failure of growth and migration of mesenchyme to form the alveolus and lip, not because an embryological line of fusion fails to close. In contrast, cleft palate develops because of failure to close the cleft during development.

The main types of cleft are summarised in Box 3.2. A complete cleft of the lip is one that extends into the nose, completely separating the lip into two portions. Incomplete clefts are limited to lip or lip and alveolus, and there is some continuity between the segments to stabilise the tissues.

Cleft lip and cleft palate

Cleft lip (with or without a palatal cleft) is a single condition that presents with varying degrees of severity. It is the most common craniofacial anomaly and affects approximately 1 per 1000 live births, roughly half of whom have a cleft lip alone and half of whom have cleft lip with a cleft palate. Twice as many males as females are affected, and the right side is twice as frequently involved.

There is a strong genetic background to cleft lip and palate, but the aetiology is complex. Either dominant or recessive inheritance can be found in familial cases, whereas others appear multifactorial. The risk of having such defects is considerably greater if one, and particularly if both, of the parents are affected or if the cleft is more severe. There are many candidate genes affecting different stages of palate development. Hedgehog pathway and PTCH gene variants affect growth and patterning, and TGF beta is involved in fusion. Many other genes have been implicated. IRF6 (interferon regulatory factor 6), FGFR2 (fibroblast growth factor receptor 2), MSX1 (Msh homeobox1), fibroblast growth

---

Box 3.1   Developmental defects of the jaws, mouth and face

Defects of the jaws

- Clefts of the palate and/or lip
- Cleidocranial dysplasia (Ch. 13)
- Cherubism (Ch. 13)
- Basal cell naevus syndrome (Ch. 10)
- Gardner's syndrome (Ch. 12)
- Osteogenesis imperfecta (Ch. 13)
- Craniofacial anomalies
- Hereditary prognathism

Defects of the soft tissues

- Ankyloglossia
- Cowden's syndrome
- Ehlers-Danlos syndrome (Ch. 14)
- Branchial and thyroglossal cysts (Ch. 10)
- Lingual thyroid (Ch. 36)
- White sponge naevus (Ch. 18)
- Some pigmented lesions (Ch. 26)

Defects of the teeth (Ch. 2)

Box 3.2   Clefts of lip and/or palate

Cleft lip

- Unilateral (usually on the left side), with or without an anterior alveolar ridge cleft
- Bilateral, with or without alveolar ridge clefts, complete or incomplete

Palatal clefts

- Bifid uvula
- Soft palate only
- Both hard and soft palate

Combined lip and palatal defects

- Unilateral, complete or incomplete
- Cleft palate with bilateral cleft lip, complete or incomplete

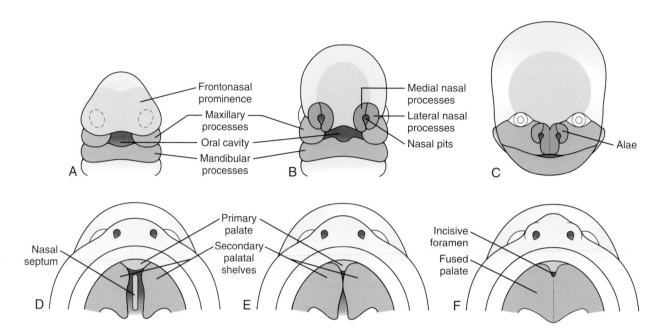

Fig. 3.1 **Development of the lip and palate.** Schematic diagrams of the development of the lip and palate in humans. (A) The developing frontonasal prominence, paired maxillary processes and paired mandibular processes surround the primitive oral cavity by the fourth week of embryonic development. (B) By the fifth week, the nasal pits have formed, which leads to formation of the paired medial and lateral nasal processes. (C) The medial nasal processes have merged with the maxillary processes to form the upper lip and primary palate by the end of the sixth week. The lateral nasal processes form the nasal alae. Similarly, the mandibular processes fuse to form the lower jaw. (D) During the sixth week of embryogenesis, the secondary palate develops in the form of bilateral outgrowths from the maxillary processes, which grow vertically down the side of the tongue. (E) Subsequently, the palatal shelves elevate to a horizontal position above the tongue, contact one another and commence fusion. (F) Fusion of the palatal shelves ultimately divides the oronasal space into separate oral and nasal cavities.

(From Dixon, M.J., Marazita, M.L., Beaty, T.H., et al. 2011. Cleft lip and palate: understanding genetic and environmental influences. Nat Rev Genet. 12(3), pp. 167-178.)

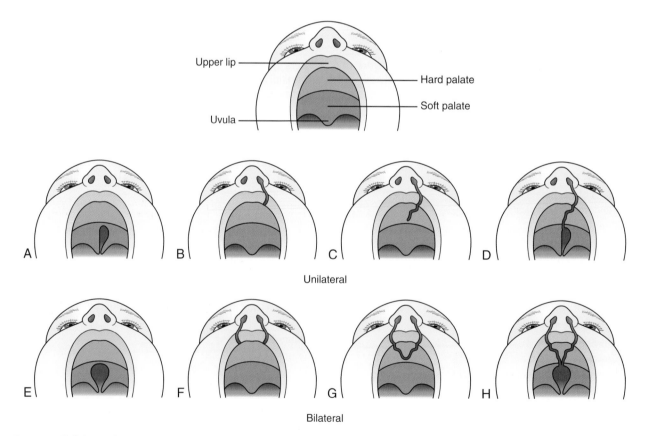

Fig. 3.2 **Cleft lip and palate types.** A set of illustrative drawings of cleft lip and palate types. A and E show unilateral and bilateral clefts of the soft palate; B, C and D show degrees of unilateral cleft lip and palate; and F, G and H show degrees of bilateral cleft lip and palate.

(From Dixon, M.J., Marazita M.L., Beaty, T.H., et al. 2011. Cleft lip and palate: understanding genetic and environmental influences. Nat Rev Genet. 12(3), pp. 167-178.)

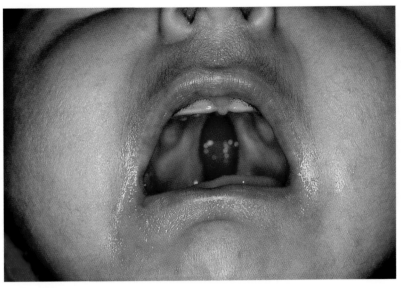

Fig. 3.3 **Cleft palate.** A broad midline defect is present. *(By kind permission of Mrs E Horrocks.)*

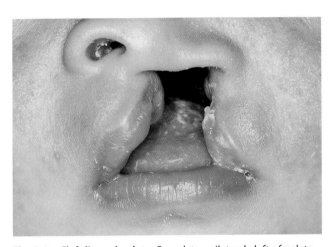

Fig. 3.4 **Cleft lip and palate.** Complete unilateral cleft of palate, alveolar bone and lip joining the oral and nasal cavities. *(By kind permission of Mrs E Horrocks.)*

Box 3.3   Management of clefts: important considerations

- Psychological support for the family and later the patient
- Provision for feeding in infancy when palatal clefts are severe
- Prevention of movement of the two halves of the maxilla or premaxilla pending surgery
- Measures to counteract speech defects
- Cosmetic repair of cleft lips
- Later closure of palate
- Monitoring for hearing loss
- Speech and language therapy
- Aggressive dental prevention regime
- Restoration of anterior teeth
- Genetic counselling if syndromic

---

factors (FGF1 and FGF8) and BMP4 (bone morphogenetic protein 4) are the most likely.

Environmental causes are also recognised and include smoking and alcohol, phenytoin and retinoids and other drugs. These environmental causes usually cause clefts combined with other developmental defects.

Review PMCID: PMC3086810

Management

The birth of a baby with a cleft lip triggers very early involvement of a multidisciplinary team. Important considerations are summarised in Box 3.3. Immediate considerations are psychological support for the family, both for the initial shock and during many years of treatment to follow. It is important to establish feeding as soon as possible. Cleft lip alone causes few problems, but a cleft palate prevents suckling, and either a feeding plate to close the defect or specially designed feeding bottles may be required.

Cleft lip is closed surgically, eliminating the cleft, repairing the continuity of the lip muscle and recontouring the philtrum and nasal aperture. Early surgery has best results with least subsequent scarring and distortion, so repair is usually performed at approximately 3 months, but earlier in some centres.

The palatal cleft is treated initially by an obturator plate that must be replaced regularly as the child grows. Surgery is performed between 9 and 12 months of age, and a bone graft may be required for wide defects. Palatal surgery leads to scarring that inhibits maxillary growth and contributes to the class III appearance of the face in later life. Re-operation may be necessary to lessen the deformity (Fig. 3.5).

Between the ages of 1 and 5 years, attention needs to be paid to hearing, for which ear grommets may be necessary to prevent otitis media and hearing loss. The distorted soft palate musculature fails to open the pharyngeal end of the Eustachian tube, predisposing to glue ear and infection. Poor hearing may interfere with development of speech, already compromised by the inability of the soft palate to effectively seal off the nose when plosive sounds (such as 'p' or 'b') are made. Speech therapy and sometimes soft palate surgery

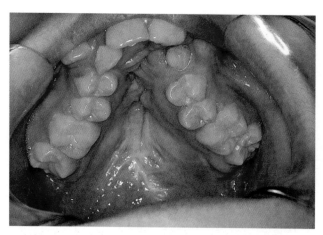

Fig. 3.5 Collapsed maxilla resulting from poorly timed surgical repair of cleft palate. Scarring and growth disturbance produce a distorted narrow maxilla. *(By kind permission of Mrs E Horrocks.)*

may be undertaken between the ages of 3 and 8 for these reasons. At approximately the age of 8 years, orthodontic treatment may start depending on need, and this and further possible surgery to reconstruct the anterior alveolus or palatal cleft may continue for several years. Thereafter, up to late teenage years, final measures are to improve appearance include excision of scars, rhinoplasty and orthognathic surgery.

More recently, observation of untreated clefts has shown that the growth potential of these tissues is virtually normal. In some centres, therefore, a soft palate cleft is repaired early, but hard palate repair is delayed until 8 or 9 years after temporary closure with an obturator. The results are good facial growth and occlusion, but speech may be impaired to some degree.

The forward rotation of the premaxilla in bilateral clefts can be managed by repositioning of this segment with bilateral bone grafts. Severe maxillary deficiency may be managed by Le Fort I internal distraction to remedy malocclusion and speech defects.

Despite several large clinical trials, controversies remain about the timing of these operations and the optimum approach.

Treatment review PMCID: PMC2884751

Dental defects

However effective the treatment, patients with clefts tend to have poor oral hygiene gingivitis and dental caries necessitating regular preventive care.

Teeth in the region of the defect are typically absent, malformed or have hypoplastic enamel. Development and eruption are delayed on the cleft side. Severe clefts are associated with absent teeth. Milder defects are peg-shaped lateral incisors and, sometimes, development of a diminutive lateral incisor on both sides of the cleft. Both deciduous and permanent dentitions are affected.

Isolated cleft palate

Clefts of the hard palate alone arise when the primary palate and lip form, but the palatal shelves fail to fuse posteriorly. The cleft is wider more posteriorly and narrow anteriorly because the shelves fuse from front to back starting at the incisive foramen.

Isolated cleft palate affects approximately 1 in 2000 births and is approximately twice as common in females. Only

occasional cases are inherited, but there is a risk of approximately 2% that a second child will be affected.

Extensive review PMCID: PMC4771933

Submucous cleft palate

Submucous clefts are clefts of the bone or muscle covered by intact mucosa, and they are thus usually visible only as a translucent area along the midline of the soft palate. They are present in approximately 1 in 1200 births but are frequently missed. A bifid uvula is a frequent sign of a submucous cleft.

On palpation the bony cleft and a notched posterior nasal spine may be felt, and the diagnosis can be confirmed by imaging. Submucous clefts cause problems through the distortion of the attachment of the muscles of the soft palate. The chief effects are slowness in feeding and nasal regurgitation. Middle ear infections and speech defects result from the defective muscle attachments and Eustachian tube function, as in overt clefts. Some symptoms are present in 90% of cases.

Operation to repair the muscle attachments is usually delayed for about 2½ years to enable the speech and degree of the defect to be assessed.

Case bifid uvula PMID: 26076543

Management

Isolated cleft palate may be missed at birth but almost immediately comes to light by causing feeding problems. Isolated cleft palate is treated in the same way as those associated with cleft lip.

Syndromic cleft lip and palate

Approximately 30% of all cases of cleft lip and palate and 50% of cases of cleft palate arise as part of a recognised syndrome. The most common of these is Down's syndrome, in which cleft lip or palate is present in approximately 1 in 200 patients (Ch. 39). Other syndromes with clefts are single gene defects, and the genes involved are often the same as those implicated in non-syndromic clefts. Different mutations, polymorphisms, variable penetrance or gene control probably account for the different presentations.

Note that a cleft can be the most prominent sign of a syndrome, and also that these syndromes are often associated with other features that affect dental treatment, such as cardiac defects, learning difficulties and dental anomalies.

Van der Woude syndrome comprises cleft lip and cleft primary and secondary palate (usually a rare combination), lower lip pits, oligodontia, a high arched palate, ankyloglossia and other features. The syndrome is inherited in an autosomal dominant pattern caused by one of several genes, but usually *IRF6*. The lip pits are characteristic, usually one each side of the midline and occasionally at the commissures or in the midline of the upper lip (Fig. 3.6). The pits extend several millimetres deep into the lip and may communicate with labial glands, but are not dilated minor gland ducts, rather a developmental groove between growth centres in the embryonic lip. Lip pits may also be seen in other syndromes but less frequently.

OTHER FACIAL CLEFTS

There are more extensive clefts that can develop along the lines of fusion of the maxillary and frontonasal processes,

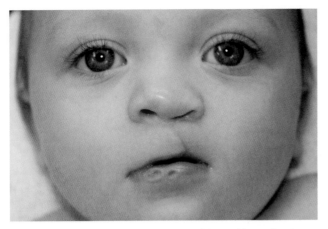

Fig. 3.6 **van der Woude syndrome. Cleft lip and lower lip pits.**
(From Hartzell L.D., Kilpatrick L.A., 2014. Diagnosis and management of patients with clefts: a comprehensive and interdisciplinary approach. Otolaryngol Clin North Am, 47, pp. 821-852.)

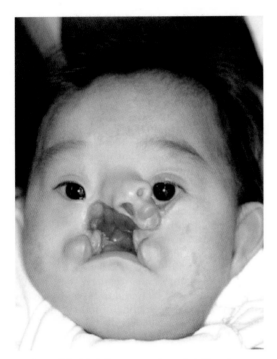

Fig. 3.7 Lateral facial cleft, a severe lateral cleft and severe bilateral cleft lip and palate. *(From Journal of Cranio-Maxillo-Facial Surgery 42 (2014) 1985e1989 42:1985-9.)*

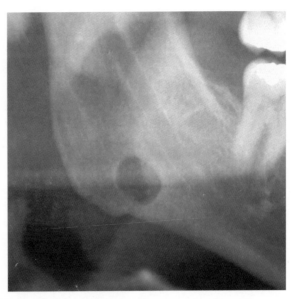

Fig. 3.8 Stafne idiopathic bone cavity.

Very occasionally one of these cavities arises in the anterior mandible, caused by inclusion of part of the sublingual gland, or ectopic salivary gland.

This condition should be diagnosed radiographically (Fig. 3.8). The cavity has a smooth rounded outline and thick even cortication and does not enlarge. Almost all are unilateral, and most patients are male. Although developmental, it appears that the cavity develops slowly in the second or third decades. Cone beam or other tomographic techniques can confirm that the mandible is indented, rather than containing a cavity. Once diagnosed, no treatment is required, and the change appears to be of no significance.

HEREDITARY PROGNATHISM

The extreme genetic form is often called 'Habsburg jaw'* and is probably a single gene disorder inherited as an autosomal dominant. Although this severe inherited form is still occasionally found, most families with a protruding mandible may simply be at one end of the spectrum of normal variation, and result from polygenic inheritance. Marked prognathism can also be seen as an acquired condition in acromegaly.

ANKYLOGLOSSIA

Ankyloglossia, or tongue tie, is caused by tethering of the tongue tip to the floor of mouth, lingual alveolar mucosa or gingiva by a short lingual fraenum (Fig. 3.9). In severe cases a broad thick fraenum effectively fuses the anterior tongue

often involving the eye and sometimes the cranium (Fig. 3.7). These are associated with severe distortion of the face, often with major tissue deficiency. Such facial clefts are usually continuous with a cleft lip and palate at their inferior end. Surgical correction of the defects is extremely difficult.

STAFNE'S IDIOPATHIC BONE CAVITY

This is a relatively common developmental anomaly caused by a lobe of the submandibular gland indenting the lingual aspect of the mandible, below the level of the inferior dental nerve canal. The cortex is invaginated into the medullary space. In a panoramic or oblique lateral radiograph the concavity appears to be a circumscribed cyst in the mandible, surrounded by a layer of cortical bone.

*Hereditary prognathism has been associated with the Habsburg dynasty. Originally a Swiss family, the Habsburgs ruled many European countries between the 11th and 18th centuries. The trait persisted for generations through interbreeding between European royal families, particularly in the Spanish branch. However, recent evaluation of portraits suggests that the family's striking appearance was caused in part by additional hypoplasia of the maxilla, accentuating the appearance. (Peacock, Z.S., Klein, K.P., and Mulliken, J.B., et al. 2014. The Habsburg jaw–re-examined. *Am J Med Genet.* 164A, pp. 2263-2269. [PubMed: 24942320])

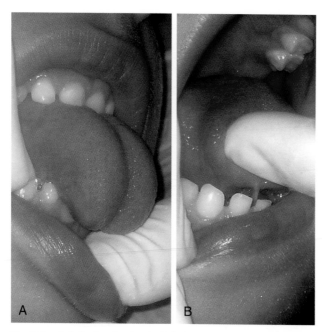

Fig. 3.9 Ankyloglossia. On the left the patient has been asked to protrude the tongue, but the tip is tethered to the lingual gingiva and the dorsum furrows along the midline. The tongue has to be displaced to see the tight lingual fraenum (*right*).

to the floor of mouth. The cause is unclear but has been associated with several genes known to cause cleft palate and clefting syndromes. However, most cases are solitary abnormalities and often have a family history suggesting an autosomal dominant inheritance. Nearly half of affected individuals will have an affected first-degree relative. When there is no family history, males are usually affected. The incidence is approximately 3%.

Reduced lingual mobility can affect feeding in the neonatal period and development of an adult pattern swallow, disturbing the soft tissue guidance for tooth position. A high frenal attachment may cause a midline diastema. Speech can be affected when the tongue tip cannot contact the upper incisors. However, patients develop compensatory speech and swallowing mechanisms, and the condition often regresses slightly during early childhood, so there may be no significant consequences. However, the inability to sweep food debris from the mouth, protrude the tongue or eat ice cream from a cone may drive adults to seek treatment.

Routine surgical treatment is therefore controversial. The fraenum is easily divided and, if there are feeding difficulties, this is appropriate and much more easily performed shortly after birth than in an older child or adult. It is also likely to be most effective before speech and swallowing are established. In general, if a fraenum is attached to the ridge rather than the floor of mouth or within 10 mm of the tongue tip and is not elastic, it is likely to cause problems.

Not all functional tongue tie is associated with an obvious fraenum. The so-called *posterior tongue tie* is a fibrous band below the mucosa tethering the centre of the tongue. It is posterior to the usual site, but still in the anterior tongue, and best thought of as a *deep tongue tie*. The band may only be palpable or noticed because the tongue dimples centrally on movement or will not protrude. Posterior ties also cause feeding problems.

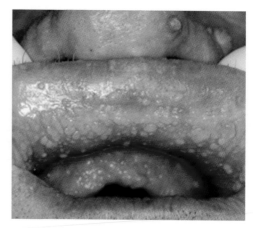

Fig. 3.10 Cowden's syndrome. Multiple nodules and papillomatous nodules on labial mucosa and alveolar ridge. *(From Flores, I.L., Romo, S.A., Tejeda Nava, F.J., et al. 2014. Oral presentation of 10 patients with Cowden syndrome. Oral Surg Oral Med Oral Pathol Oral Radiol, 117(4), pp. e301-e310.)*

Ankyloglossia can develop in adults as a result of scarring diseases, typically severe forms of epidermolysis bullosa, in which the sulci become gradually obliterated by fibrosis.

Feeding problems PMID: 12415069

Diagnosis and treatment PMID: 15839394

COWDEN'S SYNDROME

Multiple hamartoma or Cowden's syndrome* is a genetically diverse condition in which patients have mucosal polyps in the gastrointestinal tract, multiple skin and oral nodules and a high risk of developing malignant neoplasms. Mutations are classically in the PTEN gene, although many variants associated with other genes exist.

Inheritance is usually autosomal dominant and skin, and mucosal lesions develop in the second decade. Skin lesions are more obvious, multiple nodules 1 or 2 mm in diameter around the nose and mouth particularly (Fig. 3.10). Histologically the nodules can be found to be caused by a variety of hamartomas including trichilemmomas and neuromas. Multiple oral nodules develop on the dorsum of the tongue, gingiva and buccal mucosa. The appearance is often referred to as *papillomatosis* because of its shape, but viral papillomas are not a feature. All these nodules are benign.

Diagnosis is largely clinical because the oral lesions appear like fibroepithelial polyps and have no specific features. Suspected cases need urgent investigation because the risk of breast and thyroid carcinomas in later life is so high.

Web URL 3.1 Review: http://emedicine.medscape.com/article/1093383-overview

Web URL 3.2 Online risk assessor: http://www.lerner.ccf.org/gmi/ccscore/

OTHER CRANIOFACIAL MALFORMATIONS

There are many rare syndromes and diseases with characteristic craniofacial abnormalities. Key features are shown in Table 3.1. The craniosynostoses are caused by early fusion of sutures, distorting the shape of the skull while it grows.

---

*Cowden's syndrome is one of the few syndromes named after the patient, rather than the person who first described it.

Table 3.1 Other craniofacial malformations

Disorder	Type/cause	Dental and oral signs	Other features
Crouzon syndrome (craniofacial dysostosis)	Cranial synostosis resulting from mutation in fibroblast growth factor 2 gene. Autosomal dominant or sporadic mutations.	Small maxilla, dental crowding, high narrow palate, anterior open bite	Varied abnormal skull shape, proptosis and hypertelorism, increased intracranial pressure, hearing loss. Normal intelligence. Epilepsy in 10%
Apert syndrome	As Crouzon syndrome	As Crouzon syndrome, soft palate cleft in one-third of cases, progressive enlargement of posterior alveolus soft tissue. Delayed tooth eruption	As Crouzon syndrome with additional syndactyly and other hand and foot malformations. Learning disability, which can be reduced by early surgery
Treacher-Collins syndrome (mandibulofacial dysostosis)	Developmental anomaly of the first and second branchial arches, autosomal dominant and frequent sporadic mutations in one of three known causative genes affecting neural crest development	High arched palate and crowding. Small mandible with small coronoid process, cleft palate in one-third of cases, severe lateral facial clefts and absent parotid glands occasionally	Characteristic narrow face with small zygoma and outward slanting eyelids. Colobomas (notches) on lower eyelid and absent eyelashes, deformed outer and middle ear, deafness
Hemifacial microsomia (Goldenhaar syndrome)	A unilateral developmental anomaly of the first and second branchial arches	Cleft palate and facial clefts occasionally	Cardiac, vertebral and central nervous defects. Deformed outer and middle ear, deafness, colobomas on upper eyelids, accessory auricles in front of ears. Very variable presentation, similar to Treacher-Collins but usually unilateral

Dental caries

4

Quote: 'For sweetness and decay are of one root and sweetness ever riots to decay'.

Ou-Yang Hsiu of Lu-ling (AD 1007–1072)

Dental caries is a disease characterised initially by subsurface demineralisation of teeth by acids, created by bacterial metabolism of dietary refined sugars. Caries is one of the most common of all diseases and still a major cause of loss of teeth despite being completely preventable.

The ultimate effect of the caries process is to cause breakdown of enamel and dentine and thus open a path for bacteria to reach the pulp. The consequences of the caries process, even from its earliest stages, include inflammation of the pulp and, later, of the periapical tissues. Acute pulpitis and apical periodontitis caused in this way are the most common causes of toothache. Infection can spread from the periapical region to the jaw and beyond. Although this is nowadays extremely rare in the UK, people in other countries occasionally die from this cause.

Global burden caries PMID: 23720570

AETIOLOGY

In 1890, W. D. Miller showed that lesions similar to dental caries could be produced by incubating teeth in saliva when carbohydrates were added. Miller concluded that caries could result from decalcification caused by bacterial acid production. Miller's basic hypothesis was confirmed in 1954 when Orland and his associates in the United States showed that caries did not develop in germ-free animals.

It has become conventional to consider caries to be multifactorial (Fig. 4.1 and Box 4.1). However, although the multifactorial concept aids understanding, it is critical to understand that caries is caused by dietary sugar intake. All other factors are dependent on that or only modify its effect. The cause of caries is eating refined sugars.

Primary role sugar PMID: 24892213

Diet and caries PMID: 26261186

BACTERIAL PLAQUE

Plaque is a tenaciously adherent deposit that forms on tooth surfaces. It consists of an organic matrix containing a dense concentration of bacteria (Figs 4.2–4.3).

In microbiological terms, plaque is a biofilm of bacteria embedded in an extracellular polysaccharide matrix. In the protected environment in a biofilm, conditions are very different from those on a clean tooth surface or in saliva. Bacteria in biofilms can exhibit cooperative activity and behave differently from the same species in isolation in a laboratory culture medium. As a consequence, a biofilm may be resistant to antimicrobials or to immunological defences to which the individual bacterial species are normally sensitive. The biofilm traps and concentrates bacterial products, favouring survival and interactions between species. Bacterial plaque must therefore be regarded as a living ecosystem and not as a mere collection of bacteria. A key feature is the ability of dental plaque to concentrate and retain acid.

Clinically, bacterial plaque is a tenaciously adherent deposit on the teeth. It resists the friction of food during mastication and can only be readily removed by toothbrushing. However, neither toothbrushing nor fibrous foods will remove plaque from inaccessible surfaces or pits (stagnation areas; see Fig. 4.5). This tenacious adherence is mediated by the matrix polysaccharides.

Plaque becomes visible, particularly on the labial surfaces of the incisors, when toothbrushing is stopped for 12–24 hours. It appears as a translucent film with a matt surface

---

Box 4.1   Essential requirements for development of dental caries

1. Bacterial plaque biofilm
2. Cariogenic (acidogenic) bacteria
3. Plaque biofilm stagnation sites
4. Susceptible tooth surfaces
5. Fermentable bacterial substrate (sugar)
6. Time

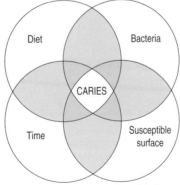

Possible interventions
Reduce intake of cariogenic sugars, particularly sucrose

Possible interventions
Reduce *Strep. mutans* numbers by:
- reduction in sugar intake
- active or passive immunisation

Diet

Bacteria

CARIES

Time

Susceptible surface

Possible interventions
Avoid frequent sucrose intake ('snacking')
Stimulate salivary flow and sugar clearance

Possible interventions
Water and other types of fluoridation
Prevention during post-eruptive maturation
Fissure sealing
Remineralising solutions
Properly contoured restorations

Fig. 4.1   The major factors in the aetiology of dental caries.

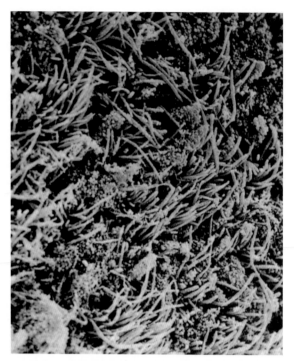

Fig. 4.2 This scanning electronmicrograph of plaque shows the large number of filamentous organisms and, in addition, many cocci clustered amongst them. *(By kind permission of Dr Sheila J Jones.)*

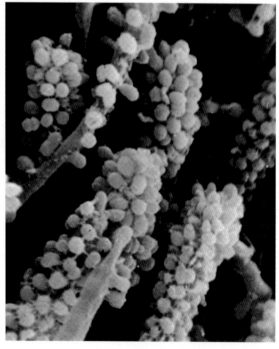

Fig. 4.3 This scanning electronmicrograph at higher power shows cocci attached to filamentous organisms to produce the corn-cob type of arrangement sometimes seen in plaque. *(By kind permission of Dr Sheila J Jones.)*

that dulls the otherwise smooth and shiny enamel. It can be made obvious when stained with disclosing agents. Little plaque forms under conditions of starvation, but it forms rapidly and abundantly on a high-sucrose diet.

In stagnation areas where plaque is undisturbed, growth of bacteria and secretion of matrix thicken the plaque. If

---

> **Box 4.2 Stages of plaque formation**
>
> * Deposition of structureless cell-free, pellicle of salivary glycoprotein
> * Further deposition of pellicle enhanced by bacterial action precipitating salivary proteins
> * Colonisation of the cell-free layer by bacteria, particularly by *Streptococcus sanguis* and *Streptococcus mutans* strains within 24 hours
> * Progressive build-up of plaque substance by bacterial polysaccharides
> * Proliferation of filamentous and other bacteria as the plaque matures

sugars are available, they are metabolised to the acid that causes dental caries.

Stages of formation of bacterial plaque

If teeth are thoroughly cleaned by polishing with an abrasive, plaque quickly re-forms (Box 4.2).

MICROBIOLOGY

Substantial evidence indicates that streptococci are associated with the development of caries, particularly of smooth (interstitial) surfaces. These include viridans streptococci, which are a heterogeneous group including *Streptococcus mutans*, *Streptococcus sobrinus*, *Streptococcus salivarius*, *Streptococcus mitior* and *Streptococcus sanguis*. These have the ability to partially lyse blood in agar culture plates to a green colour (α-haemolysis), hence the name viridans, meaning green.

Viridans streptococci vary in their ability to attach to different types of tissues, their ability to ferment sugars (particularly sucrose) and the concentrations of acid thus produced. They also differ in the types of extracellular polysaccharides that they form.

Certain strains of *S. mutans* are strongly acidogenic; at low pH, with freely available sucrose, they also store an intracellular, glycogen-like, reserve polysaccharide. When the supply of external substrate dries up, the reserve is metabolised to continue acid production for a time. Drastic reduction in dietary sucrose intake is followed by virtual elimination of *S. mutans* from plaque and reduces or abolishes caries activity. When sucrose is made freely available again, *S. mutans* rapidly re-colonises the plaque.

Completely germ-free animals do not develop dental caries when fed a sucrose-rich diet. Experiments using animals known to be colonised by only known species (gnotobiotes) have shown that the most potent causes of dental caries are a limited number of strains of the *S. mutans* group.

S. mutans strains are a major component of plaque in human mouths, particularly in persons with a high dietary sucrose intake and high caries activity (Fig. 4.4). *S. mutans* isolated from such mouths are virulently cariogenic when introduced into the mouths of animals.

Many other species of micro-organisms can also be found in plaque. However, few others are capable of causing caries in animal models and no others are as virulent. Lactobacilli and *Actinomyces* strains are also found in caries lesions, but appear to have no direct causative role. However, the complex ecosystem of plaque must include other species

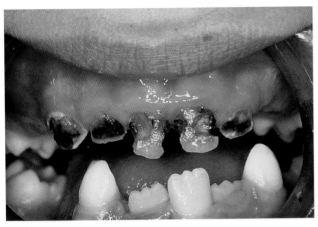

Fig. 4.4 Extensive caries of deciduous incisors and canines. This pattern of caries is particularly associated with the use of sweetened dummies and sweetened infant drinks.

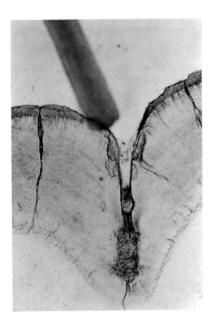

Fig. 4.5 The stagnation area in an occlusal pit. A ground section of a molar showing the size of the stagnation area in comparison with a toothbrush bristle placed above it. The complete inaccessibility of the stagnation area to cleaning is obvious.

that may interact with and contribute to *S. mutans* being able to persist in plaque when substrate is sparse.

Caries lesions tend to develop at specific sites, usually approximally or in deeper occlusal pits and fissures, and the cariogenic bacteria are found in the plaque overlying the caries, not floating free in the saliva. These sites tend to be plaque biofilm stagnation areas that are difficult for the individual patient to clean (Fig. 4.5).

Plaque microbiology ISBN-13: 978-0443101441

The ecological plaque hypothesis

Although much evidence points to *S. mutans* as the sole cause of caries, it is possible to have high *S. mutans* levels in plaque but no caries. Current research suggests that *S. mutans* can only cause caries when it is a component of a mixed plaque that fosters its virulence. *S. mutans* survives best in acidic plaque at high sucrose levels but requires other organisms to reduce the plaque pH if no sucrose is available,

and to provide a supportive ecosystem that allows it to survive. These other organisms may well benefit from the presence of *S. mutans*, so the whole plaque ecology must be seen as interdependent and cariogenic. The ecological plaque hypothesis suggests that a plaque containing other acid producing and acid resistant bacteria is important to modulate the virulence of *S. mutans*. Such other species include *Streptococcus mitis*, *Streptococcus oralis*, *S. salivarius* and *Streptococcus anginosus*, and these species are often major constituents of plaque.

This hypothesis probably explains why caries prediction tests based on *S. mutans* levels alone are poorly predictive in individual patients. It suggests that properties shared by a group of bacteria are more important (Box 4.3). The hypothesis is very similar to the current view of how periodontitis is caused by a pathogenic plaque (Ch. 7).

Ecological plaque hypothesis PMID: 20924061 and 12624191

Bacterial polysaccharides

The ability of *S. mutans* to initiate smooth surface caries and form large amounts of adherent plaque depends on its ability to polymerise sucrose into high-molecular-weight, sticky, insoluble extracellular polysaccharides (glucans) (Box 4.3). The cariogenicity of *S. mutans* depends as much on its ability to form large amounts of insoluble extracellular glucans as on its ability to produce acid.

Glucans enable streptococci to adhere to one another and to stick to and colonise the tooth surface, probably via specific receptors on the bacteria. In this way, *S. mutans* can colonise freshly cleaned sites, spread from site to site and enable a critical thickness of plaque to build up. The cariogenicity of *S. mutans* is strongly related to production of sticky, insoluble, extracellular glucan produced by some strains. The proportions of the different types of polysaccharide, and the overall amounts formed, depend both on the strains of bacteria present and the different sugars in the diet.

The importance of sucrose in this activity is explained by the high energy of its glucose–fructose bond, which allows the synthesis of polysaccharides by glucosyltransferase without any other source of energy. Sucrose is thus the main substrate used to make such polysaccharides. On a sucrose-rich diet, the main extracellular polysaccharides are glucans, glucose polymers. Other sugars are, to varying degrees, less cariogenic (in the absence of preformed plaque), partly because they are less readily formed into cariogenic glucans. Fructans formed from fructose are more soluble, produced in smaller amounts and less important in caries.

Acid-producing micro-organisms that do not produce insoluble polysaccharides do not appear to be able to cause caries of smooth surfaces. Even *S. mutans* becomes

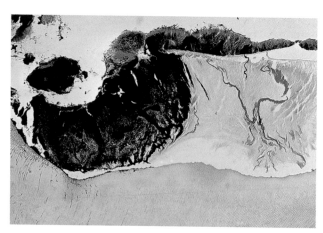

Fig. 4.6 Bacterial plaque. A decalcified section showing darkly staining plaque lying on enamel and within a carious cavity. The plaque has remained intact and adherent to the enamel throughout the processes to which the specimen was subjected in preparation for sectioning.

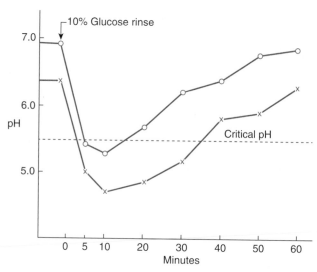

Fig. 4.7 Stephan curves showing the pH in plaque after a sucrose rinse. When the pH falls below the critical level, enamel may become demineralised. Patients with active caries tend to show a lower fall in pH, as in the lower curve as they have a more cariogenic acidogenic plaque. Note the very rapid fall in pH and the slow recovery to the normal level in spite of the very short time the sugar is in the mouth. Carbohydrates which stick to the teeth have a more prolonged effect.

Box 4.4 Microbiological aspects of dental caries

- Dental caries is a bacterial disease
- The organisms mainly associated with caries are specific strains of *Streptococcus mutans*
- The cariogenicity of *S. mutans* has been established by inoculating it into the mouths of otherwise germ-free animals (gnotobiotes)
- The presence of *S. mutans* in the human mouth is associated with caries activity
- Other bacteria are weakly cariogenic or are non-cariogenic despite being able to produce acid

---

Box 4.5 Cariogenic properties of *Streptococcus mutans*

- It produces lactic acid from sucrose
- It can live at a pH as low as 4.2
- It forms large amounts of extracellular, sticky and insoluble glucan plaque matrix
- It adheres to pellicle and contributes to plaque formation
- Produces intracellular polysaccharide reserves to survive when substrate is sparse

---

non-cariogenic when mutations cause it to produce soluble rather than insoluble polysaccharides. Polysaccharides thus contribute to the adhesiveness, bulk and resistance to solution of plaque.

Although the bacteria produce the acid that demineralises the teeth, polysaccharide is critically important to build up the thick plaque in which the acid can persist, protected from the washing and buffering action of saliva (Fig. 4.6).

Important points about microbiological aspects of dental caries are summarised in Box 4.4.

The cariogenicity of *S. mutans* depends on properties summarised in Box 4.5.

Plaque matrix PMID: 24045647

Strep mutans PMID: 14977543

Acid production in plaque

Sucrose diffuses rapidly into plaque, and acid production quickly follows. These changes can be measured directly in the human mouth by using microelectrodes in direct contact with plaque. It has been shown by this means that, after rinsing the mouth with a 10% glucose solution, the pH falls within 2–5 minutes, often to a level sufficient to decalcify enamel. Even though no more sucrose may be taken and the surplus is washed away by the saliva, the pH level remains at a low level for approximately 15–20 minutes; it returns only gradually to the resting level after approximately an hour. These changes (plotted in the so-called *Stephan curve*)

Box 4.6 Factors contributing to maintenance of low plaque pH

- Rapid production of a high concentration of acid within the plaque temporarily overcomes local buffering
- Escape of acid into the saliva is delayed by the diffusion-limiting properties of plaque and its thickness
- Diffusion of salivary buffers into plaque hampered by the diffusion-limiting properties of plaque and its thickness
- Continued acid production from bacterial intracellular storage polysaccharides after dietary sugar is exhausted

---

are shown diagrammatically in Fig. 4.7. The rapidity with which the pH falls is a reflection of the speed with which sucrose can diffuse into plaque and the activity of the enzymes produced by the great numbers of bacteria in the plaque. The slow rate of recovery to the resting pH – a critical factor in caries production – depends mainly on factors summarised in Box 4.6.

It is clear that acid production, mainly lactic acid, is responsible for caries lesions. When plaque is sampled after exposure to sucrose, lactic acid is the quantitatively predominant acid, particularly during the trough of the Stephan curve. Lactic acid has a lower pK constant and causes a greater fall in pH than equimolar solutions of acetic or propionic acids that may also be detected in plaque.

Stephan curve PMID: 23224410

Plaque minerals

In addition to bacteria and their polysaccharides, salivary components also contribute to the plaque matrix. Calcium, phosphate ions and, often, fluorides are present in significant amounts. There is some evidence of an inverse relationship between calcium and phosphate levels in plaque and caries activity or sucrose intake. The ability of plaque to concentrate calcium and phosphorus is used in mineralising mouthwashes. The level of fluoride in plaque may be high, ranging from 15–75 ppm or more, and is largely dependent on the fluoride level in the drinking water and diet. This fluoride is probably mostly bound to organic material in the plaque but, at low pH levels, may become available and active in ionic form.

SUCROSE

Ingestion of sucrose leads to a burst of metabolic activity in the plaque so that the pH may fall low enough to dissolve enamel before slowly returning to the resting level. The frequency with which substrate is made available to the plaque is therefore important. When sucrose is taken as a sweet drink, any surplus beyond the capacity of the organisms in the plaque to metabolise it at the time is washed away. If sucrose-containing drinks are taken repeatedly at short intervals, the supply of substrate to the bacteria can be sufficiently frequently renewed to cause acid in the plaque to remain persistently at a destructive level.

A similar effect may be caused by carbohydrate in sticky form, such as a caramel, which clings to the teeth and is slowly dissolved, releasing substrate over a long period. A given amount of sucrose is more cariogenic when fed to animals in small increments at intervals than when the same total amount is fed as a single dose.

In addition to acid production, providing sucrose leads to a significant increase in synthesis of extracellular polysaccharide. This prevents acid from diffusing away and being neutralised by saliva.

Colonisation by cariogenic bacteria, especially *S. mutans*, is highly dependent on the sucrose content of the diet. Sucrose is required for initial colonisation, and increasing availability increases the number of *S. mutans* in plaque. Conversely, severe reduction in dietary sucrose causes *S. mutans* to decline in numbers or disappear from plaque.

Essential features of sucrose incriminating it as the most cariogenic substrate are summarised in Box 4.7.

Primary role sugar PMID: 24892213

Diet and caries PMID: 26261186

Epidemiological studies

The importance of sucrose in human caries is seen in epidemiological studies and a few interventional studies, as summarised in Boxes 4.8 and 4.9.

Dental caries has been most prevalent in well-nourished, Westernised communities with sucrose-rich

> **Box 4.7 Factors determining the cariogenicity of sucrose**
> - Sucrose forms as much as a third of the carbohydrate content of many persons' diets
> - It promotes colonisation of teeth by *Streptococcus mutans*
> - Its disaccharide bond alone contains enough energy to react with bacterial enzymes to form extracellular dextran matrix
> - Its small molecular size allows it to diffuse readily into plaque
> - Bacterial metabolism of sucrose is rapid

> **Box 4.8 Experimental evidence for the critical contribution of sucrose to caries activity**
> - In caries-susceptible animals a sucrose-rich diet promotes caries production
> - Caries is not induced in susceptible animals if sucrose is fed only by stomach-tube; its effect is entirely local
> - Sucrose in sticky form clings to the teeth and remains available to bacteria for a longer period and is more cariogenic
> - Sucrose-containing fluids are quickly cleared from the mouth and less cariogenic
> - Frequent feeds of small quantities of sucrose are more cariogenic than the same total amount fed on a single occasion
> - Dry mouth delays clearance of sugars and enhances caries activity

> **Box 4.9 Epidemiological evidence for sucrose as the cause of dental caries**
> - Low caries prevalence in populations with low sucrose intakes
> - The decline in caries prevalence during wartime sucrose shortages
> - The rise of caries prevalence with increasing availability of sucrose
> - Archaeological evidence of low caries prevalence in eras before sucrose became freely available
> - Low caries prevalence in disorders of sucrose metabolism (hereditary fructose intolerance)

diets. Communities living on traditional diets with little or no sucrose had a low prevalence of caries, as seen, for example, in studies of parts of China and of Africa, the Seychelles, Tristan da Cunha, Alaska and Greenland. Many studies were carried out on Inuit races who were caries-free when consuming their traditional diet of seal or whale meat and fish. These non-cariogenic diets vary widely in their composition. The one common feature, and one differentiating them sharply from Westernised diets, is low or negligible consumption of refined sugar, particularly sucrose.

Britain is an example of a country where consumption of sucrose has been exceptionally high, though it has recently started to fall. In Britain and other countries, the incidence of caries has risen roughly parallel with rising

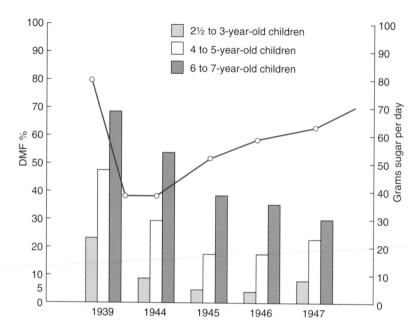

Fig. 4.8 **The wartime restrictions on diet and caries in Norway.** The continuous line shows an estimate of the individual daily sugar consumption during and after the war. The heights of the columns show the incidence of caries in children of various ages. Rationing of sugar started in 1938, but it is apparent that the incidence of caries declined slowly and continued for a short time after sugar became freely available. The greatest reduction in caries was in the youngest group of children whose teeth were exposed to the wartime diet for the shortest periods. *(From Toverud, G. 1949. Decrease in caries frequency in Norwegian children during world war 2. J Am Dent Assoc 39, p. 127.)*

consumption of sucrose. Food shortages during the 1939–1945 war largely abolished sucrose from the diet and in Britain, Norway and Japan and caries rates fell dramatically (Fig. 4.8). When sucrose became more plentiful at the end of the war, caries prevalence progressively rose. Public health measures and fluoridated toothpaste are considered the main reasons for dramatic falls in prevalence over the last decades.

In the UK in 1973, 6% of 12-year-olds had caries, with a mean DMFT (decayed, missing or filled teeth) of 5 teeth. By 2010, the percentage had dropped to 2% and the DMFT to 2. However, prevalence in the deciduous dentition remains high, and in 2013, 27% of 5-year-olds had decayed teeth.

Web URL 4.1 UK caries epidemiology: http://www.nwph.net/dentalhealth/

Sugar changed history ISBN-13: 978-0140092332

Development of caries and Westernisation of the diet are closely linked. Many countries with a previously low caries incidence still have older adults who are caries-free, but the prevalence of dental caries among children and young people has risen rapidly as a result of sweet-eating habits and processed foods with 'hidden' sugars. This effect has also been strikingly well documented in the population of Tristan da Cunha who, until the late 1930s, lived on a simple meat, fish and vegetable diet with a minimal sucrose content and had a very low caries prevalence. With the adoption of Westernised diet, the caries prevalence had risen to eightfold in some age groups by the mid-1960s, after the entire population was temporarily evacuated to the UK.

Web URL 4.2 Caries WHO data: http://www.who.int/oral_health/media/en/orh_figure7.pdf?ua=1

International increase caries PMID:19281105

Web URL 4.3 USA caries data: http://www.nidcr.nih.gov/DataStatistics/FindDataByTopic/DentalCaries/

Web URL 4.4 UK child caries survey: http://content.digital.nhs.uk/catalogue/PUB17137

Caries has become epidemic only in relatively recent decades while sucrose has become cheaper and widely available. In Britain, there was a sudden, widespread rise in sucrose consumption in the middle of the 19th century. This resulted both from the falling cost of production and, in 1861, the abolition of a tax on sugar. Evidence from exhumed skulls confirms the low prevalence of caries before sucrose became widely available and the steady rise in prevalence thereafter.

Patients unable to metabolise fructose as a result of an enzyme deficiency (hereditary fructose intolerance) cannot tolerate sucrose (a glucose-fructose disaccharide). These children avoid all sucrose-containing foods and have an unusually low incidence of caries.

Experimental studies on humans

In the Vipeholm study, more than 400 adult patients were studied in a closed institution. They received a basic low-carbohydrate diet to establish a baseline of caries activity for each group. They were then divided into seven groups that were each allocated different diets. A control group received the basic diet made up to an adequate calorie intake with margarine. Two groups received supplements of sucrose at mealtimes, either in solution or as sweetened bread. The four remaining groups received sweets (toffees, caramels or chocolate), which were eaten between meals.

The effects of sucrose in different quantities and of different degrees of adhesiveness, and of eating sucrose at different times, were thus tested over a period of 5 years. Caries activity was greatly enhanced by the eating of sticky sweets between meals (toffees and caramels) that were retained on the teeth. Sucrose at mealtimes only had little effect (Fig. 4.9). The incidence of caries fell to its original low level when toffees or caramels were no longer given, and caries activity was very slight in the control group having the low-carbohydrate diet.

Vipeholm original paper PMID: 13196991

Vipeholm revisited PMID: 2704974

In another large-scale clinical experiment in Turku (Finland), an experimental group was allowed a wide range of foods sweetened with xylitol (a sugar alcohol) but no sucrose. The control group was allowed as much sugary (sucrose-containing) foods as desired. After 2 years, the experimental group showed 90% less caries than those who had been allowed sucrose.

These two studies, though classics in their time, describe caries produced by a grossly cariogenic diet. Evidence from these studies has been important in linking frequency of intake to caries, and this is has become a fundamental underlying principle of caries prevention. However, in a more normal diet, the amount of sugar consumed may be as important as the frequency, and current evidence suggests no level of refined sugar intake can be considered safe.

Use of sugar substitutes (artificial sweeteners) in place of sucrose greatly reduces caries activity. The cariogenicity of sugars and artificial sweeteners are summarised in Table 4.1.

The Turku studies PMID: 795260

Cochrane review sugar & caries PMCID: PMC3872848

Primary role sugar PMID: 24892213

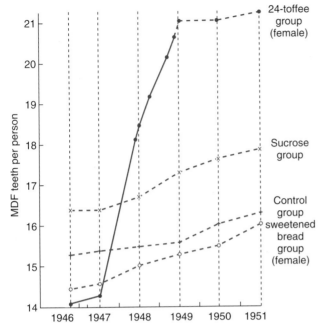

Fig. 4.9 The Vipeholm dental caries study. A simplified diagram showing the results in some of the groups of patients and, in particular, the striking effect on caries activity of sticky sweets eaten between meals when compared with the eating of sweet stuffs at mealtimes. The broken lines indicate those who consumed sugar only at meals; the continuous line shows those who consumed sugar both at and between meals. *(From Gustafsson, B.E., Quensel, C.E., Lanke, L.S., Lundqvist, C., Grahnen, H., Bonow, B.E., et al. 1954. The Vipeholm dental caries study; the effect of different levels of carbohydrate intake on caries activity in 436 individuals observed for five years. Acta Odontol.Scandi. 11, p. 232.)*

SUSCEPTIBILITY OF TEETH TO CARIES

Teeth may be resistant to decay because of factors affecting the structure of the tooth during formation. In the past it was thought that hypocalcification of the teeth or lack of calcium or vitamin D predisposed to caries. This ignored the extensive epidemiological findings that the best-nourished populations had the worst record for dental disease, but is still a common belief among patients. Heredi-

Table 4.1 Sugars and some non-sugar sweeteners*

Compound	Nature and uses	Cariogenicity
Sucrose	A disaccharide sugar (β1–4-linked glucose–fructose)	Highest of all sugars
Glucose, fructose	Monosaccharide sugars	Less cariogenic than sucrose
Lactose and galactose	Monosaccharide (lactose) and disaccharide (galactose) sugars	Less cariogenic than sucrose
Glucose syrups and maltodextrins	Hydrolysis products of starch used as bulk sweeteners	Less cariogenic than all sugars
Hydrogenated glucose syrup and lycasins	Hydrolysis products of starch which are then hydrogenated, used as bulk sweeteners	Less cariogenic than all sugars
Isomalt	Mixture of two unusual 12-carbon sugars	Low cariogenicity
Sucralose	Chlorinated disaccharide of fructose and galactose, intensely sweet, used as bulk sweetener	Non-cariogenic
Xylitol, sorbitol, mannitol, lactitol etc.	Sugar alcohols (polyols) sometimes used as bulk sweeteners	Non-cariogenic
Saccharin, aspartame, thaumatin, acesulfame K and cyclamate, Stevia glycoside (rebaudioside A)	Non-sugar intense sweeteners	Non-cariogenic
Mogrosides	Natural intense sweetener from melons and gourds, a glycoside polycarbon compound	Insufficient data, novel product, likely very low cariogenicity

*Many new medium potency natural sweeteners are known and starting to be used.

tary hypoplasia or hypocalcification of the teeth, aside from molar-incisor hypomineralisation, do not render teeth susceptible to caries. However, newly erupted teeth are generally caries susceptible until post-eruptive maturation is complete.

Effects of fluorides

Fluorides from drinking water and other sources are taken up by calcifying tissues during and after development. When the fluoride content of the water is 1 ppm or more, the incidence of caries declines substantially. Fluoride may affect caries activity by a variety of mechanisms (Box 4.10). High doses of fluoride during dental development do affect the structure of the developing teeth, as shown by mottling of the enamel. However, the lower incidence of dental caries where water is fluoridated at low level is due to its environmental effect on the teeth after eruption, reduced solubility of the enamel and promotion of remineralisation after phases of acid attack.

Although the intake of fluoride can be supplemented in many ways, water, milk, salt, toothpastes, rinses and varnish to name a few, water fluoridation is considered the most cost effective and the US Centers for Disease Control considers water fluoridation as one of the ten most important public health measures of the 20th century.

Fluoride is the only nutrient that has been proven to have this protective action, and fluoride in water and toothpastes has had a major impact on caries prevalence. Combined with a much more recent general reduction in sucrose consumption, these factors have made caries in the young largely a disease of the disadvantaged.

Web URL 4.5 Fluorides in prevention: http://www.who.int/ then search 'fluoride prevention caries' in search box

Web URL 4.6 US recommendations: http://www.cdc.gov/ then search 'fluoride dose prevent control' in search box

ADA guideline PMID: 24971851

Web URL 4.7 UK recommendations: Perform a web search for 'delivering better oral health evidence toolkit'

Role of dentist in water fluoridation PMID: 23283928

Cochrane review water fluoridation PMID: 26092033

Problems with Cochrane review fluoridation PMID: 27056513

SALIVA AND DENTAL CARIES

Saliva is critical in caries. It provides natural buffers for the acids in plaque, delivers antibacterial compounds and washes sucrose and bacterial products away. However, its effectiveness is severely limited by the plaque matrix, which prevents diffusion of saliva into the plaque.

In animals, removal or inactivation of major salivary glands leads to increased caries activity roughly in proportion to the reduction in saliva production. Dental caries may also become rampant in humans with xerostomia (Ch. 22).

Buffering power

The buffering power of saliva depends mainly on its bicarbonate content and is increased at high rates of flow. The buffering power of the saliva does increase the pH of plaque to a degree and prevents the pH from falling to very low levels. A rapid flow rate, with the greater salivary buffering power that is associated, has been found to be associated with low caries activity.

Inorganic components and enamel maturation

Calcium and phosphate ions are able to exchange in soluble form between the enamel surface, plaque and saliva, and concentrations at these three sites are in a dynamic equilibrium. Newly erupted teeth are more susceptible to caries than adult teeth. Radioactive tracer studies show that newly erupted teeth can incorporate 10–20 times as much calcium and phosphate as adult teeth while they undergo post-eruptive maturation. During this process, saliva can provide fluoride for incorporation into the enamel.

Antibacterial activities

Saliva contains thiocyanates, a lysozyme-like substance, the peroxidase system and other theoretically antibacterial peptides and substances. Nevertheless, the mouth teems with bacteria, and there is no evidence that non-specific antibacterial substances in saliva have any significant effect on caries activity.

Immunological defences

Immunological defences against *S. mutans* appear to be the main physiological mechanisms conferring caries resistance on some individuals. Immunological defences could be mediated by immunoglobulin (Ig)A in saliva or IgG in crevicular fluid. The IgG responses are the most important in resistance, but the natural immunity level varies widely between individuals. Protection is not that strong, as demonstrated by the fact that immunodeficiency does not predispose to dental caries. These defence mechanisms are easily overwhelmed if the diet is high in sucrose.

It has been shown that dripping a solution of monoclonal antibody against *S. mutans* onto the teeth prevents recolonisation by *S. mutans* in humans. For this to be effective, plaque must be removed before treatment by using chlorhexidine and effective oral hygiene. The effect of antibody lasts for several months after applications, and this 'passive immunisation' has the potential to reduce caries activity significantly. The effects are probably not mediated by traditional immune mechanisms but rather by binding to the bacteria and preventing adhesion to the forming new plaque. Once new plaque is established without *S. mutans*, the stable biofilm ecosystem prevents recolonisation long after the antibody has been washed away.

Key facts about the effects of saliva on plaque activity are summarised in Box 4.11.

The main biochemical events in dental plaque in the development of dental caries are summarised diagrammatically in Fig. 4.10.

Protective effects saliva PMID: 26701274

Box 4.12 Stages of enamel caries

- The early (sub-microscopic) lesion
- Phase of non-bacterial enamel crystal destruction
- Bacterial invasion of enamel
- Cavity formation
- Undermining of enamel from below after spread into dentine

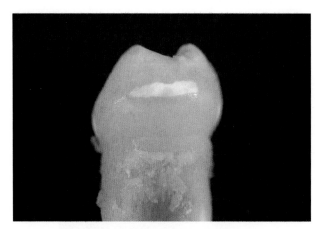

Fig. 4.11 Early enamel caries, a white spot lesion, in a deciduous molar. The lesion forms below the contact point, and in consequence is much broader than an interproximal lesion in a permanent tooth.

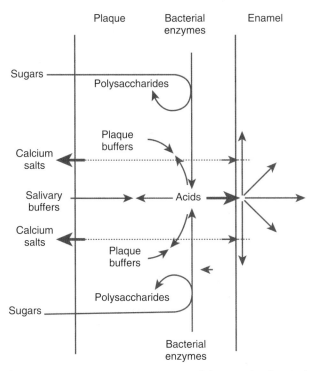

Fig. 4.10 Diagrammatic representation of the main biochemical events in dental plaque, initiating caries. *(From McCracken, A.W., Cawson, R.A. 1983.* Clinical and oral microbiology. *Washington DC.)*

PATHOLOGY OF ENAMEL CARIES

Enamel, the hardest and densest tissue in the body, consists almost entirely of calcium hydroxyapatite with only a minute organic content. It forms a formidable barrier to bacterial attack. However, once enamel has been breached, infection of dentine can spread with relatively less obstruction. Preventive measures must therefore be aimed primarily at stopping the initial attack or at making enamel more resistant.

Enamel is rendered carious by acid diffusing into it and dissolving it. The crystalline lattice of calcium hydroxyapatite crystals is relatively impermeable, but the organic matrix around the apatite crystals and in prism sheaths is permeable to hydrogen ions.

Caries is not a simple solubilisation of enamel, but a dynamic process of alternating phases of demineralisation and remineralisation. This results in a defining characteristic of enamel caries, that initially the solubilisation of enamel is a subsurface process.

Enamel caries develops in four main phases (Box 4.12). These stages of enamel caries are distinguishable microscopically and are also clinically significant. In particular, the incipient or early (white spot) lesion is potentially reversible, but cavity formation is irreversible and may require operative restorative measures to prevent progression and replace the lost tissues.

The early caries lesion

The earliest visible changes are seen as a white opaque spot that forms just below a contact point. Despite the chalky appearance, the enamel is hard and smooth to the probe (Fig. 4.11). The microscopic changes under this early white spot lesion can only be seen by using polarised light microscopy or microradiography.

The initial lesion is conical in shape with its apex toward the dentine and a series of four zones of differing translucency can be discerned. Working back from the deepest, advancing edge of the lesion, these zones consist first of a translucent zone; immediately within this is a second dark zone; the third is the body of the lesion and the fourth is the surface zone (Fig. 4.12). These changes are not due to bacterial invasion, but due to demineralisation and remineralisation in the enamel. The features of these zones are summarised in Table 4.2.

The translucent zone is the deepest zone. The appearance of the translucent zone results from formation of sub-microscopic spaces or pores where acid has dissolved apatite crystals located at prism boundaries and other areas of high organic content such as the striae of Retzius. The translucent zone is so-called because of its appearance when the

Table 4.2   Key features of the enamel zones preceding cavity formation

Zone	Key features	Comments
Translucent zone	1% mineral loss. Earliest and deepest demineralisation	Broader in progressing caries, narrow or absent in arrested or remineralised lesions
Dark zones	2%–4% mineral loss overall but a zone of remineralisation just behind the advancing front	Broader in arrested or remineralised lesions, narrow in advancing lesions
Body	5–25% mineral loss	Broader in progressing caries, replaced by a broad dark zone in arrested or remineralised lesions
Surface zone	1% mineral loss. A zone of remineralisation resulting from the diffusion barrier and mineral content of plaque. Cavitation is loss of this layer, allowing bacteria to enter the lesion	Relatively constant width, a little thicker in arrested or remineralising lesions

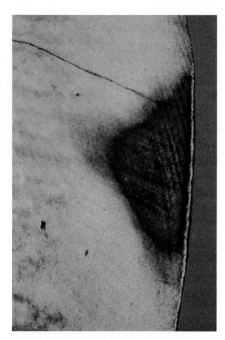

Fig. 4.12   Early approximal caries. Ground section in water viewed by polarised light. The body of the lesion and the intact surface layer are visible. The translucent and dark zones are not seen until the section is viewed immersed in quinoline.

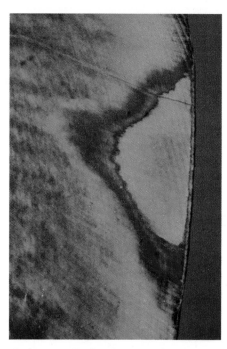

Fig. 4.13   Early approximal caries. Ground section viewed by polarised light after immersion in quinoline. Quinoline has filled the larger pores, causing most of the fine detail in the body of the lesion to disappear (Fig. 4.12), but the dark zone with its smaller pores is accentuated.

section is viewed in polarised light and mounted in quinoline, a compound with the same refractive index as enamel used in experiments on caries in vitro (Fig. 4.13).

The dark zone is fractionally superficial to the translucent zone and shows a greater degree of demineralisation and pores amounting to 2%–4% of the enamel volume. The dark zone is so-called because the quinoline technique reveals additional small pores too small to be filled by quinolone. These contain air and do not transmit light, therefore appearing dark under the microscope. These small pores are caused by remineralisation shrinking larger pores, evidence that caries has phases of repeated demineralisation and remineralisation. Caries lesions that are very slowly progressing or arrested have much larger dark zones and a smaller body, reflecting a greater degree of remineralisation.

The body of the lesion forms the bulk of the lesion and extends from just beneath the surface zone to the dark zone. The body is predominantly a zone of demineralisation. Within it, the striae of Retzius appear enhanced, particularly when mounted in quinoline and viewed under polarised light. Polarised light examination (Fig. 4.14) also shows that

the pore volume is 5% at the junction with the dark zone, but increases to at least 25% in the centre. Microradiography, which will detect demineralisation in excess of 5%, reveals radiolucent lesions that correspond closely with the size and shape of the body of the lesion, in contrast to the surface zone, which appears relatively radiopaque (Fig. 4.15). Alternating radiopaque and radiolucent lines, approximately 30 µm apart, can also be seen passing obliquely through the subsurface region. These are produced by preferential demineralisation along the striae of Retzius.

The surface zone is the most important zone in terms of prevention and management of the disease. It shows the paradoxical feature that it is much more heavily mineralised than the body and dark zones below it. It remains intact during demineralisation of the subsurface enamel and has a pore volume of only 1%. The explanation is that the surface zone is formed by remineralisation. In vitro, if the surface zone is removed and the enamel is exposed to an acid buffer, the more highly mineralised surface zone reappears by remineralisation using calcium and phosphate from the plaque or from the deeper demineralised zones.

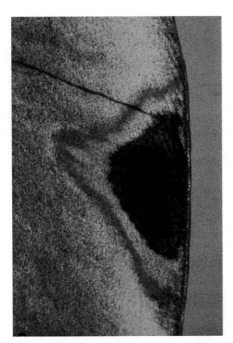

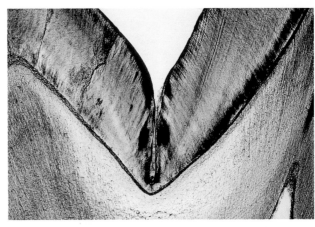

Fig. 4.16 Undecalcified section showing early enamel lesions in the enamel surrounding and deep to an occlusal pit.

Fig. 4.14 The same lesion (Figs 4.12 and 4.13) viewed dry under polarised light to show the full extent of demineralisation. (Figs 4.12–4.14) *(by Silverstone, L.M., 1983. Remineralisation and enamel caries. New concepts. Dental Update 10, 261–273.)*

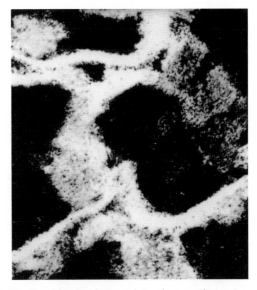

Fig. 4.17 **Demineralised enamel.** An electron photomicrograph of enamel produced after the action of very dilute acid. The crystallites of calcium salts remain intact in the prism sheaths, while the prism cores and some of the interprismatic substance have been destroyed. The same appearance is seen in early caries. *(By kind permission of Dr K Little.)*

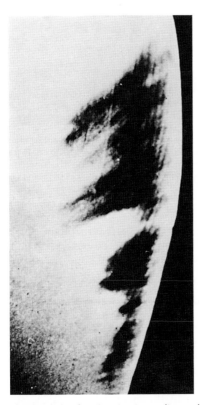

Fig. 4.15 **Early approximal caries.** A microradiograph of the same section as in Figs 4.12–4.14, showing radiolucency following the same pattern, the intact surface zone and accentuation of the striae of Retzius. *(By kind permission of the late Professor AI Darling.)*

In pit and fissure caries, the same changes take place, but the lesion forms a ring around the fissure's lateral wall. In a two-dimensional sectional view, the same zones as in smooth surface caries are seen on either side of the fissure (Fig. 4.16).

As noted earlier, the initial attack on enamel appears to be by highly mobile hydrogen ions permeating the organic matrix to attack the surface of the apatite crystals (Figs 4.17 and 4.18). The apatite crystals become progressively smaller. Microdissection of the translucent zone has shown that the apatite crystals have declined in diameter from the normal of 35–40 nm to 25–30 nm and in the body of the lesion to 10–30 nm. In the dark zone, by contrast, enamel crystals appeared to have grown to 50–100 nm and in the surface zone to 35–40 nm. These findings also support the theory that both demineralisation and remineralisation occur in phases. This changes once cavitation develops and demineralisation comes to dominate the process. Until then, bacteria cannot physically penetrate enamel because of the intact surface layer (Fig. 4.19).

Chemistry of dissolution PMID: 11132767

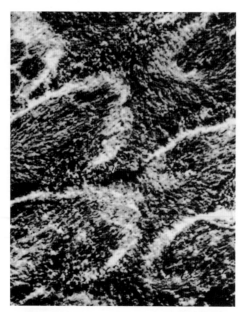

Fig. 4.18   The organic matrix of developing enamel. An electron photomicrograph of a section across the lines of the prisms before calcification showing the matrix to be more dense in the region of the prism sheaths than in the prism cores or interprismatic substance. *(By kind permission of Dr K Little.)*

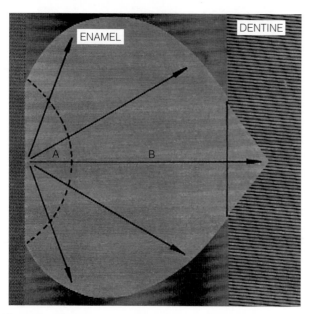

Fig. 4.19   Diagram summarising the main features of the pre-cavitation phase of enamel caries. As indicated here in this final stage of acid attack on enamel before bacterial invasion, decalcification of dentine has begun. The area (A) would be radiolucent in a bite-wing film, but the area (B) could be visualised only in a section by polarised light microscopy or microradiography. Clinically, the enamel would appear solid and intact, but the surface would be marked by an opaque white spot over the area (A) as seen in Fig. 4.11. *(From McCracken, A.W., Cawson, R.A. 1983. Clinical and oral microbiology. Washington DC.)*

Cavitation: cavity formation

While the surface layer is intact, bacteria cannot enter the enamel and caries can only progress by diffusion of acid through plaque and into the enamel. If acid attack reaches a critical level or frequency, demineralisation overwhelms

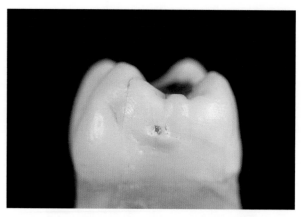

Fig. 4.20   Early cavitation in enamel caries. The surface layer of the white spot lesion has broken down, allowing plaque bacteria into the enamel.

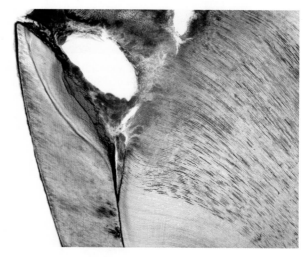

Fig. 4.21   Low-power view of caries spreading along the amelodentinal junction. Note how it spreads only a small distance in advance of caries in dentine. The amelodentinal junction is only a little more susceptible to carious spread than dentine.

the remineralising process that maintains the surface zone, and it breaks down. Once bacteria can enter the lesion, demineralisation is favoured and the caries progresses deeply toward the dentine (Fig. 4.20).

Caries first reaches the enamel-dentine junction at a small area below the centre of the lesion because of the shape of the enamel lesion. It then spreads laterally to undermine the enamel (Figs 4.21 and 4.22). This has two major effects. First, the enamel loses the support of the dentine and is therefore greatly weakened. Second, it is attacked from beneath (Fig. 4.22). Lateral spread along the amelodentinal junction is relatively limited and extends laterally only to the widest extent of the enamel lesion at the surface, which determines the area of the initial attack on the dentine.

Once dentine is destroyed and the crown weakened, enamel starts to collapse under the stress of mastication and to fragment around the edge of the (by then clinically obvious) cavity. By this stage, bacterial damage to the dentine is extensive.

The process of enamel caries is summarised in Box 4.13.

Natural rates cavitation PMID:22821238

Clinical relevance ISBN: 978-1118935828

PATHOLOGY OF DENTINE CARIES

The earliest stage of dentine caries starts deep to a carious enamel lesion *before* any clinical evidence of cavitation. At the earliest detectable stage of enamel caries radiographically (Fig. 4.23), the dentine changes cannot be seen. Diffusion of acid from the enamel lesion into the dentine causes demineralisation of the mineral component but leaves the collagenous dentine matrix intact. However, once bacteria have penetrated the enamel, they spread along the amelodentinal junction to attack the dentine over a wide area. The lesion is therefore conical with a broad base at the enamel junction and its apex toward the pulp (Fig. 4.24).

Infection of dentine is facilitated by the dentine tubules, which form a pathway open to bacteria (Fig. 4.25) once they have been slightly widened by acid attack. After deminerali-

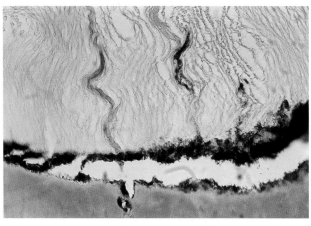

Fig. 4.22   Caries spread along the amelodentinal junction at higher power. The greater porosity and organic content here allows caries to spread preferentially laterally, though it only spreads to match the lateral extent of the surface caries, until a late stage.

Box 4.13   Process of enamel caries

- Permeation of the organic matrix by hydrogen ions causes sub-microscopic demineralisation
- Microradiography confirms that these changes represent areas of increasing demineralisation
- The dark zone is evidence that remineralisation occurs within the cavity
- The surface zone is largely formed by remineralisation
- There is alternating demineralisation and remineralisation
- When demineralisation is predominant, cavity formation progresses
- When remineralisation is predominant, caries arrests but normal enamel cannot reform
- Bacteria cannot invade enamel until demineralisation provides pathways large enough for them to enter (cavitation)

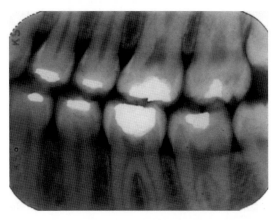

Fig. 4.23   Early enamel caries. Bitewing radiograph showing several approximal lesions, just visible. No dentine changes are seen, but they would be present microscopically.

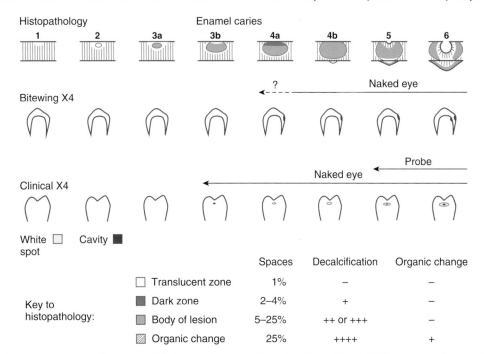

Key to histopathology:		Spaces	Decalcification	Organic change
☐	Translucent zone	1%	–	–
■	Dark zone	2–4%	+	–
▨	Body of lesion	5–25%	++ or +++	–
▨	Organic change	25%	++++	+

Fig. 4.24   This diagram summarises the sequential changes in enamel from the stage of the initial lesion to early cavity formation and relates the different stages in the development of the lesion with the radiographic appearances and clinical findings. *(Diagram kindly lent by the late Professor Al Darling and reproduced by courtesy of Darling, A.I. (Ed.), 1959. The pathology and prevention of caries. Darling. Br. Dent. J. 107, 287–302.)*

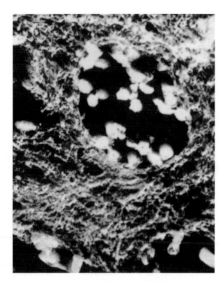

Fig. 4.25 **Infection of the dentinal tubules.** This electron photomicrograph shows bacteria in the lumen of the tubules. Between the tubules is the collagenous matrix of the dentine. *(By kind permission of Dr K Little.)*

sation, the dentine matrix is progressively destroyed by proteolytic enzymes secreted by bacteria.

Streptococci play the major role in the attack on enamel, but the bacteria present at the advancing front of dentine caries form a diverse flora of facultative anaerobes and anaerobes. Commonly isolated species include lactobacilli, *Actinomyces*, *Bifidobacterium* and *Eubacterium*, with *S. mutans* in variable amounts, the last probably contributing to more rapid progression. The flora is proteolytic and more dependent on the dentine matrix for nutrient than dietary sugars.

At first, the decalcified dentine retains its normal morphology. Once bacteria have reached the amelodentinal junction, they extend down the tubules, soon fill them and spread along any lateral branches. The tubules become distended by the expanding masses of bacteria and their products, which the softened matrix cannot confine. Later, the intervening tubule walls are destroyed, and collections of bacteria in adjacent tubules coalesce to form irregular liquefaction foci. These, in turn, coalesce to induce progressively more widespread tissue destruction (Figs 4.26 and 4.27). Eventually the dentine is completely destroyed. In some areas, bacteria-filled clefts form at right angles to the general direction of the tubules. Clinically, these clefts may allow carious dentine to be excavated in flakes in a plane parallel to the surface (Fig. 4.28).

Caries in dentine thus has zones of demineralisation, bacterial penetration and dentine destruction. The degree of destruction of the dentine is critical to restorative treatment. Even in the zone of bacterial penetration, much of the dentine structure is intact and can remineralise. It is therefore possible to restore a tooth, leaving caries and bacteria below the restoration, provided the restoration is of high quality and achieves an adequate adhesive peripheral seal. No bacterial substrate can then reach the bacteria, the caries process halts and dentine can remineralise.

Dentine caries is therefore divided into the caries-affected and caries-infected zones (Fig. 4.29). Caries-affected dentine is demineralised and its matrix only partly degraded; some of the tubular structure still remains, and bacterial numbers are low. In contrast the caries-infected zone, clinically

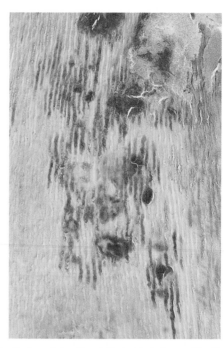

Fig. 4.26 **Caries of dentine.** Infected tubules and fusiform masses of bacteria have expanded into the softened tissue. Adjacent tubules in the demineralised dentine have been bent and pushed aside by these masses.

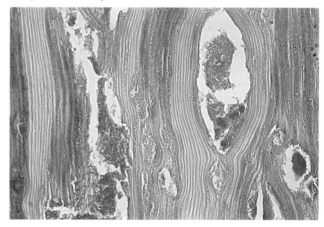

Fig. 4.27 **Advanced dentine caries.** The dentine is disintegrating (*left*). To the right is a large focus of destruction and tubules packed with bacteria.

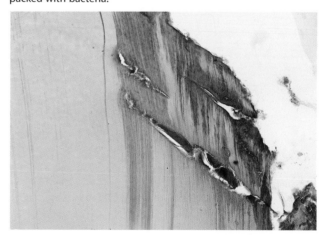

Fig. 4.28 **Clefts in carious dentine.** Infection is tracking along the tubules but has also spread across the tubules, forming heavily infected clefts. The appearances suggest that there are lines of weakness in the dentine, along which infection spreads easily.

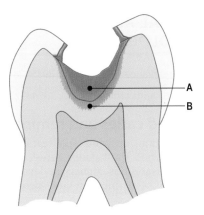
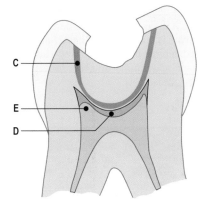

Fig. 4.29 **The zones of dentine caries and pulp-dentine defence reactions.** *Left panel*, zones of dentine caries: A, infected dentine, includes both destroyed zones and areas of bacterial penetration; B, affected dentine, demineralised dentine, with sparse bacteria only. *Right panel*, defence reactions: C, translucent dentine produced by peritubular sclerosis surrounds the lesion; D, regular reactionary dentine reduces the size of the pulp and protects it; E, pulpitis, the immunological and inflammatory reactions triggered by odontoblast damage does not help resistance to caries. *(Fig 9.4 p46, in Case 9 A large carious lesion. Banerjee A in Clinical Problem Solving in Dentistry 3rd edn 2010 Ed Odell E, Churchill Livingstone, Edinburgh).*

Box 4.14 Key events in the development of dentine caries

- Non-bacterial, pre-cavitation, acid softening of matrix
- Widening of tubules by demineralisation
- Migration of pioneer bacteria along tubules
- Development of a mixed proteolytic bacterial flora in the dentine
- Distortion of tubules by expanding masses of bacteria
- Breakdown of intervening matrix forming liquefaction foci
- Progressive disintegration of remaining matrix tissue

---

identifiable as soft, wet and brown, is largely demineralised, has no residual intact matrix to remineralise, no tubules and high numbers of bacteria. The caries-infected zone cannot remineralise effectively and provides poor support for a restoration. It usually has to be removed.

The main events in dentine caries are summarised in Box 4.14.

Infected dentine relevance PMID: 26749788

Protective reactions of dentine and pulp under caries

The extension of caries into dentine is significantly slowed by a series of defence reactions mounted by vital dentine and pulp and mediated by odontoblast activity. These reactions are not specific and may be provoked by other irritants such as attrition, erosion, abrasion and restorative procedures. Changes in dentine start even before cavity formation in enamel, but take time and so are more likely to develop prominently under slowly progressing caries. Reactionary dentine is laid down by the original odontoblasts, either as peritubular dentine or in the pulp. Once the odontoblasts die, defence reactions within the dentine cannot occur, but reactive dentine can form. This is a more rapid response by odontoblast-like cells that differentiate from pulp cells. Pulpal reactions are possible until the pulp is devitalised.

Changes in dentine in response to caries are summarised in Table 4.3.

Table 4.3 Reactionary changes in dentine

Response	Key facts
Translucent dentine	A form of reactionary dentine laid down within tubules, peritubular dentine. This reduces the diameter of the dentinal tubules, preventing bacterial penetration and generating a more heavily mineralised dentine by 'tubular sclerosis'. Translucent dentine usually forms in a band approximately halfway between the pulp and amelodentinal junction and along the sides of the carious lesion. It forms a hard more mineralised zone, that may be visible radiographically and is detectable with hand instruments when excavating caries.
Regular reactionary dentine	Forms at the pulp–dentine interface and retains the tubular structure of dentine. Forms in response to mild stimuli and may obliterate pulp horns, increasing the dentine thickness between caries and pulp. Unfortunately, it often forms most on the floor and sides of the pulp chamber where it is of little value in defence against caries. Formed by odontoblasts
Irregular reparative dentine	Forms in response to moderate or severe insult by caries and correspondingly ranges from dentine with irregular tubules to a disorganised bone-like mineralised tissue. Laid down by newly differentiated cells from the pulp
Dead tracts	Formed when odontoblasts die and their tubules become sealed off. If peritubular dentine formation was extensive before odontoblast death, the dead tract may be sclerotic and inhibit advance of caries. If not, it may allow more rapid progress.

These changes start to develop early but at best can only slow the advance of dental caries. Even the densely mineralised translucent dentine is vulnerable to bacterial acid and proteolysis, and once bacteria have penetrated the normal dentine, they can invade reactionary and reparative dentine to reach the pulp (Figs 4.30–4.34).

CLINICAL ASPECTS OF CARIES PATHOLOGY

Clinical relevance ISBN: 978-1118935828

Cochrane caries removal PMID: 23543523

Arrested caries and remineralisation

Pre-cavitation, or 'white spot' caries lesions, may become arrested when the balance between demineralisation and remineralisation is altered in favour of remineralisation (Fig. 4.35). This might follow sucrose restriction, fluoride

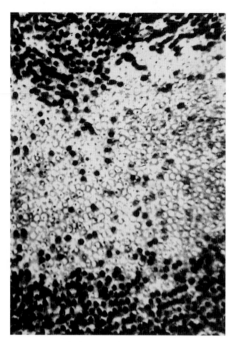

Fig. 4.30 Translucent dentine in dentine caries. The dentinal tubules are seen in cross-section. Those in the centre of the picture have become obliterated by calcification; only the original outline of the tubules remains visible, and the zone appears translucent to transmitted light. On either side are patent tubules filled with stain. *(Kindly lent by Dr GC Blake and reproduced by courtesy of the Honorary Editors, Blake, G.C., 1958. An experimental investigation into the permeability of enamel and dentine. Proceedings of the Royal Society of Medicine. 51, 678–686.)*

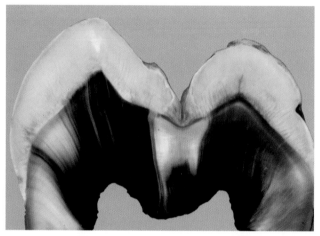

Fig. 4.31 Translucent dentine. There is early occlusal caries in the fissure, and below it peritubular dentine has sealed off the pathway to the pulp to produce a zone of translucent dentine. When dye is put into the pulp chamber, it cannot pass along the tubules in the translucent dentine as it does elsewhere. The translucent zone is thus rendered less permeable to bacteria and acid. *(From Cawson, R.H., Binnie, W.H., a Barrett, A.W, et al. 2001. Oral disease. 3rd ed. St. Louis: Mosby.)*

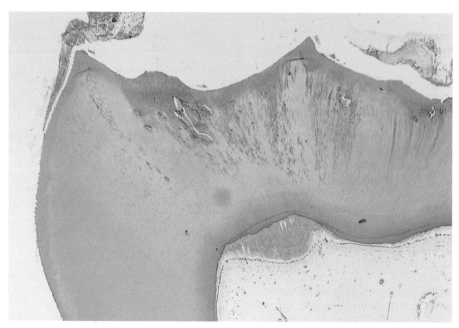

Fig. 4.32 Regular reactionary dentine below occlusal caries. Bacteria extend more than half the distance from the amelodentinal junction to the pulp, and the underlying pulp horn has been obliterated by reactionary dentine. The reactionary dentine bulges into the pulp. Note the lack of inflammation in the pulp, organised tubular structure and odontoblast layer.

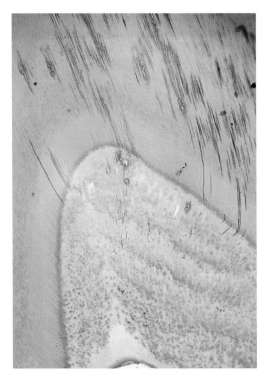

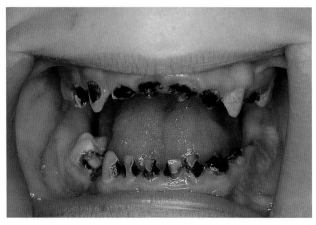

Fig. 4.35 Extensive but arrested caries following treatment for caries caused by sweetened medication.

Fig. 4.33 Regular reactionary dentine. Regular, tubular, secondary dentine has formed under a carious cavity. A line marks the junction of the primary and secondary dentine where the tubules change direction. Bacteria spreading down the tubules of the primary tissue have extended along the junction and into the tubules of the reactionary dentine.

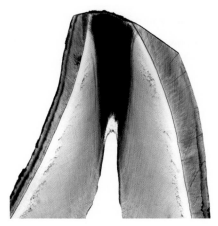

Fig. 4.34 A dead tract. The dentine below the incisal tip is 'dead'; it has no viable osteoblast processes, and dye applied to the incisal edge penetrates the tubules so that the 'dead tract' appears dark. At the proximal end of the tubules, the dead tract has been sealed off by impermeable reactionary dentine through which the stain cannot penetrate. The pulp is thus protected from irritants penetrating along the dentinal tubules, but less effectively than by translucent dentine as seen in Fig. 4.30. Note that the dye in this figure and Fig. 4.31 has been applied to opposite ends of the tubules.

application or loss of one tooth adjacent to an approximal lesion, the last uncovering a stagnation area and permitting adequate oral hygiene procedures. The source of calcium and phosphate to remineralise the lesion is saliva and plaque.

Caries progresses slowly, and even under natural conditions, approximately 50% of approximal enamel lesions may show no radiographic evidence of progression for 3 years, showing that little change may be required to favour reversal of the process. Although remineralisation may return the mineral content of an enamel lesion to close to that of the original enamel, the deposition is irregular and disorganised at the level of individual crystals, and the original enamel structure cannot be regained. Despite this, remineralised lesions that have fluoride incorporated can be less prone to carious attack than intact enamel.

Arrested enamel caries may remain opaque and white or more often becomes discoloured by incorporation of extrinsic stain – the so-called *inactive* or *brown spot lesion*.

Dentine caries may also become arrested. This may result from preventive intervention or follow collapse of overlying enamel, exposing the dentine to saliva and cleaning. Dentine caries below a completely sealed restoration will also arrest and remineralise by using mineral ions from the pulp. Remineralisation in dentine does not produce a hard material. The regrowth of crystals is less than in enamel, and the arrest process comprises cessation of demineralisation at the advancing front, cessation of dentine proteolysis by death or inhibition of bacteria in the dentine and deposition of new mineral. Remineralised arrested dentine caries does not feel like normal dentine to the probe, but is nevertheless leathery hard and dry, and not soft and wet like active caries.

The much greater natural porosity of dentine caries allows extrinsic stain to be incorporated into arrested caries, and this and bacterial products and reactions between acids and the matrix produce a dark brown colour to arrested dentine caries. If the pulp is vital, arrest of caries allows time for pulp defence reactions to produce peritubular dentine and translucent zones. These increase the mineral density of dentine below the lesion to slow its advance should the caries reactivate. Even the largest carious lesions can arrest if deprived of sucrose and exposed to saliva; caries below leaking restorations usually does not.

Preventive treatment to arrest and remineralise caries has become the paradigm of modern caries management, both for untreated caries and in placing restorations.

Caries in deciduous teeth

In adults, caries usually progresses slowly, and a small cavity may take several months to develop and several years to penetrate the enamel. By contrast, caries in children progresses quickly. Much of this can be accounted for by poor diet but, compared with permanent teeth, deciduous teeth have thinner enamel and dentine, wider flatter contact areas producing larger approximal lesions and wider dentinal tubules allowing earlier bacterial penetration.

Hidden caries

'Occult' or hidden caries describes the situation in which caries starts in an occlusal fissure and forms a very large lesion, often sufficient to destroy much of the coronal dentine and involve the pulp, despite the fact that the enamel remains reasonably intact clinically and the patient suffers little or no symptoms. Lower permanent molars are the teeth most usually affected, and the presentation is usually seen in children or young adults.

Lack of surface changes means that such lesions are often discovered radiographically, otherwise the true extent may not be revealed until the fissure is opened for exploration or to place a preventive resin restoration. However, these lesions are not truly hidden and careful examination, and transillumination will usually reveal fissure staining or subtle discolouration.

The processes of occult caries are not different from typical caries. The presentation has only become common in the UK in the last 20–30 years and may reflect increasing use of fluoride. This produces a harder more resistant enamel less likely to collapse under occlusal stress, and also more likely to remineralise using calcium and phosphate released from the underlying dentine caries.

Hidden caries PMID: 9448806

Root surface caries

Caries of the root surface is increasing in incidence while the ageing population retain more teeth. After recession of the gingival margin, cementum and root dentine are accessible to plaque. Cementum is readily decalcified and presents little barrier to infection. Root caries does not develop below the gingival margin in pockets.

Cervical cementum is very thin and invaded along the direction of Sharpey's fibres. Infection spreads between the lamellae along the incremental lines, and underlying dentine is involved almost immediately.

The causative microbial flora includes *S. mutans*, lactobacilli and several species of *Actinomyces*. Organisms such as *Actinomyces* that are unable to cause enamel caries in animal models are capable of causing root caries, but the plaque over root surface lesions is very mixed and contains many putative anaerobic periodontal pathogens too. Once the caries has invaded into dentine, the flora probably matures to one identical to coronal dentine caries.

Like enamel caries, root caries has a surface zone of remineralisation, but it is porous, and bacteria enter the tissues earlier than in enamel caries.

Root surface caries causes reactionary dentine on the pulp surface apical to the lesion because of the curvature of the dentinal tubules. This allows slowly progressing lesions to eventually penetrate to the coronal pulp without devitalising the apical pulp, which becomes closed off by the reactionary dentine.

Root surface caries is particularly seen in those with a dry mouth and those with poor oral hygiene.

Prevention root caries PMID: 23600985

Clinical aspects of reactions to caries

The pathology of dental caries may seem complex and largely irrelevant to clinical dentistry, but forms the foundation for effective prevention and restorative strategies. The mechanistic methods of tooth restoration used in the 20th century could be applied without reference to the underlying biology of disease, but modern minimum intervention or minimally invasive dentistry is entirely founded on a good understanding of the pathology of dental caries.

Examples of the clinical relevance of caries pathology are shown in Table 4.4.

Minimally invasive dentistry ISBN-13: 978-0198712091

Cochrane review treatment: DOI: 10.1002/14651858 .CD003808.pub3

Table 4.4 **The pathology of dental caries and its relevance to caries progression and treatment**

Feature	Significance
Plaque flora is a stable ecosystem	The bacterial flora is influenced by its environment, but the ecosystem will resist change in the short term. Denial of cariogenic substrate by dietary control will reduce the number of cariogenic species, but dietary change must be maintained to be effective
The early caries lesion begins as a subsurface process	Bacteria cannot enter the enamel until the surface layer is destroyed and until then can be removed by cleaning. Until cavitation, complete repair by remineralisation is possible and prevention of cavitation is critical
Enamel is permeable, pores between crystallites account for 0.1% of its volume Odontoblast processes extend to the enamel–dentine junction	Enamel is porous, acids diffuse in readily to initiate caries and diffuse to dentine to trigger pulp defence reactions early in the lesion's lifespan, well before a lesion cavitates
The translucent zone in enamel caries is present in only approximately half of caries lesions examined	The translucent zone indicates progression. Many lesions are not active much of the time
The dark zone of enamel caries is seen in almost all lesions	The dark zone indicates remineralisation. Therefore, almost all lesions undergo periodic phases of remineralisation. In a remineralised or arrested lesion, the dark zone extends to replace much of the body of the lesion
Caries lesions undergo rapid phases of demineralisation and remineralisation. Activity or arrest may be the outcome depending on the relative proportion of each	Caries may remineralise, arrest or progress only very slowly so that, initially, observation or preventive intervention rather than restoration is appropriate for most enamel lesions
The surface zone of an enamel lesion is only 30 µm thick and porous	Pressure from probing may cavitate lesions, converting an arrested or slowly progressing lesion into an active lesion. Diagnosis should not attempt to indent the surface to judge 'stickiness', only to remove plaque and feel the surface texture Fluoride and other remineralising agents may enter the lesion easily Porous enamel takes up exogenous pigments so that longstanding lesions become 'brown spot' lesions
Fissure caries spreads laterally into the walls of a fissure, not into its base	The surface layer of occlusal enamel becomes undermined but is not initially directly involved. It may not fracture or appear abnormal until the underlying lesion is large (occult caries)
The shape of the enlarging occlusal lesion is guided inwards and laterally by the prism direction	An occlusal lesion involves a much greater area of dentine than a comparably-sized smooth surface lesion
The shape of the advancing front of a caries lesion in dentine is smooth and rounded	To conserve tooth structure, cavities should have smooth rounded outlines and no sharp internal angles
Caries spreads laterally along the amelodentinal junction	Lateral extension of a cavity is often determined by clearing caries from the amelodentinal junction (ADJ). However, caries usually only spreads laterally to approximately the extent of the lesion at the enamel surface and in underlying dentine. Although leaving caries at the junction is undesirable because it leaves enamel poorly supported, removal of ADJ caries can be undertaken conservatively
Cavitation develops unpredictably in relation to the size and extent of an approximal lesion on a radiograph	Some assessment of the patient's caries risk involving dietary analysis, fluoride and other factors is required before deciding that any lesion requires operative intervention. Lesions in a high-risk patient cavitate earlier than in a low-risk patient
The pulp–dentine complex responds to caries. The dentine just before the advancing front of a caries lesion is relatively impermeable as a result of remineralisation and tubular infill	The pulp–dentine defence reactions should be preserved, and this is best achieved by non-operative intervention rather than restoration. Minimal dentine should be removed in cavity preparation. In deep lesions, removal of all softened dentine over the pulp should be avoided
Dentine caries may be divided into zones of demineralisation, penetration and destruction or into zones of infected and affected dentine	Traditionally, cavity preparation involved removal of **all** softened dentine. However, it is not necessary to remove all infected dentine to provide a successful restoration. The correct amount to remove is usually judged by the degree of softening. Discoloration is a less effective indicator. Discoloured but 'reasonably firm' (not hard) dentine may be left in situ. These zones are of little significance beyond understanding the disease process, and none can be reliably identified clinically
Peritubular dentine and remineralisation form a translucent dentine zone that walls off the lesion	Lateral spread is slowed as caries penetrates dentine. When removing softened dentine with hand instruments or a slowly revolving bur, sclerotic dentine may be felt to be harder than adjacent dentine and should be preserved

Table 4.4 **The pathology of dental caries and its relevance to caries progression and treatment** (Continued)

Feature	Significance
Peritubular dentine forms slowly	Only slowly advancing lesions are delayed by this defence reaction. A sclerotic zone visible radiographically indicates a slowly progressing or arrested lesion
Dentine tubules in mature teeth are slightly smaller than bacterial cocci	Bacterial penetration of dentine toward the pulp can only take place after some dentine demineralisation
Demineralisation precedes bacterial invasion in dentine by a small and variable distance	Not all softened dentine must be removed during cavity preparation
The advancing front of bacterial penetration into dentine is irregular at a microscopic level	The relatively large mechanical instruments used to remove softened dentine will always leave some infected dentine behind. However, if sealed effectively below restorations, these bacteria will be rendered inert
Superficial infected dentine is denatured and cannot remineralise. Deeper affected dentine will remineralise even though it contains bacteria	It is not necessary to remove all infected dentine to place a restoration, only the dentine that cannot remineralise if sealed below the restoration. Therefore, caries removal should be more conservative / minimally invasive below a well-sealed adhesive restoration
Dentine matrix is denatured by bacteria in the superficial layers of the zone of destruction	This renders the dentine susceptible to chemomechanical caries removal using proprietary mixtures of sodium hypochlorite. This procedure removes only the most damaged carious dentine, a conservative approach that preserves the deeper layers that can remineralise
Dentine splits transversely along incremental lines of growth in the zone of destruction	Dentine caries in the outer zone of destruction is easily removed in large flakes with hand instruments
Caries indicator dyes stain softened as well as infected dentine They stain collagen	Adhering strictly to the dye protocol will remove remineralisable dentine that should be left *in situ*. Caries indicator dyes promote overcutting
Reactionary dentine forms slowly and varies markedly in amount, quality and permeability and is found below only half the lesions in permanent teeth (more frequent in primary teeth)	Reactionary dentine provides little protection below rapidly progressing lesions
Formation of reactionary dentine requires a good blood supply and healthy pulp	Less is formed in older individuals. Once the pulp is inflamed, the quality of any reactionary dentine is poor and it is unlikely to be of much benefit
Symptoms of pulpitis do not correlate well with caries activity, lesion size, pulpal inflammation or even direct pulp involvement	Pulp vitality may be lost without symptoms or with only mild symptoms. An assessment of the state of a pulp is desirable to plan restoration of a deep carious lesion but, if based on symptoms alone, is unlikely to be accurate
Lesions of root caries also have a surface remineralised layer	Avoid hard probing of apparently intact though discoloured surfaces, as for enamel caries
Bacteria penetrate dentine early in root caries lesions but are accessible to non-operative preventive measures	Removal of infected dentine is not always necessary to treat early root caries
Deciduous teeth have approximately half the thickness of enamel of permanent teeth, larger pulps, longer pulp horns and, at least initially, larger dentinal tubules	Caries progresses faster in primary teeth than in permanent teeth

Pulpitis and apical periodontitis | 5

PULPITIS → Summary charts 5.1 and 5.2, pp. 79, 80

Pulpitis, inflammation of the dental pulp, is the most common reason for dental pain in younger persons. The usual cause is caries penetrating the dentine, but there are other possibilities (Box 5.1). Exposure during cavity preparation allows bacteria to enter the pulp and also damages it mechanically (Fig. 5.1). Fracture may either open the pulp chamber or leave so thin a covering of dentine that bacteria can enter through the dentinal tubules. A tooth may crack from masticatory stress, usually after weakening by restoration, and bacteria penetrate along the crack (Fig. 5.2). Thermal damage can trigger pulpitis following cavity cutting with insufficient cooling or following intermittent low-grade thermal stimuli conducted to the pulp by large unlined metal restorations. Chemical damage can result from older types of acidic restoration materials used without a cavity lining.

Pulpitis, if untreated, is often followed by death of the pulp and spread of infection through the apical foramen into the periapical tissues to cause periapical periodontitis.

Clinical features

The pulps of individual teeth are not precisely represented on the sensory cortex. Pain from the pulp is therefore poorly localised and may be felt in any of the teeth of the upper or lower jaw of the affected side. Rarely, pain may be referred to a more distant site such as the ear. Pulp pain is not provoked by pressure on the tooth. The patient can chew in comfort unless there is a large open cavity allowing food to distort or stimulate the dentine.

Acute pulpitis   In the early stages the tooth is hypersensitive. Very cold or hot food causes a stab of pain that stops as soon as the irritant is removed. While inflammation progresses, pain becomes more persistent after the stimulus, and there may be prolonged attacks of toothache. The pain may start spontaneously, often when the patient is trying to get to sleep.

The pain is partly due to the pressure on the irritated nerve endings from oedema within the rigid pulp chamber and partly due to release of pain-producing mediators from the damaged tissue and inflammatory cells. The pain at its worst is excruciatingly severe, sharp and stabbing in character. It is little affected by simple analgesics.

The outcome of acute pulpitis is unpredictable. Acute pulpitis may be deemed irreversible on the basis of various features (see Table 5.1), but even then the pulp may sometimes survive. Although pulp death is the likely outcome, acute pulpitis may progress to chronic pulpitis, and early treatment can still preserve pulp vitality. A diagnosis of

---

Box 5.1   Causes of pulpitis

- Dental caries
- Traumatic exposure of the pulp
- Fracture of a crown or cusp
- Cracked tooth
- Thermal or chemical irritation

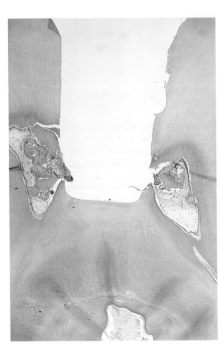

Fig. 5.1   Traumatic exposure. The pulp has been exposed during cavity preparation, and dentine chippings and larger fragments have been driven into the pulp. The tooth was extracted before a strong inflammatory reaction has had time to develop, but it is clear that some inflammatory cells have already localised around the debris, which will have introduced many bacteria to the pulp.

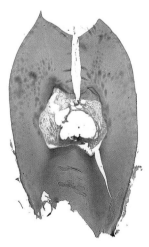

Fig. 5.2   Cracked tooth. The pulp died beneath this crack, which was undetected clinically. Decalcification of the tooth and shrinkage on preparation of a section has revealed the crack.

Table 5.1 Features of 'reversible' and 'irreversible' pulpitis

Reversible pulpitis	Irreversible pulpitis
Pain in short, sharp stabs	Constant throbbing pain with sharp exacerbations
Stimulated by hot and cold or osmotic (sweet) stimuli	Spontaneous exacerbations, as well as hot and cold or osmotic (sweet) stimuli. In late stages cold may relieve the pain
Pain resolves after stimulus removed in seconds or a few minutes	Pain persists several minutes or hours after an exacerbating stimulus

irreversible pulpitis is considered an indication for extirpation of the pulp, but it must be recognised that the diagnostic criteria are poorly defined.

Chronic pulpitis may develop with or without episodes of acute pulpitis. However, many pulps under large carious cavities die painlessly. The first indication is then development of periapical periodontitis, either with pain or seen by chance in a radiograph. In other cases, there are bouts of dull pain, brought on by hot or cold stimuli or occurring spontaneously. There are often prolonged remissions, and there may be recurrent acute exacerbations.

Pathology

Pulpitis caused by early caries results from penetration of acid and bacterial products through the dentine, and later from a mixed bacterial infection penetrating to the pulp. There is no relationship between the severity or type of pain and the histological features. Histology shows all degrees of inflammation and even progression to pulpal necrosis regardless of pain.

Acute closed pulpitis Closed pulpitis refers to inflammation inside an intact closed pulp chamber. Histologically, there is initial hyperaemia limited to the area immediately beneath the irritant (Fig. 5.3). Infiltration by inflammatory cells and destruction of odontoblasts and adjacent pulp follow. A limited area of necrosis may result in formation of an abscess, localised by granulation tissue (Figs 5.4–5.7). Later, inflammation spreads until the pulp is obliterated by dilated blood vessels and acute inflammatory cells (Fig. 5.8). Necrosis follows when pressure occludes the apical vessels.

Chronic closed pulpitis The main features are a predominantly mononuclear cell infiltrate and inflammation more limited in extent. A small area of pulpal necrosis and pus formation may be localised by a well-defined wall of granulation tissue, and a minute abscess may thus form. The remainder of the pulp may still appear normal.

Given time for the pulp to mount a reaction, as for instance beneath a relatively uncontaminated exposure, inflammation may become well localised. A partial calcific barrier may wall off the exposure with reactionary dentine around the margins, as seen following pulp capping. Calcific barriers can be seen radiographically as 'dentine bridges' and may also form apically following use of calcium hydroxide to induce apex closure. Unfortunately, the calcified layer is frequently incomplete and forms less of a barrier than might be thought (Figs 5.9 and 5.10). However, in successful cases, formation of a complete barrier of tubular reactionary dentine may allow preservation of the remainder of the pulp.

The chief factor hampering pulpal survival is its enclosure within the rigid walls of the pulp chamber and, in fully

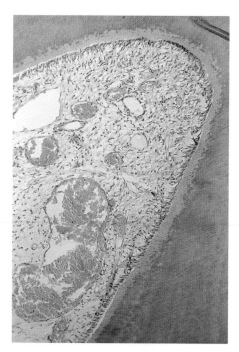

Fig. 5.3 Pulpal hyperaemia. While bacteria are still some distance from the pulp, acid permeating along the dentinal tubules gives rise to dilation of the blood vessels, oedema and a light cellular inflammatory infiltrate in the pulp.

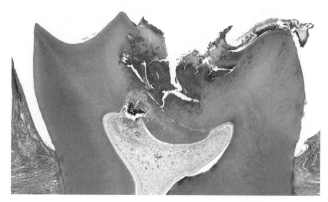

Fig. 5.4 Acute pulpitis. Low-power view showing occlusal caries penetrating to the pulp through a layer of reactionary dentine. There is a focus of acute inflammatory cells beneath the carious exposure in the pulp horn.

formed teeth, the limited aperture for the apical vessels. In acute inflammation, these vessels can readily be compressed by inflammatory oedema and thrombose. The blood supply of the pulp is thus cut off and it dies. This may be rapid in the case of acute pulpitis, or delayed in chronic lesions. The relatively prolonged survival of chronically inflamed pulps is shown by the persistence of symptoms during a long period. However, pulp death is usually the end result unless treatment is provided.

Open pulpitis Necrosis of the pulp from oedema compressing the blood supply is more likely when the walls of the chamber are intact. When there is a wide exposure or other drainage, or when there are incompletely formed open apices or multiple apices, the balance is tipped in favour of host defences, and a chronically inflamed pulp can survive despite heavy infection (Fig. 5.11).

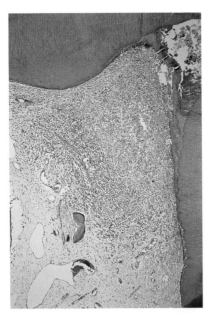

Fig. 5.5   Acute pulpitis. Beneath the carious exposure (*top right*) a dense inflammatory infiltrate is accumulating. More deeply, the pulp is hyperaemic, with dilated blood vessels.

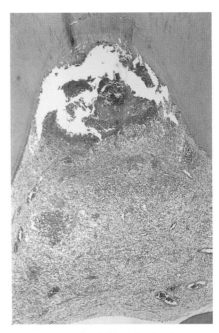

Fig. 5.7   Acute caries and pulpitis. Infection has penetrated to the pulp. Part of the pulp has been destroyed, and an abscess has formed, containing a bead of pus.

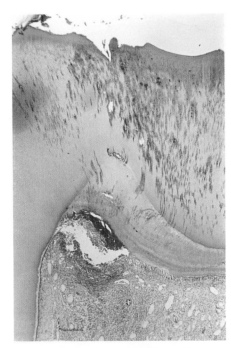

Fig. 5.6   Acute pulpitis. Infection (*dark lines of bacteria along tubules*) has penetrated a thin layer of reactionary dentine on the roof of the pulp chamber causing inflammation throughout the pulp and pus to form in the pulp horn.

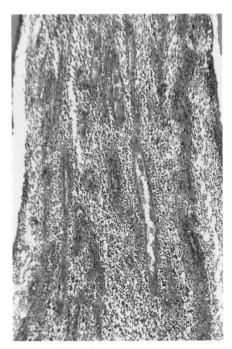

Fig. 5.8   Acute pulpitis: terminal stage. The entire pulp has been destroyed and replaced by inflammatory cells and dilated vessels.

Chronic hyperplastic pulpitis (pulp polyp)   In this rare condition, despite wide pulpal exposure, the pulp not merely survives but proliferates through the opening to form a pulp polyp.

A pulp polyp appears as a dusky red or pinkish soft nodule protruding from the pulp to fill a carious cavity. It is painless but may be tender and bleed on probing. It should be distinguished from proliferating gingival tissue extending over the edge of the cavity by tracing its attachment (Fig. 5.12). When a pulp polyp forms, the pulp itself becomes replaced

by granulation tissue (Fig. 5.13). The surface of the polyp eventually becomes epithelialised and covered by a layer of well-formed stratified squamous epithelium. This protects the granulation tissue and allows inflammation to subside and the granulation tissue to mature into fibrous tissue. The same degree of pulpal proliferation can occasionally be seen in teeth with fully formed roots (Fig. 5.14) but is most common in children. As in open pulpits, this is because open apices provide a better blood supply and prevent the pulp from dying as a result of pulpal oedema.

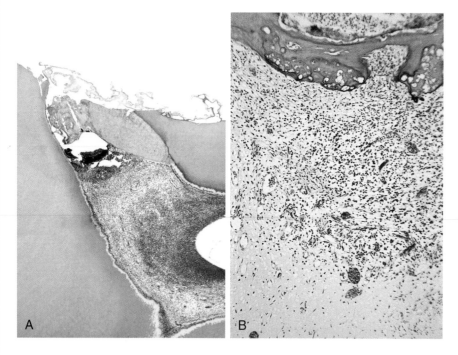

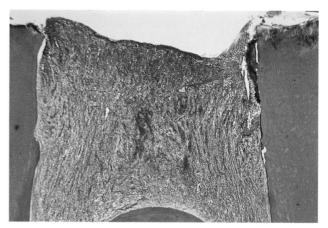

Fig. 5.9   Calcific barriers. (A) Pulpitis with formation of a barrier of thick reactionary dentine in the pulp horn, but with an abscess immediately below it. The rest of the pulp is inflamed. (B) Higher-power view of a calcific barrier induced by calcium hydroxide direct pulp capping. In this case the barrier is thin, inflammation in the underlying pulp has not subsided and the pulp cap has failed.

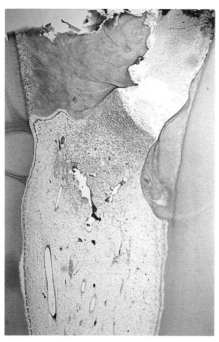

Fig. 5.11   Open pulpitis. Beneath the wide exposure the pulp has survived in the form of granulation tissue, with the most dense inflammatory infiltrate immediately beneath the open surface.

Fig. 5.10   Pulp capping. This pulp capping has induced a thick layer of reactionary dentine (with regular tubules, best seen on the left hand side of the pulp chamber wall coronally) and reparative dentine with a more irregular structure (on the right of the pulp wall). Unfortunately these reactions do not produce a complete barrier, and failure of the procedure is indicated by the inflammatory cells concentrated below a gap in the barrier.

Management

The chances of an inflamed pulp surviving are poor, and treatment options are limited (Box 5.2). As noted previously, the concept of irreversible pulpitis is considered useful for treatment planning, but criteria are poorly defined.

Open pulpitis is usually associated with gross cavity formation, and it is rarely possible to save the tooth, despite the vitality of the pulp.

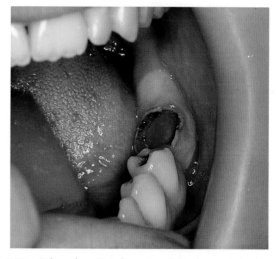

Fig. 5.12   Pulp polyp. An inflamed nodule of granulation tissue can be seen growing from the pulp chamber of this broken down first permanent molar.

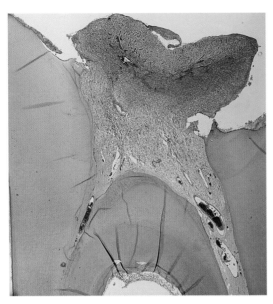

Fig. 5.13 Pulp polyp. A hyperplastic nodule of granulation tissue is growing out through a wide exposure of the pulp. The surface is ulcerated, and the loose pulp has been replaced by the proliferation of fibrous tissue and vessels with inflammatory cells.

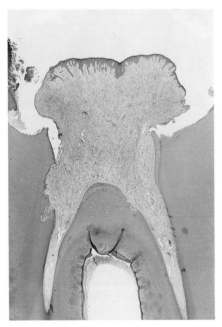

Fig. 5.14 Pulp polyp. In this broken-down molar, granulation tissue is proliferating from the pulp cavity and has acquired an epithelial covering over much of its surface, probably by shed epithelial cells from the mucosa seeding onto the surface. Note also the internal resorption (*left*) as a result of pulpal inflammation.

Box 5.2 Treatment options for pulpitis

- If fractured or cracked, stabilise fracture and seal pulp temporarily
- Removal of caries, obtundent or steroid dressing
- Removal of caries and pulp capping
- Pulpotomy in deciduous teeth
- Endodontic treatment
- Extraction
- Analgesics are largely ineffective

Box 5.3 Key features of pulpitis

- Pulpitis is caused by infection or irritation of the pulp, usually by caries
- Severe stabbing pain in a tooth, triggered by hot or cold food or starting spontaneously, indicates acute irreversible pulpitis
- Pulp pain is poorly localised
- Chronic pulpitis is often symptomless
- Untreated pulpitis usually leads to death of the pulp and spread of infection to the periapical tissues

---

Key features of pulpitis are summarised in Box 5.3, and the sequelae of pulpitis are shown in Summary chart 5.1.

PULP CALCIFICATIONS

Pulp stones, rounded masses of dentine that form within the pulp, can be seen in radiographs as small opacities. In the past, they were thought to cause symptoms but do not. They are common in normal teeth but have an increased frequency in teeth affected by caries, trauma, orthodontic movement and other potential irritants.

For unknown reasons, they are common in the teeth of patients with Ehlers-Danlos syndrome (Ch. 14), dentinal dysplasia type II (Ch. 2) and the rare disease tumoral calcinosis.

Histologically, pulp stones consist of dentine with normal or incomplete tubule formation (Fig. 5.15). A distinction used to be drawn between free and attached pulp stones. However, this is frequently an illusion caused by a plane of section which fails to pass through the connection between the pulp stone and the pulp wall. Most are large rounded irregular calcifications, often based on a central nidus of unknown material. Others, referred to as diffuse calcifications, lie parallel with the pulp wall and are thought to be an age-related degenerative change.

Pulp stones and diffuse calcification are of no clinical significance except insofar as they may obstruct endodontic treatment.

PERIAPICAL PERIODONTITIS, ABSCESS AND GRANULOMA → Summary chart 5.2, p. 80

Periapical inflammation is due to spread of infection, bacterial products or other irritants through the apex into the periodontal ligament following death of the pulp (Box 5.4). It characteristically causes tenderness of the tooth in its socket. Pulpal infection following caries is by far the most common cause (see Summary chart 5.2).

Sometimes a necrotic pulp is sterile, as for instance following trauma that damages the apical vessels. In such cases, periapical periodontitis results from irritants and mediators from the necrotic tissue.

Endodontic procedures can trigger periapical inflammation by perforation or pushing infected material or irritants such as hypochlorite through the apex. Provided the canal is clean and sealed, such acute episodes usually resolve quickly, unless large amounts of filling material remain beyond the apex.

Occlusal trauma from an over-contoured restoration will also cause an acute but usually transient sterile apical

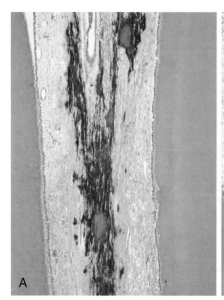
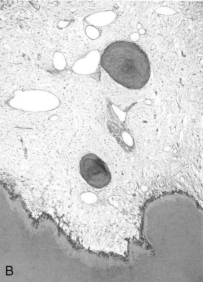

Fig. 5.15 Pulp stones. (A) The dystrophic or diffuse pulp mineralisations often found as an age change. (B) Rounded nodules of calcified tissue, in this case resembling bone rather than dentine.

Box 5.4   Causes of apical periodontitis
- Infection
- Trauma
- Chemical irritation

---

periodontitis. This will subside as the periodontal ligament remodels to accommodate the changed position of the tooth and the occlusal forces cause orthodontic movement of the tooth.

The diagnosis of pulpal, periodontal and other pain in the teeth and alveolus is summarised in Summary chart 5.2.

ACUTE APICAL PERIODONTITIS

→ Summary chart 5.1, p. 79

Spread of infection through the apex brings the causative bacteria from a protected site into an environment where the host can mount an effective host response. Acute inflammation and an immune reaction are triggered.

Clinical features

The patient may give a history of pain due to previous pulpitis, and the associated tooth may be carious, restored or discoloured due to death of the pulp. Formation of inflammatory exudate in the periodontal ligament causes the tooth to be extruded by a minute amount and the bite to fall more heavily on it. The tooth is at first uncomfortable, then increasingly tender, even to mere touch. Hot or cold substances do not cause pain in the tooth unless some viable pulp remains, as it may in a multirooted tooth.

Radiographs give little information because bony changes have had too short a time to develop. Immediately around the apex, the lamina dura may appear slightly hazy and the periodontal space may be slightly widened. When acute periodontitis is due to an acute exacerbation in a periapical granuloma (see later in this chapter), the granuloma can be seen as an area of radiolucency at the apex.

While apical periodontitis remains a localised apical inflammatory change, no facial oedema or alveolar tender-

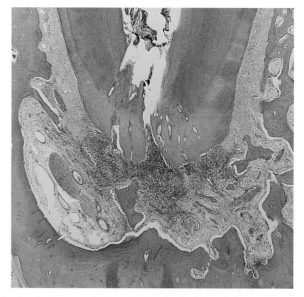

Fig. 5.16   Acute apical periodontitis. In this early acute lesion, inflammatory cells, mainly neutrophil polymorphonuclear leucocytes, are seen clustered around the apex of a non-vital tooth. The inflammatory cells are spreading around and into bone, and there has only been time for a small amount of bone resorption to develop. This would be seen radiographically only as slight fuzziness of the apical lamina dura.

ness or other reactions develop. Their onset indicates progression to apical infection.

Pathology and sequelae

Acute apical periodontitis is a typical acute inflammatory reaction with engorged blood vessels and packing of the tissue with neutrophils (Fig. 5.16). These changes are initially localised to the immediate vicinity of the apex.

At this stage periapical periodontitis is usually treated, triggered by the severe toothache. Extraction of the causative tooth or extirpation of the pulp and root filling eliminates the source of infection and drains the exudate. These are the simplest and most effective treatments. Antibiotics should not be given for simple acute periodontitis if immediate dental treatment is available.

Summary chart 5.1 Sequelae of pulpitis.

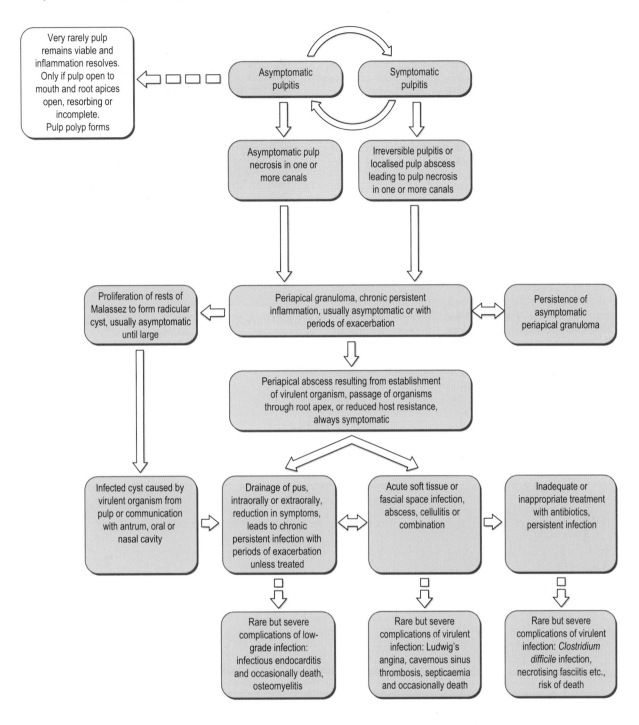

If untreated, there are two possible outcomes depending on the balance between the virulence of the bacteria and the host defences. The usual outcome is that a chronic periapical granuloma forms (later in this chapter). However, if the bacterial load is high, species are virulent or host response is inadequate, the infection will progress to an apical (or dentoalveolar) abscess (Box 5.5).

ACUTE APICAL (DENTOALVEOLAR) ABSCESS

The bacterial flora in the pulp chamber is virulent and anaerobic and can readily induce an abscess if sufficient

bacteria pass through the apex. The bacteria trigger acute inflammation, and pus starts to form and pain becomes intense and throbbing in character. At this stage, the gingiva over the root is red and tender, but there is no swelling while inflammation is confined within the bone. Unlike pulpitis, the pain of an apical abscess is accurately localised by the patient because periodontal ligament proprioceptors are triggered.

An established abscess will usually either drain through a sinus and become chronic or, much more rarely, progress to osteomyelitis or cellulitis. Usually pus and exudate will burrow a sinus tract to an adjacent pocket, the alveolar mucosa or skin. Once infection escapes into the medullary cavity of the bone, oedema may develop in the soft tissues of the face (Fig. 5.17).

Escape of pus to the skin is not common, but a classical presentation is the tracking of a sinus onto the skin near the chin as a result of a traumatically devitalised lower incisor (Figs 5.19–5.20). The regional lymph nodes may be enlarged and tender, but systemic symptoms are usually slight or absent.

Escape of pus takes a few days after the onset of pain; this relieves the pressure and pain quickly abates. If the exudate cannot escape, it may distend the soft tissues elsewhere to form a soft tissue abscess or cellulitis as described in Chapter 9.

Apical abscesses are polymicrobial infections and frequent cultivable isolates include *Veillonella sp.*, *Porphyromonas sp.*, *Streptococcus sp.*, *Fusobacterium sp.* and *Actinomyces sp.* Despite the mixed nature of the infection, penicillins remain the most effective antibiotics, with metronidazole reserved for those allergic to penicillin. However, an apical abscess cannot be treated by antibiotics alone; the causative tooth or its pulp must be dealt with because bacteria in the pulp chamber are inaccessible to the drug.

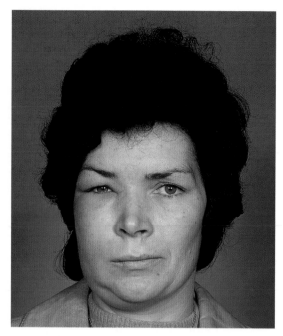

Fig. 5.17   Oedema due to acute apical periodontitis. An acute periapical infection of a canine has perforated the buccal plate of bone causing oedema of the face; this quickly subsided when the infection was treated.

Summary chart 5.2   Diagnosis of pulpal, periodontal and other pain in the teeth and alveolus.

Toothache or pain felt in teeth or alveolus								
Pain of pulpal origin			Pain of periodontal ligament origin				Neurological or vascular pain	Neuralgic or psychogenic pain
Sensitivity to sweet, hot or cold, poorly localised			Pain on biting or pressure on tooth, usually well localised to one or more teeth					
Dentine hypersentivity	Pulpitis	Cracked tooth or cusp	Periapical periodontitis	Periodontal abscess	Sinusitis		Neurological or vascular pain	Neuralgic or psychogenic pain
	Tooth is vital or partially vital and may be hypersensitive to testing							
Pain of short duration more or less limited to period of stimulus, particularly cold	Reversible pulpitis	Irreversible pulpitis	Shooting or electric shock-like pain on biting, often only on one cusp or in one direction, also when a fracture line involves periodontal ligament	Pain on pressure to single tooth, caries or other cause of pre-existing pulpitis may be present, periapical, lateral canal or furcation radiolucency only in longstanding cases	Pain on pressure to single tooth, tooth vital, abscess in ligament visible or revealed by probing furcation or deep pocket	Tenderness on pressure to teeth with apices near sinus, usually concurrent or recent nasal or sinus symptoms, not usually severe pain	Teeth vital unless previously devitalised for other reasons	Unusual localisation trigger or perceived cause, associated with depression, anxiety or delusional states, teeth vital unless previously devitalised for other reasons
	Symptoms may be limited to duration of stimulus or persist for varying period afterward, caries or other cause may be evident	Poorly defined entity, usually identified by severe continuous or spontaneous pain						
Confirm diagnosis by identifying exposed dentine or tooth wear and applying appropriate treatment	May resolve on treating cause but once established may progress to irreversible pulpitis, even after an asymptomatic period	Responds most reliably to extirpation of pulp or extraction	Confirm by identifying crack	Resolves on drainage or extirpation of pulp or extraction	Resolves on drainage and local treatment or extraction	Resolves on treatment of sinusitis	Consider mimics of pulpitis such as trigeminal neuralgia and the prodromal symptoms of facial Herpes zoster infection	Consider atypical odontalgia, atypical facial pain, 'phantom tooth' etc., but only after excluding organic causes

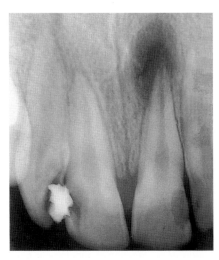

Fig. 5.18 Chronic apical abscess. Periapical bone resorption has developed as a result of inflammation. The area of radiolucency corresponds with the histological changes seen in figure 5.21.

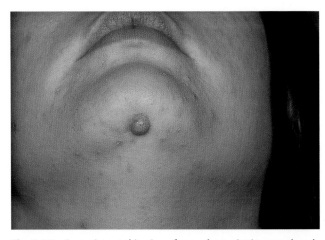

Fig. 5.19 A persistent skin sinus from a lower incisor rendered non-vital by a blow some time previously. This young woman was seen and treated unsuccessfully for 2 years by her doctor, surgeons and dermatologists before anyone looked at her teeth.

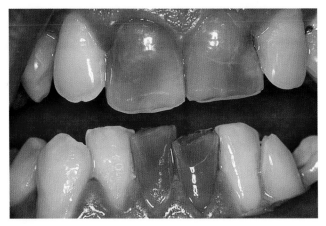

Fig. 5.20 Non-vital incisor teeth, in this case as a result of trauma. Haemorrhage and products of autolysis of the pulp discolour the dentine and darken the teeth.

Antibiotics alone fail PMID:16457000

Fatal outcome PMID:8105884

CHRONIC APICAL PERIODONTITIS AND PERIAPICAL GRANULOMA

→ Summary chart 5.1, p. 79

The most frequent outcome is for a necrotic pulp to form a chronic periapical granuloma, a focus of chronic inflammation at the root apex. Most develop without symptoms, but they can also arise from acute apical periodontitis, particularly when it has been inadequately drained and incompletely resolved.

A periapical granuloma is caused by frustrated healing. The granuloma itself is sterile in almost all cases, but bacteria and irritants from necrotic tissue remain in the pulp chamber, inaccessible to the host response. Small numbers of bacteria may occasionally pass through the apex but are quickly eliminated by the host defences. However, the continual trickle of irritants from the persistent reservoir of infection in the root canal prevents healing.

Clinical features

The tooth is non-vital and may be slightly tender to percussion, but otherwise, symptoms may be minimal.

Many periapical granulomas are first recognised as chance findings in a routine radiograph (Fig. 5.18). The granuloma forms a 'periapical area' of radiolucency a few millimetres in diameter with loss of continuity of the lamina dura around the apex. In longstanding lesions there may be hypercementosis on the adjacent root or slight superficial root resorption. The margins of the radiolucency may appear fuzzy when inflammation or infection are active, but are usually well defined and appear sharp in larger lesions. Good demarcation alone is not evidence of cyst formation.

Pathology

A periapical granuloma is a typical focus of chronic inflammation characterised by lymphocytes, macrophages and plasma cells in granulation tissue. It is important to recognise that a periapical granuloma does not contain true granulomas histologically. The term granuloma is a historic description for granulation tissue, in the same way that the word is used in pyogenic granuloma.

Inflammation is densest in the centre close to the root apex, and there is an uninflamed layer of fibrous tissue around the periphery separating the inflamed tissue from the bone. Osteoclasts resorb the bone to make space for the granuloma. There may be a central cavity with a few neutrophils, but no pus and no infection (Figs 5.21 and 5.22).

Inflammation may trigger epithelial rests of Malassez in the adjacent periodontal ligament to proliferate (Fig. 5.23), and this is the mechanism by which radicular cysts develop (Ch. 10).

Treatment and sequelae

A periapical granuloma will resolve if the causative necrotic pulp is removed, so extraction or endodontic treatment are the two options. Persistence after root canal treatment indicates treatment failure and retreatment or apicectomy may be required (Fig. 5.24).

Without treatment, the most likely outcome for a periapical granuloma is that it will persist largely unchanged.

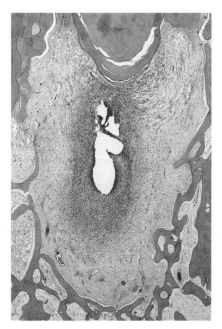

Fig. 5.21 **Chronic periapical abscess.** At the apex of the non-vital tooth (*top centre of picture*) is an abscess cavity surrounded by a thick fibrous wall densely infiltrated by inflammatory cells, predominantly neutrophils. Periapical bone has been resorbed and the trabeculae reorientated around the mass.

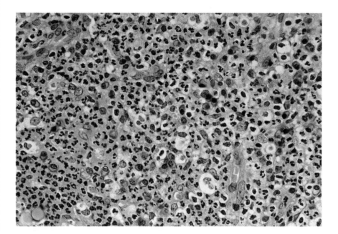

Fig. 5.22 High-power view of an apical granuloma showing neutrophils, lymphocytes and plasma cells in loose oedematous fibrous tissue.

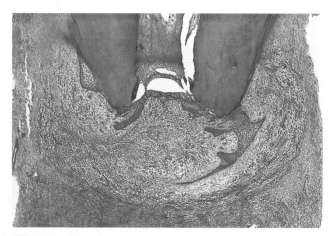

Fig. 5.23 **Epithelial proliferation in an apical granuloma.** Inflammation induces proliferation of odontogenic epithelium in rests of Malassez in the periodontal ligament. This change may lead to cyst formation (Ch. 10).

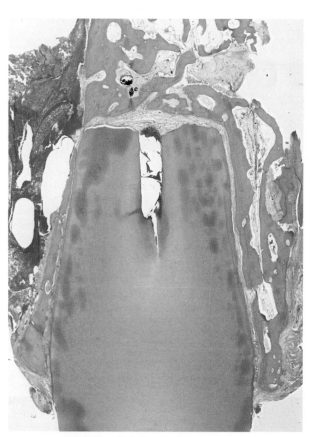

Fig. 5.24 **Low-power detail shows the effects of apicectomy.** The chronic inflammatory reaction has entirely cleared. New bone has formed to replace the excised apex with a new continuous periodontal ligament. The root filling material at the apex has been lost in preparing the section because it is too hard to cut.

There may be acute inflammatory exacerbations with symptoms from time to time, often insufficient to cause a patient to seek treatment.

The risk of leaving an untreated periapical granuloma is that it will develop into an acute periapical abscess. This is unpredictable, and granulomas that have been asymptomatic for decades may suddenly develop into an abscess. During any of these acute abscess exacerbations, a sinus may form. Sinus formation reduces pressure and usually allows the infection to persist as a chronic low-grade infection. Sinuses will normally heal when the cause is treated and do not require excision. Otherwise, they may drain intermittently and heal after each acute exacerbation.

Successful treatment is followed by resolution of inflammation, reforming of the lamina dura and periodontal ligament and bone around the apex. In rare cases, there is healing only by fibrosis. This is more frequent in the maxilla than mandible and when inflammation has resorbed the overlying cortical bone. Fibrous healing to produce an apical scar is seen radiographically and appears similar to a persisting granuloma, causing a potential problem in diagnosis.

Persistence of a periapical granuloma following root treatment is very occasionally due to the presence of bacteria within the granuloma. Although most periapical granulomas are sterile, in a very small number of cases *Actinomyces* or other organisms can form a biofilm on the outer root surface or free-floating colonies in the centre of the granuloma. This must be distinguished from an acute periapical abscess. The organisms in 'extraradicular infection' remain localised, cause persistent low-grade inflammation but do not form pus or cause a spreading infection. Extraradicular infection usually has to be eliminated by apicectomy or extraction.

Outcomes are summarised in Box 5.6 and Summary chart 5.1.

> **Box 5.6 Possible outcomes of chronic apical periodontitis**
> - Periapical granuloma formation
> - Radicular cyst formation
> - Suppuration, sinus formation or spread
> - Periodic acute exacerbations of inflammation of infection
>
> Spontaneous resolution does not occur.

Tooth wear, resorption, hypercementosis and osseointegration

6

TOOTH WEAR

Tooth wear is a widely used although rather non-specific and somewhat misleading term that includes the processes of non-carious tooth damage or 'tooth surface loss'. The processes of attrition, abrasion and erosion cause tooth wear. In any one affected patient, more than one of these processes is often active.

Multifactorial aetiology PMID: 24993256

Attrition

Attrition is wear from tooth-to-tooth contact and affects the tips of cusps and incisal edges most severely (Fig. 6.1). Attrition is a normal physiological process, and wear increases with age. Mamelons are soon lost from incisors, and by middle age attrition will have worn through the enamel on many male individuals' incisal edges and canine cusp tips. Attrition is increased when fewer teeth take the masticatory load or when the enamel is malformed. Attrition is enhanced in those with bruxism and on teeth in premature occlusion.

Attrition is often said to be worse with a coarse diet, but if the diet itself is abrasive, the effect is mixture of attrition and abrasion.

Reactionary dentine forms in response to this slow process and protects the pulp (Figs 4.32 and 4.33). Dentinal tubular sclerosis prevents dentine hypersensitivity resulting from pure attrition.

Pure attrition almost never needs treatment; if wear is significant, abrasion or erosion should be suspected.

Abrasion

Abrasion is wear of the teeth by an abrasive external agent. The most common form is occlusal wear from an abrasive diet and is frequent in developing countries and in ancient skulls.

Abrasion of the necks of the teeth buccally is seen mainly in the elderly as a consequence of overly vigorous tooth brushing or use of an abrasive dentifrice. A horizontal brushing action is often blamed, but the evidence is slim, and once a groove develops, the brush bristles are deflected into it regardless of technique. Abrasion affects both enamel and root dentine, but the softer dentine is abraded more easily. The exposed dentine is shiny and smooth, polished by the abrasive. Eventually, grooves worn into the necks of the teeth can be so deep as to extend into the site of the original pulp chamber, by then obliterated by reactionary dentine to protect the pulp (Figs 6.2 and 6.3). The crown of the tooth may even break off without exposing the pulp. Cervical abrasion can hamper endodontic treatment by causing pulpal obliteration just below cervical level. A switch to a minimally abrasive toothpaste is essential.

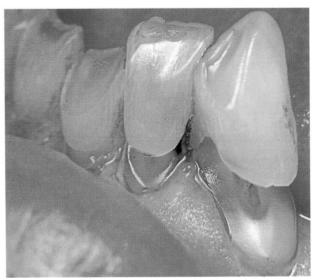

Fig. 6.2 Attrition and abrasion. Chronic physical trauma to the teeth produced by chewing and over-vigorous use of a toothbrush. The incisal edges of the teeth have worn into polished facets, in the centres of which the yellowish dentine is visible. The necks of the two nearest teeth have been deeply incised by tooth brushing, also exposing dentine. The pulp has been obliterated by secondary dentine formation, but its original site can be seen in the centre of the exposed dentine.

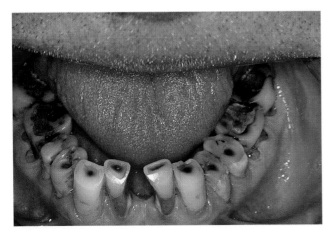

Fig. 6.1 Attrition. Excessive wear of the occlusal surfaces of the teeth, as a result of an abrasive diet. The site of the pulp of several teeth is marked by reactionary dentine which is porous and stained. Teeth remain vital.

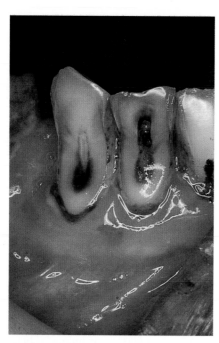

Fig. 6.3   Mixed pattern tooth loss. In this case, elements of erosion and abrasion are present. Note the shiny polished surface produced by abrasion.

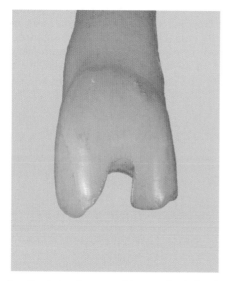

Fig. 6.4   Localised abrasion caused by opening hair grips.

A variety of habits may also cause localised abrasion such as pipe smoking and opening hairpins or holding pins (Fig. 6.4). These take years to develop because such items are not very abrasive.

When abrasion appears extensive, it is important to ensure that there is not an element of erosion.

Erosion

Erosion is progressive solubilisation of tooth substance by exposure to acid. Enamel is completely dissolved and dentine demineralised, softened and rendered prone to abrasion and attrition. Erosion is an increasing problem, and when tooth wear is severe, there is usually a significant erosive component.

The most common cause is dietary acids from over-consumption of carbonated soft drinks or fruit juices, or both (Fig. 6.5). Carbonated drinks are buffered to maintain their acidity, and this enhances the solubilisation effect. Cola-type drinks and red wine have a pH of approximately 2.5, and fruit juices approximately 3.5. Carbonated water is acid but with minimal buffering capacity and so is not damaging. Health concerns are reducing consumption of these drinks, but the focus is on calorie content rather than acidity. The average UK citizen drinks 100 litres of such drinks a year. Erosion tends to be in those with high consumption, but there is concern about erosion in children and the effects of lifelong low-level exposure. Approximately half of the fruit juice in the UK is drunk by children, and a third of 6-year-olds and a quarter of 12-year-olds have some degree of erosive tooth wear. In the United States, consumption of carbonated drinks has been in slow decline for 10 years while consumers switch to fruit juices for health reasons, but these can be even more damaging in excess.

Chronic regurgitation of gastric secretions, typically as a consequence of chronic pyloric stenosis, is a potent erosive challenge. The affected tooth surfaces are often but not always the palatal surfaces of the upper teeth (see Fig. 34.1). Similar damage can result from self-induced vomiting. The latter is characteristic of bulimia, a psychological disorder (see Ch. 40).

In the past, industrial exposure to corrosive chemicals was a significant cause of dental erosion. This is now of only historical interest, but exposure to wine in wine tasters and acid swimming pool water can all induce erosion as an occupational hazard. Some tooth-whitening products have an acid pH (most are alkaline) and are best avoided because prolonged application in trays can be very damaging.

Saliva has a protective effect, and dry mouth increases the risk of erosion. Patients should not brush their teeth until 1 hour after an acid exposure to avoid abrasion contributing to the tooth wear.

Erosion is worse on maxillary teeth, on occlusal, palatal and labial surfaces. Minor degrees are easily missed. Cusp tips are lost and become dimpled; the curvature of buccal and palatal surfaces is flattened and then rendered concave. Palatal enamel loss leaves the incisal labial enamel as a thin, sharp ridge with abnormal translucency and colour and a tendency to chip away in small fragments.

Once enamel is lost, exposed dentine wears away much faster by the combination of erosion and abrasion. Eventually the clinical crowns of all teeth are short, and vertical dimension is reduced.

Treatment should be conservative. Identifying the cause and instituting a preventive regime through diet analysis and medical history determines the intervention. Wear is slow. Study models, photographs and follow up can be used to assess treatment effect, and restorative intervention may only be required for cosmetic reasons. Dentinal hypersensitivity is a common finding because erosion opens exposed dentinal tubules. This is reduced by fluorides and removal of the cause. If patients cannot stop acid drinks, a reduced intake can be rendered safer by drinking through a straw. If interocclusal space is reduced, a Dahl-type appliance may generate space required for restorations when wear is very severe. Those with regurgitation or bulimia need medical referral.

Diagnosis and treatment PMIDs: 22240686, 22281629, 22322760, 22361546

Erosion intrinsic causes PMID: 24993266

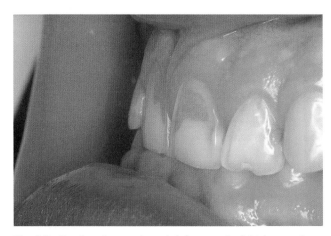

Fig. 6.5 Erosion. Saucer-shaped defects on the labial enamel resulting from acid drinks being trapped between the upper lip and teeth. See also Fig. 34.1.

Abfraction

Abfraction is a theoretical concept that has never been proven to apply to human teeth in normal function. The hypothesis is that occlusal stress is concentrated around the cervical region of the tooth, flexing and microfracturing the cervical enamel. The enamel is supposed to be weakened as a result, prone to fracture away, and predisposed to abrasion. It is difficult to see how such a mechanism could contribute to abrasion of the more elastic dentine.

Abfraction PMID: 24250083

BRUXISM

Bruxism is the term given to periodic repetitive clenching or rhythmic forceful grinding of the teeth. Some 10%–20% of the population report the habit, but the incidence rises to 90% when intermittent subconscious grinding is included. Bruxism has an equal sex incidence, is more common in children and young adults and uncommon after middle age. The aetiology is unknown but probably multifactorial. Bruxism is also common in those with disability (Ch. 39). Grinding the teeth is often a subconscious response to frustration and, although usually then brief, may be acquired as a more prolonged habit and damage the teeth.

Bruxism is divided into nocturnal and daytime types. In nocturnal bruxism, the teeth are clenched or ground many times each night but for only a few seconds at a time. Bruxism is performed during light sleep, and the movement is a grinding movement that can be heard by a bystander. The forces exerted and the total time of occlusal contact are much longer than physiological occlusal contact.

Those who indulge in bruxism during the day may grind, clench, or perform other parafunctional habits such as cheek, tongue or nail biting or tongue thrusting in addition. The last of these can be seen to cause a crenellated lateral border of the tongue. The daytime bruxing movement tends to be clenching rather than grinding and is not usually audible. Symptoms, if any, worsen while the day progresses. Daytime bruxism is seen more frequently in females. Whether it is a response to stress is controversial.

Bruxism is often performed in a protrusive or lateral excursion so that the forces are borne on few teeth and in an unfavourable direction. The resulting attrition can be deeply destructive, particularly in a Class II division 2 incisor relationship. The signs of bruxism are shown in Box 6.1.

Box 6.1 Features and effects of bruxism

- Noise during grinding (nocturnal bruxism)
- Attrition, wear facets and occasionally sensitivity
- Fracture of cusps and restorations
- Increased (adaptive) mobility of teeth
- Hypertrophy of masseter and anterior temporalis muscles
- Sometimes, although rarely, myalgia and limitation of jaw movement
- Sometimes, although rarely, tenderness on palpation of masticatory muscles

Only the grinding itself is diagnostic and may be unknown to the patient. The attrition caused could look like that of physiological wear. Bruxism is variably associated with muscle pain and headaches. The muscle pain of bruxism is felt in the morning and is the same as muscle pain after exercise. However, most 'bruxists' experience no pain, and pain does not correlate with the severity of the grinding or clenching.

Bruxism is often considered to be linked to pain dysfunction syndrome, but the association is not strong (Ch. 14). It has also been suggested that bruxism may result from occlusal interference, but bruxism may even be carried out with complete dentures.

Bruxism has been linked to a number of medical conditions. It is common in learning disability, Down's syndrome, cerebral palsy, Parkinson's disease and autism, but causative associations are difficult to prove in such a common condition. A number of drugs are associated with bruxism, or at least with repetitive mandibular movements, including dopamine antagonists, tricyclic antidepressants, amphetamines, caffeine and drugs of abuse, particularly ecstasy (MDMA).

Management

Bruxism should be treated conservatively, and any intervention should be reversible. Reassurance and explanation are often all that are required, and stress management such as relaxation, hypnosis or sleep advice may be tried.

Any restorative or implant treatment must be planned taking the extra occlusal load into account because bruxism is associated with high failure rates of restorations such as veneers and also predisposes to cusp fractures.

Appliances are widely prescribed, but there is no firm evidence to support their use. Claims that appliances act by changing the vertical dimension, relieving occlusal interference, repositioning the condyles, changing mandibular posture or preventing periodontal ligament proprioception are unproven, and their mechanisms of action are unknown. Nevertheless, appliances frequently appear to be effective, and they can be useful to protect against severe attrition. Appliances may be attached to upper or lower arches, including flat posterior bite planes and various types of occlusal splints. All should be worn at night only and initially for 1 month. If there is no improvement, treatment should be discontinued to prevent adverse effects on the soft tissues and occlusion.

If effective, the appliances may be worn intermittently during exacerbations. Soft vacuum-formed appliances are inexpensive and readily fitted as a short-term diagnostic aid but are quickly worn out by a determined bruxist. Any type of appliance can occasionally worsen bruxism. If bruxism appears related to anxiety, a short course of an anxiolytic may help break the habit. Occlusal adjustment has been shown to be ineffective and should be avoided.

Appliances probably do not help daytime bruxism.

Botulinum toxin to reduce the power of the masticatory muscles is an as yet unproven treatment.

Sleep bruxism PMID: 26758348

RESORPTION OF TEETH

Teeth can be resorbed by osteoclasts in the same way as bone. The cells are often referred to as *odontoclasts*, although they develop from the same precursors as osteoclasts and are differentiated only because they resorb teeth and are slightly smaller. Precursor cells are present in the periodontal ligament and in the dental pulp and can be triggered to migrate to the tooth surface and differentiate into odontoclasts by specific mediators.

Odontoclasts resorb and remove dentine by the same mechanisms as osteoclasts resorb bone (Fig. 6.6), excavating Howship's lacunae along the resorbed surface. Resorption is intermittent, and odontoclasts may not always be present as they disappear during inactive periods. Whenever resorption takes place, there is usually some attempt at repair by apposition of cementum or bone and resorption follows a cyclical progression.

The pattern of intermittent resorption and repair can occasionally lead to ankylosis, in which a tooth becomes fused to the surrounding bone. This may be seen in both permanent and deciduous teeth but causes more problems in the deciduous dentition because the jaw is still growing. Ankylosis will markedly delay shedding of the tooth and eruption of the permanent successor. The ankylosed tooth submerges as the alveolus grows around it, and there may be space loss as distal teeth tip into the space. Submerged

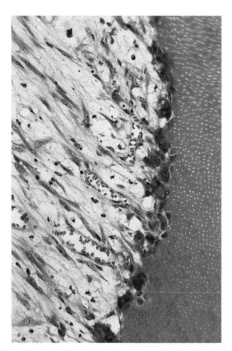

Fig. 6.6 Resorption during periapical periodontitis. Active osteoclastic resorption of dentine is continuing in the presence of inflammatory exudate. This is a common change but usually minor in extent.

teeth need to be removed surgically. Ankylosis in the permanent dentition is often associated with replacement resorption, leading to eventual loss of the tooth.

Resorption of deciduous teeth

The deciduous teeth are progressively loosened and ultimately shed by resorption as a physiological process. The cyclical nature of resorption causes the looseness of the teeth to vary before they are shed. It used to be thought that pressure from the permanent successor induced resorption, but it is now known that the follicle of the permanent successor produces soluble factors that control the resorption of both the bone and deciduous tooth root in the path of eruption. When a permanent successor is absent, resorption of deciduous tooth root starts later than normal and progresses much more slowly. However, it does usually progress until eventually the tooth is lost.

The main complication of resorption of deciduous teeth is ankylosis and submergence (see previous text). Occasionally resorption from the lateral aspect of the root cuts off a fragment that remains buried. This can either be resorbed or may eventually exfoliate like a small sequestrum of bone.

Resorption of permanent teeth

All teeth have microscopic areas of resorption and repair of no significance on their root surface, but more extensive resorption of permanent teeth is pathological. There are various causes (Box 6.2). The most common are inflammation and pressure from malpositioned teeth (Fig. 6.7). A minor degree of inflammatory resorption is common on root apices associated with periapical granulomas. Occasionally, this is a prominent feature leading to concern over the diagnosis (Fig. 6.8).

Resorption of teeth by lesions such as tumours and cysts is often said to indicate malignancy. However, resorption may result from simple pressure, and benign cysts and neoplasms may cause resorption if they are present for sufficient time. The quality of the resorption is more important in defining a possible malignant neoplasm. Resorption by malignant neoplasms is typically rapid, irregular and described as 'moth-eaten' radiographically.

Cementum is most readily resorbed, whereas enamel is the most resistant tissue, but sometimes the crown of an impacted tooth may be completely destroyed, although this takes many years (Fig. 6.9). Immature permanent teeth are resorbed more quickly because the dentine is less heavily mineralised and the dentine around open apices is very thin.

Box 6.2 Important causes of resorption of permanent teeth

- Periapical periodontitis. The most common cause, but is usually slight
- Impacted teeth pressing on the root of an adjacent tooth
- Unerupted teeth. During the course of years these may undergo resorption or hypercementosis, or both
- Replanted teeth. These are sometimes rapidly and grossly resorbed
- Pressure from cysts and neoplasms
- Idiopathic. External or internal

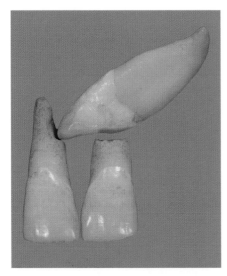

Fig. 6.7 Gross root resorption of two upper central incisors induced by an unerupted canine that has migrated across the midline.

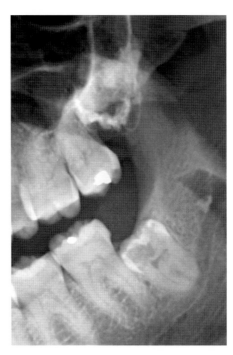

Fig. 6.9 Resorption of unerupted third molars. The crowns are hollowed out, and little more than the enamel of the upper molar remains. *(By kind permission of Mrs J Brown.)*

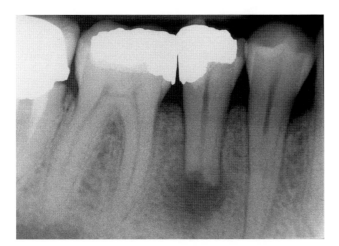

Fig. 6.8 Inflammatory resorption of the root apex induced by periapical periodontitis resulting from the non-vital pulp.

Idiopathic resorption

Idiopathic resorption of permanent teeth may start from the pulpal surface or the external surface. Either can produce the clinical feature of 'pink spot', a rounded pink area where the vascular pulp has become visible through the enamel overlying the resorbed dentine. A pink spot centrally in the crown suggests internal resorption, and one close to the gingival margin suggests external resorption. Idiopathic resorption often affects several teeth, sometimes many, and additional lesions should be sought radiographically when one is found.

Mechanisms and diseases PMID: 20659257

Internal resorption is an uncommon condition in which dentine is resorbed from within the pulp. Resorption tends to be localised, producing the characteristic sign of a well-defined rounded area of radiolucency in the crown or midroot (Fig. 6.10). Resorption is often detected by chance in a routine radiograph.

The cause is unknown, but it may occasionally follow trauma, caries or restoration. Inflammation is often present in the pulp, and some consider this presentation a type of inflammatory resorption.

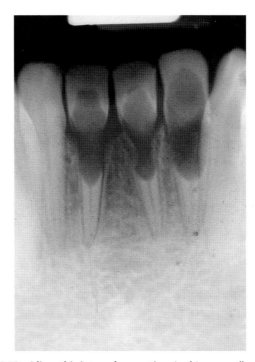

Fig. 6.10 Idiopathic internal resorption. In this unusually severe example, resorption affects the roots of three lower incisors. Note the smooth outline and process centred on the pulp.

Treatment is to remove the pulp and fill the root before too much dentine is lost, the root is perforated or the crown fractures off.

External resorption may be localised to one tooth or generalised, the latter often affecting a group of teeth but sometimes the whole dentition. The cause is unknown, although a mild degree of inflammation is often suspected. Usually, a limited area of the root is attacked from its external surface near the amelocemental junction (Figs 6.11 and

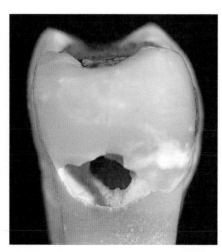

Fig. 6.11 Idiopathic external resorption. Resorption frequently starts at the amelocemental junction. In this case, the pulp is exposed.

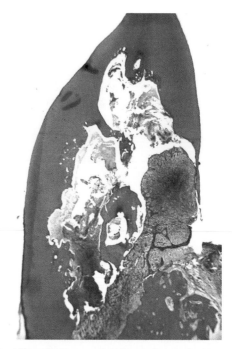

Fig. 6.13 Idiopathic resorption. A grossly resorbed central incisor with a widely perforated pulp wall. The pulp has been replaced by granulation tissue, and bony repair tissue has been laid down more deeply.

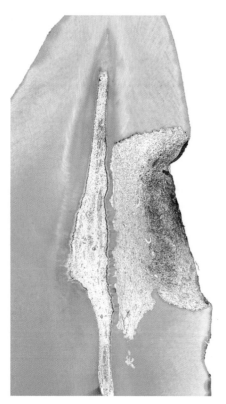

Fig. 6.12 Idiopathic external resorption. A localised area of destruction of dentine produced by osteoclastic activity. The cavity is filled with fibrous tissue containing some inflammatory cells superficially. The pulp shows no reaction, and the sparing of the circumpulpal dentine until a late stage is a characteristic feature of external resorption.

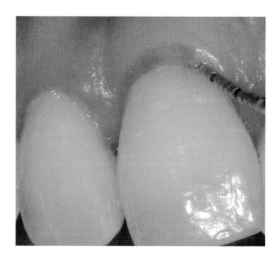

Fig. 6.14 Pink spot. External resorption has resorbed dentine below the cervical enamel, producing a pink spot by the probe tip. This is a subtle and early lesion. The crowns in Fig. 6.10 would be obviously pink. *(By kind permission of S Patel and D Vaz de Souza. From Patel, S., Harvey, S., Shembesh, et al., 2016. Cone beam CT in endodontics. Quintessence Int.)*

6.12) and resorption penetrates almost to the pulp. A very thin band of circumpulpal dentine may be preserved, but if the resorption defect communicates with a pocket or the crevice, bacteria may enter the pulp. Resorption may extend up into the crown (Fig. 6.13), producing a pink spot (Fig. 6.14). Accessible defects may be amenable to restoration with mineral trioxide or other materials, but long-term success is unpredictable.

Generalised resorption usually starts either at the amelodential junction or near the apex. Over the course of years, the roots of multiple teeth may be destroyed. The lost tissue is partially repaired by bonelike tissue. Devitalising teeth does not slow progress, and no treatment is effective.

A minor degree of external resorption is common around the apex following orthodontic treatment, particularly when fixed appliances are used to move the root apex or high forces are used.

Replacement resorption is a form of slow progressive external resorption in which the tooth is gradually replaced by bone. Replacement resorption follows ankylosis, luxation injuries and avulsion and re-implantation. Following injury there is a short period of inflammatory resorption proportional to the severity of the injury. This can often be treated by using calcium hydroxide dressings if the resorption is apical. However, when the injury to the periodontal ligament is severe, healing occurs by recruitment of precursor cells from the adjacent bone marrow causing ankylosis. If more than a small area of the root surface is involved by the ankylosis, the tooth effectively becomes part of the bone, and the normal physiological mechanisms of continuous bone turnover lead to progressive replacement of dentine by bone. The resorption progresses relentlessly and traumatised incisors in children can be completely lost in less than 5 years. In adults the process is slower but still essentially irreversible.

Replacement resorption is always associated with ankylosis. Teeth have an abnormal percussive note, no mobility and loss of lamina dura and periodontal ligament radiographically.

After trauma PMID: 7641622

HYPERCEMENTOSIS

Cellular cementum has a low turnover rate to maintain the fibre attachments of the periodontal ligament. Cementoblast precursor cells lie in the periodontal ligament and are recruited for normal turnover and to repair root fractures or resorption defects. New cementum is added to the surface without significant resorption so that the normal thickness of the cementum increases slightly with age.

Cementum is essentially bone, but unlike bone has no vascular supply and no innervation because it has no medullary spaces.

Apposition of excessive amounts of cementum is not uncommon and has several possible causes (Box 6.3), of which inflammation is probably the commonest pathological cause (Fig. 6.15). Acromegaly and calcinosis are also reported to cause hypercementosis, but the effect is rare and not significant.

Hypercementosis is usually noted radiographically, with widening of roots, usually in their apical third to produce a blunt root tip. The periodontal ligament space and lamina dura is intact around the cementum. Hypercementosis is not associated with ankylosis.

Increased thickness of cementum is not itself a disease, and no treatment is necessary. If hypercementosis is gross, as in Paget's disease, extractions become difficult (Fig. 6.16). The cementoblastoma (Ch. 11) is a benign neoplasm

of cementoblasts that can appear like hypercementosis radiographically, but there is root resorption and a characteristic presentation. Cemento-osseous dysplasia (Ch. 11) is also a distinct condition easily confused with hypercementosis.

The lesions previously called cementomas are dealt with in Chapter 11.

Concrescence is hypercementosis that causes fusion of the roots of adjacent teeth (Figs 6.17 and 6.18). It is rarely noticed until an attempt is made to extract one of the teeth. The two teeth are then found to move in unison and surgical intervention becomes necessary.

PATHOLOGY OF OSSEOINTEGRATION

Osseointegrated implants have revolutionised dentistry and are also used to retain facial prostheses, obturators and bone-conduction hearing aids.

Osseointegration is defined as a direct structural and functional connection between viable bone and the surface of a load-bearing implant. This is possible only by using

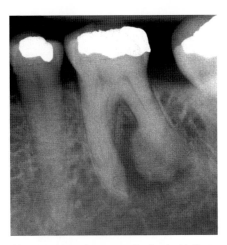

Fig. 6.15 Hypercementosis as a result of apical inflammation.

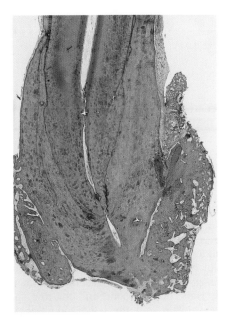

Fig. 6.16 Hypercementosis in Paget's disease. An irregular craggy mass of bonelike cementum has been formed over thickened regular and acellular cementum.

Box 6.3 Causes of hypercementosis

- Ageing
- Increased occlusal load
- Over-erupted teeth
- Periapical periodontitis. A common cause but minor in amount. Close to the apex there is usually a little resorption, but coronally cementum is laid down, forming a shoulder
- Functionless and unerupted teeth. Hypercementosis and resorption may both be present
- Paget's disease. Alternating, irregular apposition and resorption, with apposition predominating, produce an irregular mass of cementum on the root with a histological 'mosaic' pattern
- Cementoblastoma and cemento-osseous dysplasia are distinct diseases (Ch. 11)

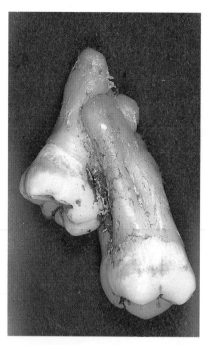

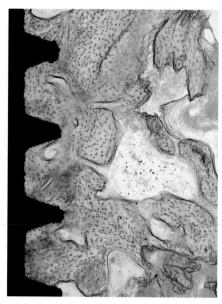

Fig. 6.19 **Successful osseointegration.** Bone (*unstained right*) in contact with implant thread (*left*). The tiny gap between the two is not appreciated with light microscopy.

Fig. 6.17 **Concrescence.** Two upper molars fused together by cementum.

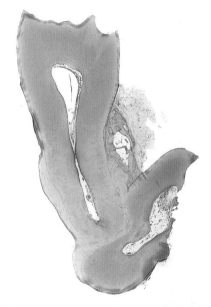

Fig. 6.18 **Concrescence.** Histological section of fused teeth reveals that the teeth are joined by cementum and not dentine.

implants made from a limited number of metals, principally titanium, niobium and some of their alloys. The correct implant shape is also necessary to provide maximum surface area and transmit load effectively to the bone.

Successful osseointegration is achieved by bone growing to contact or almost to contact the implant. No periodontal membrane is present, and the implant is held tightly by friction and a thin layer of collagen and proteoglycan bone matrix about 100 nm thick (Fig. 6.19). The implant surface does not itself induce bone formation but, in medullary bone, both trabeculae of bone and marrow spaces may contact the implant and the bone and implant become chemically bonded together.

When an implant is placed into bone, much of the initial resistance to movement comes from tight apposition of the

thread in the cortical bone. In the medulla, the implant is surrounded by blood and platelets are activated as in a normal healing response. The healing response recruits new osteoblasts from the surrounding bone and marrow and new blood vessels from the marrow. These form woven bone from the edge of the trephine hole toward the implant (distance osteogenesis), stopping just short of the implant. Bone precursors also attach to the implant, lay down bone matrix on it and form bone in direct contact with it (contact osteogenesis). Both types of healing occur around any one implant, but it is considered that the greater the area of contact osteogenesis, the better. Contact osteogenesis requires migration of the bone precursor cells through the organising clot to the implant surface, and fibrin adhesion to the implant is critical for this process. Once bone is formed, it undergoes a process of slow remodelling and increases the bonding of bone to the implant. The cortical bone support is important to stabilise the implant through the early healing phase, and it is helpful that this bone remodels very slowly. The force required to remove implants increases over several months after placement as healing and remodelling progress.

Because there is no periodontal ligament, there are no proprioceptive or pain fibres. There is no possibility of implant movement to cushion acute impact or to allow movements to adapt to functional forces. Thus, implants placed in growing jaws submerge like ankylosed teeth or move unpredictably, and orthodontic movement is not possible. However, bone trabeculae do remodel around an implant in response to stress transmitted directly to the bone.

Implants pass through the mucosa without allowing bacteria into the tissues because they develop a periodontal cuff that bears some similarity to the normal gingiva. Again, there are no collagen fibres joining the soft tissue to the implant. Instead, a dense cuff of collagen fibres runs circumferentially around the implant or its abutment. A non-keratinised junctional epithelium forms against the titanium surface, and a gingival sulcus of variable depth may be present. This epithelium is derived from the surrounding mucosa and adheres to the implant through hemidesmosomes in the same way as normal junctional epithelium adheres to tooth.

There are said to be no absolute contraindications to implant placement, but the factors listed in Box 6.4 should be considered potential problems because they are associated with a higher rate of implant failure. The infective endocarditis risk is unknown. Implant placement is a sterile procedure of lower risk than manipulating teeth and, provided the implants are well maintained, the risk of infection is very low.

Review osseointegration PMID: 12959168

Implant failure and peri-implantitis

Failure of implants is defined by progressive bone loss and increasing mobility and usually manifests shortly after placement or initial loading. Increased probing depths are often also present. Failure of integration during the healing period may be caused by movement, such as from that from early loading, or placement outside the cortex with perforation or dehiscence.

Failure in the longer term is principally from bone loss as a result of excessive loading or peri-implantitis.

Excessive loading may result from bruxism, non-axial forces from poorly designed superstructures or having too few implants to resist normal occlusal forces. Excessive loading tends to cause deep angular bone loss around the implant. The mechanisms are unclear, but may involve microfractures of the superficial bone around the implant. Fracture of the implant itself is rare.

Plaque-induced inflammation and bone loss around implants is called *peri-implantitis*, and the microbial flora and host responses are similar to those in gingivitis and periodontitis. Infrabony pockets do not develop because there are no contact points or interdental papillae to form a local plaque trap. Bone loss is horizontal or forms a broad saucer-shaped defect that affects the entire implant circumference (Fig. 6.20). Peri-implant disease affects approximately 6% of all implants placed, rising to 20% after 10 years. Peri-implantitis is preceded by peri-implant mucositis, the equivalent of gingivitis with inflammation limited to the surface. Some degree of mucositis is found in 80% of individuals with implants, but in most patients this does not progress to bone loss.

It is also possible, although much rarer, for implants to develop an apical peri-implantitis. This affects approximately 1%–2% of all implants placed, more commonly in the mandible. It presents as an apical radiolucency similar to a periapical granuloma, sometimes with pain, swelling and a sinus tract. The likely cause is persistence of apical inflammation from the pre-existing tooth.

Other causes of failure are listed in Box 6.4. In addition, implants are more likely to fail in the maxilla than the mandible, if there is movement during healing, or if the bone is overheated by the drill during placement. Poor quality bone is often blamed for failure, often on grounds of minimal cortical thickness. However, implants can be successful in medullary bone with little cortex. Relatively avascular or sclerotic bone that heals poorly is probably a greater risk.

> **Box 6.4 Factors associated with implant failure and relative contraindications to implant placement**
>
> - Incomplete facial growth
> - Uncontrolled diabetes
> - Contraindications to surgery, e.g. bleeding tendencies
> - Smoking
> - Patients prone to osteomyelitis
>   - Sclerotic bone or bone disease at site
>   - Previous radiotherapy to the jaws
>   - Previous intravenous bisphosphonate treatment
> - Poor quality bone at site
>   - Thin cortex
>   - Sparse trabeculation
>   - Osteoporosis
> - Active periodontal disease or poor oral hygiene
> - Mucosal disease
> - Possibly, high-risk patient for infective endocarditis?

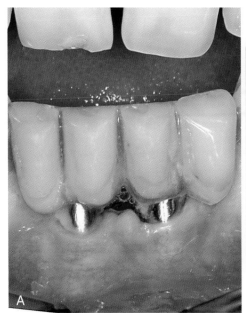

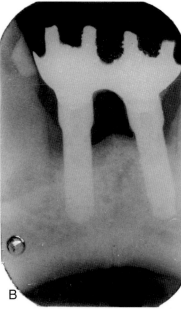

Fig. 6.20 Peri-implantitis. There is pocketing with a bead of pus exuding onto the gingival margin and a broad ring of bone loss evident radiographically. These older cylindrical coated implants were prone to peri-implantitis. *(Courtesy of Professor R Palmer.)*

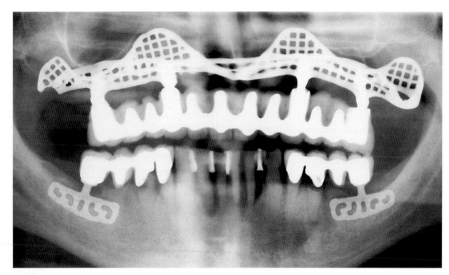

Fig. 6.21 **Gross infection around old types of implant.** There is a subperiosteal implant in contact with almost all the maxillary alveolus. Note the extensive bone loss below it, visible most clearly at the left tuberosity. There are two blade implants in the mandible, both with bone loss extending down the stem to involve the blade. The patient is at risk from severe infection and continued bone destruction until the implants are removed. *(Courtesy of Professor R Palmer.)*

The question of whether it is possible to mount a true allergic reaction to titanium dental implants is a controversial issue. Implants are made of alloys containing aluminium, vanadium or other metals to increase the strength. Cases of implants being associated with skin reactions and a peri-implantitis like inflammation are recorded, but the mechanisms are unclear. Titanium, in pure form, appears an unlikely allergen.

Occasionally, patients are seen with non-osseointegrated implants such as blade implants or pins of various metals. These older types of implant usually failed rapidly as a result of infection (Fig. 6.21).

Box 6.5   Complications of implant placement

- Incorrect placement
  - Perforation of cortex, haematoma
  - Antral or nasal perforation, sinusitis
  - Damage to inferior dental neurovascular bundle
- Infection, acute and chronic
  - Consequent alveolar bone loss
- Complications of associated surgery
  - Oroantral communication following sinus lift procedures

Gingival and periodontal diseases

7

THE NORMAL PERIODONTAL TISSUES

The periodontal tissues have a complex anatomy specialised to resist masticatory forces and seal around the teeth (Box 7.1).

The epithelium of the free and attached gingiva is stratified squamous and thinly parakeratinised. The *epithelial attachment* is made by the junctional epithelium adhering to enamel (Fig. 7.1), achieved by the cells secreting a basement membrane onto the enamel and attaching to it by hemidesmosomes. The attachment to the enamel appears histologically as a clear cuticle (Fig. 7.2). It forms an effective seal, protecting the underlying connective tissues. The epithelial attachment is so firmly adherent to the tooth surface that tension tears through the epithelium itself rather than pulling the epithelium from the tooth (see Fig. 7.2). Junctional epithelium has a high turnover rate, and the epithelial attachment is constantly reformed as the basal cells divide, mature and move upward. This results in higher permeability than other parts of the gingiva, potentially allowing the passage of molecules to and from the connective tissues.

When periodontitis develops, the attachment migrates apically and attaches to cementum by the same mechanisms. The junctional epithelial cells are believed to have an important role in regulating and modulating local immunological and inflammatory responses.

The *attached gingiva* is firmly bound down to the underlying bone to form a tough mucoperiosteum. Its stippled

---

Box 7.1 Anatomical regions of normal healthy gingival tissue

- *Junctional epithelium*. Extends from the amelocemental junction to the floor of the gingival sulcus and forms the epithelial attachment to the tooth surface
- *Sulcular epithelium*. Lines the gingival sulcus and joins the epithelial attachment to the free gingiva
- *Free gingiva*. Coronal to the amelocemental junction and attached gingiva and includes the tips of the interdental papillae
- *Attached gingiva*. Extends apically from the free gingiva to the mucogingival junction and is bound down to the superficial periodontal fibres and periosteum

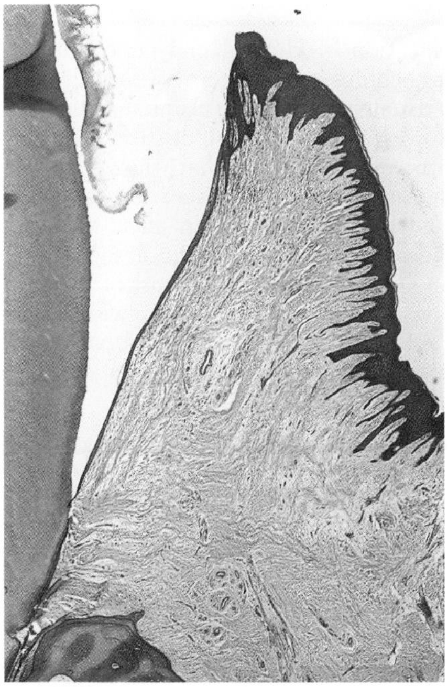

Fig. 7.1 Gingival sulcus and epithelial attachment. This sagittal section of a specimen from a woman of 27 years shows the normal appearances. Enamel removed by decalcification of the specimen has left the triangular space. The epithelial attachment forms a line from the top of the papilla to the amelocemental junction; its enamel surface, the actual line of attachment, is sharply defined. The gingival sulcus, minute in extent, is formed where the papilla curves away from the line of the enamel surface. There is hardly any inflammatory infiltrate.

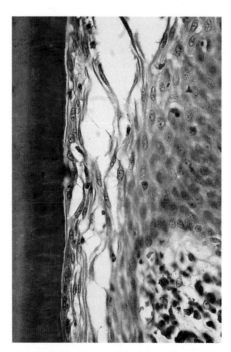

Fig. 7.2 The strength of the epithelial attachment. On this tooth the epithelial attachment has migrated on to the surface of the cementum as a result of periodontal disease. The epithelium has been torn away from the tooth, but the tear is within the junctional epithelium, leaving some of its cells still adherent to cementum and attached by a clear cuticle. A similar strength is seen when the junctional epithelium is attached to enamel.

- *Oblique fibres* form a suspensory ligament from socket to root in coronal to apical directions
- *Horizontal fibres* form a dense group attaching neck of tooth to rim of socket
- *Transeptal fibres* of the horizontal group are not attached to alveolar bone but pass superficial to it and join adjacent teeth together. They protect the interdental gingiva by resisting forces that would otherwise separate the teeth and open the contact points
- *Gingival fibres* form a cuff round the neck of the tooth supporting the soft tissues. They resist separation of the gingivae from the tooth and help to prevent formation of pockets

Table 7.1   Simplified international workshop classification of periodontal diseases

Dental plaque-induced gingival diseases
  Gingivitis associated with dental plaque only
  Gingivitis modified by systemic factors
    puberty-associated gingivitis
    menstrual cycle-associated gingivitis
    pregnancy-associated gingivitis
    diabetes mellitus-associated gingivitis
  Gingivitis associated with leukaemia and other blood disorders
Gingival diseases modified by medications
  Drug-modified gingival enlargement
Gingival diseases modified by malnutrition
  Ascorbic acid-deficiency gingivitis
Non-plaque-induced gingival lesions
  Infections, bacterial, viral fungal
  Hereditary gingival fibromatosis and other genetic conditions
  Gingival manifestations of dermatological disease
    Mucocutaneous disease
    Allergic reactions
Traumatic lesions, factitious, iatrogenic, accidental
Foreign body reactions
Chronic periodontitis, plaque induced, localised or generalised
Aggressive periodontitis, localised or generalised
Periodontitis as a manifestation of systemic disease
    haematological disorders
    associated with genetic disorders
Necrotising gingival diseases
Combined periodontal-endodontic lesions
Local predisposition to plaque-induced gingival diseases/ periodontitis

appearance is due to the intersections of its underlying epithelial ridges at the junction with the connective tissue and the bundles of collagen inserted into it.

The *alveolar mucosa* is the thin mucosa extending from the sharply-demarcated mucogingival junction into the sulcus. It has a smooth surface, darker colour and overlies loose mobile fibrous tissue. Underlying blood vessels can often be seen through the epithelial layer. It should not be confused with *alveolar ridge mucosa*, the gingiva of an edentulous ridge.

Classic description anatomy PMID: 5005682

Anatomy of periodontium ISBN-13: 978-0723438120

Gingival and periodontal fibres

The periodontal ligament comprises densely packed bundles of collagen fibres running from tooth to bone interspersed by loose connective tissue containing wide blood vessels and nerves. Compression of the ligament forces blood out through channels in the lamina dura into adjacent medullary bone, producing a viscoelastic cushion against compression and tension. The normal thickness of the periodontal ligament is approximately 0.1–0.3 mm.

The principal fibres are arranged in a series of fairly well-defined groups (Box 7.2).

The periodontal ligament fibres are embedded in cementum at their inner ends and in the lamina dura at their outer ends. New fibres replacing those that have aged, or forming in response to new functional stresses, are attached by apposition of further layers of cementum, which becomes thicker with age. The lamina dura is a layer of cortical bone continuous, at the margin of the sockets, with the cortical bone of the alveolus.

Gingival crevicular fluid (exudate)

In health, a minute amount of fluid can be collected from the gingival margins. Crevicular fluid is an inflammatory exudate, and the amount increases greatly with the degree of inflammation. Its composition changes while inflammation develops, initially being more of a transudate of tissue fluid, but in established inflammation containing more immunoglobulin (Ig), IgM, other serum proteins and neutrophils and macrophages. Crevicular fluid is not a secretion (there are no glands in this region).

Even in apparent health, there are always a few inflammatory cells in the gingiva and a very minor degree of inflammation.

CLASSIFICATION OF PERIODONTAL DISEASES

The classification of gingival and periodontal diseases is complex and confusing. The terms *gingivitis* and *periodontal disease* usually refer only to plaque-related inflammatory disease. However, there are also diseases that predispose to periodontitis and conditions that, though not induced by plaque, are worsened by it. Other diseases as diverse as tuberculosis or lichen planus may affect the gingivae occasionally. Classifications are often designed for research rather than clinical use and lose most of their value in the need to leave nothing out. Currently, a widely accepted classification is that of the 1999 International Workshop for a Classification of Periodontal Diseases, a simplified version of which is shown in Table 7.1.

Classification PMID: 10896458

CHRONIC GINGIVITIS

Chronic gingivitis is asymptomatic, low-grade inflammation of the gingivae, induced by bacterial plaque growing along the gingival margin. The cause is inadequate oral hygiene, sometimes exacerbated by local plaque traps. Gingivitis should be cured by effective oral hygiene.

Chronic gingivitis always precedes development of chronic periodontitis, but not all gingivitis will progress. The distinguishing feature between chronic gingivitis and the onset of periodontitis is loss of bone at the alveolar crest. Until this happens, and probably for a short period afterward, chronic gingivitis can generally be cured by plaque control. By contrast, loss of bone in periodontitis is essentially irreversible.

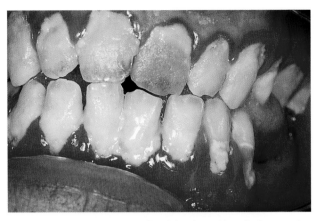

Fig. 7.3 **Severe gingivitis.** A florid, bright-red band of gingival inflammation results from very poor oral hygiene. Thick accumulations of plaque are visible on all tooth surfaces.

Box 7.3 Factors contributing to or exacerbating chronic gingivitis

Local

- Poor tooth cleaning technique
- Dental irregularities providing stagnation areas
- Restorations or appliances causing stagnation areas

Systemic

- Pregnancy
- Down's syndrome
- Poorly controlled diabetes mellitus

Clinical features

The gingivae become red and slightly swollen with oedema along the gingival margin (Fig. 7.3). *Chronic hyperplastic gingivitis* is a term sometimes given to chronic gingivitis in which the gingiva appears to enlarge. This is a result of inflammatory oedema rather than genuine tissue hyperplasia and largely resolves with treatment.

Both local and systemic factors can exacerbate chronic gingivitis (Box 7.3).

Pathology

By definition, inflammation in gingivitis is restricted to the gingival margins and does not affect the periodontal ligament or bone (Fig. 7.4).

The development of gingivitis has been arbitrarily divided histologically into 'initial', 'early' and 'established' phases (Boxes 7.4 and 7.5), whereas the fourth 'advanced' stage refers to chronic periodontitis. It must be appreciated that these stages are artificially distinguished, being largely based on animal studies and experimental gingivitis studies in humans. They simply reflect the stages of development of chronic inflammation as would be seen at any body site. By the standard of the very slow rate of disease progression in a patient, all these stages are very rapid early events.

Microbiology

Although gingivitis and periodontitis are caused primarily by microbial plaque, these diseases are not simple infections. The causative organisms remain largely outside the

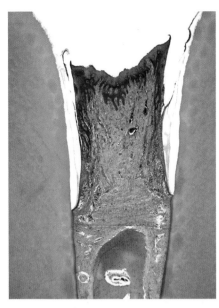

Fig. 7.4 **Chronic gingivitis.** The epithelial attachment remains at the level of the amelocemental junction, and inflammatory cells are concentrated below the junctional epithelium and extend into the deeper gingiva, around the interradicular fibres. The alveolar crest is not resorbed.

Box 7.4 'Initial stage' chronic gingivitis

- Develops within 24–48 hours of exposure to plaque
- Plaque related to gingival sulcus
- Vasodilatation
- Infiltration predominantly of neutrophils
- Leakage of exudate into gingival sulcus
- Clinically appears healthy

After 1 week, the 'early' phase starts with epithelial hyperplasia and development of a deepened crevice. Inflammation is then visible clinically.

Box 7.5 Established chronic gingivitis

- Develops after 2–3 weeks
- Dense, predominantly plasmacytic infiltrate
- Infiltrate fills but limited to interdental papillae
- Destruction of superficial connective tissue fibres
- Deepened gingival crevice
- Epithelial attachment remains at or near amelocemental junction
- Alveolar bone and periodontal ligament remain intact

After about 3 weeks, the advanced stage is characterised by extension of plaque into the crevice, loss of bone and disruption of the periodontal ligament and pocketing.

---

tissues and induce inflammation by soluble factors and triggering immune responses. There is a complex host-microbial balance in which the largely commensal organisms survive but have their growth limited by the host response. In achieving this, the host responses induce bystander damage of the periodontium. The biofilm of plaque has been considered by some to be the equivalent of one enormous organism; it is more than the sum of many individual bacterial species stuck together by polysaccharide.

The key pathogenic features of dental plaque are shown in Box 7.6.

Traditionally, plaque has been investigated by microbiological culture. Over the past several decades, this technique has allowed identification of more than 300 organisms in plaque and provided data to propose many as potential pathogens for periodontitis. However, many organisms in plaque are not cultivable. Data on these species have been obtained by molecular methods, identifying new and uncultivable species by nucleic acid sequencing. This has revealed a much greater complexity than was appreciated by even the most careful culture techniques and has led to the concept that disease is most closely related to the overall microbial flora at any site, rather than its constituent species. This led to the concept of dysbiosis, in which changes in inflammation and flora are interdependent, and change together to promote tissue destruction.

The concept of the microbiome, the total of all organisms at any site, has particular value in periodontitis, where the flora can differ markedly between sites only a millimetre or two apart, and the metabolism of the same organisms can differ in different sites in the plaque. The microbiome is defined and characterised entirely by nucleic acid sequencing, and specific organisms are often described together in groups with similar metabolic requirements or with similar characteristics. This approach is enhanced by sequencing the bacterial RNA to identify what proteins the bacteria are synthesising, providing further information on what individual species are actually doing in plaque. Using these techniques, more than 1100 species are found in the mouth but only approximately a quarter are characterised named species and more than two-thirds have never been cultivated. Organisms not previously considered to be found in the mouth are frequently detected, including pathogens from other body sites.

Healthy (uninflamed) gingivae. The plaque is supragingival and thin (10–20 cells thick). Gram-positive bacteria predominate and include *Actinomyces* species, *Rothia*, viridans streptococci and *Streptococcus epidermidis*. In elderly patients in periodontal health, Gram-positive bacteria, particularly streptococci, form the largest single group (50% of the predominant cultivable flora), whereas Gram-negative bacteria only account for 30%. The latter include Porphyromonas and Fusobacterium species.

Early (and experimental) gingivitis. If toothbrushing is neglected for several days, plaque grows in thickness and is typically 100–300 cells thick. In the earliest stages, bacteria proliferate, but the plaque remains Gram positive in character, and *Actinomyces* species become predominant.

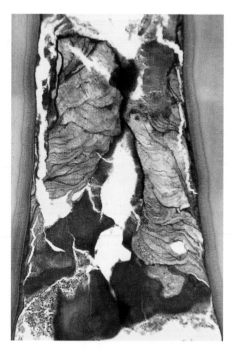

Fig. 7.5   Large deposits of subgingival calculus, showing the layered structure resulting from incremental deposition, adhering to the tooth roots on each side of the picture. The calculus has a brown colour as a result of blood and bacterial pigment within it. A thick layer of plaque, stained dark blue, adheres to the deep surface of the calculus.

Chronic gingivitis. With time, Gram-negative organisms become increasingly prominent and the plaque becomes more anaerobic. *Veillonella*, *Fusobacterium* and *Campylobacter* species become conspicuous, and the Gram-negative anaerobes normally considered to be associated with disease appear. These change the metabolic nature of the whole plaque as discussed later in this chapter, and chronic inflammation results.

Oral microbiome   PMID: 27857087

Biofilm ecology PMID: 26120510

Calculus   Calculus is calcified plaque. The calcification is less significant than the adherent biofilm of plaque on its surface. However, calculus distorts the gingival crevice and, by extending the stagnation area, promotes retention of greater amounts of plaque (Fig. 7.5). In gingival health and gingivitis, calculus is almost exclusively supragingival and forms opposite the orifices of the major salivary glands in the lower incisor and upper first molar areas. It cannot be removed by the patient and provides a rough, plaque-retentive surface. Several compounds, such as pyrophosphates, added to dentifrices have been shown to reduce calculus formation to variable degrees.

Management

Chronic gingivitis is readily recognisable from the clinical features already described, supported by probing to assess bleeding and exclude loss of attachment. Radiographs show intact crestal alveolar bone. The diagnosis is confirmed by resolution of gingivitis when effective oral hygiene measures (including calculus removal, effective toothbrushing and interdental cleaning habits) become established (Figs 7.6 and 7.7). Any local exacerbating factors must be dealt with if possible.

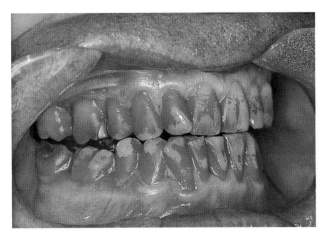

Fig. 7.6 Accumulation of plaque stained after 24 hours by disclosing solution.

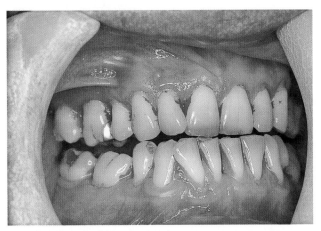

Fig. 7.7 **The effects of tooth brushing in the same patient.** Plaque remains interdentally in most areas, explaining why gingivitis is often localised here.

Systemic predisposing factors

Pregnancy

Pre-existing gingivitis may become more severe from the first 2 months of pregnancy (see Fig. 36.8). If oral hygiene is poor, inflammatory erythema, bleeding and oedema can be very florid. Swelling accentuates false pocketing. These changes are considered to result from the effects of oestrogens and progesterone on gingival vessels, but there is also evidence of an altered bacterial flora, probably due to these and other pregnancy-related compounds being bacterial nutrients. Pregnancy gingivitis can be much ameliorated or abolished by a strict oral hygiene regimen and improves after parturition.

The most florid presentation is a localised pyogenic granuloma (see Fig. 36.9) or 'pregnancy epulis'. These develop and grow very rapidly but respond to simple excision after parturition. A pregnancy epulis always develops in a background of pregnancy gingivitis.

Other conditions

A number of predisposing factors to periodontitis are discussed later in the chapter. All of these also predispose to gingivitis.

CHRONIC PERIODONTITIS

Periodontitis is present once inflammation extends beyond the gingiva to involve the periodontal ligament and resorb the crestal bone. Periodontitis is always preceded by gingivitis, and gingivitis persists in the presence of periodontitis.

Chronic periodontitis is the chief cause of tooth loss in later adult life, but symptoms are typically minimal. Many patients remain unaware of the disease until teeth become loose. Despite generally improving oral health, severe periodontitis still affects 10%–15%, and moderate periodontitis affects approximately half of the adult population in the UK.

Clinical features

Chronic periodontitis is initially asymptomatic. In the early stages patients may complain only of gingival bleeding or an unpleasant taste. Periodontitis is a potent and common cause of halitosis.

The clinical presentation depends on the level of oral hygiene. When hygiene is moderately good, the gingiva may not appear significantly inflamed, and there are few visible clues to the destruction hidden below the surface. When hygiene is poor, the additional plaque present subgingivally incites intense inflammation; the congested gingival margins become purplish-red, flabby and swollen.

Loss of attachment leads to pocketing so that a probe can be passed between teeth and gingiva. In untreated or severe disease, the interdental papillae detach from the teeth. As pockets deepen, the papillae are destroyed and the gingival margin tends to become straight with a swollen, rounded edge. Calculus forms in pockets, trapping more plaque, and bone loss renders the teeth mobile. Teeth tend to drift out of alignment and are dull to percussion and eventually become increasingly loose. In a florid untreated case, bleeding follows minimal pressure, pus may be expressed from pockets and teeth may eventually exfoliate spontaneously.

In some patients, recession is the predominant sign, especially where the gingival tissues are thin. Pocket formation may be limited, but the gingival margin migrates apically with loss of attachment, tooth support and a similar outcome.

Radiography

The earliest change is loss of definition and blunting of the tips of the alveolar crests. Bone resorption usually progresses in a predictable manner. In early periodontitis bone levels remain the same along a row of teeth (horizontal bone loss; Fig. 7.8). Later complex patterns of bone loss may develop as more bone is lost at sites of greater inflammation, localised by the underlying anatomical features of teeth and bone, local plaque traps and calculus. Thus, horizontal bone loss predominates where bone is thin, but vertical or angular bone defects develop where alveolar bone is thicker.

Aetiology

The aetiology of periodontitis appears to be primarily the long-term persistence of gingivitis. Lack of treatment, poor oral hygiene and local plaque traps preventing plaque removal are key. Persistence of inflammation leads to a vicious cycle in which swelling and false pocketing promote plaque retention, and the more protected subgingival environment fosters development of a more anaerobic plaque. As more of the gingival soft tissues become inflamed, the inflammation extends close to the crestal bone, causing bone loss and migration of the epithelial attachment onto

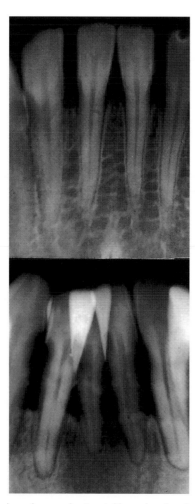

Fig. 7.8 Early and severe horizontal bone loss in advanced chronic adult periodontitis.

> **Box 7.7 Pathological processes in chronic periodontitis**
>
> - Chronic inflammation
> - Destruction of periodontal ligament fibres
> - Resorption of alveolar bone
> - Migration of the epithelial attachment toward the apex
> - Formation of pockets around the teeth
> - Formation of subgingival plaque and calculus

> **Box 7.8 Bacterial species associated with chronic periodontitis**
>
> - *Aggregatibacter* (Actinobacillus) *actinomycetemcomitans*
> - *Fusobacterium nucleatum**
> - *Porphyromonas gingivalis**
> - *Prevotella intermedia**
> - *Prevotella melaninogenica**
> - *Eikenella corrodens*
> - *Tannerella forsythia**
> - *Treponema denticola, Treponema socranskii*, and other spirochaetes*
> - *Parvimonas micra**
> - *Prevotella nigrescens**
> - *Campylobacter rectus**
> - *Eubacterium nodatum**
>
> *anaerobes

cementum. Chronic periodontitis, once established, is self-perpetuating.

For reasons that are unclear, there is wide individual variation in susceptibility.

The main features of the pathology of chronic periodontitis are summarised in Box 7.7.

Microbiology

As noted previously, the microbial flora in gingivitis is a highly complex and stable ecosystem of interdependent bacterial species in a matrix of polysaccharides, forming an adherent biofilm.

In comparison, the environment in a pocket has a lower oxygen concentration and fewer salivary nutrients and cannot be colonised by many of the bacterial species in supragingival plaque. The pocket is first colonised by facultative anaerobic Gram-positive organisms, cocci, then rods and filaments. Once these are established, Gram-negatives and true anaerobes, which are less adherent, can colonise the plaque. Eventually a 'climax community' of organisms is established, adapted to anaerobic conditions and nutrients from the pocket exudate. This takes months or years. No organism is ideally adapted to the environment and to survive all must form an interdependent ecosystem in which they can exchange nutrients and avoid the toxins bacteria secrete to gain an advantage over their competitors.

At the tooth surface the bacteria are mainly Gram positive and adherent. By contrast, plaque related to the pocket wall is less densely packed but involves many Gram-negative bacteria, including anaerobes and spirochaetes and those thought to be associated with disease (Box 7.8).

In the past there have been three hypotheses about how the plaque bacteria cause disease. The non-specific plaque hypothesis suggested that the total bulk of plaque present rather than the particular species was important. Conversely, the specific plaque hypothesis proposed that the individual species were important. Microbiological culture studies often associate particular species with disease, but also show that all implicated species can be found in healthy sites. No simple answer emerges from culture studies, leading to the multiple pathogen theories that implicate combinations of specific organisms, particularly *Porphyromonas gingivalis*, *Tannerella forsythia* and *Treponema denticola*. While these and other bacteria are clearly associated with pockets that show progressive disease, it may be simply because they are well adapted to the environment provided by the inflammation and tissue destruction. Despite a huge literature, whether these organisms are actually important remains controversial, and constant reclassification complicates their terminology. Several species listed in Box 7.8 were listed in the previous edition of this book under different names.

Non-specific plaque theory PMID: 3540019

Specific plaque theory PMID: 15143484

Newer hypotheses based on microbiome sequencing data and in vitro experiments support an even more complex theory. It is suggested that the colonisation of plaque by these disease-associated species changes the plaque ecosystem. All the bacterial species implicated in periodontitis have many virulence factors and compete with other species in plaque for nutrients such as iron. The less virulent species, which might be found normally in healthy or slowly progressing sites, start to express their own virulence factors to survive. As a result, the nature of the whole plaque metabolism may shift to a more pathogenic ecosystem in which many of the bacterial species adapt and become pathogenic. One important implication of this theory is that plaque might be returned to a non-pathogenic form by treatment targeted at specific species.

Ecological plaque hypothesis PMID: 12624191 and 16934115

Porphyromonas gingivalis PMID: 24741603

Aggregatibacter actinomycetemcomitans PMID: 20712635

A further complication arises from the detection of viruses in periodontitis. It is now thought that viral infections in the tissues synergise with the bacterial flora in disease. Similar synergy is thought to occur in other bacterial diseases such as sinusitis following viral infection. Some viruses produce cytokine analogues and viruses can interfere with neutrophil, macrophage and complement activity.

Epstein–Barr virus, cytomegalovirus and other herpesviruses are particularly associated with localised and generalised aggressive periodontitis and acute necrotising ulcerative gingivitis but are also found in chronic periodontitis. In such cases, the virus may be infecting lymphocytes in the gingiva (reflecting prior systemic infection and latency) or the epithelium, but virus is also found in the subgingival plaque. Although their role is controversial, possible mechanisms by which viral infection of lymphocytes could alter inflammatory processes are known.

Viruses in periodontitis PMID: 26980964

Not only does the flora induce inflammation, but the flora depends on the inflamed environment. Treating periodontitis with anti-inflammatory drugs alone alters the flora, excluding anaerobes that depend on blood as a nutrient when inflammation and bleeding subside.

Microbial virulence factors

Many potential virulence factors are known to be produced by periodontal micro-organisms (see Table 7.2). These include enzymes, toxins and bone-resorbing factors, but individually these are of only theoretical importance. It is probably the total production by the plaque biofilm that is important and, as noted earlier in this chapter, it may require specific circumstances to switch on synthesis of these factors. In general, it is the organisms listed in Box 7.8 that are known to produce the widest range and largest amounts of such virulence factors. Some are highly specific in action, such as the *Aggretibacter actinomycetemcomitans* leukotoxin, whereas others such as endotoxin or lipoteichoic acid are cell wall components with a broad range of proinflammatory activity, including activation of phagocytes, complement and bone resorption.

Pathology

A number of fundamental pathological principles of periodontitis are important in understanding the disease and its treatment:

Table 7.2 Possible virulence factors of plaque bacteria

Type of factor	Examples
Enzymes	Collagenase, trypsin, fibrinolysin, hyaluronidase, chondroitin sulphatase, heparinase, ribonuclease and deoxyribonuclease. Immunoglobulin proteases
Cytotoxic metabolic products	Indole, ammonia and hydrogen sulphide
Specific toxins	Powerful leukotoxins (particularly that of *Aggregatibacter actinomycetemcomitans*), epitheliotoxins (*Porphyromonas gingivalis* and *Prevotella intermedius*)
Endotoxin	From all Gram-negative bacteria, more potent from some species than others
Bone-resorbing factors	*Actinomyces viscosus* bone-resorbing factor

Bacteria remain largely in the pocket. The vast majority of the bacteria in periodontitis and gingivitis are in the subgingival plaque. Here organisms have a relatively protected environment outside the body, plentiful nutrients and a protective plaque ecosystem of interdependent species. It is usually assumed that the inflammation in the pocket wall is mediated by soluble bacterial factors penetrating the tissues and by bystander damage resulting from immune reactions.

Bacteria can penetrate the tissues. However, it is known that bacteria can penetrate the tissues, and this is best demonstrated by the bacteraemias associated with toothbrushing and tooth movement. It seems likely that the bacteria that are pushed into the tissues would elicit a much more intense inflammatory reaction and so bacterial penetration may be associated with periods of tissue damage. Some bacteria also have the ability to invade the tissues, both into the epithelial cells of the junctional epithelium and beyond. Species including *P. gingivalis*, *T. forsythia*, *F. nucleatum*, *A. actinomycetemcomitans* and *T. denticola* can be found in tissues in small numbers, and some have developed mechanisms to invade the epithelial cells, downregulate their virulence factors and survive and even multiply inside the cell, where there are plentiful nutrients and the bacteria are protected from the host immune system. The invading bacteria are able to develop a new commensal balance with the host cells, move from cell to cell and develop resistance to the antibacterial mechanisms inside the epithelial cell. Only a tiny minority of the plaque flora has this invasive capability, and it is possible that invasion happens only from time to time. However, the intracellular bacteria would be protected from antibiotics and removal by root debridement and so potentially become important. Bacterial invasion can be found in healthy, as well as diseased gingival sites, and its importance is unclear.

Subgingival calculus Calcification of plaque in a pocket produces subgingival calculus. The deposits are thin, more widely distributed, harder, darker and more firmly attached than supragingival calculus. Calculus appears laminated histologically, reflecting incremental mineralisation. The colour is caused by incorporated of blood breakdown products into the plaque before calcification. Subgingival calculus helps perpetuate chronic periodontitis. It retains a reservoir of bacteria, helping to sustain inflammation, and acts as a barrier to healing. Effective removal also acts

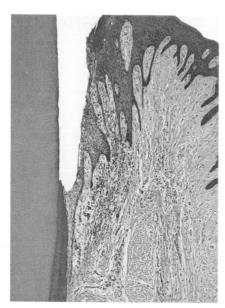

Fig. 7.9 **Transition from chronic gingivitis to periodontitis.** No pocket has yet formed, but the epithelial attachment has extended on to the cementum and inflammation has induced epithelial hyperplasia, as evidenced by development of rete processes, normally absent in junctional epithelium.

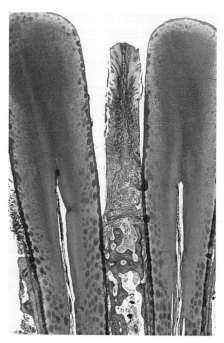

Fig. 7.10 **Established chronic periodontitis.** In this woman of 33 years, periodontal pockets have extended onto cementum and inflammatory cells fill the interdental gingiva.

as a surrogate marker for thorough root surface decontamination and is important in achieving good treatment outcomes.

Chronic inflammation Neutrophils migrate continually into pockets though junctional epithelium, probably rendering it permeable to bacterial products as a result. Plasma cells typically predominate in the tissues, accompanied by lymphocytes. Inflammatory cells infiltrate the gingival connective tissue and spread between the bundles of collagen fibres (Figs 7.9 and 7.10). Dense sheets of these cells accumulate, especially under the pocket lining epithelium, close to the plaque and calculus.

Pocketing depends on the thickness of the gingival tissues. When plaque extends along the tooth surface and the overlying gingiva is thin, the gingiva is lost, producing recession. Thick gingiva is more resilient and becomes undermined by the destruction extending down the root, producing pocketing (Fig. 7.11). Pockets protect the plaque from removal by abrasion or tooth cleaning and expose a large surface area of tissue to irritation by bacteria and their products. Pockets also favour the growth of anaerobic pathogens.

Pockets surround the teeth. One wall is formed by cementum, there may be three bone walls or soft tissue walls depending on size and bone loss. The pocket lining epithelium is continuous with the gingival epithelium at the pocket mouth and is often hyperplastic but very thin. At the base of the pocket the epithelium forms the epithelial attachment. 'Ulceration' of the lining is often described but rarely seen histologically. If it develops, it seems likely that it heals rapidly.

Epithelial migration The epithelial attachment migrates from enamel on to cementum, forming the floor of the pocket (Figs 7.12 and 7.13). The attachment to cementum is strong, and a clear refractile cuticle formed by the epithelium can sometimes be seen joining the epithelium to the root surface (see Fig. 7.2). The length of the epithelial attachment is variable but may extend over several

millimetres. It probably detaches and re-forms intermittently depending on the degree of inflammation.

Destruction of periodontal fibres Collagen fibres are destroyed progressively from the gingival margin down to the level of the floor of the pocket, but only in a localised zone around the pocket. Beyond this, there is fibrosis resulting from inflammation, but the extra collagen is not organised into functional bundles to support the tooth or gingiva.

Destruction of alveolar bone starts at the alveolar crest. The bone crest recedes just in advance of the floor of the pocket. The zone of inflammation in the gingiva or around the pocket is invariably separated from the underlying bone by a thin zone of uninflamed fibrous tissue (see Fig. 7.12). Inflammatory cells are never in contact with the bone and resorb it remotely using soluble factors or other cell signalling mechanisms to activate normal osteoclastic resorption. It has been suggested that the inflammatory cells may extend to alveolar bone and periodontal ligament during periods of active disease, but histological evidence for this is lacking. Osteoclasts are rarely seen, probably because their action is intermittent and the rate of bone destruction extremely slow. The result of bone loss is deep pockets and loss of attachment (Fig. 7.14).

Innate immune mechanisms are thought to be critically important, particularly the non-specific responses of neutrophils and macrophages to bacteria. These are probably responsible for preventing bacterial invasion of the tissues, and their importance is seen in the rapid destruction associated with neutrophil deficiency diseases such as Papillon-Lefèvre syndrome, Down's syndrome and diabetes mellitus. Neutrophils secrete many potent antibacterial compounds, in the pocket often as 'neutrophil extracellular traps', complexed with DNA.

Adaptive immune mechanisms are involved in periodontal disease, as they are in every microbial disease. However, effective responses are hampered by the fact that the target bacteria lie outside the body in the pocket, where the environment is controlled by the bacteria and not the host.

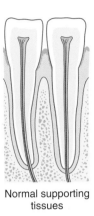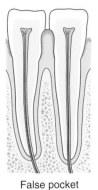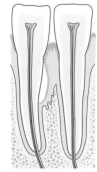

Normal supporting tissues · False pocket · Infrabony pocket (vertical or angular bone loss)

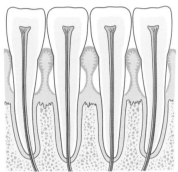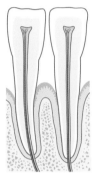

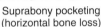

Suprabony pocketing (horizontal bone loss) · Gingival recession

Fig. 7.11 Pocket formation in periodontal disease. A simplified diagram to show the relationship between periodontal soft tissues and alveolar bone in the different presentations of periodontal disease.

It seems likely that humoral responses are the most important, cell-mediated immunity playing a role only within the tissues in maintaining and controlling inflammation. Antibodies produced against plaque bacteria may mediate opsonisation and killing of bacteria by neutrophils and macrophages in the pocket and can also activate complement in the pocket, though probably with little effect. The bacteria in the biofilm on the tooth are protected by the matrix. Unattached bacteria near the pocket wall may be more susceptible.

Overall, it is clear that the immunological reactions in chronic periodontitis are protective. The importance of the immune responses is seen in HIV infection, in which periodontal destruction may be greatly accelerated and acute invasive infections develop.

Bystander damage always accompanies inflammatory diseases. It may be more prominent when excessive activation of neutrophils, macrophages, complement and other inflammatory and immunological mechanisms is triggered by bacterial factors. Cytokines secreted by inflammatory cells often have damaging effects, such as bone resorption triggered by interleukin 1 and 6 and tumour necrosis factor alpha. However, damage by these host mechanisms is minor, and disease progression is very slow; inflammation and immunity are overall protective. When inflammation is suppressed, as for instance in smokers, periodontitis progresses more quickly.

Episodic and chronic nature of destruction A remarkable feature of periodontal disease is that tissue destruction is so slow, despite the presence of huge numbers of bacteria in periodontal pockets. In an otherwise healthy person, it is not uncommon for half a century to pass before 1 cm of alveolar bone is lost. Although overall slow, it is clear that

destruction progresses in rapid spurts. These may be triggered by reduction in host defences or perhaps by poorly understood ecological and virulence changes in the plaque flora driven by changes in the subgingival environment.

Review pathology of periodontitis PMID: 24762896

Review host defence PMC: 4510669

Neutrophil NETs PMID: 26442948

Systemic predisposing factors

Many diseases and habits are said to predispose to gingivitis and periodontitis. The role of pregnancy has been noted in the section on gingivitis. More are discussed later in the section on systemic disease. However, few cause accelerated periodontitis. Most are immunosuppressive and cause acute infection around the teeth, and a few are structural and cause early exfoliation of teeth, but the mechanisms and clinical picture are quite different from plaque-induced disease in normal individuals. Two factors that do genuinely appear to represent a more severe form of the typical disease are smoking and diabetes. Others are shown in Box 7.14.

Smoking

Smokers have greater susceptibility to periodontitis but, paradoxically, less inflammation is evident clinically. The reasons for this are not understood, but smoking is known to interfere with inflammatory and immune reactions, probably by activating endothelial and inflammatory cells in the lungs and circulation, and by inducing them to secrete cytokines and other compounds inappropriately. Also, nicotine is a vasoconstrictor, although its effects on the gingiva

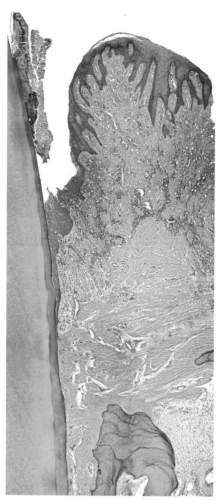

Fig. 7.12 Chronic periodontitis. The amelocemental junction lies at the top of the picture covered by plaque and calculus that extend into the upper pocket. The epithelium of the pocket wall is hyperplastic and irregular, but at the base of the pocket, the lining epithelium forms an epithelial attachment tightly apposed to the cementum. The alveolar bone crest shows resting and reversal lines indicating remodelling during phases of bone loss and recovery. A broad band of uninflamed densely fibrous tissue, almost scar tissue, separates the bone from the inflamed tissue.

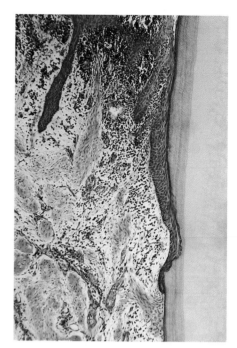

Fig. 7.13 Chronic periodontitis. Higher-power view showing the epithelial attachment lying against cementum. Note how collagen has been lost from the areas containing inflammatory cells.

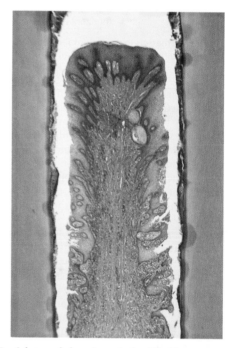

Fig. 7.14 Advanced chronic periodontitis. The cementum on the pocket walls is covered with a thin layer of plaque. The epithelium of the pocket lining is hyperplastic, and the pocket extends beyond the lower edge of the picture.

have proved difficult to measure. Overall, smokers have greater loss of attachment, early tooth loss and respond less well to treatment. The relative risk is high, even if only a few cigarettes are smoked each day. It has been estimated that one cigarette a day produces as much attachment loss as 1 year of untreated disease in a non-smoker. All forms of tobacco smoking have the effect, and continuing to smoke reduces the effectiveness of treatment.

Smokeless tobacco use also promotes periodontal destruction but by direct vascular and abrasive effects.

Smoking and periodontitis PMID: 9722693 and 11021635

Diabetes mellitus

Diabetes increases the risk of periodontitis approximately threefold. Disease severity is directly related to hyperglycaemia and poorly controlled diabetics, particularly those with glycosylated haemoglobin levels above 9%, suffer worst. Both type 1 and type 2 diabetes predispose. In well-controlled diabetes, acceleration of gingivitis may not be noticeable. The links between periodontitis and

diabetes are probably explained by a reduction in neutrophil function and excessive cytokine responses to bacteria by macrophages.

In recent years, it has become clear that diabetics with periodontitis are also more at risk of other diabetic complications such as nephropathy and ischaemic heart disease. It has been suggested that periodontal inflammation or pathogenic bacteria may account for these links, and it has been shown that periodontitis can predict the other complications. Several studies have shown that effective periodontal disease treatment can improve diabetic control, though the effect is small.

There is a role for dental practitioners to identify patients with undiagnosed diabetes on the basis of their periodontitis and refer them for diagnosis.

Diabetes and periodontitis PMID: 16881798

Osteoporosis

It seems logical that reduced bone mineral density in osteoporosis would predispose to alveolar bone loss in periodontitis, but the relationship has proved difficult to investigate, and the association remains contentious and any effect must be small. The association may be difficult to show because the reduced bone density mostly affects women after the menopause, and periodontitis is a very slowly progressing disease.

General principles of management of chronic periodontitis

The main components of the management of periodontal disease are summarised in Box 7.9.

Management largely depends on time-honoured, manual methods of plaque control.

Effective daily plaque removal by the patient is imperative for success. Conscientious toothbrushing and interdental cleaning with aids such as floss (if there is minimal disease), wooden sticks or small interproximal brushes, as necessary, are required. These simple measures will bring about complete resolution of simple gingivitis as mentioned earlier.

Anything hampering plaque control, particularly calculus and faulty restorations, should be dealt with. Other conditions promoting stagnation (Box 7.10) may be more difficult to eliminate.

Treatment of periodontal pockets

The initial aim is to produce a root surface to which the pocket wall and gingival tissue may reattach. This requires a clean root and resolution of inflammation in the pocket wall. The key methods are therefore thorough plaque control and subgingival scaling or root debridement, which remove all (or almost all) calculus and some superficial cementum to ensure elimination of plaque from any surface irregularities. Root debridement cannot remove subgingival plaque entirely, but it reduces bacterial bulk, disturbs the plaque environment, renders the pocket more aerobic and changes the composition of the plaque flora. It is not intended to 'plane' the root surface and remove absorbed toxins.

Following these procedures, inflammation reduces, the tissues shrink and the pocket lining junctional epithelium reattaches to the cementum and enamel surface to produce a 'long epithelial attachment' extending from the level of the old pocket floor to the gingival margin. The long epithelial attachment is firm, shallower probing depths result, and it is sufficiently robust to remain in place for the life of the patient provided supragingival plaque is controlled. However, reattachment of connective tissue to the tooth with a reformed periodontal ligament cannot be expected with these treatments. Bone loss will remain, collagen fibres will not reattach to cementum and the functional periodontal ligament is reduced in length. Some recession also usually results from reduction of gingival inflammation, reducing pocket depth from the coronal end.

Successful reduction in probing depths and bleeding can be expected if the initial pocket was less than 5 mm in

> **Box 7.9 General principles of management of periodontal disease**
>
> - Prevention is most effective
> - Control of bacterial plaque
> - Establishment of healthy gingival contour accessible to plaque control
> - Minimisation of periodontal tissue loss
> - Use of antibiotics in selected cases
> - Mucogingival surgery in selected cases

> **Box 7.10 Factors promoting stagnation and persistence of plaque**
>
> - Calculus
> - Overhanging restorations
> - Food packing due to faulty contact points
> - Irregularities of the teeth
> - Mouth breathing
> - Pocketing
> - Extension to the furcation

> **Box 7.11 Factors compromising subgingival plaque removal**
>
> - Excessive pocket depth
> - Convoluted root morphology, furcations
> - Inaccessible root surfaces (e.g. distal surfaces of posterior teeth)
> - Operator competence
>
> Failure of benefit from root debridement is shown by:
>
> - Bleeding or exudation of pus on probing the depth of pocket
> - Increasing probing depths
> - Deterioration of bone levels seen radiologically

depth. Failure to achieve clinical improvement is usually due to either a lapse in plaque control by the patient or failure to remove all subgingival plaque (Box 7.11). If this happens, more aggressive treatment may be required, but will still only be effective if plaque is controlled by excellent oral hygiene.

When root debridement fails, a variety of surgical and other adjunctive techniques are available. The earliest form of resective surgery was gingivectomy. This is still a useful procedure, particularly in patients with false pockets due to fibrous gingival hyperplasia or drug-associated gingival overgrowth who may be unresponsive to non-surgical treatment. However, simple gingivectomy causes loss of attached gingiva and is poor cosmetically.

Flap operations Surgical approaches usually depend on elevation of flaps and are designed to facilitate cleaning of the root. Inflamed tissue is curetted away, and the root surfaces are cleaned. The flaps are then sutured back around the necks of the teeth. The flap can be replaced at or near the preoperative level, or it can be repositioned apically so that it just covers the alveolar crest. The former approach requires that the flap must reattach to the denuded root surface by a long epithelial attachment. Apical placement of the flap may produce a poor cosmetic result and expose complex root forms, but removes the pocket.

Reattachment ('regenerative') surgery The goal of this technique is formation of cementum to anchor periodontal fibres to the root surface. This ideal result ('new attachment') would obviously be the most satisfactory method of treatment. A new connective tissue attachment can only form if cells from the remaining healthy periodontal ligament repopulate the root surface. In practice, the pocket lining epithelium proliferates quickly and grows and attaches to the root before new attachment can form. Insertion of a barrier membrane between the flap and root surface may prevent epithelial and gingival connective tissue ingrowth ('guided tissue regeneration'). Many membrane types, both resorbable and non-resorbable can be used. Guided tissue regeneration is more effective than simple flap surgery in reducing probing depths and forming bone, but there is considerable variation in results, little or no histological evidence of new functional periodontal ligament being formed and no evidence of clinical benefit.

Additional bone-inducing graft materials such as demineralised freeze-dried bone allograft, enamel matrix derivatives and recombinant human platelet-derived growth factor are not yet considered reliable at inducing attachment, but may have some value in reduction of pocket depths in selected cases.

Limitations of periodontal surgery Meta-analyses show that both surgical and non-surgical treatment have similar outcomes when the standard of plaque control is high. Surgery in shallow pockets causes further attachment loss, and surgery is not beneficial until probing depths reach 6 mm. Even scaling and root debridement in shallow pockets less than 3 mm causes attachment loss.

Role of antibiotics

Antibiotics can disturb the bacterial flora but cannot eliminate it. The biofilm is mostly dead bacteria and matrix; only viable and unattached bacteria would be susceptible. The stable ecosystem of plaque protects bacteria from antibiotics but also prevents them recolonising the plaque if they can be eliminated, providing a potentially long term beneficial effect. Bacteria in a biofilm tolerate antibiotics better, but they are not intrinsically resistant. However, biofilms harbour so-called *persister* cells, non-growing bacteria that are unaffected by antibiotics and can re-establish infection once the antibiotic treatment ceases.

Antibiotics are usually reserved for disease responding poorly to conventional treatment, usually with deep pockets. Overall, tetracyclines or a combination of metronidazole and amoxicillin seem to be the most effective.

Tetracycline-containing plastic fibres and other antibiotic slow release systems have been placed in the gingival sulcus for direct delivery of a high local concentration but the former are no longer available and there is limited evidence to support use of the latter, perhaps because the agents are washed away by the flow gingival crevicular fluid. Tetracyclines are particularly effective in aggressive periodontitis (later in this chapter).

Current evidence suggests that a 7–14 day course of metronidazole and amoxicillin after completion of debridement provides additional benefit for pocketing over 6 mm in depth. The benefit is 0.5–1 mm probing depth, and it is still detectable many months after treatment. Reductions of up to 3 mm are claimed for the deepest pockets.

A strategy of 'full mouth disinfection' comprises topical intraoral applications of chlorhexidine with complete subgingival debridement in 1 day to attempt to change the whole flora at once and prevent reinfection from untreated sites. There appears to be little enhanced benefit from this approach.

Risks from antibiotic adverse effects and bacterial resistance must be weighed against their benefits and routine use for periodontitis cannot be justified.

Antibiotic use PMID: 26427574

Box 7.12	Factors affecting prognosis of periodontal disease

- Oral hygiene status and motivation
- Degree of attachment loss
- Age
- Gender, worse in males
- Smoking
- Furcation involvement
- Residual pocketing after treatment
- Tooth vitality
- Host resistance
- Intensive maintenance treatment
- Poorly defined genetic factors

Treatment of advanced periodontal disease

Once pocketing has extended beyond the point where treatment can be beneficial, the teeth should be extracted. Deep pockets are a source of sepsis that may have remote effects such as infective endocarditis. Making an early planned decision to extract teeth preserves bone for implants or dentures.

Prognosis in periodontal disease

Predictions about the results of treatment are not completely accurate, especially in multirooted teeth, but some factors are known to be associated with tooth loss after treatment (Box 7.12). However, overall treatment is very effective if completed and maintained. Most teeth that are lost are extracted in the 5 years after treatment, and these are usually teeth that had adverse features at initiation of treatment.

Much depends on the level of oral hygiene maintained by patients and whether they are sufficiently strongly motivated in the long term, together with factors affecting individual teeth, such tooth type, root length, root anatomy and degree of furcation involvement (Figs 7.15 and 7.16).

Despite intensive investigation, there remains, for no clear reason, a 'high-risk' group for periodontitis who suffer more extensive bone loss than others of similar age.

Complications of chronic periodontitis

Complications can be local or systemic (Box 7.13).

Some systemic complications arise from the transient bacteraemia associated with mastication and tooth brushing. Bacteraemia is most severe when pockets are deep and inflamed, but it is still detectable in near heathy mouths. Infective endocarditis is the most significant complication and is discussed in Chapter 32.

Severity of periodontitis is clearly associated with cardiovascular disease, mediated by the overall bacterial burden and not specific species. However, it remains unclear whether this association might be caused by smoking or

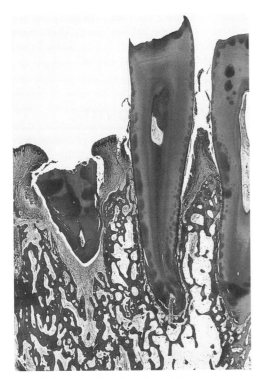

Fig. 7.15   Infrabony pocket. A neglected dentition with a retained carious root and teeth with periodontitis. The middle tooth has an angular infrabony defect on one side, but only horizontal bone loss on its opposite side.

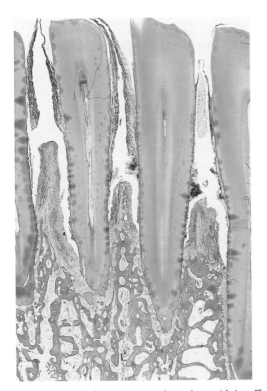

Fig. 7.16   Severe bone loss. Extensive bone loss with insufficient bone support for effective treatment. The tooth to the left of centre has infrabony pocketing extending almost to the apex, though the pulp remains vital.

Box 7.13   Complications and possible complications of chronic periodontitis

Local
- Periodontal abscess
- Tooth mobility
- Tooth loss through exfoliation

Systemic
- Infective endocarditis
- Atherosclerosis and cardiovascular disease
- Poor diabetic control
- Preterm birth

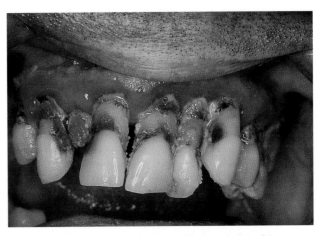

Fig. 7.17   Advanced periodontitis with recession. In this neglected mouth, deposits of plaque and supragingival calculus adhere to the exposed roots, which have active root caries. Probing depths are minimal despite disease progression.

other risk factors that are common to both diseases. A number of systemic infections are thought to contribute to atheroma through lipopolysaccharide and activation of systemic inflammatory mechanisms. Immune cross-reactivity between tissues and bacteria is often cited as a possible mechanism. Whether periodontal treatment can reduce atheroma or its complications is unclear and probably unlikely.

The suggestion that periodontitis affects diabetic control can now be considered proven, and treatment of periodontitis appears to improve diabetic complications, at least as measured by surrogate blood markers.

Periodontitis has also been associated with elevated risk of preterm birth and low birthweight. However, the numerous other potential confounding factors make this association difficult to investigate, and studies of periodontal treatment have failed to show any protective effect.

GINGIVAL RECESSION

Recession of the gingivae and exposure of the roots is common (Figs 7.17 and 7.18). It is progressive and so worsens with age, but it is not a feature of ageing itself and susceptibility varies. The major predisposing factor is thinness of the gingival tissue, so recession is worst around upper canines, lower incisors and lingual to lower molars. Loss of attachment in areas of thick tissue produces pockets whereas thin tissue is destroyed entirely. Recession cannot be reversed.

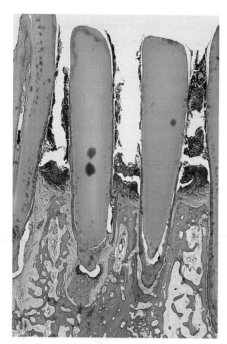

Fig. 7.18 Periodontitis with recession. In this case, gingival destruction is almost as great as the degree of bone resorption so that excessively long clinical crowns have been produced. Supragingival calculus and a dense inflammatory infiltrate in the gingiva can be seen. The tooth to the left of the midline appears non-vital. Although the pulp cannot be seen, there is a periapical granuloma and apical inflammatory hypercementosis.

The exact cause of recession is unclear, but the most common association is with plaque-induced inflammation. One hypothesis suggests that epithelial proliferation of the junctional epithelium in inflammation results in an epithelial 'bridge' of rete processes extending to the external gingival epithelium across the narrow band of inflamed connective tissue. This is followed by remodelling of the gingival margin to preserve a normal epithelial thickness. Whether cervical abrasion caused by a stiff brush and abrasive toothpaste follows recession or causes it is impossible to ascertain, but the two are closely linked. Recession at the papilla, as opposed to in the thin buccal or lingual aspect of teeth is always associated with prior periodontitis.

Other hypothetical causes include acid regurgitation and minor tooth movements. It is clear that the thin tissue is not resistant to any insult and recession often follows direct trauma from factitial injury, trauma from oral piercings, topical tobacco and betel quid.

Receded gingival margins often appear relatively uninflamed.

Treatment of gingival recession

Recession itself is asymptomatic and primarily of cosmetic concern. It is often self-limiting, no longer advancing once thicker bone is reached. Effective atraumatic cleaning is required to prevent additional inflammatory destruction. In most cases, recession is not associated with gingival inflammation because cleaning is effective.

Free gingival grafting or connective tissue grafting combined with advanced buccal flaps can be used to cover the exposed root, but success requires good height of adjacent bone and soft tissues. Sometimes when recession extends past the mucogingival junction a graft may anchor the softer alveolar mucosa to bone and prevent rapid extension toward the apex.

The second significant problem with recession is dentine hypersensitivity from the exposed root. This results from additional demineralisation and can be tackled using fluoride or dentinal tubule blocking agents.

Recession review PMID: 21941318

AGGRESSIVE PERIODONTITIS

Aggressive periodontitis is defined as periodontitis characterised by rapid attachment loss and bone destruction in otherwise healthy patients. Often the destruction seems out of proportion to the small amounts of plaque present and there seems to be a clear association with the periodontal pathogens *A. actinomycetemcomitans* or *P. gingivalis*. *A. actinomycetemcomitans* leukotoxin-producing strains are claimed to be closely associated and can be isolated specifically from the sites of destruction. High concentrations of antibodies are found in the serum and gingival fluid. There is often a familial background to aggressive disease, and patients have slightly impaired neutrophil function, both chemotaxis and phagocytosis, or hyperreactive macrophages that produce excessive cytokines. However, these underlying factors do not cause other diseases or predispose to other infections and have been suggested to be induced by the periodontal flora.

Although aggressive periodontitis is recognised by its rapid onset and progression, it seems to be self-limiting. After a period of rapid attachment loss, the disease process often slows and becomes indistinguishable from chronic periodontitis. Diagnosis is based on clinical and radiological features. The microscopic features are the same as in chronic periodontitis, and biopsy is not helpful in diagnosis.

Localised aggressive periodontitis

This condition was previously known as *localised juvenile periodontitis*, and the changed name reflects that it may develop in adults, although almost all cases seem to start around puberty. It is uncommon, having a prevalence of approximately 1:1000, with those of African or Afro-Caribbean descent more frequently affected.

The characteristic feature is rapid breakdown of attachment on permanent first molars and incisors, often in a strikingly symmetrical pattern and in individuals younger than 30 years old. By definition, no more than two teeth other than incisors or first molars can be affected. Gingival inflammation is minimal or absent, and the main feature is drifting and loosening of teeth (Fig. 7.19). Deep, angular bone loss and displacement of the anterior teeth are typical findings (Fig. 7.20), and teeth may exfoliate spontaneously.

Generalised aggressive periodontitis

When the disease process involves more than two teeth other than incisors and first molars, it is defined as generalised. These patients often lack the prominent antibody response to the typical periodontal pathogens, and while similar organisms to those in the localised form are present, there is a more mixed flora typical of late chronic periodontitis. It is unclear how many patients with the generalised form have progressed from the localised form.

Treatment of aggressive periodontitis

Treatment must be aggressive because severely affected teeth may lose attachment rapidly and require extraction. Currently, early aggressive root debridement and antibiotic

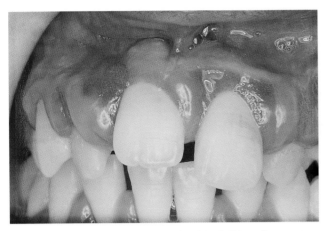

Fig. 7.19 Localised juvenile periodontitis. Drifting of upper central incisors due to gross loss of attachment. There is some marginal inflammation, but oral hygiene is good and the clinical appearance belies the periodontal destruction visible radiographically or on probing.

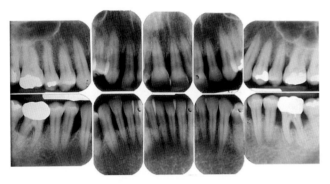

Fig. 7.20 Juvenile periodontitis. Young adult patient aged 20 years, showing severe bone destruction around three first permanent molars and upper and lower incisors. Probing depths exceeded 10 mm. *(Courtesy Dr R Saravanamuttu.)*

administration is the most successful approach and may be dramatically successful in the early stages of the disease. *A. actinomycetemcomitans* is particularly sensitive to tetracyclines and minocycline has been the traditional choice of antibiotic. However, better results are claimed with combination treatments of penicillins and metronidazole. Culture of subgingival flora has been suggested to tailor the antibiotic selection but is rarely available.

Persistent pocketing often requires surgical treatment, and maintenance therapy is critical to prevent relapse. Because the disease has a strong genetic background, siblings should be screened for the disease.

Aggressive periodontitis: DOI 10.1111/prd.12013 and other articles in the same issue

'PREPUBERTAL' PERIODONTITIS

Severe periodontitis in children is very unusual, and it is now thought that all periodontitis affecting the deciduous dentition has an underlying systemic cause, almost always a host defence defect and usually leucocyte adhesion deficiency. Leukocyte adhesion deficiency results from lack of functional surface adhesion receptors on neutrophils, macrophages or both, preventing these inflammatory cells from emigrating into inflamed or infected tissues. This causes recurrent skin and fungal infections and delayed wound

---

> **Box 7.14 Premature periodontal tissue destruction associated with systemic disease**
>
> **Immunodeficiencies**
> - Down's syndrome (Ch. 39)
> - Neutropaenia (Ch. 27)
> - Leukaemias (Ch. 27)
> - Leukocyte adhesion deficiency
> - Severe diabetes mellitus
> - HIV infection (Ch. 29)
> - Papillon–Lefèvre syndrome
> - Rare defects of neutrophil function
>   Chediak Higashi syndrome
>   Chronic granulomatous disease
>
> **Genetic syndromes**
> - Hypophosphatasia (Ch. 13)
> - Ehlers–Danlos syndrome type VIII (Ch. 14)

healing in addition to periodontitis. Periodontitis becomes evident soon after tooth eruption, and while the underlying deficiency persists, treatment is ineffective. The only effective treatment is bone marrow transplantation.

Other causes of childhood periodontitis that might cause similar presentations include neutropenia, leukaemia, hypophosphatasia, Papillon–Lefèvre syndrome, HIV infection and acrodynia (heavy metal poisoning).

Prepubertal periodontitis PMID: 9673168

PERIODONTITIS AS A MANIFESTATION OF SYSTEMIC DISEASE

A diverse range of diseases can present with periodontal destruction, some simply predisposing to conventional periodontitis and others causing distinctive patterns of destruction. Predisposing conditions such as diabetes have been previously dealt with and others fall into the category of aggressive periodontitis. All except Down's syndrome are uncommon or rare, but are important to distinguish from early-onset periodontitis in that the underlying disorder may threaten the patient's health or life.

Recognised causes of premature periodontal destruction are summarised in Box 7.14 and are discussed in more detail in separate sections elsewhere.

Agranulocytosis and acute leukaemia may also be associated with necrotising gingivitis and periodontal tissue destruction. Agranulocytosis is mainly a disease of adults, whereas the common childhood type of acute leukaemia (acute lymphocytic leukaemia) typically produces gingival enlargement rather than periodontal destruction. The importance of cyclic neutropenia has been greatly exaggerated. It is little more than a pathological curiosity, and early-onset periodontitis is by no means always associated. All these immunodeficiency disorders are typically associated with abnormal susceptibility to non-oral infections.

Down's syndrome

In Down's syndrome, gingivitis is exacerbated by excessive plaque formation and difficulties in establishing effective toothbrushing habits. Progress to periodontitis between age 15 and 25 was usual in the past and early tooth loss was a frequent consequence (see Fig. 39.4), but enhanced

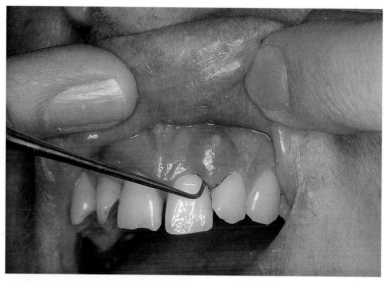

Fig. 7.21 **Periodontal abscess.** The abscess is pointing on the alveolar mucosa well above the attached gingiva. The probe is inserted deeply in the pocket communicating with the abscess.

preventive regimes have proved effective and patients with Down's syndrome now retain more teeth into adulthood. Multiple immunodeficiencies and 'early ageing' of the immune system contribute, and there is early colonisation by periodontal pathogens. Small teeth with short roots predispose to tooth loss. Calculus used to be considered prevalent, but recent data suggests this is simply a reflection of oral hygiene and not a feature of the syndrome.

Papillon–lefèvre syndrome

Papillon–Lefèvre syndrome is an exceedingly rare autosomal recessive disorder. The main features are, typically, hyperkeratosis of palms and soles starting in infancy and early-onset periodontal destruction caused by a loss-of-function mutation in the cathepsin C gene. Those with the disease are homozygous for the mutation and completely lack cathepsin C activity. Parents and carriers are heterozygous and have low cathepsin C activity but suffer no ill-effects.

Cathepsin C is a lysosomal protease that plays an essential role in activating antibacterial compounds stored in an inactive form in neutrophils. Lack of activation impairs host responses to bacteria. Patients may also have intellectual impairment, intracranial calcifications, hyperhidrosis and recurrent skin infections. Diagnosis is by genetic screening.

PERIODONTAL (LATERAL) ABSCESS

A periodontal abscess results from acute infection of a periodontal pocket. The alternative name of lateral abscess indicates that the abscess lies at the side of the tooth rather than apically. The causes are uncertain but probably related to factors that tip the host-bacterial balance in favour of the bacteria. Thus, it sometimes follows treatment such as root debridement when trauma to the pocket lining implants bacteria into the tissues or damage by a foreign body such as a fish bone or toothbrush bristle trapped in a pocket. Food packing down between the teeth with poor contact points may contribute. More often the cause is obscure and may be a change in the pocket flora or host defences. Pericoronitis is a form of periodontal abscess beneath the operculum of a partially erupted molar. More generalised chronic periodontitis is usually associated.

Drainage through the pocket mouth is prevented by inflammatory oedema and soft tissue swelling.

Clinical features

The onset is rapid. Gingival tenderness progresses to throbbing pain. The tooth affected is vital and tender to percussion. The overlying gingiva is red and swollen. Pus may exude from the pocket, but a deeply sited periodontal abscess may point on the alveolar mucosa, forming a sinus. The vitality of the tooth and its less severe tenderness usually distinguish a lateral abscess from acute apical periodontitis. The great depth of the pocket, from which pus may exude, helps make the diagnosis clear (Fig. 7.21).

Radiographic changes are not visible until after approximately a week. A radiolucent area may then be seen beside the tooth.

Pathology

The bony wall of the pocket is actively resorbed by many osteoclasts. There is dense infiltration by neutrophils and pus formation (Figs 7.22 and 7.23). The pocket deepens rapidly by destruction of periodontal fibres, sometimes to the apex of the tooth. Alveolar bone in the floor of the original pocket is destroyed, and the pocket extends rapidly. Occasionally, pus tracks apically or from a deeply sited pocket so that a facial abscess or cellulitis results.

Treatment

A periodontal abscess should be drained, ideally through the pocket, by subgingival curettage and the root surfaces thoroughly debrided. Incision through the overlying gingiva is best avoided unless drainage through the pocket fails, as a permanent soft tissue fenestration may result. However, if periodontal disease is severe and widespread, it may be more appropriate to extract the affected tooth. After treatment, the site will have suffered a significant acute attachment loss.

ACUTE PERICORONITIS

Incomplete eruption of a wisdom tooth produces a large stagnation area under the gum flap that anatomically

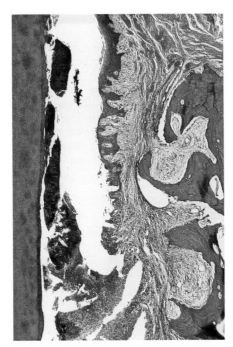

Fig. 7.22 Acute periodontal abscess. There is well-advanced chronic periodontitis, but acute inflammatory changes have developed in this pocket with destruction of periodontal ligament and alveolar bone with formation of an abscess and a deep intrabony pocket (from a man of 55 years).

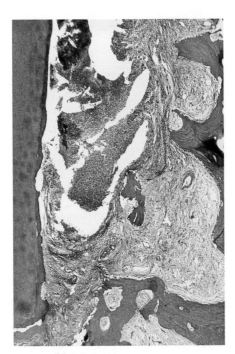

Fig. 7.23 Periodontal abscess. Higher-power view of the floor of the pocket shows the purulent inflammation and gross resorption of alveolar bone extending to the apex.

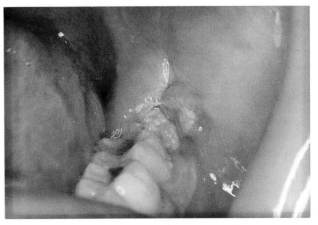

Fig. 7.24 Pericoronitis. A pocket has formed between the gingiva and the crown of a partially erupted third molar, which is overlaid by the operculum.

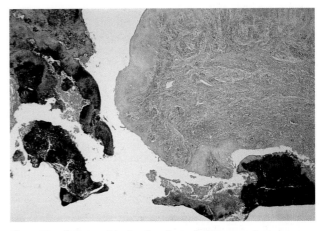

Fig. 7.25 Pericoronitis. Section through the operculum shows the heavy deposits of microbial plaque beneath it and along its anterior edge (*left*) (Gram stain).

> **Box 7.15 Factors contributing to pericoronitis**
> - Impaction of food and plaque accumulation under the gum flap
> - An upper tooth biting on the gum flap
> - Acute ulcerative gingivitis (rarely)

mimics a pocket. It can easily become infected, causing pericoronitis. Several factors (Box 7.15) may contribute.

Pericoronitis is caused by a mixed infection with various potential periodontal pathogens, particularly anaerobes.

Clinical features

Young adults are affected. The main symptoms are soreness and tenderness around the partially erupted tooth (Figs 7.24

and 7.25). There is pain, swelling, difficulty in opening the mouth, lymphadenopathy, sometimes slight fever and, in severe cases, suppuration and abscess formation. Swelling and difficulty in opening the mouth may be severe enough to prevent examination of the area.

Management

Food debris should be removed from under the gum flap by irrigation. The position of the affected tooth, its relationship to the second molar and any complicating factors should be determined by radiography.

In mild cases, it may be enough for patients to keep the mouth clean and to use hot mouth rinses whenever symptoms develop, until the inflammation subsides. This may happen naturally by further eruption or by extraction of the tooth after the infection has been overcome.

If radiographs show that the third molar is badly misplaced, impacted or carious, it should be extracted after inflammation has subsided. Spread of infection (cellulitis or osteomyelitis) may follow extraction of the tooth while infection is still acute, but is rare.

When an upper tooth is biting on the flap, it is often preferable to extract it, especially if the lower tooth is ultimately to be removed. If there are strong reasons for retaining the upper tooth, the cusps can be ground sufficiently to prevent it from traumatising the flap. In the past, caustic agents such as trichloracetic acid were commonly used to reduce the operculum. This was very effective but carries a risk of accidental burns to adjacent mucosa or skin. Electrocautery may also be used. In severe cases, particularly when there is fever and lymphadenopathy, penicillin or penicillin and metronidazole should be given.

Pus may track posteriorly from the operculum to cause serious fascial space infection as described in Chapter 9. In the pre-antibiotic era, acute infection from pericoronitis was a relatively common cause of death in young adults.

Both treated and untreated acute pericoronitis may become chronic if the operculum remains. In the absence of further acute episodes, there is extensive bone loss around the partially erupted tooth and its neighbours so that the second molar can be compromised.

ACUTE NECROTISING ULCERATIVE GINGIVITIS

Acute ulcerative gingivitis is a distinct and specific disease that can cause significant periodontal tissue destruction. The disease is also a complication of HIV infection as discussed in Chapter 29.

Clinical features

The incidence of ulcerative gingivitis has declined sharply in the Western world in the last 60 years. It typically affects apparently healthy young adults, usually those with neglected mouths.

Typical features are summarised in Box 7.16.

Crater-shaped or punched-out ulcers form initially at the tips of the interdental papillae. Ulcers are sharply defined by erythema and oedema; their surface is covered by a greyish or yellowish tenacious slough. Removal of the slough

causes free bleeding. The severe halitosis, likened to rotting hay, is characteristic.

Lesions remain restricted to the gingivae and supporting tissues. They mainly spread along the gingival margins and deeply, destroying interdental soft and hard tissues, but rarely spreading to alveolar mucosa. Deep spread can cause rapid destruction of both soft tissues and bone, producing triangular spaces between the teeth (Fig. 7.26).

If treatment is delayed, the end result is distortion of the normal gingival contour, promoting stagnation and possibly recurrences or chronic periodontal disease.

Aetiology

The bacteria responsible are a complex of spirochaetes and fusiforms (Fig. 7.27). These organisms are present in small numbers in the healthy gingival flora. With the onset of ulcerative gingivitis, both bacteria proliferate until they dominate the local bacterial flora. This, together with invasion of the tissues by spirochaetes seen by electron microscopy, and the sharp fall in their numbers with effective treatment indicate that they are the responsible agents. Nevertheless, it is still uncertain whether this

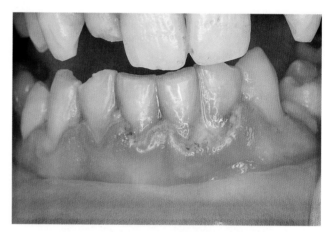

Fig. 7.26   Acute necrotising ulcerative gingivitis. Characteristic features, a crater-shaped ulcer starting at the tips of the interdental papillae, and covered by an ulcer slough.

Box 7.16   Typical features of acute necrotising ulcerative gingivitis

- Young adult males mainly affected
- Often cigarette smokers and/or with minor respiratory infection
- Cratered ulcers starting at the tips of the interdental papillae
- Ulcers spread along gingival margins
- Gingival soreness and bleeding
- Foul breath
- No significant lymphadenopathy
- No fever or systemic upset
- Smears from ulcers dominated by Gram-negative spirochaetes and fusiform bacteria
- Responds to oral hygiene and metronidazole in immunocompetent patients

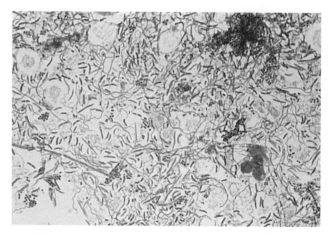

Fig. 7.27   A smear from an ulcer of acute necrotising ulcerative gingivitis shows the dense proliferation of *Treponema vincentii* and *Fusobacterium nucleatum*.

Box 7.17   Bacteria implicated in acute ulcerative gingivitis

- *Treponema vincentii*
- *Fusobacterium fusiformis*
- *Prevotella intermedia*
- *Porphyromonas gingivalis*
- *Selenomonas sputigena*
- *Leptotrichia buccalis*

Box 7.18   Differential diagnosis of acute necrotising ulcerative gingivitis

- Primary herpetic gingivostomatitis (see page 235)
- HIV-associated acute ulcerative gingivitis (see page 113)
- Gingival ulceration in acute leukaemia or aplastic anaemia (see page 115)

Box 7.19   Causes of gingival enlargement

Fibrous gingival hyperplasia

- Hereditary gingival fibromatosis
- Drug-associated
  - Phenytoin
  - Calcium-channel blockers
  - Cyclosporin

Inflammatory gingival swelling

- Chronic 'hyperplastic' gingivitis
- Pregnancy gingivitis
- Leukaemic infiltration
- Wegener's granulomatosis
- Sarcoidosis
- Orofacial granulomatosis
- Scurvy

'fusospirochaetal complex' is the sole cause of ulcerative gingivitis and other bacteria have been implicated (Box 7.17).

Despite doubts about the precise identity of the bacterial cause of acute ulcerative gingivitis, it is clearly an anaerobic infection and responds rapidly to metronidazole.

Host factors Ulcerative gingivitis is a disease of otherwise healthy young adults usually with neglected, dirty mouths. However, ulcerative gingivitis may also develop in children having immunosuppressive treatment and in patients with HIV infection.

Local factors appear to be important and ulcerative gingivitis does not appear to be transmissible. Ulcerative gingivitis ('trench mouth') was almost epidemic among soldiers in the 1914–1918 war and civilians subjected to bombing in the 1939–1945 war. Other evidence also suggests that stress may be a predisposing factor in this infection. Smoking and upper respiratory infections have also been implicated. However, ulcerative gingivitis is relatively rarely seen in the UK now (Box 7.18).

Treatment

Oral hygiene and debridement are essential. A 3-day course of metronidazole or penicillin greatly accelerates resolution. Once the acute phase has subsided, the oral hygiene and other associated risk factors must be addressed to lessen the risk of recurrence.

HIV-ASSOCIATED PERIODONTITIS

HIV-associated ulcerative gingivitis is a severe form of acute ulcerative gingivitis associated with soft-tissue necrosis and rapid destruction of the periodontal tissues. It is typically intensely painful. There is little deep pocketing, because soft tissue and bone are destroyed virtually simultaneously. More than 90% of the attachment can be lost within 3–6 months, and the soft-tissue necrosis can lead to exposure of bone and sequestration.

The pain of HIV-associated periodontitis is usually aching in character and felt within the jaw rather than in the gingivae. It may be felt before tissue destruction becomes obvious. HIV-associated gingivitis and periodontitis are usually generalised but are sometimes localised to one or more discrete areas.

Bacteriologically, HIV-associated periodontitis resembles classical periodontitis in HIV-negative persons, but poor control of viral infections may also contribute. It is typically associated with a low CD4 count and a poor prognosis for the patient.

Management

Debridement and removal of any sequestra under local anaesthesia, chlorhexidine mouth rinses, systemic metronidazole and analgesics may be effective. Additional broad-spectrum antibiotics have been recommended by some, but increase the risk of thrush to which these patients are particularly susceptible. If thrush is present or develops, antifungal treatment is required. For persistent pain, oral analgesics are indicated.

The condition of linear gingival erythema in HIV infection is caused by candidal infection in the gingival crevice and on the free gingiva.

GINGIVAL ENLARGEMENT

Gingival swelling may be due to fibrous hyperplasia, inflammatory swelling or infiltration by other types of cells (Box 7.19).

Hereditary gingival fibromatosis

Gingival fibromatosis is a feature of several heritable syndromes and is rare. As an isolated condition, hereditary gingival fibrosis is associated with mutation in the SOS1 gene, a signalling pathway protein.

Gingival enlargement may precede eruption of the teeth or may not develop until later in childhood. The gingivae may be so grossly enlarged as completely to bury the teeth or prevent eruption. The tissue is pale, firm and smooth or stippled in texture (Fig. 7.28).

Histologically, the gingival tissue consists of thick bundles of collagenous connective tissue with little or no inflammatory exudate (Fig. 7.29). When it develops as part of a syndrome, the most common association is hypertrichosis

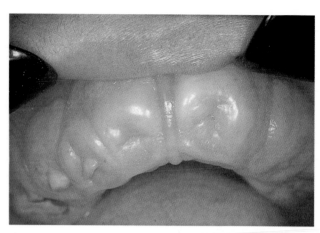

Fig. 7.28 **Hereditary gingival fibromatosis.** Fibrous overgrowth of the gingiva has covered the crowns of the teeth and almost buried them.

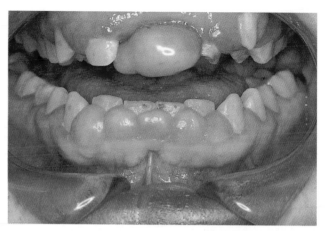

Fig. 7.30 **Gingival hyperplasia due to phenytoin.** Characteristically (and unlike Fig. 7.28), the fibrous overgrowth has originated in the interdental papillae, which become bulbous but remain firm and pale. Localised gross enlargement such as that around the upper central incisor may result and forms a plaque trap.

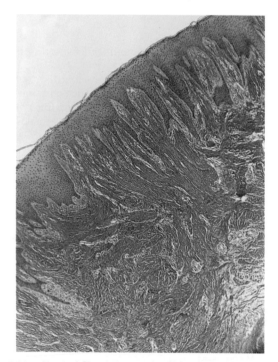

Fig. 7.29 **Gingival fibromatosis.** Both the genetic and drug-induced types share this histological picture of gross fibrous overgrowth. In this image the tissue has been stained with a Van Gieson stain that highlights the collagen red. Note the absence of inflammation.

Other syndromes with generalised gingival enlargement due to other causes must be distinguished, such as hyaline fibromatosis and glycogen storage diseases.

Fibrous enlargement of the tuberosity is a poorly understood bilateral fibrous growth of the maxillary alveolus posterior to the premolar teeth. Some cases may have mild forms of hereditary gingival fibromatosis, but onset and growth is usually in adulthood.

Review PMID: 17189459

Drug-induced gingival overgrowth

The antiepileptic drug phenytoin (Epanutin), calcium-channel blockers such as nifedipine and diltiazem (for hypertension or angina) and the immunosuppressive drug cyclosporin can cause hyperplasia of gingival fibroblasts. Phenytoin is the most potent stimulus with half of long term users affected to some degree. All drug-induced enlargement affects primarily the papillae, whereas hereditary forms are diffuse.

The interdental papillae become bulbous and overlap the teeth (Fig. 7.30); they may eventually overgrow the occlusal or incisal level. Typically, the gingivae are firm and pale, and the stippled texture is exaggerated, producing an orange-peel appearance. Gingivitis contributes, and overgrowth of the gingivae can sometimes be prevented or kept under control by rigorous oral hygiene. Frequently, however, gingivectomy becomes necessary to allow cleaning or for cosmetic reasons. Management can be problematic if the epilepsy is associated with learning disability or when nifedipine and cyclosporin are combined, as in patients with renal transplants. Early changes can be seen after only 3 months of drug treatment, allowing intervention to prevent the condition. The mechanisms are unknown, and there may be a genetic predisposition.

Histologically the tissues are densely fibrous.

Web URL 7.1 Review: http://emedicine.medscape.com/article/1076264

PMID: Drugs and gingival overgrowth: 25680368

PMID: Management gingival overgrowth: 16677333

and mental disability. In other syndromes a range of features may coexist, including coarse and thickened facial features, simulating acromegaly, epilepsy or deafness, and cherubism.

The excess gingival tissue can only be removed surgically but is likely to re-form. Gingivectomy should be delayed as long as possible, preferably until after puberty, when the rate of growth of the tissues is slower. Maintenance of oral hygiene is important to prevent infection becoming established in the deep false pockets. However, inflammation is frequently insignificant.

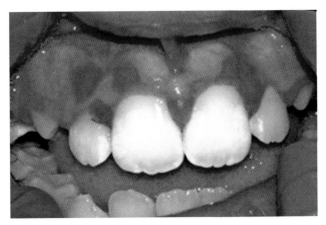

Fig. 7.31 **Localised juvenile spongiotic gingivitis.** In this patient there are several patches, but often there is only one. Note how they do not necessarily involve the gingival margin. *(Fig. 18-13 from Law, C.S., Silva D.R., Duperon, D.F, et al., 2014. Gingival disease in Childhood. In: Newman, M.G., Takei, H.H., Klokkevold, P.R., et al. (Eds.), Carranza's clinical periodontology, twelfth ed. Saunders, Philadelphia, pp. 252-260.)*

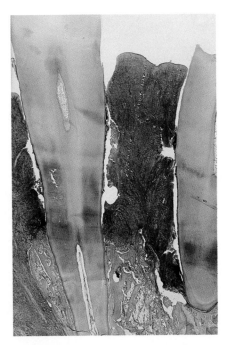

Fig. 7.32 **Acute myelomonocytic leukaemia.** The gingival swelling can be seen to be due to packing of the gingivae with leukaemic cells, immature and abnormal neutrophils or monocytes, stained dark blue. The periodontal tissues have broken down as a result of the poor resistance to infection.

LOCALISED JUVENILE SPONGIOTIC GINGIVITIS

This recently described condition is rare, distinctive and does not respond to improvement in oral hygiene. The features are sessile rounded nodules of bright red, sharply demarcated and soft stippled or slightly papillary mucosa extending from the gingival margin to the mucogingival junction or beyond, a few millimetres in diameter (Fig. 7.31). The buccal gingiva, usually maxillary, are most frequently involved, and most patients are female and between the ages of 6 and 18 years. The tissue bleeds easily. Most patients have a single focus.

The histological appearances are also distinctive, resembling inflammation of the junctional epithelium with a slightly papillary hyperplasia of the epithelium.

The true nature of this condition remains to be determined. One suggestion is that it is a zone where junctional epithelium extends to the gingiva. Lesions usually do not recur on excision, but whether they require any intervention or not is unclear. It can occasionally be found in adults.

Description PMID: 18602289

PLASMINOGEN DEFICIENCY GINGIVITIS

This rare inherited deficiency has a distinctive gingival presentation as described in Chapter 28.

OTHER INFLAMMATORY GINGIVAL SWELLINGS

Chronic 'hyperplastic' and pregnancy gingivitis and drug induced overgrowth have been discussed previously.

Wegener's granulomatosis is an uncommon, vasculitic disease described in Chapter 33. Occasionally, the first sign is a characteristic form of proliferative gingivitis, bright or dusky red in colour and with a granular surface, to which the term 'strawberry gums' has been applied. Early recognition may be life-saving.

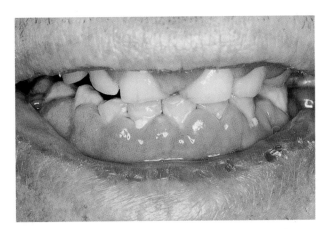

Fig. 7.33 **Acute myelomonocytic leukaemia.** The gingival margins are swollen and soft due to the leukaemic infiltrate.

Sarcoidosis and orofacial granulomatosis can give rise to generalised nodular gingival enlargement. These are discussed in Chapters 30 and 34, respectively.

Acute leukaemia, particularly acute myelomonocytic leukaemia, causes gingival swellings. The abnormal white cells are unable to perform their normal defensive function and cannot control infection at the gingival margins. The abnormal leucocytes pack the area until the gingivae become swollen with leukaemic cells (Fig. 7.32). These cells are so defective that infection progresses, leading to ulceration and breakdown of the tissues. Clinically, the gingivae are swollen, shiny, pale or purplish in colour and frequently ulcerated (Fig. 7.33). Other signs of leukaemia (pallor,

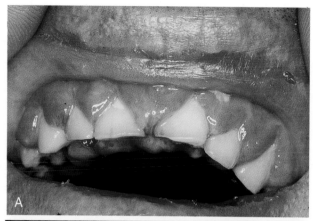

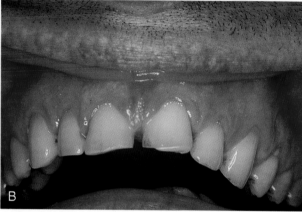

Fig. 7.34 Acute leukaemia. (A) Gross leukaemic infiltration has caused the gingival margins to reach the incisal edges of the teeth. (B) The benefits of plaque control with an antibiotic mouth rinse and oral hygiene have restored the normal appearance, showing that these gingival manifestations are dependent on oral hygiene.

purpura or lassitude) may also be seen. Topical antibiotics or chlorhexidine and improved oral hygiene may lead to regression of the swelling (Fig. 7.34).

Other features of leukaemia are discussed in Chapter 27.

Scurvy causes grossly swollen and congested gingivae, and early tooth loss. Features are described in Chapter 35.

Infections of the jaws

8

Severe infections of bone are uncommon despite the numerous pathogenic bacteria in the mouth and the easy access to the medullary cavity through tooth roots and extraction sockets. Indeed, the bone of the jaws appears remarkably resistant to osteomyelitis. Oral and perioral soft tissue infections almost always originate in teeth or periodontium and in the past particularly, but occasionally today, they can be life-threatening or fatal by direct or haematogenous spread. Infection has been considered curable for decades, but the rise of antibiotic resistance poses a threat to the population, and dentists have important roles to play in antibiotic stewardship.

The processes of frustrated healing in a periapical granuloma are described in Chapter 5. Although the periapical granuloma is normally sterile, bacteria may enter the apical tissues sporadically to seed an infection. Dental extraction is often the precipitating factor in osteomyelitis, so understanding the normal healing processes is fundamental for prevention.

NORMAL HEALING OF AN EXTRACTION SOCKET

Stages in the normal healing of a single-rooted tooth extraction socket are shown in Fig. 8.1.

The first stage of healing is the formation of a clot. Normal clotting mechanisms produce a loose clot that fills the bony and soft tissue socket. Activated platelets trigger retraction of the clot, expressing fluid so that it becomes harder and shrinks below the level of the adjacent soft tissues, pulling any mobile soft tissue inward to reduce the area of the clot exposed. Clot retraction is usually complete in 4 hours, and the surface of the clot changes from shiny to matt. After retraction, the clot continues to stabilise by fibrin cross-linking, so avoiding rinsing is usually recommended for 24 hours. A socket containing early clot is shown at the top of Fig. 8.1(A). Much of the clot (1) is bright red from trapped erythrocytes, and the periodontal ligament can still be seen around the socket periphery (2).

Lysis of the clot begins within 2 days, caused primarily by the fibrinolytic enzyme plasmin, generated by activation of plasminogen in the clot. A 2-day-old socket is shown in (B) and (C). In (B), the section is stained with haematoxylin and eosin and in (C) with a stain that shows fibrin in yellow, bone in red and the periodontal ligament in turquoise. The ligament is still sharply defined but, at higher power, the emigration of inflammatory cells into the clot would be seen. It is at this stage, when fibrinolysis has started but the clot is not well anchored to the wall, that the risk of dry socket from clot lysis or loss is highest.

At 4 days, capillaries and fibroblasts (granulation tissue) are growing into the blood clot from the periphery so that it is now firmly fixed to the socket wall. Macrophages migrate into the clot and start to demolish it ready for replacement by granulation tissue. The surface of the clot is white and porous clinically. Bacterial enzymes have lysed the surface fibrin, and there are bacteria in the superficial fibrin, which gradually disintegrates. Epithelium at the gingival margin undergoes hyperplasia and starts to grow over the intact clot, below the surface debris.

At 8 days (D), the socket is filled by granulation tissue (3) and the superficial layers contain inflammatory cells (4). The granulation tissue is soft or gelatinous and contains little collagen. It appears red if exposed ('socket granulations'). The periodontal ligament is no longer clearly identifiable. The lamina dura of the socket (5) is intact but, at higher power, osteoclasts would be seen on its surface. There is early surface resorption. Depending on the surface area of the socket mouth, epithelial migration is complete between 7 and 10 days; in this socket it is delayed and there is inflammation at the surface.

At 18 days (E), the socket is filled by granulation tissue and the fibroblasts within it have laid down a collagen network. The outline of the lamina dura is still visible (6) and woven bone is forming around the periphery of the socket. On the left, there is a thick layer of woven bone trabeculae (7) and a blue rim of cellular osteogenic tissue at the bone-forming front (8).

By 6 weeks (F), the woven bone has filled the socket and is remodelling to lamellar bone (9). The outline of the lamina dura (10) persists for a very variable length of time, depending on the bone turnover rate. By 3 months, it is usually not detectable radiographically, but socket outlines may persist for years in the elderly.

Wound healing review PMID: 20139336

ALVEOLAR OSTEITIS

Alveolar osteitis ('dry' socket) is by far the most frequent painful complication of extractions. It is not really an infection but leads to superficial bacterial contamination of exposed bone and can progress to osteomyelitis, though extremely uncommonly. Osteitis simply means inflamed bone, not infection. Alveolar osteitis develops after 1%–2% of extractions, more frequently for lower-third molar extractions.

Aetiology

Alveolar osteitis is frequently unpredictable and without any obvious predisposing cause, but numerous possible aetiological factors exist (Box 8.1).

Alveolar osteitis is more likely to follow difficult disimpactions of third molars or traumatic extractions than uncomplicated extractions. However, the blood supply to the area often appears to be the critical factor. In healthy persons, alveolar osteitis virtually only affects the lower molar region, where the bone is more dense and less vascular than elsewhere. Alveolar osteitis is also an expected complication of extractions when the alveolar bone is sclerotic, as in Paget's disease, after radiotherapy and where vascular disease causes ischaemia of the bone. Alveolar osteitis is also more

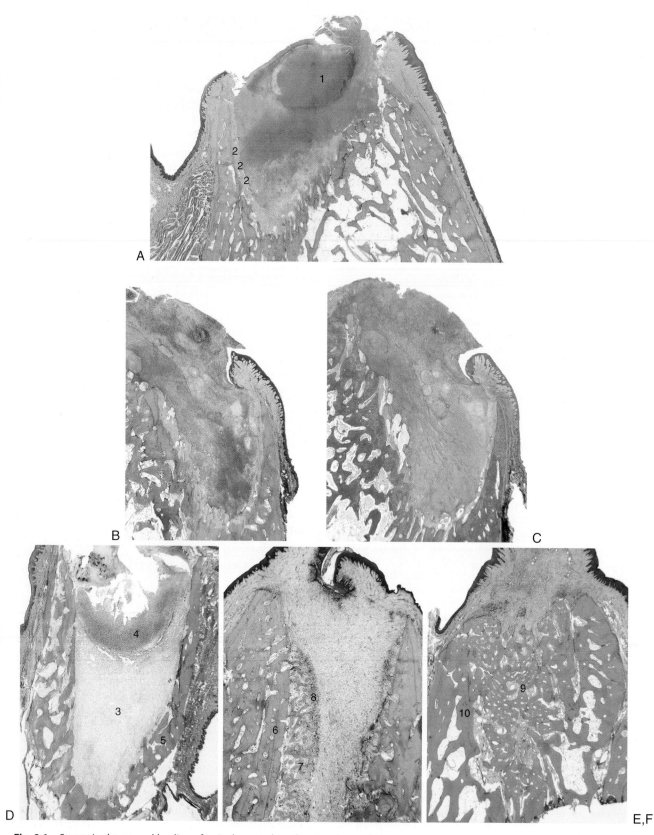

Fig. 8.1 Stages in the normal healing of a single-rooted tooth extraction socket.

Box 8.1   Predisposing factors for alveolar osteitis

- Excessive extraction trauma
- Limited local blood supply
- Gingival infection such as acute ulcerative gingivitis, pericoronitis or abscess
- Local anaesthesia with vasoconstrictor
- Smoking
- Oral contraceptives
- Osteosclerotic disease: Paget's disease, cemento-osseous dysplasia
- Radiotherapy
- History of previous dry socket

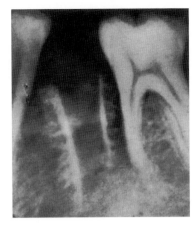

Fig. 8.3   Sequestration in a severe dry socket. Almost the whole of the lamina dura and attached trabeculae have become necrotic, forming a sequestrum. Healing is delayed while the sequestrum remains in place. Most dry sockets are not associated with sequestration, or with only small sequestra.

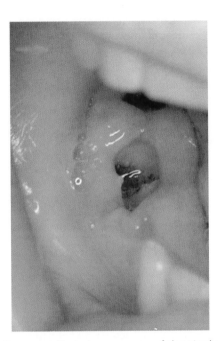

Fig. 8.2   Dry socket. Typical appearances of chronic alveolar osteitis; the socket is empty, and the bony lamina dura is visible.

frequent in susceptible patients when local anaesthesia is used, as a result of vasoconstriction.

The immediate cause is early loss of clot from the extraction socket due to excessive local fibrinolytic activity. The alveolar bone and gingiva have a high content of fibrinolysin activators (plasmin), that are released when the bone is traumatised, degrading the clot and leaving the socket empty. Once the clot has been destroyed, bacterial colonisation from the mouth is inevitable, and bacterial enzymes contribute to clot lysis.

The oestrogen component of oral contraceptives enhances serum fibrinolytic activity and interferes with clotting, and its use is associated with a higher incidence of alveolar osteitis.

Clinical features

Patients aged 20–40 years are most at risk, and women are more frequently affected. Pain usually starts a few days after the extraction, but sometimes may be delayed for a week or more. It is deep-seated, severe and aching or throbbing. The mucosa around the socket is red and tender. There is no clot in the socket, which contains, instead, saliva and often decomposing food debris (Fig. 8.2). When debris is washed

away, whitish, dead bone may be seen or may be felt as a rough area with a probe and probing is painful. The appearance of an empty socket and exposed bone is diagnostic. Sometimes the socket becomes concealed by granulations growing in from the gingival margins, narrowing the opening and trapping food debris. Pain often continues for a week or two, or occasionally longer. Sequestration of the socket wall may sometimes be seen radiographically (Fig. 8.3), but a radiograph performs no useful purpose except to exclude retention of a root fragment.

Pathology

Infected food and other debris accumulates in direct contact with the bone. Bone damaged during the extraction, particularly the dense bone of the lamina dura, dies. The necrotic bone and socket lodge bacteria which proliferate freely in the avascular spaces unhindered by host defences. In the surrounding tissue, inflammation prevents spread of infection beyond the socket walls. Dead bone is gradually separated by osteoclasts, and sequestra are usually shed in tiny fragments. Healing is slow. Granulation tissue cannot grow in from the socket walls and base until the necrotic bone is removed.

Although there is no infection within the tissues, the colonisation of the socket and sequestra by oral bacteria probably contributes to pain and slow healing. Anaerobes are thought to be significant and can produce fibrinolytic enzymes. However, antibiotics including metronidazole have not been shown to either prevent dry socket or speed healing reliably. Only chlorhexidine rinsing preoperatively has been shown to reduce incidence.

Prevention

Preventive measures are shown in Box 8.2. Because damage to bone is an important predisposing factor, extractions should be carried out with minimal trauma. Immediately after the extraction the socket edges should be squeezed firmly together and held for a few minutes until the clot has formed.

In the case of disimpactions of third molars, where alveolar osteitis is more common, prophylactic antibiotics are sometimes given. Their value is unproven, and there is no indication for using antibiotics for routine dental extractions. However, in patients who have had irradiation for oral cancer or have sclerotic bone disease, postoperative antibiotic cover should be given and the tooth removed surgically to cause as little damage as possible to surrounding bone. Antibiotics are given primarily to prevent osteomyelitis rather than dry socket.

There remain a few patients especially prone to alveolar osteitis, which follows every extraction under local anaesthesia including regional blocks. In such patients, dry socket may be preventable if general anaesthesia is used, although this is difficult to justify clinically.

Treatment

It is important to explain to patients that they may have a week or more of discomfort. It is also important to explain that the pain is not due, as patients usually think, to a broken root. Local conditions strongly favour persistence of infection, and the aim of treatment is to control symptoms until healing is complete, usually after approximately 10 days.

Treatment is to keep the open socket clean and to protect exposed bone from excessive bacterial contamination. The socket should be irrigated with mild warm antiseptic or saline to remove all food debris. Chlorhexidine must not be used; allergy to chlorhexidine in this situation can be fatal. It is then traditional to place a dressing into the socket to deliver analgesia and close the opening so that further food debris cannot enter the socket. Many socket dressings have been formulated and should be antiseptic, obtundent, adhere to the socket wall, and be absorbable. Whatever is used, the minimum dressing to close the socket opening is used because dressing packed hard into the socket will delay healing. Non-absorbable dressings must be removed as soon as possible to allow the socket to heal. A dressing may only last 1–2 days, and the whole process needs repeating until pain subsides, normally after one or two dressings. Frequent hot saline mouthwashes also help keep the socket free from debris.

Key features of alveolar osteitis are summarised in Box 8.3.

Dry socket review PMID: 18755610 and 12190139

OSTEOMYELITIS OF THE JAWS

Unlike the long bones, osteomyelitis in the jaws is almost always of local origin and not caused by blood-borne infection. The classification of osteomyelitis is somewhat confusing, with a range of overlapping conditions. Their names are more descriptions of their clinical presentation based on the chronicity of the infection and effects on the bone.

There are no strict definitions, and not all cases can be easily categorised.

Syphilitic, actinomycotic and tuberculous osteomyelitis of the jaws are distinct entities, but largely of historical interest.

ACUTE OSTEOMYELITIS

→ Summary charts 5.1 and 13.1 pp. 79, 222

In acute osteomyelitis bacteria and inflammation spread through the medullary bone from a focus of infection.

By far the most common cause is spread of infection from a periapical infection, but there are other potential sources of infection (Box 8.4). The jaws are resistant to osteomyelitis, and most patients have a predisposing cause. These may be local factors, usually causing sclerosis and reducing the vascularity of the bone, or systemic predispositions to infection. The most important are summarised in Box 8.5.

The effect of immunodeficiency is variable, and acute osteomyelitis of the jaw is uncommon in HIV infection.

Clinical features

Most patients with osteomyelitis are adult males, who have more dental infections than females. Almost all cases affect the mandible, which is less vascular than the maxilla.

Early complaints are severe, throbbing, deep-seated pain and swelling with external swelling due to inflammatory oedema. Later, distension of the periosteum with pus and, finally, subperiosteal bone formation cause the swelling to become firm. The overlying gingiva and mucosa is red, swollen and tender.

Associated teeth are tender. They may become loose, and pus may exude from an open socket or gingival margins. Muscle oedema causes difficulty in opening the mouth and swallowing. Regional lymph nodes are enlarged and tender and anaesthesia or paraesthesia of the lower lip, caused by pressure on the inferior dental nerve, is characteristic.

Box 8.5 Important predisposing conditions for osteomyelitis

Local damage to or disease of the jaws

- Radiation damage
- Causes of osteosclerosis
  - Paget's disease
  - Fibro-osseous lesions, particularly cemento-osseous dysplasia
  - Osteopetrosis

Impaired immune defences

- Poorly controlled diabetes mellitus
- Sickle cell anaemia
- Chronic alcoholism or malnutrition
- Drug abuse
- Tobacco smoking
- Malignant neoplasms and their treatment

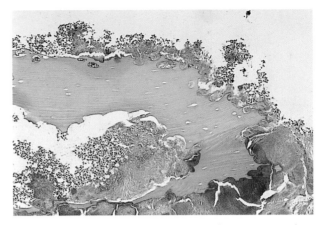

Fig. 8.5 High-power view of a sequestrum showing non-vital bone (the osteocyte lacunae are empty) and eroded outline with superficial lacunae, produced by osteoclastic resorption, and a dense surface growth of bacteria.

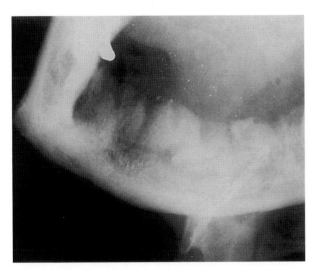

Fig. 8.4 Osteomyelitis of the mandible following dental extractions. The outlines of the extraction sockets can be seen, together with dense sequestra of bone lying in a poorly circumscribed radiolucency.

Frequently, the patient remains surprisingly well but, in the acute phase, there may be fever and leucocytosis.

Radiographic changes do not appear until after at least 10 days, and radiographs can provide little useful information before this time except to identify a local predisposing cause. Later, there is loss of trabecular pattern and areas of radiolucency indicating bone destruction and sometimes widening of periodontal ligament. Affected areas have ill-defined margins and a moth-eaten appearance similar to a malignant neoplasm (Fig. 8.4). Areas of dead bone appear as relatively dense areas which become more sharply defined as they are progressively separated as sequestra. Later, in young persons particularly, subperiosteal new bone formation causes a buccal swelling and appears as a thin, curved strip of new bone below the lower border of the jaw in lateral or panoramic radiographs.

Osteomyelitis of the newborn is a distinctive variant affecting the maxilla shortly after birth and is potentially fatal. The cause is either birth injuries or uncontrolled middle ear infection. Other than in children, the maxilla is very rarely affected.

Osteomyelitis of newborn PMID: 15125285

Pathology

Acute osteomyelitis is a suppurative infection with a mixed bacterial flora, much of which forms a biofilm on sequestra of bone. Oral bacteria, particularly anaerobes such as *Bacteroides*, *Porphyromonas* or *Prevotella* species, are important causes. Staphylococci may be responsible when osteomyelitis follows an open fracture and the bacteria enter from the skin.

The mandible has a relatively limited blood supply and dense bone with thick cortical plates. Infection and acute inflammation cannot escape, and the pressure spreads infection through the marrow spaces. It also compresses blood vessels confined within the rigid boundaries of the vascular canals. Thrombosis and obstruction then lead to further bone necrosis. Dead bone is recognisable microscopically by lacunae empty of osteocytes and medullary spaces filled with neutrophils and colonies of bacteria that proliferate in the dead tissue (Fig. 8.5).

Pus, formed by liquefaction of necrotic soft tissue and inflammatory cells, is forced along the medulla and eventually penetrates the cortex to reach the subperiosteal region by resorption of bone. Distension of the periosteum by pus stimulates subperiosteal bone formation, but perforation of the periosteum by pus and formation of sinuses on the skin or oral mucosa are rarely seen in developed countries and after effective treatment.

At the boundaries between infected and healthy tissue, osteoclasts resorb the periphery of the dead bone, which eventually becomes separated as a sequestrum (Fig. 8.6). Once infection starts to localise, new bone forms around it, particularly subperiosteally.

Where bone has died and been removed or shed as sequestra, healing is by granulation tissue with formation of woven bone in the proliferating connective tissue. After resolution, woven bone is gradually replaced by compact bone and remodelled to restore normal morphology.

Osteomyelitis early diagnosis PMID: 21982609

Management

The key factor is to assess whether the infection is limited to the jaws or may be spreading systemically. A severely ill or very pale patient and a very high temperature suggest possible systemic spread and indicate a need to check for an underlying predisposing disease and consider blood

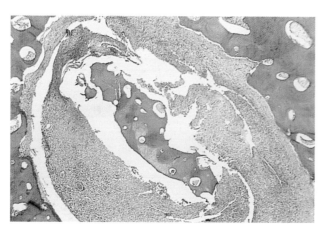

Fig. 8.6 Late-stage chronic osteomyelitis. A sequestrum trapped in a cavity within the bone. It is surrounded by fibrous tissue containing an infiltrate of inflammatory cells. Surgical intervention is needed to remove an infected sequestrum such as this.

Box 8.6   Summary of management of acute osteomyelitis

Essential measures

- Bacterial sampling and culture
- Vigorous (empirical) antibiotic treatment
- Drainage
- Analgesics
- Give specific antibiotics once culture and sensitivities are available
- Debridement
- Remove source of infection, if possible

Adjunctive treatment

- Sequestrectomy
- Decortication if necessary
- Resection and reconstruction for extensive bone destruction

---

culture to exclude septicaemia. The main requirements are summarised in Box 8.6.

Bacteriological diagnosis   A specimen of pus or a swab from the depths of the lesion must first be taken for culture and sensitivity testing, ideally by using an anaerobic sampling technique.

Antimicrobial treatment   Immediately after a specimen has been obtained, vigorous antibiotic treatment should be started. Initially, penicillin, 600–1200 mg daily can be given by injection (if the patient is not allergic), with metronidazole 200–400 mg every 8 hours. Clindamycin penetrates avascular tissue better and is frequently effective. The regimen is adjusted later in the light of the bacteriological findings.

Debridement   Removal of foreign or necrotic material and immobilisation of any fracture are necessary if there has been a gunshot wound or other contaminating injury.

Drainage   Pressure should be relieved by tooth extraction. Local analgesia is usually impossible in the presence of acute infection, but the earlier any causative tooth can be removed the better. Drainage may be achievable through the root canal as a temporary measure. If so, it may be possible to retain and restore the tooth at a later date. Alternatively bur holes through the cortex or decortication, as

---

Box 8.7   Acute osteomyelitis of the jaws: key features

- Mandible mainly affected, usually in adult males
- Infection of dental origin; anaerobes are important
- Pain and swelling of jaw
- Teeth in the area are tender: gingivae are red and swollen
- Sometimes paraesthesia of the lip
- Minimal systemic upset
- After about 10 days, radiographs show moth-eaten pattern of bone destruction
- Good response to prompt antibiotic treatment and debridement

---

necessary, allow the exudate to drain out into the mouth or externally, reducing the pressure and preventing infection from being pushed further through the medullary bone. Such surgical drainage is rarely used now that high-dose and high-potency antibiotic regimes are available.

Removal of sequestra   Dead bone should not be forcibly separated, and vigorous curetting is inadvisable but, in the late stages, a loosened sequestrum may have to be removed. Teeth should be extracted only if loosened by tissue destruction. With effective antibiotic treatment, areas of non-vial bone may not sequestrate and will be incorporated back into the healing bone. However, sequestra colonised by a bacterial biofilm will always eventually be shed.

Adjunctive treatment   Decortication or hyperbaric oxygen therapy, or both, may be attempted, particularly in radiation-associated osteomyelitis, although the effectiveness of hyperbaric oxygen is unproven. However, these are usually performed for chronic disease after other measures have failed.

Complications and resolution

Acute osteomyelitis usually resolves fully following aggressive treatment. Anaesthesia of the lower lip usually recovers with elimination of the infection. Rare complications include pathological fracture caused by extensive bone destruction, chronic osteomyelitis after inadequate treatment, cellulitis due to spread of exceptionally virulent bacteria or septicaemia in an immunodeficient patient.

Key features of acute osteomyelitis of the jaws are summarised in Box 8.7.

Review treatment PMID: 8229407

CHRONIC OSTEOMYELITIS → Summary charts 5.1 and 13.1 pp. 79, 222

Chronic osteomyelitis is much more common than acute osteomyelitis and arises from infection by weakly virulent bacteria or in avascular bone. Most cases develop without a prior acute phase, and only rarely does acute osteomyelitis lead to chronic osteomyelitis. When it does, it usually follows inadequate treatment.

Like the acute condition, there are usually predisposing factors such as those listed in Box 8.5. However, local bone sclerosis or irradiation are factors much more likely to predispose to chronic osteomyelitis than acute.

Clinical features

The picture is often dominated by persistent ache or pain, often relapsing, during a long period with a bad taste from

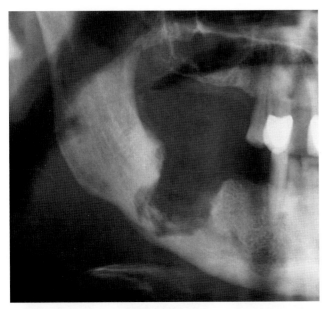

Fig. 8.7   Chronic osteomyelitis. The extent of destruction is much more readily apparent than in acute osteomyelitis. Note the sequestra lying close to the lower border and the peripheral sclerosis. A slight convexity of subperiosteal new bone formation is evident below the lower border.

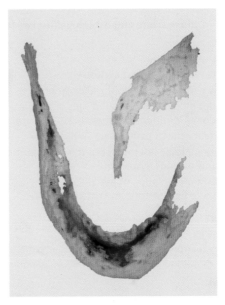

Fig. 8.8   Sequestration of the entire mandible following chronic osteomyelitis of odontogenic origin.

pus draining to the mouth through sinuses. In more active phases there is swelling, increased pain and discharge, and increased tooth mobility. There may be exposed bone. Initially the original focus of infection can be identified, but chronic osteomyelitis may persist after its removal and the chronic infection becomes self-perpetuating in the bone.

Radiographic appearances are variable but sometimes distinctive (Fig. 8.7) with patchy and poorly defined radiolucency and sclerosis, sometimes resembling a malignant neoplasm. Sequestra may be identified, and there may be a periosteal new bone layer (see proliferative periostitis later in this chapter).

Pathology

Chronic osteomyelitis is a suppurative infection, but suppuration is generally limited and may cease in quiescent periods.

Persistent low-grade infection is associated with chronic inflammation, activation of osteoclastic bone destruction and granulation tissue formation. Healing is frustrated by inability of the inflammation and immune response to access bacteria in dead avascular bone and by the slow separation of dead bone as sequestra. Sequestra will usually separate spontaneously during months or years and may be several centimetres in length. If antibiotic treatment is effective, sequestra may be sterilised and become reincorporated into healing bone. Conversely, infection may spread widely through abnormal bone or in a debilitated host but never develop the florid features of acute osteomyelitis (Fig. 8.8).

Chronic osteomyelitis is resistant to treatment and must be treated aggressively to overcome the factors noted previously that favour persistence of infection. The source of infection must be removed. Prolonged antibiotic treatment is the mainstay of treatment and must continue for at least 6 weeks and be tailored to the sensitivity of the microorganisms. If sequestra are large, they must be removed surgically, and ideally all non-vital bone should be removed. Sometimes this requires corticectomy, which has the added

> **Box 8.8   Chronic osteomyelitis of the jaws: key features**
> - Mandible mainly affected
> - Infection of dental origin
> - Low-grade pain
> - Sclerosis or avascular bone often a predisposing factor
> - Resistant to treatment
> - Prolonged antibiotic treatment required
> - Role for surgery to remove sequestra and sclerotic bone

advantage of opening the bone to healing from the periosteum. Thus, surgical intervention plays a much greater role in chronic than acute osteomyelitis. The response is slow, and antibiotics may be required for several months. If infection persists despite treatment, implantation of antibiotic-impregnated plastic beads provides a local slow release of antibiotic in high concentrations.

Key features of chronic osteomyelitis are shown in Box 8.8

DIFFUSE SCLEROSING OSTEOMYELITIS

This is an even lower intensity of infection, without formation of pus, in which low-virulence organisms or repeated inadequate antibiotic treatment may lead to longstanding widespread osteomyelitis. The presence of infection is not obvious, and chronic low-level dull pain and swelling are often not severe enough to immediately suggest osteomyelitis. The main features are radiographic. There is extensive patchy sclerosis of the mandible, poorly localised and without a clear focus of radiolucent infection.

Diffuse sclerosing osteomyelitis is a controversial condition. In the past it has been confused with florid cemento-osseous dysplasia, and this confusion is understandable. The radiological features are similar, and the sclerosis of cemento-osseous dysplasia predisposes to infection. Diagnosis is difficult and should only be made when it is

Box 8.9   Diffuse sclerosing osteomyelitis: key features

- Affects adults
- No sex predilection
- Affects mandible almost exclusively
- Patchy diffuse sclerosis in the alveolar process
- Changes more marked around sites of periapical or periodontal chronic inflammation
- Persistent ache or pain but no swelling
- Radiographically resembles but is distinct from florid cemento-osseous dysplasia
- May be a presentation of the SAPHO (synovitis, acne, pustulosis, hyperostosis and osteitis) syndrome

Pathology

- Bone sclerosis and remodelling
- Scanty marrow spaces and little or no inflammatory infiltrate, although adjacent to areas of inflammation

Treatment

- Elimination of originating source of inflammation, but sclerotic areas remain radiographically

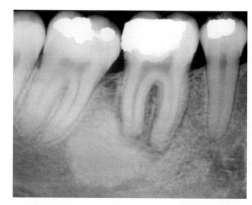

Fig. 8.9   Sclerosing osteitis. A focal zone of sclerosis associated with periapical inflammation from a non-vital lower first molar. *(Courtesy of Mr EJ Whaites.)*

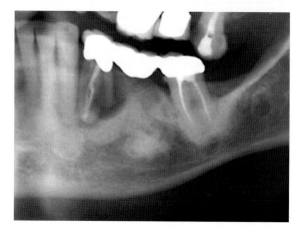

Fig. 8.10   Sclerosing osteitis. Multiple foci of sclerosis around non-vital teeth, superficially resembling florid cemento-osseous dysplasia. *(Courtesy of Professor MP Foschini.)*

clear that there is infection present and not on the basis of radiological features alone. Biopsy may confirm inflammation in medullary spaces but is best avoided because of the risk of introducing further infection into the sclerotic bone.

Some cases may be part of syndromes of 'primary chronic osteomyelitis', syndromic combinations of synovitis, acne, pustulosis, hyperostosis and osteitis (SAPHO syndrome) or its childhood form of chronic recurrent multifocal osteomyelitis (CRMO). These cause zones of patchy radiolucency and sclerosis without clinical infection. These conditions are difficult to diagnose and require specialist investigation.

It is not always clear whether the presentation is infectious at all. It has been suggested that the condition is due to tendon and periosteal inflammation rather than infection.

Treatment is to deal with any possible foci of infection with local measures and antibiotics. The key features of diffuse sclerosing osteomyelitis are shown in Box 8.9.

Review of causes PMID: 3171740

SAPHO syndrome PMID: 24237723

Tendoperiostitis PMID: 1437057

CHRONIC LOW-GRADE FOCAL OSTEOMYELITIS AND SCLEROSING OSTEITIS → Summary charts 5.1, 13.1 and 12.2 pp. 79, 222, 203

In some cases, a focus of osteomyelitis is so small or caused by such low-virulence organisms that the clinical presentation is dominated by the local bone reaction to the infection rather than the infection itself. Focal sclerosing osteomyelitis is commoner in the young because their bone is better vascularised and produces more reactive bone deposition around the infection. Suppuration and widespread infiltration of marrow spaces by inflammatory cells are absent, and bacteria are not readily cultivable. The key feature is a poorly defined zone of bony sclerosis. Centrally there is a nidus of infection, but it can be impossible to see it on plain

radiographs, although it may be visualised on cone beam computed tomography (CT).

Sclerosing osteitis is a term given to a localised area of sclerosis without evidence of infection. These are probably a reaction to inflammation rather than infection and are frequently seen around the roots of non-vital teeth (Fig. 8.9), if multiple resembling lesions of cemento-osseous dysplasia (Fig. 8.10). No treatment is required for the bone, but the causative tooth will usually prove to be non-vital and may be extracted or root-filled.

Key features of sclerosing osteomyelitis are listed in Box 8.10.

Sclerosing osteitis PMID: 23880262

OSTEORADIONECROSIS

When the predisposing cause for any type of osteomyelitis is radiotherapy, the condition is called *osteoradionecrosis*. Radiotherapy induces endarteritis of vessels causing a marked reduction in bone vascularity, inhibiting an effective host response to infection and reducing the sclerotic response to infection. The risk of osteoradionecrosis rises with the radiation dose. At the normal doses of radical radiotherapy given for most oral carcinomas, approximately 60–65 Gy, approximately 5% of patients may suffer this distressing complication. Only directly irradiated bone is at

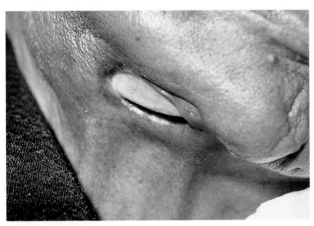

Fig. 8.11   Chronic osteomyelitis secondary to radiotherapy. Part of the necrotic portion of the mandible is visible, having ulcerated through the skin.

risk, and it is almost always the mandible affected, following irradiation of oral or major salivary gland cancers.

The causative bacteria are oral flora and periodontal pathogens, which gain entry to the bone after minor trauma, dental infection or tooth extraction. The mucosa is atrophic and heals poorly after radiotherapy. Infection spreads rapidly and is difficult to treat. The clinical and radiographic features are those of chronic osteomyelitis (see Fig. 8.11) except that healing is impaired, sequestra separate much more slowly and there is no periosteal reaction. The course is often prolonged, and surgical intervention and aggressive antibiotic therapy are usually required. Pentoxifylline, a tumor necrosis factor antagonist, and hyperbaric oxygen are claimed to aid healing, but results are variable and the latter is very expensive and not widely available. Unfortunately treatment is not always successful, and low-grade grumbling osteomyelitis may persist for the rest of a patient's life.

Prevention is key, and the dentist plays an important role (Box 8.11).

Treatment PMID: 23108891

Risk of development PMID: 22669065

Prevention after extraction PMID: 21115324

PROLIFERATIVE PERIOSTITIS

Proliferative periostitis is not an infection, but a response to it. Inflammation or infection causes the periosteum of the surrounding bone to become active and lay down layers of new bone around the cortex as a healing response. This new bone is rapidly formed and less well-mineralised than the normal cortex and may expand the bone by up to a centimetre or more in thickness. The process is intermittent, producing multiple layers that can be seen radiographically as 'onion-skinning'.

The ability to produce large amounts of periosteal new bone is more or less limited to children and adolescents. In older patients it forms more slowly and during a longer period. Chronic osteomyelitis in children and adolescents is often dominated by the periosteal reaction, which can be florid enough to cause facial asymmetry.

Proliferative periostitis develops over malignant neoplasms and foci of osteomyelitis, so the underlying cause must be identified. When it is osteomyelitis, vague pain is typical, and the focus of infection or a small sequestrum may only be detected on cone beam CT.

Key features are listed in Box 8.12.

Clinical description PMID: 289735

Signs and causes PMID: 9768431

MEDICATION-RELATED OSTEONECROSIS OF THE JAWS (MRONJ)

Previously called *bisphosphonate-related osteonecrosis*, this condition is now known to be induced by a variety of drugs that inhibit either osteoclast activity or angiogenesis. It is also known as *antiresorptive-related osteonecrosis* (Box 8.13).

The majority of patients affected are elderly and have metastatic malignant disease because this is the main indication for the causative drugs (Box 8.14). Steroid use and smoking can also contribute.

Bisphosphonates are prescribed to prevent osteoclastic bone resorption and thus the enlargement of bony metastases and development of pathological fractures. The drugs are concentrated in osteoclasts and bound into bone matrix

Box 8.12   Proliferative periostitis key features

- Children and adolescents mainly affected
- Usually associated with periapical but sometimes other inflammatory foci
- Periosteal reaction affecting lower border of mandible causing 'onion skin' thickening and swelling of bone
- Sometimes incorrectly called Garrè's osteomyelitis*

Pathology

- Parallel layers of highly cellular woven bone interspersed with scantily inflamed connective tissue
- Small sequestra sometimes present

Treatment

- Eliminate focus of infection
- Bone gradually remodels after 6–12 months

*Garrè's (note correct accent and spelling) osteomyelitis is a misnomer. In his original description he made no mention of proliferative changes in the lesion, X-rays had not then been invented, and he provided no histological back-up. This historic term has no place in current usage. Reference PMID: 3041342

Box 8.13   Drugs associated with jaw osteonecrosis

- Antiresoptive
  - Bisphosphonates
    Alendronate
    Pamidronate
    Risendronate
    Zolendronate
    And other high potency types
  - Denosumab (antibody RANKL inhibitor)
- Antiangiogenic
  - Tyrosine kinase inhibitors
    Sorafenib
    Sunitinib
  - Bevacizumab (vascular endothelial growth factor inhibitor)
  - Rapamycin (mTOR [mechanistic target of rapamycin] inhibitor)

Box 8.14   Risk factors for bisphosphonate-induced osteonecrosis

- Intravenous high-dose bisphosphonate treatment usually for bone metastases or hypercalcaemia of malignancy
- Immunosuppression from chemotherapy or steroids
- Anaemia
- Dental surgery or sepsis, ill-fitting dentures and poor oral hygiene
- Female patients
- Elderly patients
- Smoking

by osteoblasts, where they remain active in bone for many years, being slowly released on bone turnover*. The osteoclast inhibition also delays bone healing.

Osteonecrosis is associated with the most potent bisphosphonates administered intravenously, and oral doses for osteoporosis carry a much lower risk. Exactly why bisphosphonates cause areas of bone to become non-vital is unclear. It has been thought that the drugs cause sterile necrosis, which then becomes infected. However, it is also possible that the effect is an osteomyelitis from the outset, modified by reduced healing capacity of the bone. The jaws are particularly at risk because of their poor blood supply in the elderly, potential foci of dental infection and covering of thin easily traumatised mucosa, but other bones have been affected.

Bisphosphonates inhibit osteoclasts and also inhibit angiogenesis and are frequently used to treat metastases to bone, particularly from multiple myeloma, breast and prostate carcinoma. This is highly effective, constraining growth of metastases and inhibiting pathological fractures and their consequences, particularly nerve injury from spinal collapse. Risk is associated with high-potency bisphosphonates such as alendronate, pamidronate and zoledronate, especially when administered long term and in high doses intravenously. Osteonecrosis affects approximately 1% of patients on these regimes, although occasional cases have also been reported following oral administration for osteoporosis. The risk of developing MRONJ following a single extraction in a patient who has had intravenous high potency bisphosphonates is 0.5%.

In two-thirds of patients a dental extraction is the precipitating factor, and in most of the remainder there is no identifiable trigger. A striking presentation is painless exposed bone (Figs 8.12 and 8.13); some patients may experience no acute symptoms or infection for prolonged periods. Once infection is introduced, the condition develops into acute or chronic osteomyelitis depending on the virulence of the organism and resistance of the patient. The drugs cause reduced bone turnover so that sequestra of necrotic bone separate very slowly and healing is inhibited. Later complications can include oroantral and cutaneous fistulas with suppuration.

The organisms colonising the dead bone are a mixed flora of oral bacteria in a biofilm. Common species are *Actinomyces*, streptococci, *Serratia*, and enterococci, and facultative anaerobes predominate. As noted previously, it is unclear whether infection or necrosis is the primary disease process.

Review PMID: 16243172 and 20508948

Management

Prevention of infection is paramount. Potential problems should be eliminated before bisphosphonate treatment, infective foci eliminated and teeth of dubious prognosis removed. Some authorities also suggest removal of tori and sharp ridges if prone to denture trauma.

*Bisphosphonate-induced osteonecrosis resembles the toxic necrosis of bone called *phossy jaw*, a scourge of match factory workers in Victorian times who ingested white phosphorus (P_4). They frequently died or lost a whole jaw from osteonecrosis. Public outrage and a famous strike in East London forced improvements in factory conditions and the introduction of the (slightly) safer red phosphorus match. Both white phosphorus and the two phosphonate groups in bisphosphonate drugs mimic pyrophosphate and act as inhibitors of enzymes that act on it.

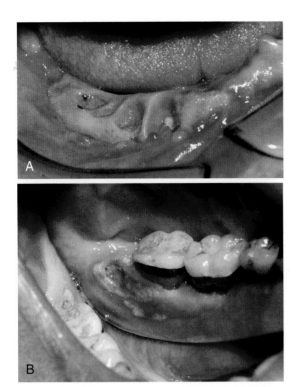

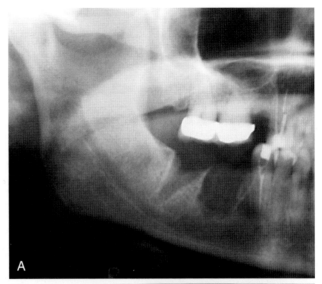

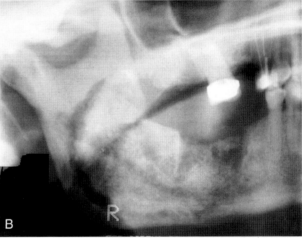

Fig. 8.12 **Exposed necrotic bone in bisphosphonate-induced osteonecrosis, (A) following extraction and (B) apparently spontaneous.** Despite exposure of large areas of necrotic bone, there is no overt infection in these early lesions. *(From Ruggiero, S.L., Fantasia, J., Carlson, E. 2006. Bisphosphonate-related osteonecrosis of the jaw: background and guidelines for diagnosis, staging and management. Oral surg oral med oral pathol oral radiol 102, pp. 433–441.)*

After drug treatment, patients at risk are identified through their medical history. Additional predisposing factors will help gauge their risk (Box 8.5). Caries and periodontitis must be controlled. Ideally, all surgical dentistry should be avoided for as long as possible after drug administration. There is a role for attempting what might otherwise be considered heroic restorations and endodontics to avoid extractions. If extractions cannot be delayed, they are probably best followed by postoperative antibiotics and chlorhexidine rinses until the sockets are fully epithelialised. Unfortunately, these precautions are not always successful, and sometimes extraction of a tooth reveals an apparently already non-vital socket that does not bleed. Discontinuation of the bisphosphonates either before extractions or long term does not appear to help because their effects last at least a year after administration and may be permanent.

Management of established MRONJ is largely empirical. There is no reproducibly successful treatment, and the aim is to manage pain and favour the very slow healing that will take place if infection can be controlled. When bone is exposed but symptoms are minimal, long-term chlorhexidine mouth rinses reduce pain and the risk of infection. Attempts to remove necrotic bone surgically usually worsen the condition, and sequestra should only be removed when mobile. Uncomfortable sharp edges may be reduced with a bur. If there is infection or soft tissue swelling, aggressive and long-term antibiotic therapy based on the results of antibiotic culture and sensitivity is required to restore a stable chronic condition that can be controlled with topical treatments. If infection cannot be controlled, then more aggressive antibiotic regimes combined with surgery may be necessary. Severe complications including extraoral sinuses

Fig. 8.13 **Bisphosphonate-induced osteonecrosis.** Non-healing extraction sockets in a breast cancer patient receiving bisphosphonate treatment. (A) There are minimal changes initially, but 12 months later, (B) there is a large sequestrum still incompletely separated extending from the premolar region, just above the lower border cortex and involving most of the ramus. *(From Ruggiero, S.L., Fantasia, J., Carlson, E. 2006. Bisphosphonate-related osteonecrosis of the jaw: background and guidelines for diagnosis, staging and management. Oral surg oral med oral pathol oral radiol 102, pp. 433–441.)*

and pathological fractures may require surgical intervention. Many patients remain surprisingly asymptomatic, but managing pain may require potent analgesics in the short term.

Management PMID: 25234529

Management Cochrane DOI: 10.1002/14651858.CD008455 .pub2

TRAUMATIC SEQUESTRUM

This is a rare but well-described oddity that often causes confusion in clinical diagnosis. It is also known as mylohyoid ridge sequestrum because the most common site is on the posterior part of a sharp mylohyoid ridge, inferior to the third molar (Fig. 8.14). Here the mucosa is thin and prone to trauma, and a traumatic ulcer can lead to devitalisation of a small area of the underlying cortical bone. This slows ulcer healing, but the dead bone eventually separates and the ulcer heals spontaneously. The sequestrum is usually only 1–2 mm in size. Mandibular tori may be similarly affected.

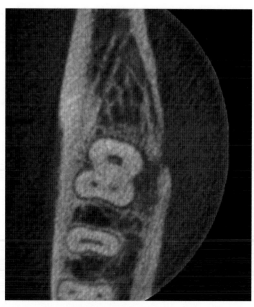

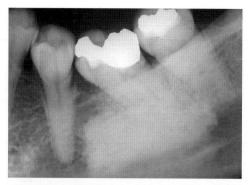

Fig. 8.15 **Sclerotic bone island in the posterior mandible, a relatively dense example.** The periphery may be sharply or less well-defined. *(Courtesy Mr EJ Whaites.)*

Fig. 8.14 **Traumatic sequestration.** Cone beam computed tomography axial view through lower molars showing loss of a small fragment of cortical bone lingual to the distal root of the last molar, caused by sequestration following trauma to the posterior edge of the mylohyoid ridge.

No treatment may be required. Once the sequestrum is loose, it may be removed to speed healing.

Case series PMID: 8515988

SCLEROTIC BONE ISLANDS

These areas of sclerosis, also known as *dense bone islands*, *enostoses* or *idiopathic osteosclerosis*, are found in all bones including the jaws. They are sometimes seen by chance in routine, particularly panoramic, radiographs (Fig. 8.15). They appear to be a normal anatomical variant and should not be mistaken for a low-grade bone infection (particularly if first noticed after a surgical procedure). They resemble sclerosing osteitis but are not associated with a focus of infection or inflammation. Histologically, they comprise an island of normal but dense cortical bone within the medullary cavity.

Operative interference should be avoided. Repeat radiographic follow up will confirm the diagnosis as the appearance will not change.

Large case series PMID: 21912499

Major infections of the mouth and face 9

Although there are many types of facial infection, the vast majority are odontogenic, that is, they arise by spread of infection from a tooth or the periodontium.

PERIAPICAL (DENTOALVEOLAR) ABSCESS

Usually a non-vital pulp produces no more consequence than an asymptomatic and sterile periapical granuloma. Untreated, these may produce intermittent pain in periods of acute inflammation and persist as chronic inflammation with periods of exacerbation of symptoms. However, infection may eventually develop into an acute periapical infection with abscess formation.

In an abscess, bacteria cause localised tissue necrosis, and pus forms by the action of neutrophil proteolytic enzymes. The process is localised by granulation tissue forming the abscess wall. The surrounding soft tissues become oedematous with inflammatory exudate. Once an apical abscess is established, it is unlikely to resolve spontaneously.

It might be expected that the infection and oedema would spread through the path of least resistance into medullary bone and cause osteomyelitis, but this is unusual. For reasons that are not clear, the exudate usually tracks toward the adjacent cortex and perforates it, through the action of osteoclasts activated by the inflammation, and drains into the mouth.

The oedema in the periodontal ligament causes slight extrusion of the tooth, which comes into premature occlusion, is painful on biting and tender to percussion. There is throbbing intense pain, distinct from the sharp excruciating pain of any acute pulpitis that preceded pulp necrosis. Drainage of pus and exudate into the mouth, usually through the alveolar mucosa or gingiva, releases pressure, and the pain reduces to a dull ache.

The regional lymph nodes may be enlarged and tender, but systemic symptoms are usually slight or absent.

Apical abscesses are polymicrobial infections and frequent cultivable isolates include *Veillonella*, *Porphyromonas*, *Streptococcus*, *Fusobacterium* and *Actinomyces* species. Despite the mixed nature of the infection, penicillins remain the most effective antibiotics, with metronidazole reserved for those allergic to penicillin. However, an apical abscess cannot be treated by antibiotics alone; the causative tooth or its pulp must be dealt with because bacteria in the pulp chamber are inaccessible to the drug. Local dental treatment is usually effective without the addition of antibiotics.

Review and sequelae PMID: 21602052

COLLATERAL OEDEMA

Even while the infection is limited to the bone, and continuing after it drains intraorally, there is oedema of the adjacent soft tissues (Fig. 9.1). Oedema is a purely inflammatory reaction, and the swollen tissues contain no bacteria. In children oedema is very prominent and gives the impression of cellulitis of the face, but the oedema is soft, unlike the firm brawny swelling of spreading infection, and there is no pyrexia. No specific treatment is required for a face enlarged by oedema. It resolves quickly when the causative tooth is dealt with.

'FASCIAL' OR TISSUE SPACE INFECTIONS

When pus from an apical abscess or pericoronitis breaks out into soft tissue, its path is guided by muscle attachments and fascia. These can divert the path of drainage away from the mouth into the tissues of the face, where pus and spreading infection can localise in the 'fascial spaces'. Anatomical descriptions of these spaces imply that fascia is a well-organised fibrous sheet dividing the face and neck into defined compartments and spaces. In reality, there are no spaces, but the inflammation and infection tend to localise reproducibly in tissue planes bounded by subcutaneous tissue, the masticatory muscles and muscles of the neck and the carotid sheath (Box 9.1). The fascial spaces are only potential spaces enlarged by accumulation of exudate or pus. Because the spaces have a large volume, pressure in the exudate is reduced, and it tends to accumulate rather than burrow onward to the surface. When the space is distended, its blood supply is disrupted, and the environment becomes avascular and anaerobic, favouring infection and inhibiting host defences.

Nature of fascial spaces PMID: 23913739

Health services implications PMID: 22819453

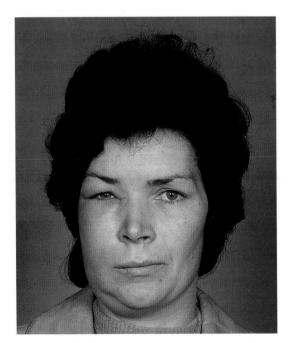

Fig. 9.1 **Oedema due to acute apical periodontitis.** An acute periapical infection of a canine has perforated the buccal plate of bone causing oedema of the face; this quickly subsided when the infection was treated.

The fascial spaces extend from the base of the skull to the mediastinum, and the inflammatory exudate acts as a vehicle to spread the infection into potentially life-threatening sites. The large volume of exudate and bacterial load produce pyrexia, toxaemia and symptoms of pain and trismus. There is a risk of spread to remote sites through lymphatics or blood vessels.

Once an infection penetrates into the tissue planes, it may spread or become localised depending on the causative bacteria and the resistance of the host. Infection from teeth tends to localise reproducibly in the spaces listed in Table 9.1, but it will be noted that these spaces intercommunicate and infection may involve several of them (Figs 9.2 and 9.3).

> **Box 9.1   The main structures directing spread of infection in the face and neck**
>
> - Muscles
>   - Buccinator
>   - Mylohyoid
>   - Masseter
>   - Medial pterygoid
>   - Superior constrictor of the pharynx
> - Fascia
>   - Investing layer of fascia
>   - Prevertebral fascia
>   - Pretracheal fascia
>   - Parotid fascia
>   - Carotid sheath

FACIAL CELLULITIS → Summary charts 5.1 and 34.1 pp. 79, 461

The great majority of fascial space infections are in the form of cellulitis in which, unlike a localised abscess, bacteria spread through the soft tissues (Fig. 9.4). Cellulitis causes gross inflammatory exudate and tissue oedema, associated with fever and toxaemia. Before the advent of antibiotics, the mortality was high. If treatment is delayed, the disease can still be life-threatening through airway compromise or erosion of the carotid sheath when the lateral pharyngeal space is involved. In Ludwig's angina particularly, airway obstruction can quickly result in asphyxia.

Table 9.1   Tissue spaces commonly involved by dental infection*

Space	Anatomy	Usual sources of infection
Submental	Between mylohyoid and the skin, platysma and investing layer of fascia. Contains the submental lymph nodes	Lower incisors
Submandibular	Between mylohyoid, and the skin, platysma and investing layer of fascia and between the hyoglossus and body of mandible. It contains the submandibular gland and submandibular lymph nodes and communicates anteriorly with the submental and posteriorly and upward into the sublingual space	Lower canine, premolar and molar teeth, when their apices lie below the mylohyoid attachment
Sublingual	Between hyoglossus and the tongue muscles medially and mylohyoid and the body of mandible laterally. Contains the sublingual gland. Communicates posteriorly with the submandibular space around the posterior free edge of the mylohyoid around the submandibular gland and duct	Lower incisor and canine teeth. Molars less frequently when apices are above the mylohyoid attachment
Buccal	Between buccinator muscle and the overlying skin, platysma and fascia. Posteriorly limited by ramus of mandible and masseter. Contains the buccal pad of fat. Communicates posteriorly with the pterygomandibular space	Usually upper molar and premolar teeth, sometimes lower molars when their apices lie below the buccinator attachment
Submasseteric	Between the lateral surface of the ramus of the mandible and the periosteum with masseter muscle	Rarely involved, usually from pericoronitis around the lower third molar
Parotid	Contains the parotid gland, bounded by superficial fascia and base of skull	Only involved by spread from other spaces
Pterygomandibular	Between the medial surface of the ramus of the mandible and the medial pterygoid muscle with the lateral pterygoid forming its roof and the parotid gland posteriorly. Contains the lingual and inferior dental nerves and communicates upward with the infratemporal fossa	Pericoronitis around distally inclined lower third molars or upper third molars
Lateral pharyngeal	Between superior constrictor with the styloid muscles and medial pterygoid or submandibular gland. Limited posteriorly by the vertebral fascia. Contains the carotid sheath, along which infection can track to the mediastinum. Anteriorly there is communication along styloglossus with the sublingual and submandibular spaces	Pericoronitis around the lower third molar (and infections in the tonsil)
Canine fossa	In the canine fossa, bounded by the muscles of lips and face	Upper lateral incisors, canines or first premolars, including periodontal abscesses
Palate	Between the mucosa with periosteum and palatal bone	Upper molars

*The canine fossa and palate are not classed as tissue spaces, but pus frequently collects at these sites.

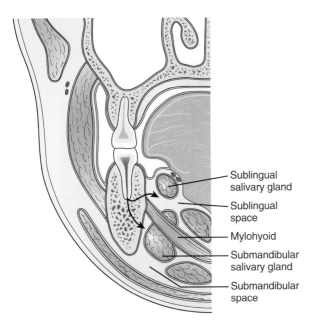

Fig. 9.2 **Paths of infection spread from lower molars.** By penetrating the lingual plate of the jaw below the attachment of mylohyoid infection immediately enters the submandibular space. Below the mylohyoid is the main body of the submandibular salivary gland with its deep process curving around the posterior border of the muscle; infection from the third molar can follow the same route to enter the sublingual space.

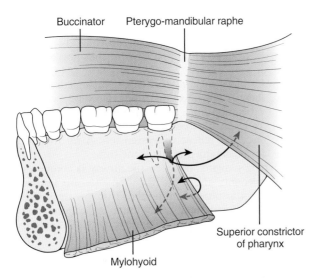

Fig. 9.3 **Paths of infection from the third molar.** The diagram shows the lingual aspect of the jaw and indicates how infection penetrating from the lingual plate of bone can enter the sublingual space above, or the submandible space below, the mylohyoid muscle, which forms the major structure of the floor of the mouth. Moreover, because this point is at the junction of the oral cavity and pharynx, infection can also spread backward to reach the lateral surface of superior constrictor, the lateral pharyngeal space.

The characteristic features are diffuse swelling, pain, fever and malaise. The swelling is tense and tender, with a characteristic board-like firmness. The overlying skin is taut and shiny. Pain and oedema limit opening the mouth and often cause dysphagia. Systemic upset is severe with worsening fever, toxaemia and leucocytosis. The regional lymph nodes are swollen and tender.

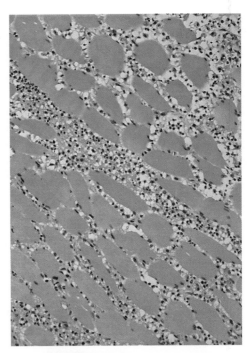

Fig. 9.4 **Cellulitis.** Infection spreading through the tissues is accompanied by a dense infiltrate of neutrophils, macrophages and fibrin exudate, here separating muscle bundles in a facial muscle. The muscle bundles are normally closely packed with minimal space between them.

Pathology

The bacterial flora is similar to the dentoalveolar abscess from which it is derived, but with a greater proportion of anaerobes such as *Porphyromonas*, *Prevotella* and *Fusobacterium* and anaerobic streptococcal species.

Infection spreads mainly from mandibular third molars, whose apices are closely related to several fascial spaces. In the early stages the infection does not localise, but after antibiotic treatment or time for a host response to develop, and depending on the organisms, small locules of pus develop scattered in the tissues.

Cellulitis, as opposed to abscess, is more frequent in patients with immunocompromise.

Ludwig's angina

Ludwig's angina* is a severe form of cellulitis that usually arises from the lower second or third molars. It involves the sublingual and submandibular spaces bilaterally, almost simultaneously, and readily spreads into the lateral pharyngeal and pterygoid spaces and can extend into the mediastinum.

The main features are rapidly spreading sublingual and submandibular cellulitis with painful, brawny swelling of the upper part of the neck and the floor of the mouth on both sides (Fig. 9.5). With involvement of the parapharyngeal space, the swelling tracks down the neck (Figs 9.6 and 9.7) and oedema can quickly spread to the glottis.

---

*Wilhelm Friedrich von Ludwig described the condition in 1836. He was physician to the royal family of King Wilhelm I, King of Prussia and the first German emperor. Although sometimes considered to have died of the condition that bears his name, this appears unlikely. PMID: 16696873

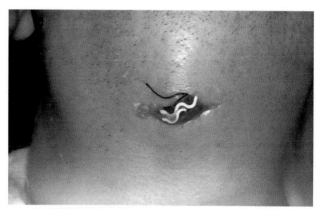

Fig. 9.5 Ludwig's angina. Incision and drainage of the front of the neck to relieve the pressure of exudate which compromises the airway. The neck is grossly swollen, shiny and dusky in hue; the edges of the wound have pulled apart, indicating the distension of these normally lax tissues.

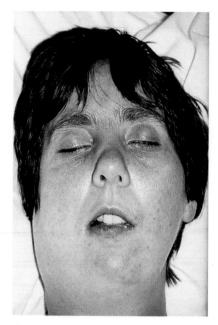

Fig. 9.7 Ludwig's angina. There is cellulitis and gross oedema of the right submandibular and sublingual spaces extending on to the left side and into the neck and parapharyngeal space. *(By kind permission of Professor JD Langdon.)*

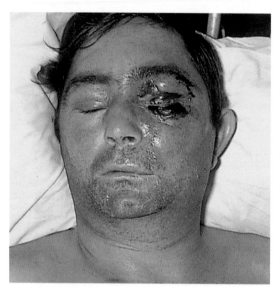

Fig. 9.6 Facial cellulitis arising from an infected upper tooth. The tissues are red, tense and shiny, and the patient is incapacitated by the systemic effects of infection. *(By kind permission of Professor JD Langdon.)*

Swallowing and opening the mouth become difficult, and the tongue may be pushed up against the soft palate. Oral obstruction or oedema of the glottis causes worsening respiratory obstruction. The patient soon becomes desperately ill, with fever, respiratory distress, headache and malaise.

Management

The principles of treatment for cellulitis are to provide immediate aggressive antibiotic treatment to prevent further spread of infection and to remove the causative tooth or deal with pericoronitis as soon as possible. Teeth with apical infection are usually removed, draining any pus localised in the bone. Teeth can sometimes be preserved by obtaining drainage through the pulp chamber, but teeth cannot be left open for more than 48 hours because this will compromise the success of subsequent root treatment, making retention pointless. For this reason, many teeth are extracted, and emphasis must be on effective drainage. Impacted teeth with pericoronitis must be dealt with after the infection has resolved because surgery cannot be performed in an infected field without risking further spread. General anaesthesia

may be required for extractions as local anaesthetic may not be effective in the inflamed tissues.

Antibiotic treatment is empirical initially with high-dose penicillins, but a sample for culture and sensitivity must be obtained before commencing treatment in case a change of antibiotic is required subsequently. Occasionally bacterial species unresponsive to first-line antibiotics are found.

Drainage plays little role in treatment of pure cellulitis because there is no collection of pus. However, when there is potential compromise of the airway or a suggestion that pus may be localising (see later in this chapter), then drains may be placed to relieve tissue tension. A microbiological sample can be obtained at the same time.

In Ludwig's angina, or when the airway is compromised by any infection, the main requirements are immediate admission to hospital, securing the airway by tracheostomy if necessary, procurement of a sample for culture and sensitivity testing, aggressive antibiotic treatment and drainage of the swelling to reduce pressure.

Key features of fascial space infections are summarised in Box 9.2.

Ludwig's in children PMID: 19286617

Fatal outcome PMID: 17828174

Airway compromise PMID: 10326823

FACIAL ABSCESS

Depending on the micro-organisms and effectiveness of host defences, pus from an apical abscess or pericoronitis may localise in the tissues to form a discrete abscess rather than spreading. Systemic signs are less marked and inflammation and swelling less extensive in abscess than in cellulitis. The collection of pus is surrounded by compressed fibrous and granulation tissue, which prevent spread but also natural drainage. Eventually an abscess will point to a surface and drain spontaneously, but this is best prevented by early intervention because formation of a sinus to the skin is usually followed by disfiguring scarring.

When pus starts to collect in the tissues, the brawny diffuse swelling of oedema and cellulitis can still be present, but a localised zone of softening develops over the pus, with a darker red zone of inflammation. Pyrexia increases. If left too long before drainage, the overlying skin becomes fluctuant just before the abscess drains spontaneously.

The principles of management of abscess are the same as for cellulitis, except that early surgical drainage of pus is essential. Small abscesses may resolve with high-dose antibiotics alone, but better and more rapid resolution will follow surgical drainage in most cases.

ANTIBIOTIC ABSCESS

The antibiotic abscess or 'antibioma' is an abscess that has been controlled but not eliminated by antibiotic treatment. This may arise after inadequate, often prolonged intermittent antibiotic treatment, particularly at insufficient dose. It may also arise from effective antibiotic treatment provided without ensuring that a collection of pus has been drained. The pus can be rendered sterile or nearly so, and the surrounding granulation tissue matures to dense scar tissue, producing a thick zone of fibrosis around the pus.

The patient has a hard mass, with puckering of the skin if superficially located, and either mild symptoms of intermittent pain and swelling or no symptoms at all. Treatment may be conservative, but resolution takes many months, and it is usually better to excise the whole mass. Drainage alone removes any residual infection, but the main signs arise from the fibrosis. Antibioma is commoner in countries where antibiotics are available without prescription.

Microbiology antibiotic choice PMID: 16916672

NECROTISING FASCIITIS → Summary chart 5.1 p. 79

Necrotising fasciitis is an uncommon, rapidly spreading, potentially lethal infection causing necrosis and rapid dissolution of subcutaneous tissues and fascia with loss of attachment of the overlying skin. Muscles are relatively spared. Rarely, the infection can have a dental source and may threaten the airway. Most patients are of middle age or older, and the majority have some kind of predisposing factor such as immunosuppression, steroid use, chronic disease or smoking.

The virulence factors of the causative organisms seem to be the key factor. Many types of bacteria, both aerobic and non-aerobic, can be responsible. Samples usually reveal mixed infections; a quarter of cases are caused by single organisms, usually Group A streptococci or staphylococci, particularly methicillin-resistant *Staphylococcus aureus*. The remainder have a mixed flora including anaerobic pathogens such as *Porphyromonas* and *Prevotella* species.

Clinically, there is initially a rapidly spreading area of erythema of the skin. The margins soon become ill defined. Thrombosis and necrosis cause the skin to become painful and oedematous, dusky red then purplish and black. Undermining of the skin causes separation from the underlying connective tissue and accumulation of subcutaneous gas, which may be visible on radiographs.

The airway may need protection by tracheostomy, and immediate admission to hospital is required. Unusually in an infection, aggressive surgery is required as soon as the condition is recognised. The extent of undermining of the skin should be explored and widely opened to drainage, debridement and for removal of necrotic tissue. Penicillin and metronidazole or clindamycin should be given empirically until bacteriological findings dictate alternatives. Hyperbaric oxygen provides additional benefit, if available.

Untreated or ineffectively treated, necrotising fasciitis proceeds to systemic spread of infection with toxic shock and death.

Case report PMID: 23821623

Microbiology and management PMID: 10760723

CAVERNOUS SINUS THROMBOSIS
→ Summary chart 5.1 p. 79

Cavernous sinus thrombosis is an uncommon life-threatening complication of infection that can sometimes originate from an upper anterior tooth, the sinuses or nose. The path of infection from the anterior teeth is to the canine space, and then by retrograde flow through the low-pressure venous system around the eye to the cavernous sinus. Infection may also spread to the cavernous sinus from the posterior aspect following infection in the infratemporal fossa, again via the venous system. Skin abscesses on the face are another source of infection.

Clinically, gross oedema of the eyelid is associated with pulsatile exophthalmos due to venous obstruction. Cyanosis, proptosis, a fixed dilated pupil and limited eye movement develop rapidly. There is pain around the eye, over the maxilla and headache with vomiting in late stages. The patient is seriously ill with rigors, a high swinging fever and deteriorating sight.

Early recognition and treatment of cavernous sinus thrombosis are essential. The main measures are use of prolonged intravenous antibiotics, drainage of pus and removal of any causative tooth. Anticoagulation is no longer used. In developed countries, aggressive antibiotic treatment has reduced the mortality to 20%, but spread to the contralateral sinus followed by meningitis or clotting in the cerebral sinuses are potentially fatal complications. Without antibiotics, almost all cases are fatal. As many as half of survivors may lose the sight of one or both eyes, even when correctly treated. Progression is often very rapid, with death in less than 24 hours if untreated.

Case report PMID: 2685213

Treatment PMID: 22326173

NOMA (CANCRUM ORIS, NECROTISING STOMATITIS)

Noma** is a severe oral infection, starting in the gingiva as acute necrotising ulcerative gingivitis and extending onto and destroying part of the jaw or face. It progresses rapidly and may be fatal if inadequately treated.

Noma is so widespread in sub-Saharan Africa as to have become a subject for a World Health Organization project, which has estimated the overall incidence in Africa to be nearly 150,000 cases a year. Smaller numbers of cases have been reported from South America and the Far East.

The main bacteria isolated are anaerobes including *Fusobacterium necrophorum*, *Prevotella intermedia* and spirochaetes. *F. necrophorum* is a commensal in the gut of herbivores and also a cause of necrotising infections in animals. It may play an important role in noma in Africa as a result of patients living in close proximity to and often sharing drinking water with cattle. The flora is often referred to as a 'fusospirochaetal complex' because no particular species alone appears to account for the disease, which is a true polymicrobial infection.

Malnutrition due to poverty and climatic disasters is the major factor in the aetiology. Other factors are poor oral hygiene and other infections, particularly measles and herpesviral diseases. Noma affects children younger than 10 years. The few cases in adults are likely to be secondary to HIV infection, but it remains a rare complication despite the immune deficiency.

Noma starts within the oral cavity from an acute necrotising ulcerative gingivitis or a painful, small, reddish-purple spot or indurated papule that ulcerates. There is extensive oedema. The infection and necrosis extend outward, rapidly destroying soft tissues and bone (Fig. 9.8). Diffuse oedema of the face, foetor and profuse salivation are associated. While the overlying tissues become ischaemic, the skin turns blue-black.

The gangrenous area becomes increasingly sharply demarcated and ultimately sloughs away. Muscle, invaded by the micro-organisms, undergoes rapid necrosis associated with only a weak inflammatory response (Fig. 9.9). The slough is cone-shaped, with its apex superficially so that the underlying destruction of hard and soft tissues is more extensive than external appearances suggest. The slough separates, the bone dies; sequestration and exfoliation of teeth follow. A gaping facial defect is left (Fig. 9.10) that heals poorly with scarring and distortion of tissues (Fig. 9.11).

Management

Malnutrition and underlying infections must be treated. A combination of penicillin or an aminoglycoside and metronidazole will usually control the local infection, but light surgical debridement of necrotic soft tissue is also needed. After control of the infection and recovery of health, reconstructive surgery is usually required to prevent permanent disfigurement. However, there is a significant mortality, almost all cases if untreated and 5%–10% if treated.

Noma mechanisms PMID: 12002813

Noma review PMID: 16829299

**Noma was first described in 1595 in Holland where, as in other parts of Europe, severe malnutrition and debilitating diseases were widespread. The term 'noma' was coined in 1680. Since then, noma has virtually disappeared from Europe.

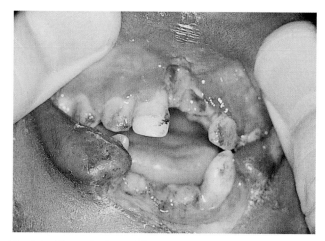

Fig. 9.8   Noma. In the maxilla there is extension of necrotising gingivitis into the alveolar process and in the lower arch anteriorly, resulting in destruction of much of the lower lip.

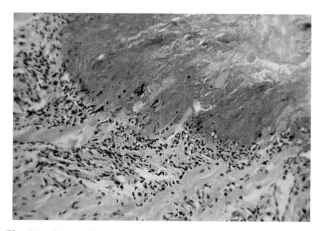

Fig. 9.9   Noma. Muscle has been invaded by spirochaetes and fusiforms. There is rapid necrosis and only a light inflammatory response of neutrophils.

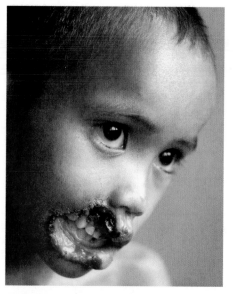

Fig. 9.10   Noma. A six-year-old child with noma extending onto the lips and cheek. *(From Srour, M.L., Wong, V., Wyllie, S. 2014. Noma, actinomycosis and nocardia. In: Farrar, J., White, N.J., Hotez, P.J., et al. eds. Manson's tropical diseases. St. Louis: Elsevier, pp. 379-384.e1.)*

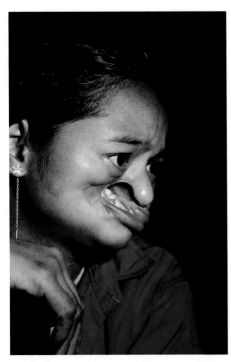

Fig. 9.11 **Noma.** A sixteen-year-old showing the long-term effects of facial tissue loss following noma at age 4 years. *(From Srour, M.L., Wong, V., Wyllie, S. 2014. Noma, actinomycosis and nocardia. In: Farrar, J., White, N.J., Hotez, P.J., et al. eds. Manson's tropical diseases. St. Louis: Elsevier, pp. 379-384.e1.)*

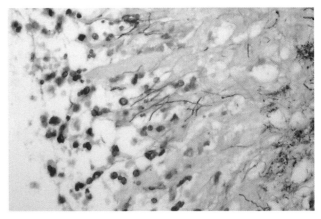

Fig. 9.12 **Actinomycosis.** Individual branching filaments of *Actinomyces* seen at high power as blue threads in the edge of this sulphur granule stained with Gram stain. The red objects on the left are inflammatory cells on the surface of the colony.

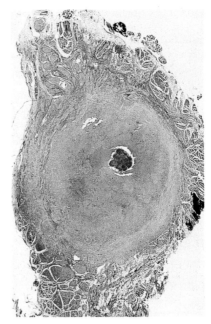

Fig. 9.13 **Actinomycosis.** This single, complete loculus was from an early case of actinomycosis that followed dental extraction. The colony of actinomyces with its paler staining periphery (a 'sulphur' granule) is in the centre; around it is a dense collection of inflammatory cells, surrounded in turn by proliferating fibrous tissue. It will be apparent that an antibiotic cannot readily penetrate such a fibrous mass and must be given in large doses to be effective.

ACTINOMYCOSIS

Actinomycosis is a chronic, suppurative infection caused by *Actinomyces sp.* Although common in the past, it has become rare. Half of all cases of actinomycosis affect the face and neck.

Clinically, men are predominantly affected, typically between the ages of 30 and 60 years. A chronic soft tissue swelling near the angle of the jaw in the upper neck is the usual complaint. In the past this would progress to a dusky-red or purplish, firm and slightly tender swelling with multiple discharging sinuses. Pain is minimal. In the absence of treatment, a large fibrotic mass can form, covered by scarred and pigmented skin, on which several sinuses open.

However, such a florid picture is rarely seen now. Currently, the usual clinical features are a persistent subcutaneous collection of pus or a sinus, unresponsive to conventional, short courses of antibiotics.

Pathology

The key microbiological signature is the presence of *Actinomyces israelii* or *Actinomyces gerencseriae* in a mixed infection with aerobic and anaerobic organisms. These are slow-growing aerobic organisms, and simple conventional cultures may only grow the accompanying organisms, usually coagulase-negative staphylococci, *S. aureus* and both α- and β-hemolytic streptococci. This may lead to a false-negative diagnosis, and pus samples for culture must be sent to the laboratory with a form indicating a suspicion of actinomycosis; otherwise the true nature of the infection may be missed.

A. israelii is a long filamentous Gram-positive bacterium, not a fungus as its name suggests. The classification of this genus of bacteria is complex, and many so-called oral *Actinomyces* are now reclassified and not thought pathogenic. However, pathogenic species can still be isolated from the mouth and are the likely source for actinomycosis of the head and neck. Injuries, especially dental extractions or fractures of the jaw, can provide a pathway and sometimes precede infection but, in fact, rarely do so. Most patients will have been previously healthy.

Actinomycosis spreads by direct extension through the tissues and does not follow tissue planes or spread to lymph nodes like other odontogenic infections. The infection is chronic and suppurative. In the tissues, colonies of *Actinomyces* form rounded colonies of filaments with peripheral, radially arranged club-shaped thickenings (Fig. 9.12). Neutrophils mass round the colonies, pus forms, chronic inflammatory cells surround the pus and an abscess wall of fibrous tissue forms (Fig. 9.13).

The abscess eventually points on the skin, discharging pus in which so-called *sulphur granules* (colonies of *Actinomyces*) may be visible with the naked eye as yellow flecks. The abscess continues to discharge, infection spreads laterally to cause further abscesses and surrounding tissues become fibrotic. Untreated, the area can become honeycombed with abscesses and sinuses, in widespread fibrosis.

Microbiology PMCID: PMC4094581

Management

Actinomycosis should be suspected if a skin sinus fails to heal after a possible focus has been found and eliminated. A fresh specimen of pus is needed. A positive diagnosis can rarely be made without 'sulphur granules', which may be found by rinsing the pus with sterile saline. The laboratory should be warned that actinomycosis is suspected to enable appropriate media to be used and the culture maintained long enough for these slow-growing organisms to be detected.

Frequently, penicillins will have been given but in doses insufficient to control the infection. This makes subsequent bacteriological diagnosis difficult. In the correct clinical setting, empirical treatment as actinomycosis is logical even if bacteriological confirmation is not forthcoming.

The mainstay of treatment is penicillin, which should be continued for a minimum of 4–6 weeks, renewed as necessary, because pockets of surviving organisms may persist in the depths of the lesion to cause relapse. Abscesses should be drained surgically as they form and sinuses excised. Combined surgical and antibiotic treatment is most effective. For patients allergic to penicillin, erythromycin can be given.

Healing leads to scarring and puckering of the skin at the sites of sinuses, and these often have to be excised for cosmetic reasons.

The key features of actinomycosis are given in Box 9.3.

Review PMID: 9619663

Treatment PMID: 25045274

Biopsy diagnosis PMID: 24870370

Other 'actinomycoses'

Infections with other non-pathogenic filamentous Gram-positive bacteria can be misclassified as actinomycosis. Examples are extraradicular infection in periapical granulomas, in which a colony of bacteria very occasionally grows beyond the root apex. The colony is like a sulphur granule, but isolated in the cavity where it may remain localised for a long period to cause failure of root canal treatment. Similar colonies may be found in tonsil crypts and growing around sequestra as they exfoliate into the mouth. However, none are spreading infections, none require intensive antibiotic treatment and none are true actinomycosis.

Extraradicular actinomycosis PMID: 12738954

THE SYSTEMIC MYCOSES

Deep tissue oral mycoses are rare in Britain but may be seen in immunocompromised patients or in those from endemic areas such as South America and other tropical regions (Box 9.4). Cryptococcosis is the most common mycosis in AIDS and is sometimes the presenting disease. Clinically, most of the systemic mycoses can cause oral lesions at some stage, and often then give rise to a nodular and ulcerated mass, which can be tumour-like in appearance (Fig. 9.14). The most characteristic oral infection is the nodular mulberry-like gingival hyperplasia and ulceration of paracoccidioidomycosis, or South American blastomycosis, a fungal infection of lungs, lymph nodes, bone and mucosa that is endemic in Brazil (Fig. 9.15). Clinically, this has a superficial resemblance to gingival lesions of Wegener's granulomatosis.

Microscopically, most systemic mycoses give rise to granulomas similar to those of tuberculosis, but there may also be abscess formation. Characteristic yeast forms or hyphae may sometimes be seen with special stains such as periodic acid–Schiff (PAS) (Fig. 9.16). However, microscopy may not be diagnostic, and culture of unfixed material may be

> **Box 9.4 Some systemic mycoses that can affect the mouth**
>
> - Histoplasmosis
> - Rhinocerebral mucormycosis
> - Rhinocerebral aspergillosis
> - Cryptococcosis
> - Paracoccidioidomycosis (South American blastomycosis)

> **Box 9.3 Actinomycosis: key features**
>
> - Rare chronic infection by filamentous bacterium, usually *Actinomyces israelii*
> - Infection spreads through the tissues to produce multiple abscesses and sinuses, in severe cases
> - More usually now, there is only a localised subcutaneous collection of pus
> - Microscopy shows large radially arranged colonies of actinomyces
> - Pus forms centrally and connective tissue forms an abscess wall
> - Sulphur granules (colonies of *Actinomyces*) from the pus are best for culture
> - Responds to prolonged treatment with penicillin
> - Surgical drainage of locules of pus may be needed

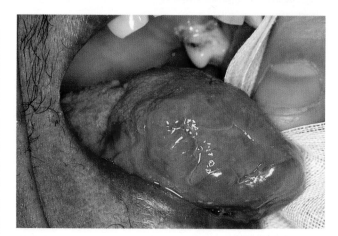

Fig. 9.14 Histoplasmosis. The gross nodular swelling of the tongue and ulceration are typical of many of the systemic mycoses.

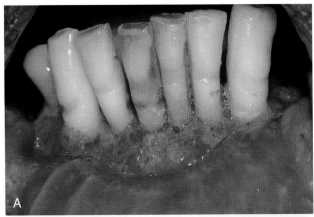

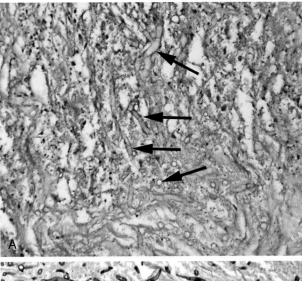

Fig. 9.15 South American blastomycosis. Characteristic nodular enlargement of gingiva seen in the upper image (A); note extension to labial mucosa. The lower figure (B) shows nodular lesions and erythema extending onto the palate. *(Courtesy of Dr RS Gomez and Dr BC Durso.)*

Fig. 9.17 Mucormycosis. The tissue is necrotic and infiltrated by the very pale, broad, knobbly branching hyphae of *Mucor* spp., seen as broad ribbons or circles in cross-section (*arrowed*). These are difficult to see in routine stains (A) but revealed by Grocott staining, which stains their cell walls black (B).

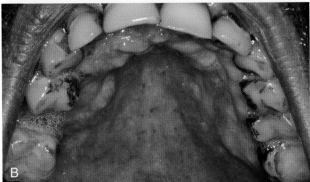

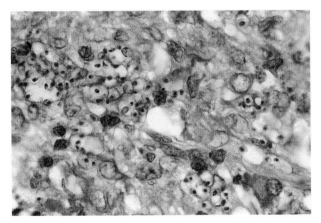

Fig. 9.16 Histoplasmosis. Part of an oral biopsy under high power, showing numerous typical round yeast forms with their clear haloes (periodic acid–Schiff stain).

necessary. Treatment requires systemic antifungal drugs, which have significant adverse effects.

Systemic mycoses in HIV PMID: 1549312

Histoplasmosis case reports PMID: 23633697 and 23219033

Paracoccidioidomycosis PMID: 8164159 and 8464610

Mucormycosis

This rare disease is the most significant deep mycosis of the head and neck because of its rapid progression and frequently fatal outcome. The causative fungi are environmental, often soil saprophytes that can only infect a debilitated or immunocompromised host. Many unrelated genera and species, including *Mucor sp.* and *Rhizopus sp.*, can cause the infection, and the name of the condition is difficult to align with the organisms; mucormycosis and zygomycosis are considered synonymous.

Most patients have poorly controlled diabetes, iron overload or a cause for immunosuppression. The infection often starts in the sinuses or nose from inhaled spores. The fungi invade blood vessels and so cause rapidly spreading tissue necrosis and large tissue defects (Fig. 9.17). Treatment requires surgical clearance and aggressive antifungal treatment, but a third of patients have a fatal outcome.

Review PMID: 8464609 and 18248590

SYSTEMIC INFECTIONS BY ORAL BACTERIA

The mouth harbours a great variety of microbes and virulent pathogens, particularly in periodontal pockets, but high levels of immunity and the fact that many of these organisms can only thrive in a mixed bacterial ecosystem keep the infection localised. It is almost always in the immunocompromised that oral commensals can spread and cause septicaemia or remote infections.

Infective endocarditis

A special example of a systemic infection of dental origin is infective endocarditis, which can occasionally follow dental operations, particularly extractions, and cause irreparable damage to heart valves (Ch. 32).

Lung and brain abscesses

Some of these abscesses are due to oral anaerobic bacteria that are probably aspirated during sleep to cause a lung abscess and then a secondary brain abscess. Isolated brain abscesses caused by oral bacteria are recognised but difficult to explain.

Cysts in and around the jaws

10

Cysts are the most common cause of chronic swellings of the jaws. A cyst comprises a wall of fibrous tissue and a central lumen, or space, lined by epithelium. Cysts are more common in the jaws than in any other bone because only the jaws contain epithelium, remaining after tooth formation.

> **Definition** Cysts are pathological fluid-filled cavities lined by epithelium.

CLASSIFICATION OF CYSTS

There are many types of cyst, and those in the head and neck are difficult to classify neatly and comprehensively. There is not currently a complete classification that is accepted internationally. A classification based on the current WHO classification is given in Box 10.1.

Cysts can be classified into two groups based on the origin of the epithelium that lines the central cavity. **Odontogenic cysts** are lined by odontogenic epithelium derived from the dental lamina. This epithelium originates by proliferation of rests of Serres, reduced enamel epithelium or rests of Malassez. Odontogenic cysts, therefore, can only affect the tooth-bearing regions of the jaws. Odontogenic cysts account for most cysts of the jaws. By far the most common is the radicular cyst, and this and the dentigerous cyst are common enough to present regularly in general dental practice (Box 10.2).

Odontogenic cysts can be further divided into inflammatory and developmental types depending on their cause. In reality, most of the developmental cysts are of unknown cause, and the developmental aetiology is assumed. Some of the developmental cysts are caused by specific gene mutations.

Non-odontogenic cysts are lined by other types of epithelium, and they are usually developmental in origin.

Some of the odontogenic tumours also contain cystic spaces lined by epithelium and need to be taken into account in differential diagnosis (Ch. 11).

Although the classification of cysts provides a logical way to list and understand them, it has little bearing on diagnosis and treatment, which are determined by the individual cyst type. It is not possible to identify odontogenic epithelium under the microscope unless it has basal cells resembling ameloblasts or fortuitously forms Rushton bodies (hyaline bodies), an enamel matrix-like secretory product that can only be formed by odontogenic epithelium (Fig. 10.11).

Web URL 10.1 Odontogenic epithelium residues: http://obm.quintessenz.de/obm_2004_03_s0171.pdf

Incidence of cysts PMID: 23766099

There are many other causes of circumscribed areas of radiolucency in the jaws that mimic cysts (Box 10.3).

General reference work ISBN-13: 978-1405149372

Box 10.1 Cysts of the jaws, face and neck

ODONTOGENIC CYSTS

Cysts of inflammatory origin
Radicular cyst
   Residual radicular cyst
Inflammatory collateral cysts

Cysts of developmental or unknown origin
Dentigerous cyst
   Eruption cyst
Odontogenic keratocyst
Orthokeratinised odontogenic cyst
Lateral periodontal cyst
   Botryoid odontogenic cyst
Glandular odontogenic cyst
Calcifying odontogenic cyst
Gingival cysts
   Gingival cyst of infants
   Gingival cyst of adults

NON-ODONTOGENIC CYSTS

Incisive canal cyst
Nasolabial cyst
Sublingual dermoid cyst
Thyroglossal duct cyst
Branchial cyst
Foregut cysts

Box 10.2 Relative frequency of different types of jaw cyst

Radicular*	45%
Residual radicular	7%
Dentigerous	16%
Odontogenic keratocyst	10%
Incisive canal	10%
Collateral	3%
Lateral periodontal	<1%

*The relative proportions of cysts are considerably affected by the incidence of non-vital teeth in a population as this determines the incidence of radicular cysts. These are UK estimates, and radicular cysts are less common than previously.

COMMON FEATURES OF JAW CYSTS

Many features are shared by all types of cysts. All cysts enlarge slowly, and there are two main mechanisms of enlargement: expansion under internal hydrostatic pressure and growth of the wall.

Hydrostatic pressure is the mechanism of cyst growth in almost all cysts. The luminal contents are under pressure for a variety of reasons. There is poor lymphatic drainage from the cavity, the wall and lining have partial properties of a semipermeable membrane and the lumen contains many degraded inflammatory proteins and dead lining cells. These and other factors produce an osmotic pressure that expands the cyst. The pressure is probably intermittent and of the order of 70 cm of water and therefore higher than the capillary blood pressure, able to compress veins and lymphatics in the wall so that fluid cannot escape. Expansion is slow. It takes 5 years for a cyst in the mandible to enlarge to a few centimetres diameter in an adult (Fig. 10.1), but growth is faster in children because bone turnover is more rapid and the bones less dense, providing less resistance to enlargement. Enlargement resorbs bone around the periphery and then pushes the periosteum outward.

Box 10.3   Radiographic mimics of cysts

- Anatomical structures (maxillary antrum and foramina)
- Large periapical granulomas
- Odontogenic tumours, particularly ameloblastoma (Ch. 11)
- Solitary bone cyst and aneurysmal bone 'cyst' (Ch. 13)
- Giant cell lesions (Ch. 12)
- Cherubism (Ch. 13)

Growth of the wall is a less common mechanism, seen primarily in odontogenic keratocysts. In this cyst the epithelial lining has a high mitotic rate, and the lumen is filled with keratin, which is resistant to degradation, insoluble and thus exerts little osmotic pressure. Instead the wall enlarges by growing, budding and insinuating finger-like processes or developing outpouchings that extend into adjacent bone. Glandular odontogenic cyst grows in a similar way.

Growth pattern and effects on adjacent structures differ with the mechanism of enlargement. Hydrostatic pressure acts equally in all directions, and all cysts that grow this way enlarge equally in all directions until surrounding structures restrict them. Initially they will enlarge like a balloon, forming a hollow sphere by resorbing medullary bone. Later, enlargement is restricted by cortical bone, tooth roots or the cortical layer around the inferior dental canal. The pressure will then push out the cyst in other directions, but pressure is exerted on these resisting structures, and eventually the cyst will move teeth orthodontically, resorb the cortex and push the inferior dental canal out of the way. Over a longer period tooth roots may be resorbed. Conversely, the odontogenic keratocyst, without any internal pressure, burrows along the path of least resistance in the medullary bone, around the teeth without displacing them.

Expansion of the jaw results from resorption of the cortex and pushing out of the periosteum. The periosteum is a tough resistant elastic layer that the cyst cannot penetrate. As it expands, it forms a new cortical bone layer around the cyst. There is not time to form a well-organised lamellar bone layer, and the 'periosteal new bone layer' is mostly soft woven bone. Palpation of the new bone layer can cause it to crack, and the fragments rubbing together give rise to the clinical sign of 'egg shell crackling'. Cysts expand the cortex closest to their site of origin first. Cysts arising in the

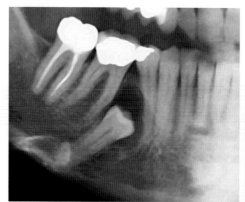
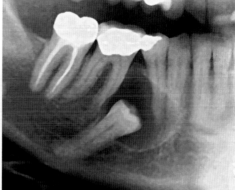
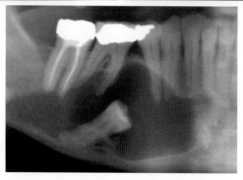

Fig. 10.1   Growth of an untreated cyst. This dentigerous cyst was identified at the size shown *upper left*. After 15 months it had grown to the size shown *upper right*. It took a further 5 years and 4 months to grow to the size in the lower radiograph. Generally cysts enlarge slowly, but more quickly when inflammation is present. *(By kind permission of Mr O Obisesan.)*

alveolus expand buccally first, except in the lower molar region where the lingual cortex is closer and thinner. The periosteal new bone layer can be seen in radiographs.

Expansion is rarely seen in odontogenic keratocysts until very large because their lack of internal hydrostatic pressure renders them unable to resorb the cortex. Expansion is seen, but it is a late sign in cysts that have reached a comparatively large size or in children where the bone is less dense and growing.

Tooth vitality is not affected by cysts. The radicular cyst is caused by a non-vital tooth, but the adjacent teeth may be tipped and resorbed without loss of vitality. The neurovascular bundles to their apices are either displaced to the periphery of the cyst or run across the lumen where they are prone to damage on surgical treatment.

A bluish colour is characteristic of cysts that have expanded beyond the cortex and results from their fluid content. It may be possible to transilluminate cysts or demonstrate fluctuance if they expand through the cortex in two places.

Radiological features are common to most cysts. All produce sharply defined evenly radiolucent lesions with a smooth rounded outline. The surrounding bone forms a reactive thin cortical or sclerotic layer around any cyst that grows slowly enough, and this is seen as cortication, a distinct white line around the edge of the lesion. Cysts may be unilocular (one cavity) or multilocular (many cavities). Multilocular cysts have a scalloped outline, and septa may be visible dividing the locules from one another. The radiological appearances provide an opportunity to assess the growth pattern and effects on cortex, teeth and other structures that give clues to diagnose individual types of cyst.

Clinical presentation. Cysts in bone may enlarge without signs or symptoms for a long period, and approximately one-third of cysts are chance radiographic findings. A further third present with painless expansion or displacement of teeth. The remaining third become infected, either through communication with a non-vital tooth or by rupturing into the soft tissues. Cysts may therefore present as abscesses, and their cystic nature may not be immediately evident. A 'cyst abscess' has a fuzzy rather than a corticated outline radiographically. Very large cysts may precipitate a pathological fracture.

Fluid content. Aspiration of cyst fluids for diagnosis is obsolete as an investigation, but thick white paste found in a cyst is probably keratin and indicates a likely diagnosis of odontogenic keratocyst. Most cyst fluids are watery and opalescent but sometimes more viscid and yellowish, and they sometimes shimmer with cholesterol crystals (see later in this chapter). A smear of this fluid may show typical notched cholesterol crystals microscopically (Fig. 10.8). In infected cysts, an aspirate of pus should be taken for bacterial culture and sensitivity.

Key features of jaw cysts are shown in Box 10.4.

TREATMENT OF JAW CYSTS

Most types of cyst are treated in the same way, the exceptions being odontogenic keratocyst and a few other rare types that have a risk of recurrence. Their special treatment is discussed later in this chapter with each entity. The remaining types of cyst have limited treatment options.

It may seem odd to be discussing treatment before definitive diagnosis, but in clinical practice, treatment is often performed on the basis of a differential diagnosis based on clinical and radiological features. The dentist therefore needs sufficient knowledge to be suspicious of features of

---

Box 10.4 Key features of jaw cysts

- Form sharply-defined radiolucencies with corticated smooth borders
- Aspiration can confirm fluid contents, excluding a solid lesion
- Cysts close to the mucosal surface may be transilluminated and appear bluish
- Grow slowly, displacing rather than resorbing teeth
- Symptomless unless infected and frequently chance radiographic findings
- Rarely large enough to cause pathological fracture
- Form compressible and fluctuant swellings if extending into soft tissues

---

Box 10.5 Advantages and limitations of enucleation of cysts

Advantages

- The cavity usually heals without complications
- Little aftercare is necessary
- The complete lining is available for histological examination

Possible disadvantages

- Infection of the clot filling the cavity
- Recurrence due to incomplete removal of the lining
- Serious haemorrhage (primary or secondary)
- Damage to apices of vital teeth projecting into the cyst cavity
- Damage to the inferior dental nerve
- Opening the antrum when enucleating a large maxillary cyst
- Fracture of the jaw if an exceptionally large mandibular cyst is enucleated

---

cysts that might recur, as these require a biopsy to plan treatment. Otherwise, if a confident differential diagnosis is made, and if the cyst is small, it may be treated and the final diagnosis confirmed by histopathology subsequently.

Enucleation and primary closure is the usual method of treatment and is usually entirely effective (Box 10.5). A mucoperiosteal flap over the cyst is raised and a window is opened in the bone large enough to give adequate access. The soft tissue of the cyst wall is then separated from the bony wall. In thick-walled cysts it separates cleanly with a blunt instrument and scoops out easily; in thinner-walled cysts more care is needed. The entire cyst is removed intact and should be sent for histological examination. If there is a non-vital tooth associated, as in a radicular cyst, this is treated as described later in this chapter. If there are apices of other teeth extending into the cavity, these teeth are usually either root treated preoperatively or on cyst removal by a retrograde approach. Alternatively they may be extracted.

The edges of the bone cavity are smoothed off, free bleeding is controlled and the cavity is irrigated to remove debris. The mucoperiosteal flap is replaced and sutured in place on sound bone around the margin of the bony window. The cavity fills with blood and organises. The sutures should be left for at least 10 days.

Box 10.6 Advantages and limitations of marsupialisation of cysts

Advantages

- Shrinkage before enucleation
  - may allow preservation of teeth
  - reduce the operative risk to inferior dental nerve
  - reduce the risk of mandibular fracture
- Shrinkage allows easier enucleation of residual cyst
- Enucleation may not be possible in a compromised patient

Possible disadvantages

- Shrinkage is very slow, over weeks and months
- Tendency for the opening to shrink faster than the cavity
- Close follow up required
- Patient must keep the cavity clean
- No complete lining for histological examination

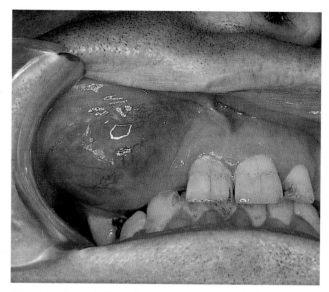

Fig. 10.2 Typical clinical appearance of a large cyst. This radicular cyst in the right maxillary alveolar process forms a rounded swelling with a bluish colour.

Any disadvantages are largely theoretical, and in competent hands even very large cysts can be enucleated safely. Recurrence is remarkably rare unless the cyst has been misdiagnosed. There are few contraindications, and they are relative rather than absolute.

Marsupialisation Marsupialisation, or decompression, was a largely outmoded treatment but has regained popularity for very large odontogenic keratocysts. The cyst is opened essentially as for enucleation, but the lining is left in place and sutured to the oral mucous membrane at the margins of the opening to produce a wide communication into the mouth. The aim is to decompress the cavity and make it into a pouch continuous with the oral mucosa. The cavity gradually closes by ingrowth of bone from the periphery and replacement of the lining epithelium by ingrowth of the oral epithelium.

However, considerable aftercare is needed to keep the cavity clean. The cavity is initially packed with ribbon gauze and, after the margins have healed, a plug or extension to a denture is made to fill the opening. Food debris has to be regularly washed out, and the opening shrinks with healing. A further disadvantage is that the complete lining is not available for histological examination.

The main application of marsupialisation is for temporary decompression of exceptionally large cysts where fracture of the jaw is a risk. When the cyst has shrunk and enough new bone has formed, the remaining lining can be enucleated. Occasionally, retention of the tooth in a dentigerous cyst is needed and marsupialisation may allow it to erupt.

Advantages and limitations are given in Box 10.6.

Case series marsupialisation PMID: 25631867

Curettage Curettage is the scraping of the bony cavity after enucleation or piecemeal removal of a lesion. It is not necessary in most cysts because the soft tissue separates easily from the smooth bony wall of the cavity. When the lining is friable, as in odontogenic keratocyst, a light curettage may help dislodge any remaining small fragments that could seed recurrence, but is only a precautionary measure after attempting removal of the entire lining.

Infected cysts Cysts that become secondarily infected must have the infection treated first by antibiotics and drainage to avoid performing surgery in an infected field. Once the infection is controlled, the cyst is removed.

TREATMENT OF SOFT TISSUE CYSTS

Soft tissue cysts are almost always benign. Unlike cysts in bone, they need to be removed with a small amount of surrounding normal tissue to avoid bursting them or leaving small fragments in the tissues to seed a recurrence. Soft tissue cysts are therefore excised (removed by cutting around them) with a small margin of normal tissue, shaped to allow easy wound closure.

ODONTOGENIC CYSTS

RADICULAR CYST → Summary chart 10.1 p. 163

Radicular cysts, or periapical cysts, are the most common type of cyst in the jaws and also the most common cause of major, chronic swellings. They are odontogenic and inflammatory in type. The radicular cyst is defined by its location at the apex of a non-vital tooth.

Definition A radicular cyst is a cyst on the apex of a non-vital tooth.

Clinical features

The age at presentation is wide, ranging from 20–60 years. Radicular cysts are more common in males than females, roughly in the proportion of 3 to 2. The maxilla is affected more than three times as frequently as the mandible. These features reflect the frequency and location of non-vital teeth. Although deciduous teeth are often devitalised by caries, radicular cysts are rarely seen before the age of 10 years, probably because of the time required for them to form.

There is a slowly progressive painless swelling, with no symptoms until the cyst becomes large enough to be noticed (Fig. 10.2). The swelling is rounded and at first hard. Later, when the bone has been reduced to eggshell thickness, a crackling sensation may be felt on pressure. Finally, part of the wall is resorbed entirely away, leaving a soft fluctuant swelling, bluish in colour, beneath the mucous membrane. The dead tooth from which the cyst has originated is (by

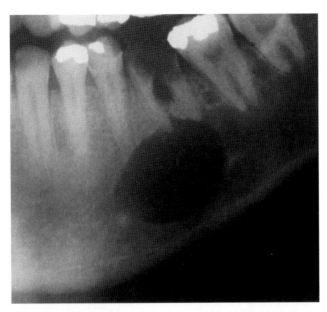

Fig. 10.3   A radicular cyst on a grossly carious and non-vital first permanent molar. A rounded and sharply defined area of radiolucency is associated with the apices of the roots.

definition) present, and its relationship to the cyst will be apparent in a radiograph (Fig. 10.3). Infection may supervene because of the associated non-vital tooth, and the swelling becomes painful and may rapidly expand, partly due to inflammatory oedema.

Key features of radicular cysts are summarised in Box 10.7.

Radiography

A radicular cyst appears as a rounded, radiolucent area with a sharply defined outline. A condensed radiopaque corticated periphery is present only if growth is slow and is usually more prominent in longstanding cysts. The dead tooth from which the cyst has arisen can be seen and often has a large carious cavity or other cause evident. Adjacent teeth may be tilted or displaced a little and can become slightly mobile as their bony support is reduced.

Pathogenesis

Epithelial proliferation A non-vital tooth is present by definition. Most non-vital teeth persist in a symptomless state for many years, causing no more than a periapical

granuloma. However, inflammation in the granuloma is sufficient to induce proliferation in the epithelial rests of Malassez, the network of strands of epithelium that remain after breakdown of the root sheath of Hertwig. Rests of Malassez are more frequent around the apical third of the root and vary in number between individuals, perhaps explaining why some individuals suffer multiple radicular cysts.

Cavitation When the epithelial rests proliferate, they grow into larger islands of epithelium that break down to form a cavity in the centre. This is because the proliferating cells lie peripherally in the basal cell layer and move toward the centre of the island as they mature. Eventually they die and autolyse, producing a central cavity.

Fluid accumulation As soon as a cavity forms, tissue fluid collects and debris from dead epithelial cells and inflammatory exudate produce the hydrostatic pressure that causes cyst expansion. Radicular cysts enlarge in a balloon-like fashion producing the signs noted earlier, expansion and pressure effects on bone and teeth.

Secondary inflammation The wall becomes inflamed because of the non-vital tooth. Lymphocytes, plasma cells and macrophages collect in foci in the fibrous wall. There is always inflammation somewhere in the wall of a radicular cyst. Leakage from inflamed blood vessels allows erythrocytes to pass into the wall and cyst cavity. Unlike most other cell types, red cells have free cholesterol in their membranes. When the red cells in the cyst lumen or wall degenerate, their membranes release their cholesterol, which crystallises and induces a foreign body inflammatory reaction with giant cells and macrophages. The other lipid from the membrane is taken up by macrophages that develop a foamy cytoplasm of engulfed fat droplets. Clusters of crystals and inflammatory cells form nodules in the wall ('mural nodules') that hang into the cyst cavity. Inflammation induces the cyst lining epithelium to become hyperplastic.

Bone-resorbing factors Experimentally, cyst tissues in culture release bone-resorbing factors. These are predominantly prostaglandins E2 and E3. Different types of cysts and tumours may produce different quantities of prostaglandins, but it is unclear whether this aids growth of the cyst in vivo.

Histopathology

The smallest and earliest cysts are no more than a periapical granuloma containing a few strands of proliferating epithelium (Figs 10.4 and 10.5). Later, a well-organised thick cyst wall with epithelial lining and dense inflammatory infiltrate develops.

The fibrous wall consists of collagenous connective tissue with variable inflammation, usually plasma cells and macrophages. Mural nodules of cholesterol clefts (Figs 10.6 and 10.7) and cholesterol crystals are found in the wall and lumen (Fig. 10.8). Peripherally, osteoclasts resorb the inner aspect of the bony cavity to allow expansion. Beyond that, in the adjacent medullary cavity, osteoblasts react to the inflammation by increasing bone deposition, producing the line of cortication seen radiographically.

The lumen is lined by a non-keratinising epithelium of variable thickness. More inflamed cysts have a more hyperplastic epithelium that appears net-like (Fig. 10.9), forming rings and arcades (Fig. 10.10). Hyaline bodies may be seen in the epithelium, confirming that it is odontogenic in origin (Fig. 10.11), and mucous cells may be present as a result of metaplasia (Fig. 10.12).

Longstanding cysts typically have a thin flattened epithelial lining, a thick fibrous wall and less inflammatory infiltrate.

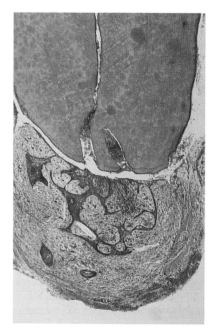

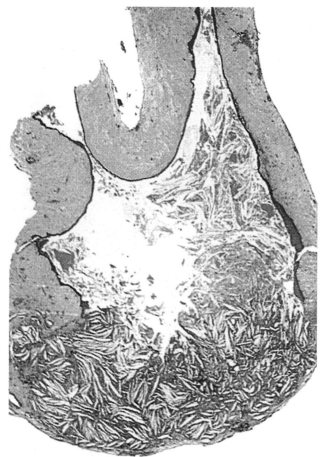

Fig. 10.4   The earliest stages of formation of a radicular cyst. Some periapical granulomas, such as this, contain proliferating strands of odontogenic epithelium. In places the epithelium has broken down centrally to form small epithelium-lined spaces.

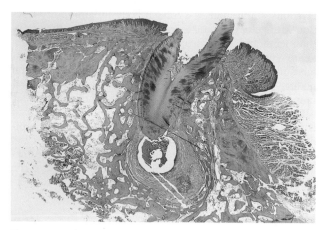

Fig. 10.5   A developing radicular cyst. An epithelium-lined cavity has formed in this large periapical granuloma. There is a thick fibrous capsule infiltrated by chronic inflammatory cells. The alveolar bone has been resorbed and remodelled to accommodate the slowly expanding swelling.

Fig. 10.6   Cholesterol clefts in a cyst wall. This low-power view shows the relationship of cholesterol clefts to the cyst. Cholesterol crystals are formed in the fibrous wall. The epithelium overlying this focus has broken down, and the cholesterol has leaked into the cyst lumen. Elsewhere the lumen is lined by a flattened layer of squamous epithelium.

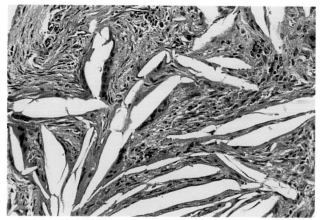

Fig. 10.7   Cholesterol clefts. Cholesterol has been dissolved out during preparation of the section, leaving clefts. The crystals are treated as foreign bodies, and flattened multinucleate foreign body giant cells are seen along the edges of several clefts.

Differential diagnosis

Radicular cysts are usually readily recognised by their clinical and radiographic features, so a confident preoperative diagnosis makes biopsy unnecessary unless there are unusual features such as root resorption or a poorly defined margin.

Histological examination is essential to confirm diagnosis, but because the histological features are not entirely specific, it is really undertaken to exclude unsuspected diagnoses.

Treatment

Radicular cysts are almost always treated by enucleation and primary closure (mentioned previously). The associated non-vital tooth is usually extracted because radicular cysts tend to develop in irregular dental attenders, and the tooth is often unrestorable. However, it can be preserved in most cases by placing an orthograde root filling before surgery and performing an apicectomy and retrograde filling, usually with mineral trioxide aggregate, when the cyst is enucleated. Healing may take several months before bone fills

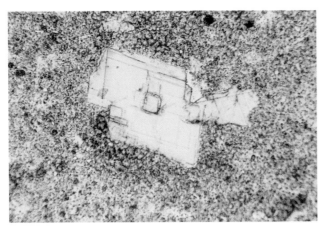

Fig. 10.8   Cholesterol crystals from a cyst aspirate indicating the presence of inflammation. The rectangular shape with a notched corner is characteristic.

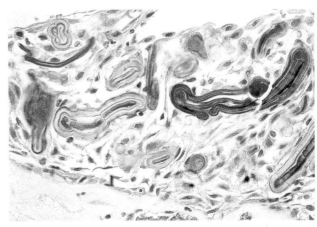

Fig. 10.11   Hyaline or Rushton bodies. These translucent or pink-staining lamellar bodies are secreted by the cyst lining epithelium and indicate the odontogenic origin of a cyst.

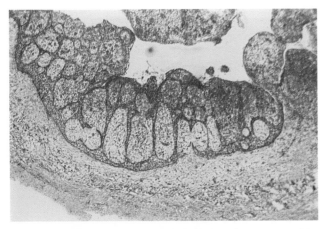

Fig. 10.9   Radicular cyst. The epithelial lining often assumes this arcading pattern with numerous inflammatory cells beneath its surface.

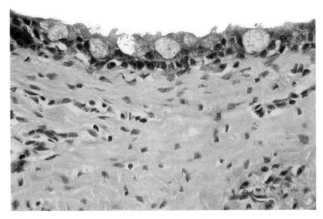

Fig. 10.12   Mucous metaplasia in a radicular cyst. This change is of no clinical significance and happens in a proportion of all cyst types, but is most typical of dentigerous cysts.

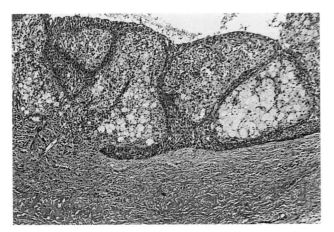

Fig. 10.10   Higher power of the lining of a radicular cyst. The arcading epithelium contains numerous neutrophils emigrating into the lumen, and there are pale-staining areas of foamy macrophages in the inner wall.

the cavity, and any cortical expansion slowly reduces with remodelling.

The treatment of suspected radicular cysts by root filling alone is somewhat contentious. Animal studies suggest that small cysts may resolve if the causative tooth is effectively

root treated. Unfortunately this is difficult to prove in humans as the presence of a cyst can only be confirmed histologically, after removal. Because periapical granulomas can also attain a significant size (several centimetres), it is never certain exactly what has been treated. Although the size of a periapical radiolucency does affect the chances of it being a cyst rather than a granuloma, there is no defined cut-off size to guide treatment. Sometimes even a lesion a few millimetres diameter can be a well-organised radicular cyst. Sharp definition of the lesion radiographically is also a poor indicator because definition is partly a function of size; larger periapical granulomas always appear better defined radiographically.

However, it is clear that what *appear* to be cysts as large as approximately 20 mm in diameter can often resolve after endodontic treatment. It is therefore worth trying conservative treatment for small suspected radicular cysts provided the patient accepts a risk of failure and will wait to assess the response. This may avoid surgery but carries some risks: infection in the cyst and failing to diagnose a completely different unsuspected lesion that just happens to be at the apex of a non-vital tooth.

General reference ISBN-13: 978-1405149372

Size cyst v granuloma PMID: 18634946 and 20171356

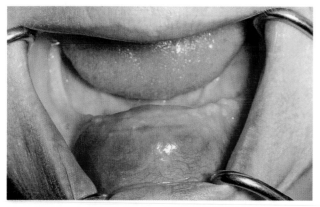

Fig. 10.13   Residual cyst. The causative tooth has been extracted leaving the cyst in situ. See also Fig. 10.14.

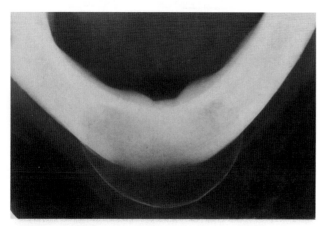

Fig. 10.14   Radiographic appearance of the residual cyst shown in Fig. 10.13. Note the thin bulging periosteal new bone layer which can give rise to the clinical sign of eggshell crackling.
(Figs 10.13 and 10.14 kindly provided by Mr P Robinson.)

Lateral radicular cyst

→ Summary chart 10.1 p. 163

A so-called *lateral radicular cyst* is a radicular cyst that forms at the side of a non-vital tooth root at the opening of a lateral branch of the root canal, rather than at the apex. They are rare and need to be distinguished from lateral periodontal cysts, a different type of cyst (later in this chapter) that forms beside tooth roots.

Residual radicular cyst

→ Summary chart 10.1 p. 163

A residual radicular cyst is a radicular cyst that has persisted after extraction of the causative tooth. The features are identical to other radicular cysts, except that the key diagnostic feature has been removed; this may complicate differential diagnosis. Residual cysts are more frequent in older persons (Figs 10.13 and 10.14) and present with expansion of the jaw. Once the causative tooth has been removed, inflammation subsides (Fig. 10.15) so that residual cysts grow very slowly.

INFLAMMATORY COLLATERAL CYSTS

These are rare cysts adjacent to the cervical area or furcation of molars, particularly mandibular molars. One presentation is buccal to erupting first permanent molars in children (often called 'mandibular buccal infected cyst'). Another is

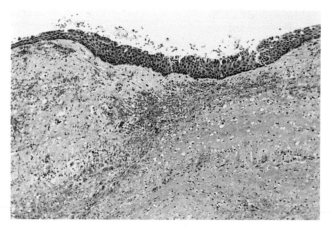

Fig. 10.15   Lining of a residual cyst. There is only a minor degree of inflammation and the epithelium forms a thin regular layer.

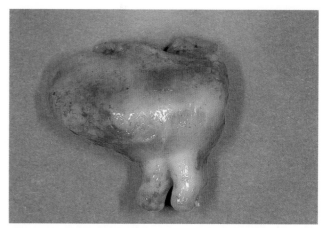

Fig. 10.16   Dentigerous cyst. This cyst has been removed together with its associated tooth. The cyst surrounds the crown and is attached at the cementoenamel junction.

a cyst as large as approximately 2 cm in diameter adjacent to the furcation in molars of young adults expanding the alveolus (paradental or bifurcation cyst). If large, they tip the roots lingually and the crown buccally. In both types, the affected tooth is vital but typically shows pericoronitis or gingival inflammation.

These cysts are poorly understood. A proportion are bilateral, and a few are associated with enamel spurs or pearls in the buccal bifurcation (Ch. 2). They expand by internal pressure similarly to a radicular cyst, which they resemble histologically. Enucleation is effective, and the tooth can be conserved. Mandibular buccal infected cysts communicating with a pocket may resolve spontaneously.

Review PMID: 15128056

Paradental type PMID: 1065342

DENTIGEROUS CYSTS

→ Summary chart 10.1 p. 163

This common cyst surrounds the crown of a tooth and is an expansion of the follicle caused by separation of the reduced enamel epithelium from the enamel (Figs 10.16 and 10.17). The cyst is therefore odontogenic. The cyst wall is

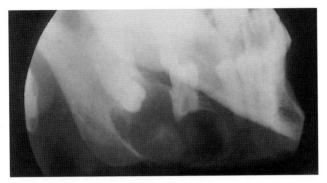

Fig. 10.17 Dentigerous cyst. The cyst has developed around the crown of the buried third molar (*left*), but has extended forward to involve the root of a vital second molar. The vitality of the second molar is a key feature in differentiating whether this is a dentigerous or radicular cyst.

attached to the neck of the tooth, prevents its eruption and may displace it for a considerable distance.

> **Definition** The dentigerous cyst is a cyst around the crown of an unerupted tooth, with the epithelial lining attached around the cemento-enamel junction.

Clinical features

Dentigerous cysts are more than twice as common in males as females, and two-thirds develop on lower third molars. Upper canines and lower premolars are also affected, reflecting the most frequently impacted teeth. These cysts present between the ages of 10 and 30 years. They grow by internal pressure and cause the same clinical features as other cysts that expand the jaw; expansion with displacement of adjacent structures. They are often a chance radiographic finding when the cause is sought for an unerupted tooth.

Radiography

The cavity is circumscribed, rounded and always unilocular and contains the crown of the tooth (Fig. 10.17). Dentigerous cysts grow slowly and have a corticated outline. Cysts may attain a very large size, larger than 10 cm, and large cysts may appear to be multilocular on radiographs (pseudoloculation) because bony ridges on the inside of the bony cavity are superimposed on the image. The affected tooth is often displaced a considerable distance, lower third molars to the lower border of the mandible or high in the ramus. In longstanding cysts, the enclosed tooth may become resorbed (Fig. 10.18).

Pathogenesis

Dentigerous cysts are considered to be developmental, but inflammation from pericoronitis or an adjacent non-vital tooth may initiate some. Multiple dentigerous cysts are seen in those with cleidocranial dysplasia (Ch. 13) who have many unerupted teeth.

The earliest event is separation of the reduced enamel epithelium from the crown to form the cyst space. The epithelium is tightly bound to the enamel during formation but more loosely attached after the normal time of eruption, but the reason for separation is unclear. As the reduced enamel epithelium stops at the cementoenamel junction, the lining epithelium is attached there and the fibrous wall is continuous with the periodontal ligament (Figs 10.19 and 10.20).

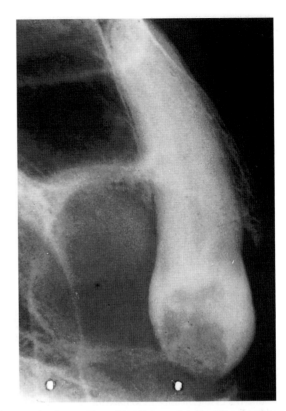

Fig. 10.18 Resorption of tooth associated with a dentigerous cyst. The crown of this buried canine within the cyst shows resorption. This is seen only in longstanding cysts, as in this otherwise edentulous patient.

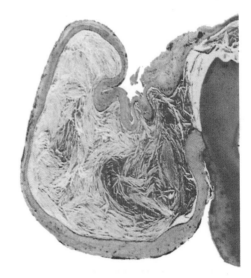

Fig. 10.19 Dentigerous cyst. The cyst surrounds the crown of this molar, and the wall is attached to its cementoenamel junction. There is a uniform, thin epithelial lining with minimal inflammatory infiltrate. Cholesterol clefts are numerous in the lumen, a result of the formation of cholesterol crystals in the wall.

The cyst enlarges by internal pressure, expanding the dental follicle, displacing adjacent structures and eventually expanding the jaw.

Histopathology

The wall of dentigerous cysts in their early stages comprises an uninflamed fibrous wall lined by a thin, sometimes

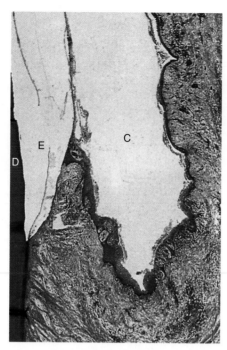

Fig. 10.20 Dentigerous cyst. To the left is the dentine (D). E is the enamel space left after decalcification and is separated from the cyst cavity (C) by a thin layer left by the inner enamel epithelium. The cyst itself appears to have formed as a result of accumulation of fluid between the inner and outer enamel epithelium and by continued proliferation of the latter to form the cyst lining, which joins the tooth at the epithelial attachment.

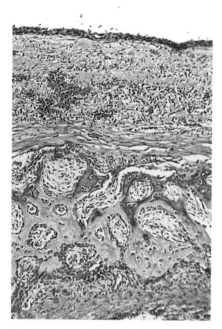

Fig. 10.21 Section through the full thickness of the wall of a dentigerous cyst. There is minimal inflammation, and the epithelium is only two or three cells thick. Beyond the fibrous tissue the outermost layer of the wall is formed by woven bone, a feature common to most types of intraosseous cyst.

bilaminar, epithelium that resembles reduced enamel epithelium (Figs. 10.21 and 10.22). While the cyst enlarges, a degree of inflammation usually develops, and inflammatory or metaplastic changes can develop to differing degrees in different cysts. There may be frequent mucous cells or focal

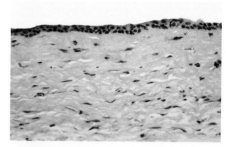

Fig. 10.22 Dentigerous cyst. In this uncomplicated cyst there is no inflammation, and the wall comprises a layer of fibrous tissue lined by a thin layer of stratified squamous epithelium two cells thick.

keratinisation. Once significant inflammation supervenes, the appearances come to resemble a radicular cyst, and the diagnosis can no longer be made on biopsy alone.

Differential diagnosis

The key diagnostic feature is the dentigerous relationship to the tooth. It is normally possible to make a confident diagnosis radiographically and proceed to treatment without biopsy, confirming the diagnosis after enucleation. However, care must be taken not to be caught out by other lesions simulating a dentigerous relationship. An odontogenic keratocyst, ameloblastoma or other radiolucent lesion may occasionally grow around the crown of an unerupted tooth to create a similar radiographic appearance (Fig. 10.32). Identifying a clear attachment at the cementoenamel junction will reduce the likelihood of this error. Because of this risk, the diagnosis should always be confirmed by histological examination, primarily to exclude other unexpected lesions.

It is also sometimes necessary to differentiate an enlarged follicle from a dentigerous cyst. The width of a normal follicle radiographically can be 2–3 mm. If there is uncertainty whether a cyst space has developed, radiographic follow up rather than intervention is appropriate.

Treatment

Dentigerous cysts are usually treated by enucleation with removal of the unerupted tooth, there usually being no reason to conserve the impacted lower third molar. However, for other teeth, such as maxillary canines that are in a favourable position, it may be possible to marsupialise a dentigerous cyst to allow the tooth to erupt, providing space and traction orthodontically if necessary. Alternatively, the tooth can be transplanted but with a risk of resorption in the long term.

It remains unresolved whether leaving disease-free unerupted third molars in situ, according to current guidelines, risks development of dentigerous cysts in later life. This would appear to be so, but the risk must be very low.

Key features of dentigerous cysts are summarised in Box 10.8.

Review PMID: 20605411

General reference ISBN-13: 978-1405149372

ERUPTION CYST

An eruption cyst is a superficial dentigerous cyst arising on a tooth during eruption. They are therefore seen in children, forming a soft, rounded, swelling on the alveolus. Trauma

Box 10.8 Dentigerous cyst: key features

- Arise in bone and contain the crown of an unerupted tooth, which is usually displaced
- Are most frequently associated with unerupted third molars and canines
- Clinical and radiographic features usually provide an accurate preoperative diagnosis but confirmation is histological
- May be mistaken radiographically for an odontogenic keratocyst or ameloblastoma
- Respond to enucleation or marsupialisation and do not recur after treatment

Table 10.1 The two types of odontogenic cysts that keratinise

Feature	Odontogenic keratocyst	Orthokeratinised odontogenic cyst
Type of keratinisation	Parakeratin	Orthokeratin
Relative frequency (%)	90	10
Male: female ratio	1.5:1	2:1
Association with impacted tooth (%)	35	70
Midline location (%)	6	16
Radiographic appearance	Usually multilocular	Almost always monolocular
Recurrence rate (%)	3–20	2

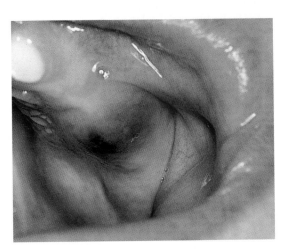

Fig. 10.23 An eruption cyst over an erupting upper molar. There has been bleeding into the cyst cavity as a result of trauma.

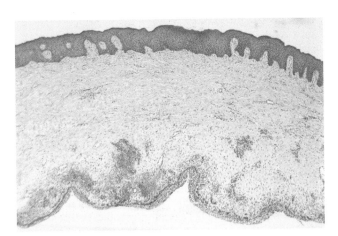

Fig. 10.24 Roof of an eruption cyst. At the upper surface is the keratinised epithelium of the alveolar ridge and, below, separated by a thin layer of relatively uninflamed fibrous tissue, the lining of an eruption cyst.

to the cyst causes internal bleeding and a dark blue colour (Figs 10.23 and 10.24).

Most eruption cysts burst spontaneously, and the tooth erupts normally, but if very large, the cyst roof may be incised or removed. Haemorrhage around an erupting tooth is much more likely to be traumatic than indicate an eruption cyst.

Case series PMID: 14969381

ODONTOGENIC KERATOCYST → Summary charts 10.1 and 10.2 pp. 163, 164

The odontogenic keratocyst is the commonest keratinising cyst in the jaws and has a characteristic clinical, radiological and histological appearance. It is important to recognise because it may recur after treatment, can grow to a very large size without symptoms and is sometimes associated with a syndromic presentation.

The name of this cyst indicates that its epithelial lining keratinises, but this alone is not specific. Another less common cyst, the orthokeratinising odontogenic cyst, also has this feature, and minor focal keratinisation can be seen in other odontogenic cysts. The differences between the two keratinising cysts are summarised in Table 10.1. Sublingual dermoid cysts are also heavily keratinised, but these are soft tissue cysts and readily differentiated.

> **Definition** The odontogenic keratocyst is a developmental odontogenic cyst with a tendency to recur, characterised by a histological appearance of parakeratinised lining epithelium with palisaded ameloblast-like basal cells.

Keratin filling the cyst lumen is bright white and when seen at operation is a useful diagnostic feature indicating these cyst types. It may be appreciated on opening a cyst for biopsy or if the cyst is punctured (Fig. 10.25), and its nature may be confirmed by histology. It should not be mistaken for pus.

Clinical features

Peak incidence is between ages 20 and 30 years, but the age range is very broad. The mandible is usually affected. At least 50% of odontogenic keratocysts form in the posterior body and lower ramus. Odontogenic keratocysts, like other jaw cysts, are symptomless until the bone is expanded or they become infected, both rare features in this cyst type.

Radiography

Odontogenic keratocysts produce well-defined radiolucent areas, with a more or less rounded or scalloped margin. Some are unilocular, but the majority are multilocular (Fig. 10.26). The margin is sharply demarcated and corticated radiographically.

The characteristic growth pattern is evident radiologically and is almost diagnostic. There is extensive spread forward

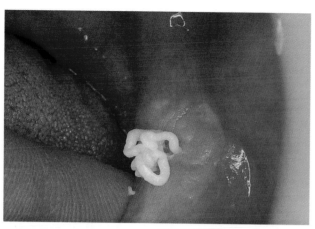

Fig. 10.25   An odontogenic keratocyst. Perforation of and pressure on the cyst roof has caused keratin, which fills the lumen, to extrude, and the characteristic appearance helps confirm the diagnosis.

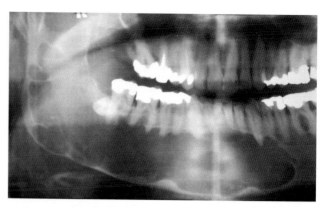

Fig. 10.27   Odontogenic keratocyst. Huge lesion extending from coronoid to the opposite molar region with minimal tooth displacement or expansion of bone.

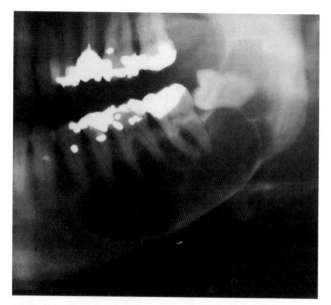

Fig. 10.26   Odontogenic keratocyst. Part of a panoramic tomogram showing typical appearances. The cyst is multilocular and has extended a considerable distance along the medullary cavity without appreciable expansion or displacement of the teeth.

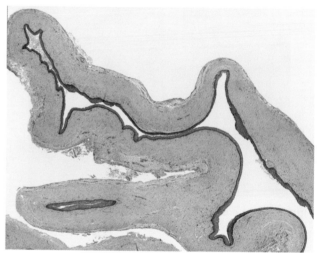

Fig. 10.28   Odontogenic keratocyst. Typical folded cyst outline with a satellite cyst lying in the wall. The fibrous tissue is uninflamed and thin.

and backward along the medullary cavity with minimal expansion until the whole of the medulla is replaced. There is minimal displacement and no resorption of teeth or the inferior dental canal (Fig. 10.27). In a minority of cases, the cyst may arise at the site of a tooth that has failed to develop.

The lack of expansion results in many odontogenic keratocysts being large at time of discovery.

Pathogenesis

Odontogenic keratocysts arise from the various rests of odontogenic epithelium that remain in the alveolus after tooth development, probably usually the rests of Serres.

Many odontogenic keratocysts are caused by mutation, deletion or other inactivation of the patched (PTCH) gene on chromosome 9q, a tumour suppressor gene. This gene is discussed in more detail in the following section. Loss of PTCH gene activity releases a brake on the cell cycle, mediated through the hedgehog pathway. Mutation of the gene

is found in a third of odontogenic keratocysts, and the remainder may have other genetic faults in this signalling pathway. Mutation results in a relatively high proliferative activity in the cyst lining epithelium. This has two consequences. First, the cysts appear to enlarge by growth of the wall rather than internal pressure. Second, epithelial proliferation probably favours recurrence if small pieces of epithelium are left after incomplete removal.

The lining becomes folded because growth of the wall exceeds that of the cavity containing the cyst (Fig. 10.28). Extensions of the lining penetrate the wall to form small daughter cysts that enlarge to produce a multilocular lesion. The cyst wall produces bone-resorbing factors that resorb the surrounding medullary bone, allowing the cyst to enlarge slowly but relentlessly along the medullary cavity.

The possible neoplastic nature of odontogenic keratocysts

There has always been a tendency to regard these cysts as 'aggressive' on grounds of recurrence and the fact that they may grow to a very large size before detection. This, together with the fact that odontogenic keratocysts are caused by inactivation of a tumour suppressor gene, has led some to classify them as benign neoplasms. The term *keratocystic odontogenic tumour* was proposed in 2005 to signify its

Table 10.2 Evidence for and against odontogenic keratocyst being a neoplasm

In favour of neoplasm	Against neoplasm
Recurrence	Recurrence is thought to follow incomplete removal
Infiltrative ('aggressive') growth pattern	Growth is relentless but not aggressive or destructive
High proliferative activity of epithelial lining	Responds to marsupialisation
Caused by mutation or deletion of PTCH tumour suppressor gene	
May contain defects of p16, p53 and other tumour suppressor genes	
Associated with other neoplasms in the basal cell naevus syndrome	
Squamous cell carcinoma may rarely develop within an odontogenic keratocyst	Squamous cell carcinoma may also develop in radicular and dentigerous cysts.

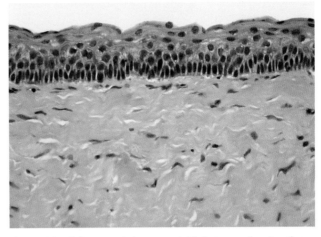

Fig. 10.29   Odontogenic keratocyst. High power, showing the typical features of the epithelial lining: a flat basement membrane; elongated palisaded basal cells with focal reserve polarity; 10–20 cells in thickness and with a corrugated parakeratotic surface.

Box 10.9   Typical histological features of odontogenic keratocyst

- Epithelial lining of uniform thickness with flat basal layer
- Thin eosinophilic layer of parakeratin with corrugated surface
- Clearly defined basal layer of tall cells, at least focally with reversed polarity (Fig. 10.29)
- Epithelial lining weakly attached to the fibrous wall
- Thin fibrous wall
- Satellite cysts in the wall (Fig. 10.28)
- Inflammatory cells typically absent or scanty

---

neoplastic status. However, this never gained wide acceptance, and the name *odontogenic keratocyst*, which has a long history, is again the official name.

Although the arguments for a neoplasm are more numerous and, in some ways, convincing, neoplasms are defined on the basis of their relentless growth and not by their molecular genetics. The odontogenic keratocyst responds well to marsupialisation provided all of the locules are opened to the surface. This is the best evidence that the cyst is not a neoplasm.

The evidence for and against a neoplastic nature is listed in Table 10.2.

Cyst or neoplasm PMID: 21270459

Histopathology

Unlike the common cysts, odontogenic keratocyst has a diagnostic histological appearance (Box 10.9) so that biopsy is the definitive diagnostic investigation (Fig. 10.29). In a typical cyst the fibrous wall is very thin and uninflamed. The lining epithelium has a corrugated thinly parakeratinised surface and a palisaded basal layer of columnar cells that show reverse polarity, at least focally. The basal cells resemble pre-ameloblasts and indicate the cyst's odontogenic origin. The epithelium often separates from the wall. In the fibrous tissue of the wall there are usually scattered islands of odontogenic epithelium. These can form small 'satellite' or 'daughter' cysts, each of which will enlarge to become a separate locule in a multilocular cyst.

However, if inflammation develops, the epithelial lining undergoes hyperplasia, loses its characteristic features and resembles that of a radicular cyst (Figs 10.30 and 10.31), making histological diagnosis more difficult. Because there is often focal inflammation in cysts, as large a biopsy sample as possible should be obtained for diagnosis.

Differential diagnosis

The odontogenic keratocyst is usually correctly identified radiologically, unless small and unilocular, in which case it may resemble any other cyst or well-defined radiolucent lesion. If the diagnosis is suspected, or if there is doubt, a biopsy is required to confirm the diagnosis. Correct preoperative diagnosis is necessary to select the special treatment given to this cyst type.

Occasionally, an odontogenic keratocyst may envelop an unerupted tooth or entrap a tooth and prevent its eruption, superficially producing a radiographic resemblance to a dentigerous cyst (Fig. 10.32). Odontogenic keratocysts with many locules may simulate an ameloblastoma radiographically (Fig. 10.33), but the relative lack of expansion identifies the cyst.

General reference ISBN-13: 978-1405149372

Treatment and recurrence

If the cyst is treated by simple enucleation, because the diagnosis was not suspected preoperatively, recurrence is likely. Recurrence has several contributing causes (Box 10.10). Historically, recurrence rates of more than 50% were reported, but with the current techniques described later in this chapter, recurrence rates of 2%–3% can be achieved.

Probably the major factor leading to recurrence is the difficulty in removing every trace of the epithelial lining, which is friable and has a complex outline. Any fragments missed may survive and grow because of their proliferative activity. Larger cysts have a higher risk of recurrence because complete removal is more difficult. When the cyst extends

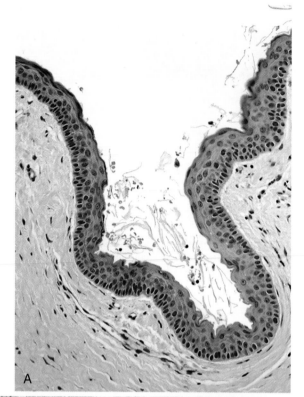

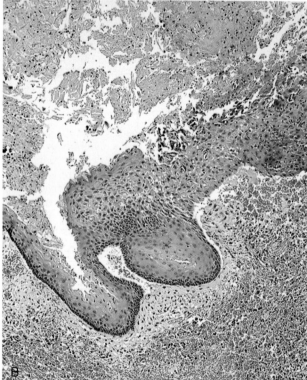

Fig. 10.30 Inflamed odontogenic keratocyst. Some areas of the lining show typical features (A), but in (B) inflammation has induced epithelial thickening and loss of the basal palisading and keratin.

around multirooted teeth, these may have to be sacrificed to ensure complete removal.

Even if effectively removed, it is possible for a completely new cyst to form from residual dental lamina rests, explaining apparent recurrence as long as 40 years after removal.

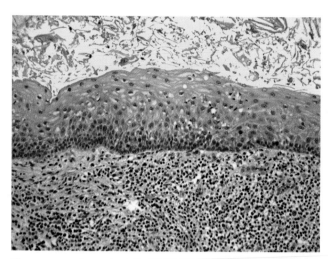

Fig. 10.31 Inflamed odontogenic keratocyst. Higher power of a more inflamed cyst with complete loss of diagnostic histological features. The epithelial lining resembles that of a radicular or inflamed dentigerous cyst with only a hint of keratin on the left to give a clue to the correct diagnosis.

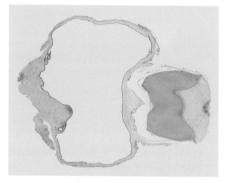

Fig. 10.32 A cyst arising in the follicle of an unerupted developing tooth. Radiographically, the cyst might have appeared to be in a true dentigerous relationship with the crown. However, this is not a dentigerous cyst; its lining does not join the tooth at the amelocemental junction (as in Figs 10.19 and 10.20). A higher-power view would reveal the characteristic lining of an odontogenic keratocyst.

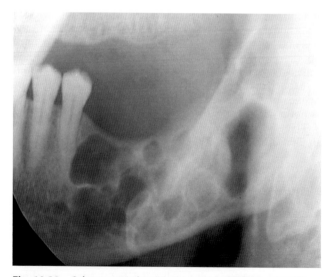

Fig. 10.33 Odontogenic keratocyst with multiple locules. Note the cortication around each cavity. The appearances resemble ameloblastoma, though the lack of expansion gives a clue to the correct diagnosis. *(Courtesy of Mr EJ Whaites.)*

Otherwise, recurrence is often within the first 5 years after treatment. Vigorous treatment is likely to reduce the risk of recurrence, but there is no absolute certainty of a cure in one operation, and patients need long-term radiographic follow up.

Ideally, therefore, diagnosis should be confirmed by biopsy to allow more thorough treatment than for other cysts.

Treatment depends largely on the extent of the cyst and the degree of multilocularity. Unilocular and small multilocular cysts can be treated conservatively and are usually enucleated and the bony cavity curetted vigorously to remove every fragment of cyst lining.

A useful additional precaution is the treatment of the cavity wall with a fixative (Carnoy's solution). This can be applied either before enucleation to kill and toughen the lining for removal or to the bony walls after curettage to destroy residual epithelial cells. It kills and denatures tissue to a depth of approximately 1–2 mm, far enough to kill the full thickness of the wall. However, it is a caustic mixture of ferric chloride in alcohol, chloroform and highly concentrated acetic acid and must be used with care near vital structures such as the inferior dental neurovascular bundle. The inclusion of chloroform makes Carnoy's solution controversial, and a modified formula without it appears to be equally effective in early analyses. Some authorities claim no added benefit versus careful mechanical removal and curettage of the cavity, but most consider that adding Carnoy's solution reduces recurrence by about half.

Recently, a more conservative approach has been proposed. It has been recognised that a low risk of recurrence is better than a mandibular resection and consequent morbidity. Although recurrences are seen as a failure of treatment, if detected early they may be easily managed by minor surgery, and a second curettage will often be effective.

Perhaps surprisingly given the so-called *aggressive* nature of this cyst and its lack of internal pressure, marsupialisation has been found to be effective. Marsupialisation is followed by slow shrinkage of the cyst, allowing enucleation of the residual cyst with preservation of teeth. Reduction in size is associated with ingrowth of oral epithelium into the cavity, replacing the typical keratinised epithelium with non-keratinising stratified squamous epithelium. This makes enucleation of the residual cyst much easier, and recurrence is less frequent than after enucleation alone. Teeth displaced by the cyst often regain an upright position.

Complete resolution after marsupialisation is possible but takes a long time, as long as 20 months, and it requires cooperative patients who will irrigate the cavity and keep it open and clean until it resolves. However, use as a primary treatment is increasing because the morbidity is considerably less than radical surgery, and the procedure is simpler than trying to enucleate the lining from a large cavity with a complex shape.

For the most extensive cysts, resection and reconstruction with a bone graft may be required. This controls recurrence but carries high morbidity. Posterior maxillary cysts may be treated more aggressively as they can be difficult to eradicate if they escape the confines of the bone and occasionally these extend to the skull base.

If an unsuspected odontogenic keratocyst is accidentally enucleated, radiographic follow up is appropriate and any recurrence can be treated appropriately.

Key features of odontogenic keratocysts are summarised in Box 10.11.

Marsupialisation PMID: 8863300

Recurrence and treatment PMID: 15883937

Basal cell naevus syndrome

This syndrome, often called Gorlin's or Gorlin-Goltz syndrome, is inherited as an autosomal dominant trait. It is defined by the triad of multiple basal cell carcinomas, odontogenic keratocysts and various skeletal anomalies.

The syndrome is caused by any one of many mutations in, or occasionally deletions in, the patched (*PTCH*) gene on chromosome 9q. This gene is important in developmental patterning, and families with the syndrome have inactivation of one allele causing the skeletal anomalies. The gene is also a tumour suppressor gene and modulates the cell cycle via the hedgehog (HH) signalling pathway. Inactivation or mutation of the second copy of the gene is associated with development of multiple basal cell carcinomas and odontogenic keratocysts. Mutations of the same gene may also be found in a variety of other neoplasms associated with the syndrome. Mutations in *PTCH* may also be found in odontogenic keratocysts in patients without the syndrome.

The main features of the syndrome are listed in Box 10.12 and the facial appearance is shown in Fig. 10.34, although a great many other abnormalities may be present. Although the gene is highly penetrant, it shows considerable variation in expressivity, so the effects vary between families and individuals. There is no clear correlation between the features seen and the particular gene mutation. One of the most consistent features, and one useful in confirming the diagnosis, is the presence of palmar pits, small round pinpoint depressions on the palms and soles of feet 1–2 mm

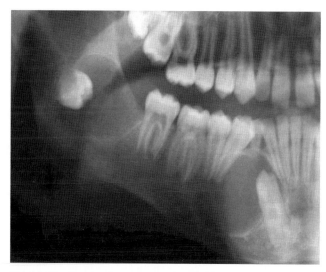

Fig. 10.35   Basal cell naevus syndrome. These two odontogenic keratocysts appear to be dentigerous but are not convincingly attached to the amelocemental junction of the teeth. Biopsy revealed odontogenic keratocysts and the presence of two in one patient, particularly a child, indicates the syndrome.

Case series PMID: 8042673

Diagnostic criteria management PMID: 21834049

Basal cell carcinomas PMID: 21834049

Web URL 10.2 Genetics: http://omim.org/entry/109400

ORTHOKERATINISED ODONTOGENIC CYST

The second type of keratinising jaw cyst is the orthokeratinised odontogenic cyst (Fig. 10.36). It is less common than the parakeratinised type and used to be thought a variant.

This cyst differs in a number of respects from the true odontogenic keratocyst, having a lower proliferative activity and no association with basal cell naevus syndrome. Differences are summarised in Table 10.1, and the most important difference is that orthokeratinised cysts are less likely

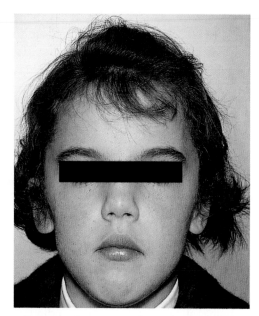

Fig. 10.34   Basal cell naevus syndrome. The typical facies with a broad nasal root and mild frontal bossing.

in diameter. These are caused by focal lack of keratin and may appear red or a dark colour as they fill with dirt. Although these may be seen in other diseases, three or more pits is a diagnostic feature for the syndrome.

In view of the great variety of abnormalities that may be present, the effects on the patient depend on the predominant manifestation.

In some cases, there are innumerable basal cell carcinomas. These are sometimes termed 'naevoid' because a linear cluster of them in their early stages looks like a birthmark and because they often present in children. The face is a common site, and they behave as conventional basal cell carcinomas.

Almost all patients have odontogenic keratocysts, necessitating repeated operations. The presence of an odontogenic keratocyst in a child or multiple cysts should raise suspicion of the syndrome (Fig. 10.35). The cysts are identical to the non-syndromic equivalents and have the same tendency to recur. *PTCH* mutations are found in more than 80% of syndromic cysts.

Cleft lip or palate or both is seen in a small proportion of these patients.

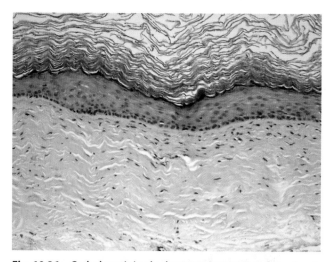

Fig. 10.36   Orthokeratinised odontogenic cyst. Uninflamed wall with a thickly orthokeratinised epithelium. Keratin fills the lumen, but the other characteristic features of odontogenic keratocyst are not present; note the lack of palisaded basal cells.

to recur than parakeratinised cysts. The cyst has no particular clinical or radiological features that would allow preoperative diagnosis. Most are thought to be dentigerous cysts radiographically because many arise in a dentigerous relationship to a lower third molar. Enucleation is curative.

Case series PMID: 20121617

LATERAL PERIODONTAL CYSTS

These uncommon developmental odontogenic cysts form in the periodontal ligament beside the mid portion of the root of a vital tooth, presumably arising from a rest of Malassez.

They affect middle-aged and elderly adults, and are usually chance radiographic findings when small. More than three-quarters arise in the lower canine and premolar region, and their location is characteristic and almost diagnostic (Fig. 10.37). Occasional examples reach several centimetres in diameter and expand the jaw and displace teeth.

This cyst has a diagnostic histological appearance, shared with its multilocular variant, the botryoid odontogenic cyst (Fig. 10.38). The lining is squamous or cuboidal epithelium that is mostly only one or two cells thick but has focal rounded thickenings or plaques (Fig. 10.39). In the plaques, the cells can have a swirling appearance, sometimes with clear cytoplasm, resembling the dental lamina. The cyst should be enucleated. If the cyst is small, the related tooth, which is vital, can be retained.

Features are summarised in Box 10.13, together with the botryoid odontogenic cyst.

Case series PMID: 8665317

Botryoid odontogenic cysts

The botryoid odontogenic cyst is a rare variant of the lateral periodontal cyst that is multilocular (Fig. 10.38). Apart from this feature, the cyst appears identical histologically (Fig. 10.39).

It typically affects the anterior mandible in adults older than 50 years and has a tendency to recur after enucleation. If the multilocularity is noted radiographically,

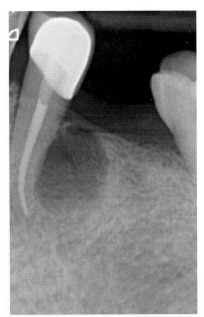

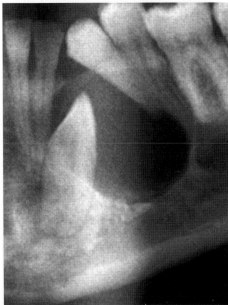

Fig. 10.37 Lateral periodontal cyst. Two typical examples of lateral periodontal cysts in the usual site adjacent to roots of lower canines and premolars.

> **Box 10.13   Key features of lateral periodontal cysts**
>
> **Lateral periodontal cysts**
>
> - Developmental cysts that form beside a vital tooth
> - Usually seen by chance in routine radiographs
> - Resemble other odontogenic cysts radiographically
> - Diagnostic histological appearance
> - Respond to enucleation
>
> **Botryoid odontogenic cysts**
>
> - Rare variant of lateral periodontal cyst
> - Affect the mandibular premolar to canine region
> - Microscopically, as lateral periodontal cyst but multilocular*
> - Have a tendency to recur after enucleation
>
> *Multilocularity not necessarily visible in radiographs

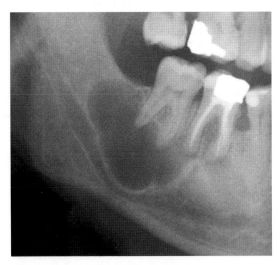

Fig. 10.38 Botryoid odontogenic cyst. There is corticated and well-defined radiolucency with a scalloped outline as evidence of possible multilocularity, but no other clue as to the cyst type.

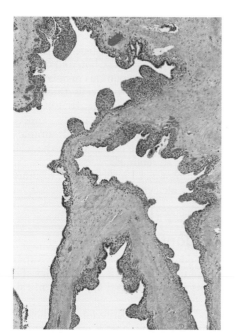

Fig. 10.39 Botryoid odontogenic cyst. A cyst with several locules and the characteristic lobular thickenings or plaques of the lining epithelium. A lateral periodontal cyst has the same appearance, but a single cyst cavity.

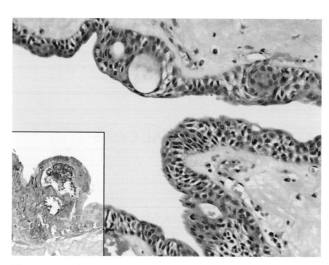

Fig. 10.40 Glandular odontogenic cyst. The epithelial lining has an occasional plaque similar to those in lateral periodontal cysts and contains small glands or duct-like spaces. *Inset*, glands contain mucin revealed by staining with alcian blue and periodic acid–Schiff producing a bright blue reaction.

the cyst is usually mistaken for an odontogenic keratocyst preoperatively.

Features are summarised in Box 10.13.

Case series PMID: 8683420

GLANDULAR ODONTOGENIC CYST

The glandular odontogenic cyst is a rare odontogenic cyst also known as the *sialo-odontogenic cyst*. Glandular odontogenic cysts are diagnosed in middle-aged patients and usually in the mandible, anterior to molars. The cysts are unilocular or multilocular and expand the jaw and displace and resorb teeth.

The cyst has a diagnostic histological appearance with small glands that are lined by mucous cells and secrete mucin and lie in thickenings of the epithelial lining (Fig. 10.40).

Approximately a third of cases recur after enucleation and additional curettage and sacrifice of teeth or conservative excision may be necessary. Clinical and radiographic misdiagnosis as odontogenic keratocyst will fortuitously result in more aggressive treatment, and this is usually sufficient to prevent recurrence. Features are summarised in Box 10.14.

Case series PMID: 7600223

Diagnosis and recurrence PMID: 21915706

Box 10.14 Glandular odontogenic cyst

- Rare developmental odontogenic cyst
- Frequently multilocular*
- Diagnostic histological appearance
- Has a strong tendency to recur
- Small lesions may be enucleated with curettage
- Large multilocular lesions are excised conservatively

*Multilocularity not necessarily visible in radiographs

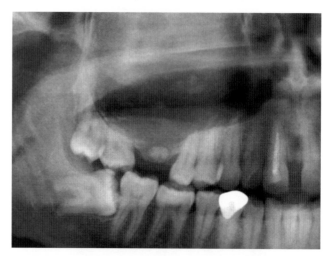

Fig. 10.41 Calcifying odontogenic cyst. This typical large corticated maxillary example is mostly radiolucent but contains some patchy mineralisation, both centrally and around the periphery, especially around the inferior margin.

CALCIFYING ODONTOGENIC CYST

The calcifying odontogenic cyst is rare. Clinically, almost any age and either jaw can be affected. The site is most often in bone anterior to the first molar but, occasionally, it can develop as a small nodule on the gingiva that indents the underlying bone.

On radiographs, the appearance is usually unilocular but may be multilocular and contain flecks or, more rarely, dense masses of calcification (Fig. 10.41). Occasionally, roots of adjacent teeth are resorbed. Unless mineralisation is present, the radiographic appearances are not diagnostic.

The lining of the cyst looks like ameloblastoma (see Ch. 11) with an epithelium with cuboidal or ameloblast-like basal cells (Figs 10.42 and 10.43) and often a thick layer of stellate reticulum. The diagnostic feature is a peculiar form of abnormal keratinisation producing clusters of pale swollen, eosinophilic cells with a hole centrally. The hole is produced by degeneration and loss of the nucleus, leaving

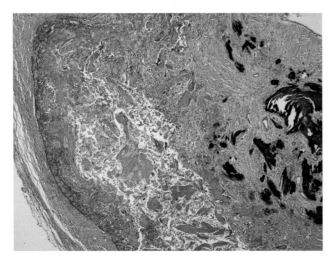

Fig. 10.42 Calcifying odontogenic cyst. The fibrous wall and epithelium run along the left with the lumen filled by ghost cells centrally. Some ghost cells have become incorporated into the fibrous wall on the right and are calcifying.

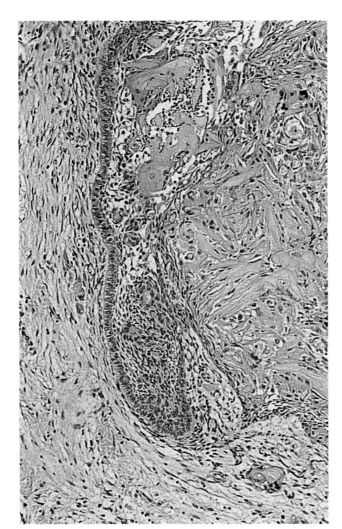

Fig. 10.43 Calcifying odontogenic cyst. There is a thin lining of epithelium with a basal layer of palisaded ameloblast-like columnar cells with stellate reticulum-like suprabasal cells. The lumen (*top right*) is filled by ghost cells shed into the cyst cavity.

a pale 'ghost' of the cell (Fig. 10.44). The ghost cells often stack up in layers and may calcify in a patchy fashion, giving the cyst its name and producing the spotty radiopacities that give a clue to the diagnosis. Where this keratin-like material comes into contact with connective tissue, it induces a dentine-like matrix or mineralised tissue called dentinoid.

Approximately 10% of calcifying odontogenic cysts are associated with odontomes or other odontogenic tumours.

The behaviour of a calcifying odontogenic cyst is benign, and enucleation is usually effective. However, very similar histological features may be found in a solid odontogenic tumour from which the calcifying odontogenic cyst must be differentiated. These solid dentinogenic ghost cell tumours have a risk of recurrence on removal, whereas the cysts usually do not.

Key features are summarised in Box 10.15.

Case series PMID: 1716354

Ghost cell lesions PMID: 18221328

> **Box 10.15 Calcifying odontogenic cyst: key features**
> * Rare odontogenic cyst
> * Wide age range
> * Radiographically unilocular often undistinguishable from other jaw cysts
> * Calcifications in the cyst wall may suggest the diagnosis
> * Forms at any site in alveolar ridge, usually posteriorly
> * Occasionally forms in soft tissue of the gingiva
> * Diagnosed by finding ghost and ameloblast-like cells histologically
> * Usually responds to enucleation
> * Solid lesions are distinct and more aggressive (page 176)

CARCINOMA ARISING IN ODONTOGENIC CYSTS

Extremely rarely, a carcinoma arises from the epithelium of a cyst lining. In such cases the cyst has usually been untreated for a long period of time. Radicular, dentigerous and odontogenic keratocysts can all undergo malignant change, and the carcinomas are usually squamous in type (Fig. 11.50).

Such cases are often diagnosed only after removal, but if allowed to progress will present with the typical features of carcinoma in the jaw.

Review PMID: 21689161

GINGIVAL CYST OF THE NEWBORN

Also known as Bohn's nodules, these small cysts of the dental lamina can be found in as many as 80% of newborn infants. They form small nodules or cysts on the alveolar ridge, each up to 2 mm diameter. Their whitish colour is caused by their content of keratin. They are considered to be due to proliferation of the epithelial rests of Serres (Fig. 10.45) but can arise on the lateral aspects of the ridge and the crest. They resolve spontaneously by rupture over a few days and are of no significance, but may be mistaken for natal teeth.

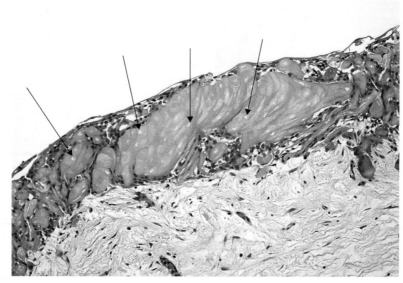

Fig. 10.44   Calcifying odontogenic cyst, fibrous wall below, lumen above. The epithelial cells in this area are inconspicuous, the epithelium being almost replaced by numerous ghost cells. *Arrows* indicate the nuclear holes that give these cells their name.

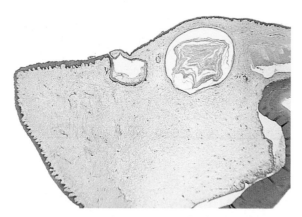

Fig. 10.45   Gingival cyst of the newborn (Bohn's nodules). This section from an embryo shows cyst formation in the rests of Serres superficial to the developing teeth. The cysts are lined by keratinising epithelium.

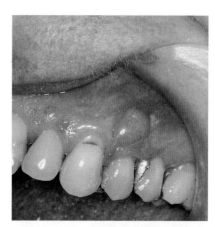

Fig. 10.46   Gingival cyst of adult. Typical presentation as a superficial cyst in the attached gingiva of a premolar tooth.

Incidence PMID: 21995277

Epstein's pearls

Epstein's pearls are similar small cysts along the midpalatine raphe in the newborn. They may enlarge sufficiently to appear as creamy-coloured swellings a few millimetres in diameter, but also resolve spontaneously in a matter of weeks or months.

GINGIVAL CYST OF ADULTS

Gingival cysts in adults are rare and present after the age of approximately 40 years, most often in the lower canine and premolar region. Clinically, they form dome-shaped swellings less than 1 cm in diameter and sometimes erode the underlying bone by pressure (Fig. 10.46). They are lined by very thin, flat, stratified squamous epithelium and may contain fluid or layers of keratin, and sometimes the epithelium forms plaques similar to those in lateral periodontal cysts. They do not recur on excision.

Case series PMID: 26233969

NON-ODONTOGENIC CYSTS

NASOPALATINE DUCT OR INCISIVE CANAL CYST

The formation of a cyst in the incisive canal is surprisingly common in some studies, accounting for around 5% of jaw cysts and making this the commonest non-odontogenic cyst of the jaws. They are also known as *incisive canal cysts*.

Clinical features

These cysts arise in the incisive canal, and the presentation depends on where in the canal they form. They may form a superficial soft tissue cyst in the incisive papilla if at the oral end (Fig. 10.47), grow primarily into the nose if at the

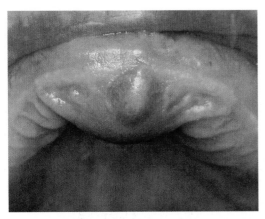

Fig. 10.47 **Nasopalatine cyst.** Typical presentation with a dome-shaped bluish enlargement overlying the incisive canal.

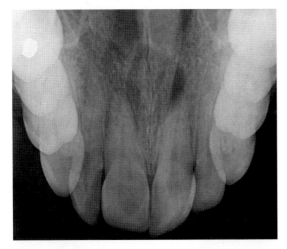

Fig. 10.48 **Nasopalatine cyst.** The usual appearance is a rounded or pear-shaped area of radiolucency, at the site of the incisive canal.

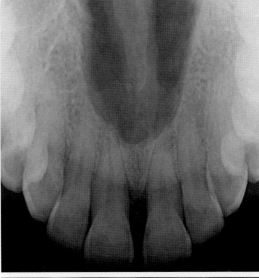

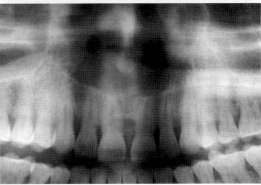

Fig. 10.49 **Nasopalatine cyst.** This example is so large that is visible on a panoramic radiograph and extends beyond the posterior limits of an occlusal view.

superior end or grow slowly in the bone of the anterior palate if they arise in the middle. Often they burst into the mouth or nose, producing intermittent salty discharge. Cysts from the middle of the canal expand the bone of the palate downward and upward, while they grow forward, over or between the central incisor apices to expand the anterior alveolus in the midline.

Radiography shows a rounded radiolucent area with a corticated outline at the site of the incisive canal (Fig. 10.48). In anterior occlusal or periapical films they may appear heart-shaped because of superimposition of the anterior nasal spine. They are usually symmetrical but become asymmetrical when large (Fig. 10.49). The root apices of the central incisors are often pushed apart.

The normal incisive canal appears as large as 10 mm in diameter radiographically because of enlargement and distortion. In deciding from a radiograph whether or not an unusually large incisive canal is a cyst or not, a cut off value of 6–8 mm is usually taken, but there may be no need for immediate surgical exploration as radiographic follow up will detect enlargement if a cyst is present.

Key features of nasopalatine duct cysts are summarised in Box 10.16.

Case series PMID: 1995816

Patent nasopalatine duct PMID: 2185448

Box 10.16 Nasopalatine duct cyst: key features
- Often asymptomatic, chance radiographic findings
- Form in the incisive canal region
- Arise from vestiges of the nasopalatine duct
- Lined by squamous or columnar respiratory epithelium
- The long sphenopalatine nerve and vessels may be present in the wall
- Can usually be recognised radiographically
- Do not recur after enucleation

Pathogenesis and pathology

The nasopalatine duct is an air passage between the mouth and the organ of Jacobson in the nasal septum of many animals, including cats and cattle. Jacobson's organ is used to sense pheromones and assess the state of sexual readiness of potential mates. Humans have no Jacobson's organ, though the duct forms in embryos and then involutes. Remnants of the vestigial duct sometimes persist and occasionally give rise to nasopalatine duct cysts.

The epithelial lining is usually either stratified squamous epithelium or ciliated columnar (respiratory) epithelium with mucous glands (resembling either oral or nasal mucosa respectively; Fig. 10.50).

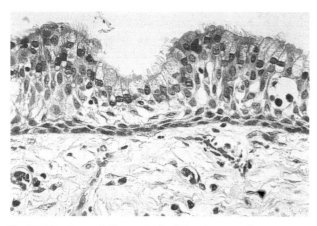

Fig. 10.50 **Nasopalatine cyst.** The lining, in part at least, may consist of respiratory (ciliated columnar) epithelium, as here. Alcian blue staining reveals blue mucin in goblet cells.

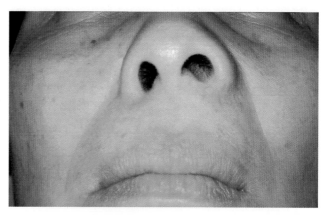

Fig. 10.52 **Nasolabial cyst.** Typical fullness of the nasolabial fold and in the lateral wall and floor of the nasal cavity caused by this cyst on the patient's left. *(Adapted from Yuen HW, et al., 2006. Nasolabial cysts: Clinical features, diagnosis, and treatment, Fig.1 British Journal of Oral and Maxillofacial Surgery, 45(4), 293-297)*

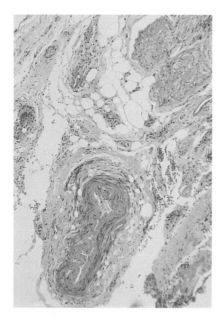

Fig. 10.51 **Nasopalatine cyst.** Nerves and blood vessels of the incisive canal in the cyst wall.

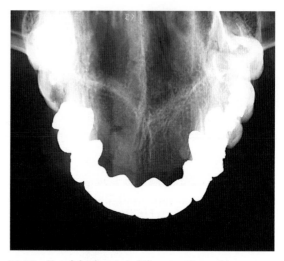

Fig. 10.53 **Nasolabial cyst.** A different patient with a cyst on their right, showing pressure resorption of the anterior lip of the nasal cavity, seen as asymmetry and a scooped out concavity to the patient's right of the anterior nasal spine.

The long sphenopalatine nerve and vessels that pass through the incisive canal are often removed with the cyst and seen histologically (Fig. 10.51), but no deficit results.

Nasopalatine duct cysts can be enucleated without recurrence.

NASOLABIAL CYST

This very uncommon cyst forms outside the bone in the soft tissues, deep to the nasolabial fold. It probably arises from the lower end of the nasolacrimal duct and is occasionally bilateral. It presents over a wide age range, mostly in middle-aged adults, and much more commonly in females. The cysts form soft tissue swellings in the upper lip, distort the nostril (Fig. 10.52) and cause pressure resorption of the anterior maxilla if large (Fig. 10.53).

The lining is pseudostratified columnar respiratory epithelium, like the nasolacrimal duct. The cyst is excised, usually from an intraoral approach through the labial sulcus.

Review and treatment PMID: 26153269

SUBLINGUAL DERMOID CYST

These are cysts above the hyoid and mylohyoid, immediately beneath the tongue (Fig. 10.54), usually in the midline, occasionally to one side (Fig. 10.55). They are lined by a keratinising stratified squamous epithelium like skin, complete with associated sebaceous glands, sweat glands and sometimes hair follicles. Those without skin adnexae are called *epidermoid cysts*.

A sublingual dermoid is more deeply placed than a ranula (Ch. 22), lacks the bluish appearance and is firmer. They are asymptomatic when small, enlarge to interfere with speech or eating and can attain a large size over many years, completely concealed by the tongue in its normal resting position. Most present in the second or third decade.

These cysts are removed by excision.

Review PMID: 20392029

Case series PMID: 15018452

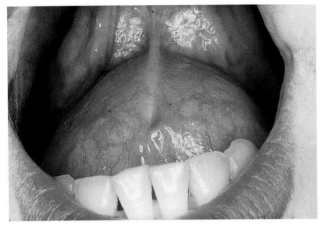

Fig. 10.54 **Sublingual dermoid cyst.** This is an unusually large specimen but appears even larger because the patient is raising and protruding her tongue. This cyst, unlike a ranula, can be seen to have a thick wall because it has arisen in the deeper tissues of the floor of the mouth.

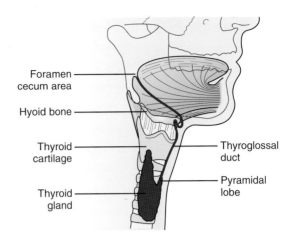

Fig. 10.56 **Path of the thyroglossal duct.** Ectopic thyroid, cysts, and occasionally thyroid carcinomas can be found anywhere along the line of the tract, but are commonest where it loops below and behind the body of the hyoid. The path of the tract is convoluted in the adult, but in the early embryo it is a short straight line.

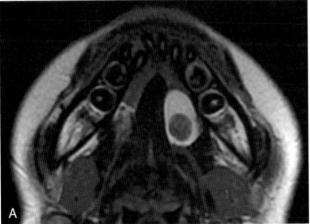

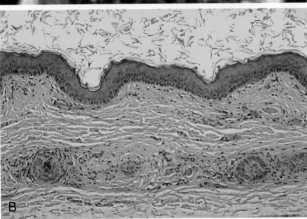

Fig. 10.55 **Sublingual dermoid cyst.** In the magnetic resonance imaging scan of a different example, the fluid contents produce a bright signal showing a circumscribed cyst to one side of the floor of mouth (A). On biopsy (B) the cyst is lined by a thin orthokeratinising epithelium like that of the skin and a few islands of glandular epithelium lie in the wall. The lumen is filled by keratin flakes.

THYROGLOSSAL DUCT CYST

Thyroglossal or thyroglossal duct cysts develop from embryological epithelial remnants of the thyroglossal duct, anywhere along its rather convoluted path from the dorsum of tongue to the site of the thyroid gland (Fig. 10.56). The duct forms at week 4 in utero and by week 8 has reached the site of the normal thyroid gland. By week 10 it has involuted, leaving only occasional small nests of epithelium in approximately 10% of individuals.

Thyroglossal cysts are the commonest neck cysts, and almost all present in the area of the body of the hyoid bone, very rarely in the floor of mouth or at the foramen caecum. Those around the hyoid bone form swellings in the midline neck skin in adolescents and young adults (Fig. 10.57). Classically the cyst rises on swallowing while the tongue moves upward.

Histologically, the cysts are lined by stratified squamous epithelium or respiratory epithelium, and there are often clusters of ectopic thyroid tissue in the wall.

These cysts are removed surgically with the body of the hyoid bone and tissue along the line of the tract down to the gland, to ensure that all remnants and any ectopic gland are removed. This prevents recurrence, development of new cysts and ensures removal of all ectopic microscopic thyroid tissue, which can rarely be the site of development of a thyroid cancer.

See also lingual thyroid in Chapter 36.

Review: PMID: 25439547

BRANCHIAL CYST

The five pharyngeal arches develop between weeks 2–6 in utero and give rise to many structures in the head and neck. Failure of fusion of the arches can leave embryological remnants in the neck that can give rise to branchial cysts. These occur at reproducible sites. By far the commonest is the second branchial arch cyst, which is visible externally at the anterior border of sternomastoid muscle (Fig. 10.58), just

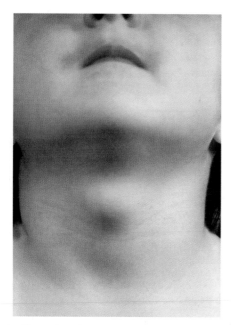

Fig. 10.57 Thyroglossal cyst. A typical thyroglossal cyst in the midline close to the body of the hyoid bone and just below the skin. *(From Chummy, S.S., 2011. Last's Anatomy: Regional and Applied, 12th edition. Churchill Livingstone, Edinburgh.)*

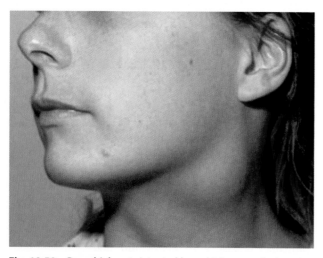

Fig. 10.58 Branchial cyst. A typical branchial cyst at the junction of level 2 and level 3 in the neck, and just anterior to sternomastoid muscle. *(From Myers, E.N., 2008. Operative Otolaryngology: Head and Neck Surgery, 2nd Edition. Elsevier, Edinburgh.)*

below the angle of the mandible. Genuine branchial cysts, as opposed to lymphoepithelial cysts arising in lymph nodes at a similar site, extend deeply, sometimes between the branches of the carotid or even as far as the pharynx, the embryological path of the second arch cleft. Sometimes the cysts open to the skin and are then known as *branchial clefts*.

Branchial cysts can attain a large size and present in adolescents or adults up to 40 years of age. They are lined by non-keratinising squamous epithelium and often have lymphoid tissue in their wall.

A branchial cyst in an adult older than 45 years would be extremely unlikely, but an identical presentation may develop when tonsil or base of tongue carcinomas metastasise to a cervical lymph node. These metastases are often cystic and can be difficult to tell from a benign cyst histologically. This is discussed further in Chapter 21.

Origin and imaging: PMC4729717

FOREGUT CYST

These very rare cysts are developmental anomalies in children and adolescents, usually in the midline ventral tongue or floor of mouth. The cyst is lined by gastric or other intestinal mucosa and is treated by excision.

OTHER CYSTS IN OTHER CHAPTERS

Ameloblastoma is an odontogenic tumour that can be unilocular or multilocular and be clinically and radiologically indistinguishable from other types of cyst (Ch. 11).

Mucous retention and extravasation cysts are considered in Chapter 22.

Malignant neoplasms can arise in radicular, dentigerous and odontogenic keratocysts, though exceedingly rarely, and this topic is covered in Chapter 11.

A further group of cysts common in the head and neck are skin cysts, epidermoid and dermoid cysts ('sebaceous' cysts) arising from inflammation or trauma to skin.

Also excluded from the earlier classification are two lesions that are cystic in their radiographic appearances but lack an epithelial lining, the solitary bone 'cyst' and aneurysmal bone 'cyst', covered in Chapter 13.

A number of other cysts are historical concepts, now abandoned. It is now considered that there is no such entity as a globulomaxillary cyst, median mandibular cyst or median palatal cyst.

Summary chart 10.1 Differential diagnosis of the common and important causes of a well-defined monolocular radiolucency in the jaws.

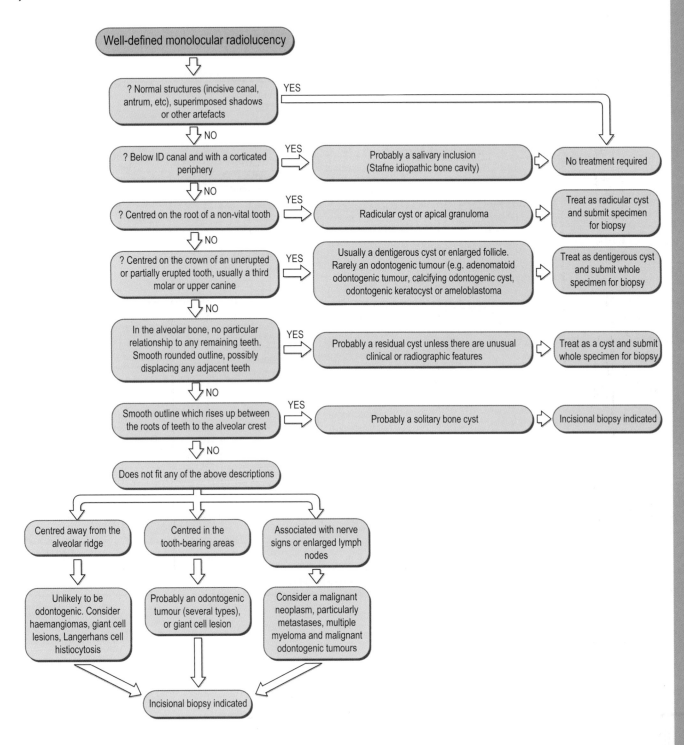

Summary chart 10.2   Differential diagnosis of a multilocular radiolucency at the angle of the mandible.

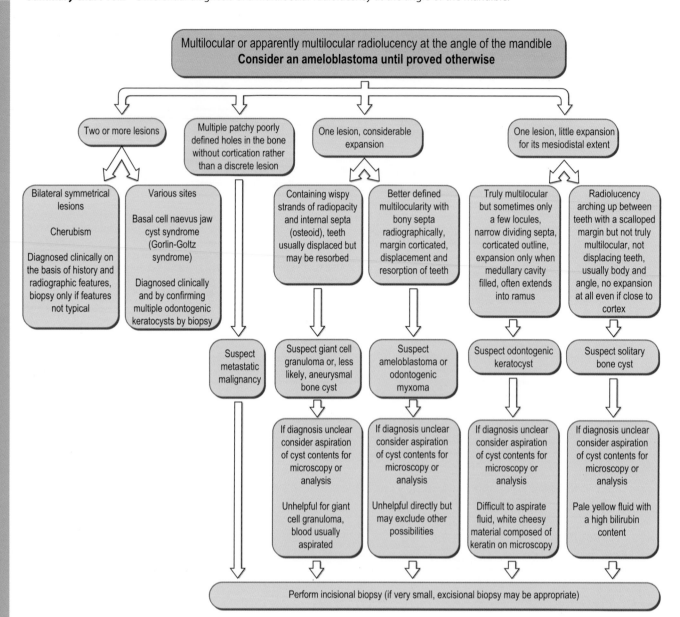

Odontogenic tumours and related jaw lesions

11

Neoplasms and other tumours affecting the jaws can be odontogenic, derived from odontogenic tissues, or non-odontogenic (Box 11.1). It is not always obvious whether a swelling is odontogenic or not clinically and, in many instances, the origin and nature of a particular lesion may be unclear until biopsy.

Odontogenic tumours are the most common neoplasms of the jaws. There are many types, and the majority are rare. Odontogenic tumours may be derived from odontogenic epithelium (dental lamina, reduced enamel epithelium, rests of Serres, rests of Malassez) or products of odontogenic mesenchyme (dental follicle, dental papilla, pulp, periodontal ligament) or both in varying proportions. The dental follicle gives rise to the inner half of the lamina dura of the socket, so lesions of bone can be odontogenic too.

The accepted standard classification of odontogenic tumours is that of the World Health Organization (WHO). A simplified version of the current classification is shown in Box 11.2, and the whole classification is given in Appendix 11.1 together with brief details of the rarer lesions. It should be noted that this is a classification of *tumours* (swellings), not only of neoplasms, and it therefore includes lesions of differing types and behaviour. To aid understanding, the tumours are classified and listed in a slightly different order here.

Box 11.1 Important causes of tumours (swellings) of the jaws

- Cysts, predominantly odontogenic cysts
- Odontogenic tumours
- Giant cell lesions
- Fibro-osseous lesions
- Primary (non-odontogenic) neoplasms of bone
- Metastatic neoplasms

Box 11.2 Simplified classification of odontogenic and jaw tumours*

Benign epithelial tumours

- Ameloblastomas
  - Ameloblastoma
  - Ameloblastoma, unicystic type
  - Ameloblastoma peripheral/extraosseous type
  - Metastasizing ameloblastoma
- Squamous odontogenic tumour
- Calcifying epithelial odontogenic tumour
- Adenomatoid odontogenic tumour

Benign mixed epithelial and mesenchymal tumours

- Ameloblastic fibroma
- Primordial odontogenic tumour
- Odontome (developing/compound and complex)
- Dentinogenic ghost cell tumour

Benign mesenchymal tumours

- Odontogenic fibroma
- Odontogenic myxoma / myxofibroma
- Cementoblastoma

Fibro-osseous lesions

- Cemento-ossifying fibromas
- Cemento-osseous dysplasia

Malignant neoplasms

- Ameloblastic carcinoma
- Primary intraosseous carcinoma NOS
- Sclerosing odontogenic carcinoma
- Clear cell odontogenic carcinoma
- Ghost cell odontogenic carcinoma
- Odontogenic carcinosarcoma
- Odontogenic sarcomas

---

*For the full classification, see Appendix 11.1

BENIGN EPITHELIAL TUMOURS

AMELOBLASTOMAS → Summary chart 10.2
p. 164

Several types of ameloblastoma are recognised. All are benign epithelial neoplasms in which the epithelium contains ameloblast-like cells and stellate reticulum-like cells, indicating its odontogenic nature.

Solid/multicystic or 'conventional' ameloblastoma

This is the most common type and the most common neoplasm in the jaws. Ameloblastomas are usually first recognised between the ages of 30 and 50 years and are rare in children and old people. Eighty per cent form in the mandible; of these 75% develop in the posterior molar region and often involve the ramus. They are symptomless until the swelling is noticed (Fig. 11.1). Ameloblastomas can grow to enormous size and cause major disfigurement.

Practical Point Ameloblastoma should be included in the differential diagnosis for any radiolucency in the posterior alveolus and lower ramus of the mandible.

Radiographically, ameloblastomas typically form rounded, cyst-like, radiolucent areas with well-defined margins. The smallest appear unilocular, larger ameloblastomas may comprise a few large clustered cysts ('soap-bubble' multilocularity) or numerous small cysts a few millimetres across ('honeycomb' multilocular pattern) or a mixture of patterns (Fig. 11.2). Expansion may be both lingual and buccal. Other multilocular lesions that may mimic ameloblastoma radiologically include odontogenic keratocyst, giant-cell granuloma and odontogenic myxoma. Ameloblastomas with a single bony cavity simulate many types of cyst and tumour radiographically.

Pathology

The cause of ameloblastomas is not known, although most have recently been shown to harbour the V600E mutation in the *BRAF* gene or mutations of the *SMO* gene. The V600E oncogenic mutation is found in many malignant and benign neoplasms and activates the MAP kinase pathway, a driver of cell division and differentiation. It is not clear yet whether this mutation is causative, but its discovery has led to apparently successful experimental use of specific inhibitors in patients with otherwise untreatable disseminated ameloblastoma. SMO mutations appear less frequent and activate the hedgehog pathway, with similar effects.

Conventional ameloblastomas are a mixture of solid neoplasm and cysts (Fig. 11.3), and either component may predominate.

The solid areas comprise fibrous tissue containing islands or interconnected strands and sheets of epithelium with a peripheral layer of palisaded preameloblast-like cells that, at least focally, have nuclei at the opposite pole from the basement membrane (reversed polarity, a feature seen in ameloblasts just before secretion of enamel matrix). There are two histological patterns.

In the *follicular* pattern, the most common and most readily recognisable type (Fig. 11.4), there are islands with an outer layer of tall, columnar, ameloblast-like cells with reversed polarity surrounding a core of loosely arranged polyhedral or angular cells, resembling stellate reticulum (Fig. 11.5). In the *plexiform* pattern the epithelium forms

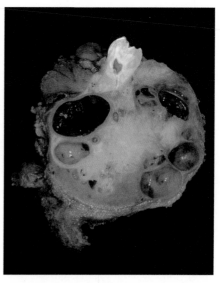

Fig. 11.3 Ameloblastoma of the conventional solid/multicystic type in a resection specimen showing multiple cysts.

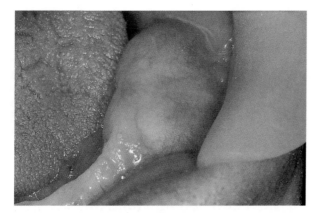

Fig. 11.1 **Ameloblastoma.** Typical presentation. There is a rounded, bony swelling of the posterior alveolar bone, body and angle of the mandible. There is no ulceration, which would be a feature only seen in very large tumours that have perforated the cortex.

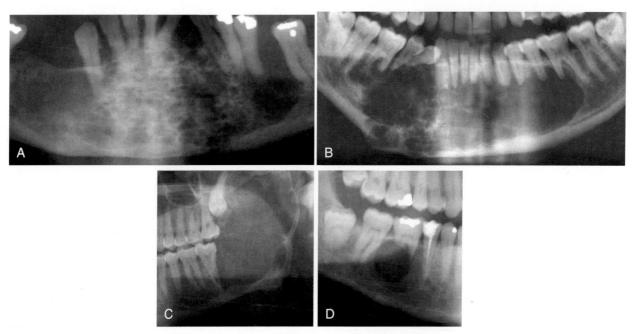

Fig. 11.2 **Ameloblastoma.** Four different ameloblastomas (A-D) showing the range of radiographic features, including honeycomb, multilocular, and apparently unicystic. All were typical solid/multicystic ameloblastoma on biopsy.

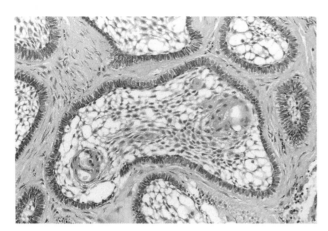

Fig. 11.4 **Ameloblastoma.** Islands of follicular ameloblastoma comprising 'stellate reticulum' and a peripheral layer of elongate ameloblast-like cells.

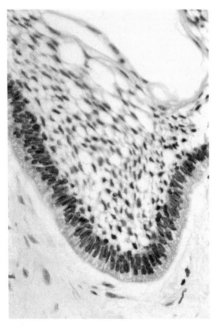

Fig. 11.5 **Ameloblastoma.** At high power in this follicular ameloblastoma, the palisaded, elongate peripheral cells with reversed polarity are seen to be very similar in appearance to ameloblasts.

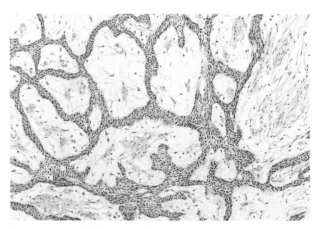

Fig. 11.6 **Ameloblastoma, plexiform type.** There are thin, interlacing strands of epithelium, but typical ameloblasts are often not seen in this pattern.

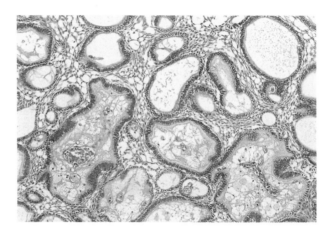

Fig. 11.7 **Ameloblastoma.** Plexiform ameloblastoma composed of interconnecting strands of epithelium surrounding islands of connective tissue. Several of the stromal islands have degenerated to form small cysts.

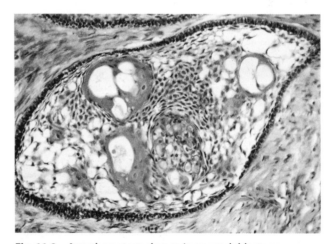

Fig. 11.8 **Acanthomatous change in an ameloblastoma.** Stellate reticulum-like cells have undergone squamous metaplasia to form keratin. This is called *acanthomatous* because it looks like prickle cells in keratinising epithelium.

strands and interconnected sheets and the ameloblast cells are often less prominent (Fig. 11.6). These two histological patterns do not reflect behaviour and are of no significance.

Cyst formation is common, and there are usually several large cysts as large as a few centimetres in diameter. Even apparently solid ameloblastomas have numerous microscopic cysts. In the follicular pattern, the cysts develop in the stellate reticulum inside the epithelial islands, whereas in the plexiform pattern the cysts are caused by degeneration of the connective tissue stroma (Fig. 11.7).

Other less common histological variants include the *acanthomatous* type, in which prickle cells replace the stellate reticulum and sometimes form keratin (Fig. 11.8). The rare *basal cell* variant and consists of more darkly staining basal cells with little evidence of ameloblasts. In the *granular cell pattern* the epithelium in the central areas of the tumour islands degenerates into sheets of large eosinophilic granular cells (Fig. 11.9).

A much more important histological feature is that islands of ameloblastoma can extend into the medullary spaces of surrounding bone. This behaviour is not expected in a benign neoplasm because it resembles infiltration by a malignant neoplasm. Only a minority of ameloblastomas

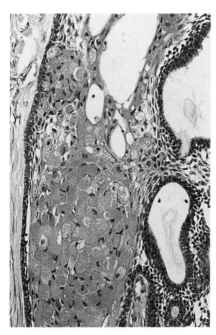

Fig. 11.9 Ameloblastoma. Granular cell change in an ameloblastoma. Ameloblastoma and stellate reticulum-like cells have undergone degenerative change to form large pink granular cells. In some tumours this change is extensive, and the term 'granular cell ameloblastoma' is applied.

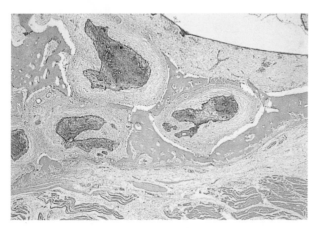

Fig. 11.10 Ameloblastoma. Islands of ameloblastoma penetrating surrounding bone at the periphery of the lesion. Such bony infiltration demands that ameloblastoma is excised with a margin rather than curetted.

have this feature, but it determines the necessary treatment. The islands of ameloblastoma may extend into bone marrow spaces for several millimetres beyond the edge of the main bony cavity. If left behind after surgery, they will seed recurrence (Fig. 11.10).

Additional types of ameloblastoma are listed in Appendix 11.1.

Key features are shown in Box 11.3.

Extensive review PMID: 7633291

Behaviour and treatment

Ameloblastomas enlarge the jaw slowly, displacing and often resorbing tooth roots, perforating the cortical bone and, if large, expanding into soft tissue constrained only by the periosteum. Although benign, they can be difficult to eradicate.

Box 11.3 Ameloblastoma: key features

- Benign neoplasm of odontogenic epithelium
- The most common odontogenic neoplasm
- Usually presents between ages 30 and 50 years
- Locally infiltrative into surrounding bone
- Typically asymptomatic and appears as a multilocular cyst radiographically
- Most commonly forms in posterior mandible
- Treated by excision with a margin of normal tissue
- Maxillary ameloblastomas can invade the cranial base and be lethal

Maxillary ameloblastomas are particularly dangerous, partly because the bones are considerably thinner than those of the mandible and present weak barriers to spread. Maxillary ameloblastomas tend to form in the posterior region and to grow backwards and upwards to invade the sinonasal passages, pterygomaxillary fossa, orbit and eventually the cranium and brain. They are thus occasionally lethal despite being benign.

The diagnosis must be confirmed by biopsy. The permeation of adjacent medullary bone previously discussed cannot usually be detected preoperatively, but if seen in a biopsy indicates a need for more aggressive treatment.

In recent years there has been a tendency to try to treat ameloblastoma conservatively to avoid the morbidity of large surgical excisions, especially in adolescents. Case selection for conservative treatment is paramount. Small mandibular lesions can sometimes be enucleated, the cavity curetted and the lower border and much of the cortex preserved. Such treatment must be undertaken in the expectation that there may be recurrence. Advocates of conservative treatment point out that, for the few recurring lesions, resection will be required but that the majority will benefit. Conversely, recurrence carries risks if ameloblastoma escapes into soft tissue or extends posteriorly into the infratemporal fossa as these are potentially fatal complications. Conservative management remains controversial. Marsupialisation is ineffective.

The standard of care for ameloblastoma therefore remains wide surgical excision, preferably removing 10 mm of apparently normal bone around the margin to ensure that any extension into the medullary bone is removed. Complete excision of a large ameloblastoma may therefore require partial resection of the jaw, often with the condyle and bone grafting. Smaller lesions may be excised, leaving the lower border of the jaw intact and extending the resection subperiosteally. Bony repair then causes much of the jaw to re-form. These more extensive operations normally guarantee cure.

Regular radiographic follow-up is essential, and recurrence may not appear for several years. Spread of ameloblastomas into the soft tissues is difficult to manage.

Key features of ameloblastomas are summarised in Box 11.3.

Literature review PMID: 7633291

Treatment PMID: 16487813

Benign but sometimes fatal PMID: 7718524

Desmoplastic ameloblastoma

The desmoplastic ameloblastoma is a distinctive variant of conventional ameloblastoma. These ameloblastomas arise

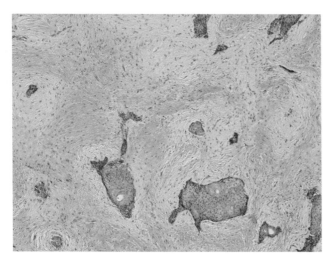

Fig. 11.11   Desmoplastic ameloblastoma. Most of the lesion is densely collagenous stroma, containing dispersed strands and spiky irregular islands of epithelium without the typical peripheral ameloblasts. They may be found focally, but they, and stellate reticulum, are sparse.

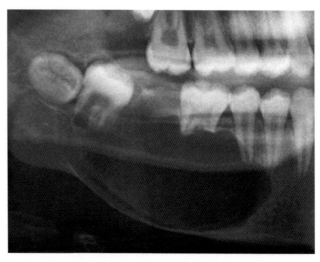

Fig. 11.12   Unicystic ameloblastoma. This ameloblastoma forms a monolocular radiolucency in a young adult, with expansion and root resorption. Its unicystic nature was confirmed after removal, but cannot be determined radiographically.

with equal frequency in both jaws and often present in the anterior regions as a fine honeycomb radiolucency resembling a fibro-osseous lesion. The islands of epithelium are sparse, do not show obvious ameloblasts and the lesion is dominated by densely collagenous ('desmoplastic') tissue (Fig. 11.11). Behaviour and treatment are the same as for the conventional ameloblastoma.

Case series PMID: 11140898

Metastasising ameloblastoma

This is a very rare curiosity, a histologically typical ameloblastoma which, although apparently benign, gives rise to distant metastases. The metastases are usually in the lung. Some cases appear to have resulted from aspiration implantation at surgery, and others follow surgical disruption at the primary site or repeated incomplete removal, suggesting that they result from surgical implantation into the circulation and are not truly malignant.

Both the primary tumour and the 'metastases' look histologically identical to conventional benign ameloblastomas, and metastasis cannot be predicted. Because the 'metastases' are really benign, local excision of the secondary deposit(s) should be curative.

Case series PMID: 20970910

Unicystic ameloblastoma

→ Summary chart 10.1 p. 163

The unicystic ameloblastoma is an ameloblastoma that has a single cyst cavity. Such ameloblastomas present at a younger age than conventional ameloblastoma, in the second and third decades and may account for 10% of all ameloblastomas. Many present in a true dentigerous relationship to an unerupted third molar. The remainder may simulate any odontogenic cyst type depending on location, but often suggestive features of root resorption, cortical perforation or large size may give clues (Fig. 11.12).

In theory, the single cyst structure should mean that these ameloblastomas could be treated by simple enucleation with a low risk of recurrence. Unfortunately, making a preoperative diagnosis of unicystic ameloblastoma is difficult, and

there remains controversy about exactly what constitutes a unicystic structure.

An ameloblastoma with only one bony cavity radiographically can be a conventional solid or multicystic ameloblastoma. This will not become apparent until the lesion has been opened or examined histologically and the multiple cysts seen. It is therefore important to bear in mind the various configurations of an ameloblastoma that could present radiologically as a single cyst. These are shown in Fig. 11.13.

An ameloblastoma where the epithelium is limited to a single layer lining the lumen is termed a *luminal type* of unicystic ameloblastoma. If there are papillary projections into the cyst lumen, but no islands within the wall, this is termed an *intraluminal unicystic* or *plexiform unicystic ameloblastoma*. In these types, ameloblastoma epithelium is limited to the lumen or inner cyst wall and the lesion may be enucleated.

The danger of making this diagnosis on radiological grounds alone is shown by the third diagram in Fig. 11.13. Here a conventional ameloblastoma has developed one very large dominant cyst. However, there is a focus of solid/multicystic ameloblastoma in one area of the wall that might penetrate its full thickness or even into surrounding bone. This has been called the *mural type* of unicystic ameloblastoma, but in reality it is a conventional ameloblastoma that could easily be misdiagnosed as a unicystic one.

The histological appearances of the true unicystic ameloblastomas are similar and are shown in Fig. 11.14. The tumour cells forming the cyst wall are often flattened and easily mistaken for those of a non-neoplastic cyst.

It is often said that unicystic ameloblastomas may be enucleated without recurrence. This may be true, but the difficulty is making the diagnosis preoperatively. The diagnosis can only be made confidently after removal because it requires detailed histological examination of the whole wall. A single biopsy of a stretched cyst lining is insufficient for diagnosis. In many cases unicystic ameloblastomas are not recognised before surgery and are enucleated on the assumption that they are dentigerous or other types of cyst. After diagnosis, it is usually sufficient to monitor radiographically,

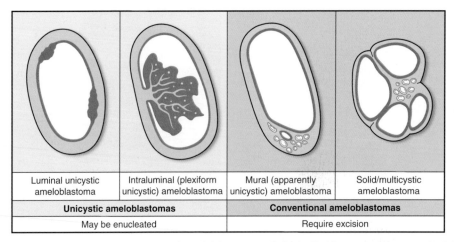

Luminal unicystic ameloblastoma	Intraluminal (plexiform unicystic) ameloblastoma	Mural (apparently unicystic) ameloblastoma	Solid/multicystic ameloblastoma
Unicystic ameloblastomas		**Conventional ameloblastomas**	
May be enucleated		Require excision	

Fig. 11.13   Explanations for a unicystic presentation of ameloblastoma radiologically. The two patterns on the left are true unicystic ameloblastomas, whereas those on the right are conventional ameloblastomas with one or more large cysts. See the text for a further explanation of the significance.

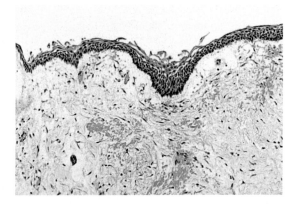

Fig. 11.14   Unicystic ameloblastoma. Part of the lining of a large unicystic ameloblastoma. The epithelium is often stretched and loses its typical features, with only a few ameloblast-like basal cells.

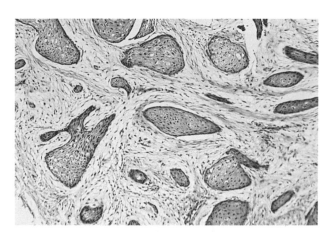

Fig. 11.15   Squamous odontogenic tumour. The lesion is composed of islands of squamous epithelium without peripheral palisaded cells.

and most will heal without problems. Any recurrence should be treated as conventional ameloblastoma.

There is insufficient evidence to give a recurrence rate for unicystic ameloblastomas, but it is clear that they do have a low rate of recurrence, approximately 10%.

Review PMID: 9861335

Treatment and recurrence PMID: 11023100

SQUAMOUS ODONTOGENIC TUMOUR

This rare tumour mainly affects young adults and involves the alveolar process of either jaw, close to the roots of teeth.

Radiographically, the squamous odontogenic tumour can mimic severe bone loss from periodontitis if high in the alveolus or produce a unilocular or multilocular cyst-like cavity if more deeply placed.

Histologically, it is composed of rounded islands of squamous epithelium with flattened peripheral cells (not elongate ameloblasts) in a fibrous stroma (Fig. 11.15). No keratin should be present in the epithelium, which may also contain laminated calcifications or globular eosinophilic structures. Unfortunately, the histology is not very specific, and

squamous odontogenic tumour is prone to overdiagnosis because there are histological mimics found next to cysts and in inflammatory lesions.

This tumour is benign and removed by curettage and extraction of any teeth involved.

Case and review PMID: 20697852

Review PMID: 8915020

CALCIFYING EPITHELIAL ODONTOGENIC TUMOUR

→ Summary chart 11.1 p. 185

This rare tumour, also known as a *Pindborg tumour* after its discoverer, is important because it can be mistaken for a carcinoma microscopically.

It arises in middle-aged and elderly adults after the age of 40 years, usually in the posterior body of the mandible, which is twice as frequently involved as the maxilla. Presentation is either with swelling or as an asymptomatic chance radiographic finding. There is a well-defined radiolucent area initially, sometimes corticated, that may develop

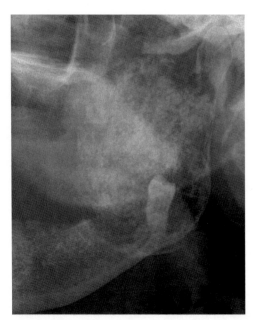

Fig. 11.16 Calcifying epithelial odontogenic tumour. This posterior mandibular lesion is a mixed radiolucency.

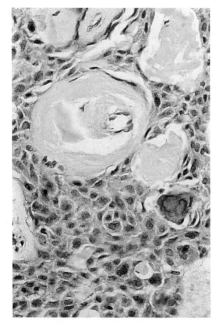

Fig. 11.18 Calcifying epithelial odontogenic tumour. At higher power the epithelial cells are seen to have sharply defined cell membranes resembling squamous epithelium and pleomorphic hyperchromatic nuclei. The pale pink material is amyloid.

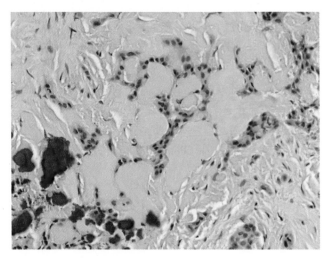

Fig. 11.17 Calcifying epithelial odontogenic tumour (Pindborg tumour). The tumour is composed of strands and sheets of polyhedral epithelial cells, in the centre with rounded deposits of secreted pale pink-staining amyloid. Toward the lower left, some of this material has mineralised, stains a darker-blue colour and gives rise to radiopacities within the lesion.

increasing internal radiopacity when it mineralises. Most present as a mixed radiolucency (Fig. 11.16).

Pathology

This unusual tumour resembles a carcinoma but is benign. It comprises sheets or strands of epithelial cells in fibrous tissue (Fig. 11.17). The epithelial cells have a prickle cell morphology with intercellular bridges and appear very eosinophilic. Their nuclei, in a proportion of cases, show gross variation in nuclear size, including giant nuclei, and hyperchromatism, mimicking malignancy (Fig. 11.18). At the periphery these cells can extend into adjacent medullary spaces, appearing to be infiltrative. Despite these alarming features, mitoses are very rare.

The diagnosis is aided by areas of amyloid deposited in the connective tissue. This amyloid material is pink,

> **Box 11.4 Calcifying epithelial odontogenic tumour: key features**
>
> - Rare neoplasm of odontogenic epithelium
> - Usually presents between ages 40 and 70 years
> - Most commonly forms in posterior mandible
> - Solid tumour, radiolucent, becoming a mixed radiolucency with time
> - Histopathologically can resemble carcinoma
> - The only odontogenic tumour to contain amyloid
> - Locally infiltrative like ameloblastoma
> - Treated by excision with a small margin

homogeneous and often mineralises, producing rounded densely mineralised masses with concentric 'Liesegang' rings. The amyloid may be sparse or a dominant feature and can be identified with Congo Red staining. It is a precipitated secretory product of the epithelial cells, a defective truncated protein called *odontogenic ameloblast-associated protein* (ODAM) that is normally found in tooth germs in small quantities, confirming the odontogenic nature of this tumour. It is the mineralisation of the amyloid that produces the dense radiopacities seen on radiographs. Because the mineralisation is dystrophic and not actively caused by the tumour cells, the amount of mineralisation is very variable. Some tumours remain completely radiolucent, most are mixed radiolucencies and some become densely radiopaque.

Calcifying epithelial odontogenic tumours extend into peripheral bone medullary spaces like ameloblastomas, and complete excision of the tumour with a border of normal bone should be curative, but recurrence will follow incomplete excision.

Key features of calcifying epithelial odontogenic tumour are summarised in Box 11.4.

Review PMID: 10889914

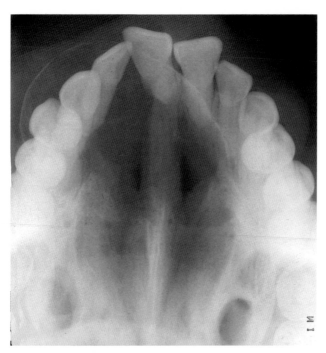

Fig. 11.19 Adenomatoid odontogenic tumour, a typical cyst-like presentation in the anterior maxilla. No mineralisation is evident in this example.

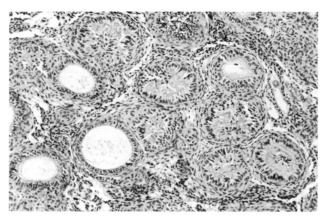

Fig. 11.20 Adenomatoid odontogenic tumour. Low magnification shows duct-like microcysts and convoluted ring structures. The stroma is scanty.

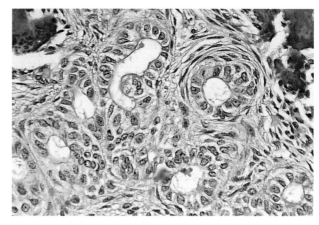

Fig. 11.21 Adenomatoid odontogenic tumour. At higher power the duct-like spaces, which give the tumour its name, are seen.

ADENOMATOID ODONTOGENIC TUMOUR → Summary charts 10.1 and 11.1 pp. 163, 185

Adenomatoid odontogenic tumour is uncommon, completely benign and a hamartoma not a neoplasm. Its name comes from its histological resemblance to a gland because it contains duct-like structures.

Adenomatoid odontogenic tumours present in late adolescence or young adulthood and are more common in females than males. Most develop in the anterior maxilla and form a very slow-growing swelling resembling a dentigerous or radicular cyst (Fig. 11.19) or are chance findings in the follicle of an extracted unerupted tooth. When in the wall of a cyst, a subtle radiographic clue is fine speckled mineralisation around the wall.

Pathology

A well-defined capsule encloses sheets, whorls and arcading strands of epithelium, among which are microcysts, resembling ducts cut in cross-section and lined by columnar cells similar to ameloblasts (Figs 11.20 and 11.21). These microcysts may contain homogeneous eosinophilic material. Fragments of amorphous or crystalline calcification may also be seen among the sheets of epithelial cells.

These lesions shell out readily, enucleation is curative and recurrence is almost unknown.

Key features of adenomatoid odontogenic tumour are summarised in Box 11.5.

Case series PMID 22869356

> **Box 11.5   Adenomatoid odontogenic tumour: key features**
>
> - Rare
> - Hamartoma of odontogenic epithelium
> - Usually presents between ages 15 and 30 years
> - Most common in the anterior maxilla
> - Often appears radiographically as a dentigerous cyst
> - Encapsulated – treated by enucleation

BENIGN EPITHELIAL AND MESENCHYMAL TUMOURS

AMELOBLASTIC FIBROMA
→ Summary chart 10.1 p. 163

Although rare, this tumour is important as one that is much more common in children and can be very destructive in the growing facial bones.

Ameloblastic fibromas affect young persons aged 7–20 years, usually in the posterior mandible. They form multi- or unilocular radiolucencies that expand the jaw slowly and displace teeth or prevent their eruption.

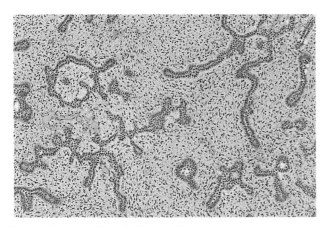

Fig. 11.22 Ameloblastic fibroma. The appearance is somewhat similar to that of ameloblastoma, but the pattern of budding strands is distinctive, and the connective tissue resembles the undifferentiated mesenchyme of the dental papilla.

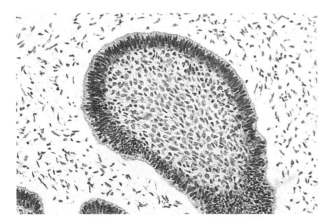

Fig. 11.23 Ameloblastic fibroma. At higher power the resemblance to dental papilla, ameloblasts and stellate reticulum is seen more clearly.

Pathology

Ameloblastic fibroma comprises interconnected strands and small islands of odontogenic epithelium in a cellular mesenchymal tissue resembling dental papilla. Unusually, it is considered that both epithelium and connective tissue are neoplastic.

The epithelial strands and islands are composed of cuboidal cells where the strands are thin, but they broaden out and have peripheral buds resembling cap stage tooth germs, with central stellate reticulum and peripheral elongate ameloblast-like cells (Figs 11.22 and 11.23).

Ameloblastic fibroma is benign and separates readily from the surrounding bone. Conservative resection is effective but, if incomplete, recurrence follows. In the maxilla, an excision margin of bone is often taken because the bones are thin and confident excision is more difficult than in the mandible.

There is a potential for malignant change following repeated incomplete removal (see odontogenic sarcomas).

Key features are summarised in Box 11.6.

Review: PMC2807540

AMELOBLASTIC FIBRODENTINOMA AND FIBRO-ODONTOME

When a tumour resembling an ameloblastic fibroma forms enamel and dentine, the lesion has been described as an ameloblastic fibro-odontome. When they form dentine alone, the term *ameloblastic fibrodentinoma* is used. These variants are now considered to be developing odontomes with a prominent soft tissue component (discussed later in this chapter).

Are developing odontomes PMID: 16202078 and 6938886

PRIMORDIAL ODONTOGENIC TUMOUR

This very rare and recently described odontogenic tumour of children and adolescents produces a large expanding radiolucency in the posterior mandible and ramus. It is often associated with an unerupted tooth and then appears radiographically as a dentigerous cyst.

Histologically, the tumour resembles a giant solid mass of dental papilla with a thin layer of ameloblasts around the periphery but no odontoblasts, dentine or enamel matrix. The few cases reported have been excised without recurrence.

Original description PMID: 24807692

ODONTOMES (ODONTOMAS*)

→ Summary charts 11.1 and 12.1 pp. 185, 202

Odontomes are developmental malformations (hamartomas) of dental tissues and not neoplasms. They are the commonest odontogenic tumours and are chance radiographic findings or present having prevented tooth eruption in children and adolescents. In their early stages they are radiolucent, developing opaque flecks and then dense opaque masses as enamel and dentine form internally (Fig. 11.24). Occasionally they may erupt and then often become infected because of their convoluted shape and because no organised epithelial attachment forms.

Case series PMID: 21840103

Review PMID: 1067549

The two common types of odontome are compound and complex odontomes. Both are easily enucleated and do not recur. If odontomes are left untreated in the jaw, cysts of

---

*In the UK, the term *odontome* is traditionally used, but the international terminology is *odontoma*. Odontoma incorrectly suggests a benign neoplasm. These lesions are hamartomatous and show no progressive growth.

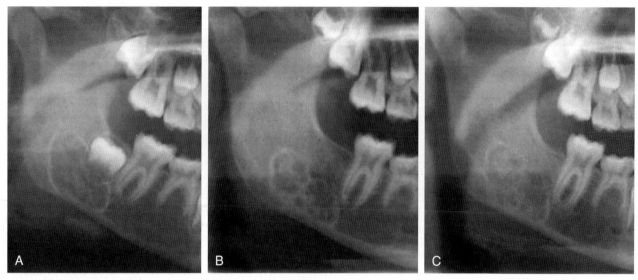

Fig. 11.24 **A developing complex odontome.** These three panoramic radiographs (A–C) were taken 2 years between each and show the progressive development and mineralisation of an odontome, which has been left in situ because of its size and close relationship to the inferior dental nerve canal. *(By kind permission of Mr D Falconer.)*

> **Box 11.7 Complex and compound odontome: key features**
>
> - Hamartomas of odontogenic epithelium and mesenchyme
> - Usually found between ages 10 and 20 years
> - Develop like teeth with initial (crypt-like) radiolucent phase, intermediate stage of mixed radiolucency, finally densely radiopaque
> - Benign, stop growing once mature
> - May be compound (many small teeth) or complex (disordered mass of dental hard tissue)
> - Most common sites are anterior maxilla and posterior mandible
> - Respond to enucleation

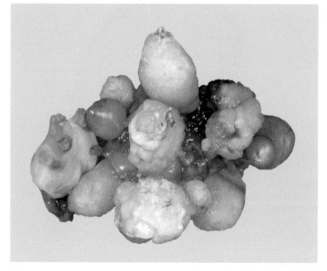

Fig. 11.25 **Compound odontome,** a cluster of small deformed teeth or denticles.

dentigerous type may form by separation of reduced enamel epithelium from enamel. Multiple odontomes are a component of Gardner's syndrome (Ch. 12).

There is an ill-defined borderland between odontomes and some malformed teeth. *Dens in dente*, invaginated odontomes, tuberculate mesiodens, dilated odontomes and connate teeth are distinctive minor tooth malformations discussed in Chapter 2.

Key features of compound and complex odontomes are summarised in Box 11.7.

Compound odontome

These are clusters of many separate, small, tooth-like structures (denticles) within one crypt, the whole lesion usually no larger than 20 mm in diameter (Figs 11.25 and 11.26). This type is usually found in the anterior maxilla and causes minimal swelling.

Histologically, the denticles are embedded in fibrous connective tissue and have a fibrous capsule around the entire lesion (Figs 11.27 and 11.28). Each denticle has an organised structure with pulp centrally and an enamel cap over the abnormally shaped dentine. The denticles develop like

normal teeth, mineralise fully and once mature, stop growing.

Complex odontome

Complex odontomes consist of a single irregular mass of hard and soft dental tissues, having no morphological resemblance to a tooth and frequently forming a cauliflower-shaped disorganised nodule of enamel and dentine. These may reach several centimetres in size and often expand the jaw.

Radiographically, when calcification is complete, an irregular radiopaque mass is seen containing areas of densely radiopaque enamel (Fig. 11.29).

Histologically, the mass consists of all the dental tissues in a disordered arrangement, but frequently with a radial structure. The pulp is usually finely branched so that the mass is perforated, like a sponge, by small branches of pulp (Fig. 11.30).

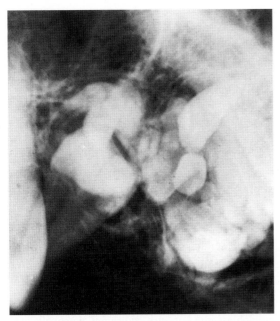

Fig. 11.26 Compound odontome. The denticles overlap each other in the radiograph but are, nevertheless, just visible as individual tooth-like structures.

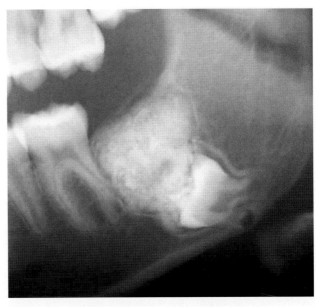

Fig. 11.29 Complex odontome. In this radiograph, the odontome overlies the crown of a buried molar and shows the typical dense amorphous area of radiopacity. Note the radiolucent rim of follicle and lamina dura of a 'crypt' extending around the lesion.

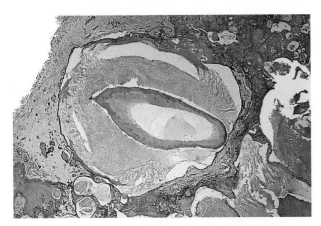

Fig. 11.27 Compound odontome. A denticle of dentine surrounded by enamel matrix is lying within more irregular calcified tissues.

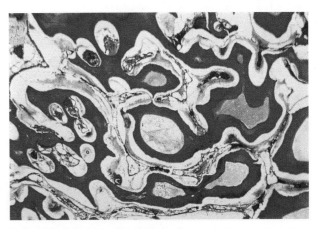

Fig. 11.30 Complex odontome. A disorganised mass of dentine, enamel and cementum penetrated by fine divisions of pulp.

Other types of odontome

Ameloblastic fibrodentinoma and *ameloblastic fibro-odontome* are mixed lesions with a component of complex odontome and a major component of soft tissue resembling ameloblastic fibroma. In the fibrodentinoma, only dentine is present, and in the fibro-odontome, both enamel and dentine are present.

Both lesions share many features with odontomes, presenting in the first and early second decade, usually in the posterior mandible. Initially radiolucent, they progressively develop radiopacity within while the hard tissues grow and mineralise (Fig. 11.31).

In the past these have been considered benign neoplasms in their own right, but it is now thought that they are just odontomes with a prominent soft tissue component and that, if untreated, they will eventually cease growing and mineralise. They can be treated by enucleation and do not recur, and may be suspected preoperatively by their radio-paque elements.

Fibrodentinoma etc. PMID: 16202078 and 6938886

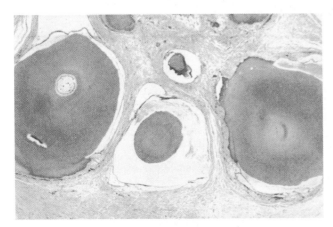

Fig. 11.28 Compound odontome. Sections from various areas of the odontome, seen in the radiograph shown in Fig. 11.26, show denticles of dentine and enamel cut in various planes, and more irregular calcified tissues, within a connective tissue capsule.

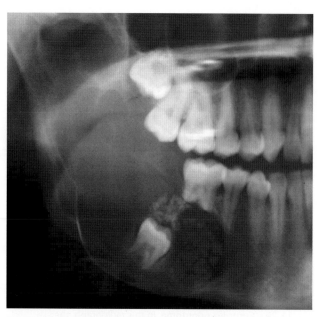

Fig. 11.31 Developing complex odontome. This large lesion has both a mineralising odontome component above and anterior to the unerupted tooth and a significant radiolucent soft tissue portion distally. The soft tissue element has the histological appearance of ameloblastic fibroma, and such lesions were previously called *ameloblastic fibro-odontome*.

CALCIFYING ODONTOGENIC CYST

→ Summary chart 11.1 p. 185

The calcifying odontogenic cyst is rare and has been considered both an odontogenic tumour and an odontogenic cyst, but it is currently classified with cysts (Ch. 10) as it rarely if ever recurs on removal. However, it is easily confused with odontogenic tumours radiographically and histologically (Box 11.8).

Box 11.8	**Calcifying odontogenic cyst: key features for differential diagnosis from odontogenic tumours**

- Forms at any site in alveolar ridge, usually posteriorly
- Radiographically unilocular
- Calcified ghost cells can be seen radiographically, the internal mineralisation suggesting an odontogenic tumour
- Ameloblastoma-like areas present histologically

DENTINOGENIC GHOST CELL TUMOUR

→ Summary charts 11.1 and 13.1 pp. 185, 222

This very rare odontogenic tumour is technically a benign neoplasm but, like ameloblastoma, infiltrates adjacent tissues and has an aggressive growth pattern. It arises most frequently in the mandibular body with swelling and a mixed radiolucency with a well-demarcated border.

Histologically, dentinogenic ghost cell tumour appears like ameloblastoma but with additional ghost cells (see calcifying odontogenic cyst (Ch. 10)) and formation of dentinoid, or dysplastic dentine. Dentinoid is an osteoid-like material formed by the connective tissue but induced by the epithelium in a similar way to dentine (Fig. 11.32). Ghost cells are found in a spectrum of lesions from the benign calcifying odontogenic cyst, the benign but aggressive dentinogenic ghost cell tumour and the extremely rare malignant ghost cell odontogenic carcinoma. Distinction between the three is based on size, cystic or solid destructive growth, mitotic activity and cytological atypia.

Surgical excision with a margin of normal tissue is recommended because of a tendency to recur.

Ghost cell lesion spectrum PMID: 18221328

Review PMID: 26341683

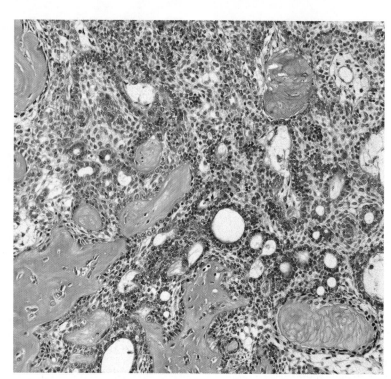

Fig. 11.32 Dentinogenic ghost cell tumour. Solid sheets of ameloblastoma-like epithelium, with stellate reticulum, two islands of ghost cells (*right*) and irregular islands of dentinoid (*left*).

BENIGN MESENCHYMAL TUMOURS

These tumours do not contain any true mesenchyme, that is an embryonic tissue, but rather are tumours of its derivatives: the fibroblasts and osteoblasts of dental follicle, pulp, periodontal ligament and cementum.

ODONTOGENIC FIBROMA

→ Summary chart 10.1 p. 163

The odontogenic fibroma is a benign neoplasm of fibrous tissue.

Clinically, odontogenic fibroma arises across a wide age range, more frequently affects the mandible and forms a slow-growing asymptomatic mass that may eventually expand the jaw. It appears as a sharply defined, rounded radiolucent area in a tooth-bearing region.

Pathology

Odontogenic fibromas consist of spindle-shaped fibroblasts and bundles of whorled collagen fibres (Fig. 11.33). Some lesions contain rests of odontogenic epithelium, apparently by chance. These islands are not required for diagnosis; they just reflect the odontogenic origin.

Odontogenic fibromas are benign, enucleate easily from surrounding bone and do not recur.

Case series PMID: 21684774

Granular cell odontogenic tumour

This odd and very rare tumour shares many features with odontogenic fibroma, but the fibroblasts become rounded and enlarged with prominent granular cytoplasm (Fig. 11.34). It is not known whether this is a degenerative change in an odontogenic fibroma or a distinct tumour in its own right. Treatment is as for odontogenic fibroma.

Case series PMID: 12424457

ODONTOGENIC MYXOMA

→ Summary chart 10.2 p. 164

The odontogenic myxoma is a benign neoplasm, the third commonest odontogenic tumour after odontomes and ameloblastoma. Most arise between the ages of 10–30 years and produce asymptomatic swellings of the jaws, usually posteriorly in the mandible.

Myxomas cause radiolucent areas with scalloped indistinct margins or a soap-bubble or honeycomb appearance (Figs 11.35 and 11.36). They displace teeth after destroying their supporting bone and are more extensive than is appreciated radiographically. Expansion is usually prominent.

Pathology

This is the odontogenic tumour that most deserves the name of a mesenchymal tumour because its appearance is exactly that of the mesenchyme of the developing dental follicle and papilla. The bulk of the myxoma is loose myxoid (mucous) ground substance, containing dispersed spindle-shaped or angular fibroblasts with long, fine, anastomosing processes (Figs 11.37 and 11.38). The ground substance is

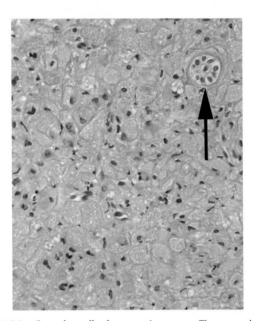

Fig. 11.34 Granular cell odontogenic tumour. There are sheets of pale, slightly grey cells with granular cytoplasm dispersed in collagen. An occasional rest of odontogenic epithelium may be found (*arrowed*), but as is the case for odontogenic fibroma, these are not required for diagnosis.

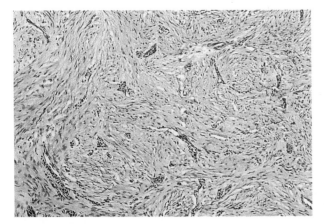

Fig. 11.33 Odontogenic fibroma. This rare mesenchymal odontogenic tumour consists of fibrous tissue containing rests and strands of odontogenic epithelium resembling those found in the periodontal ligament.

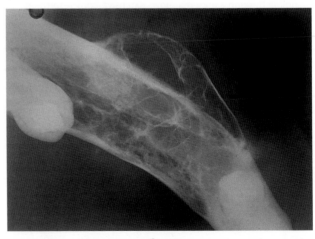

Fig. 11.35 Odontogenic myxoma. An occlusal view showing the finely trabeculated, honeycomb appearance and expansion of the mandible. Evidence of residual tumour was still present after 35 years in spite of vigorous treatment, both surgery and radiotherapy, in its earlier stages.

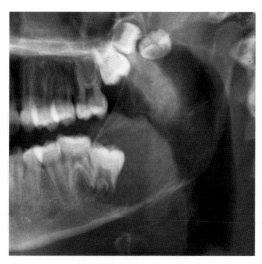

Fig. 11.36 Odontogenic myxoma. Another example from a panoramic view, this has a less honeycomb appearance, but straight septa are seen within it.

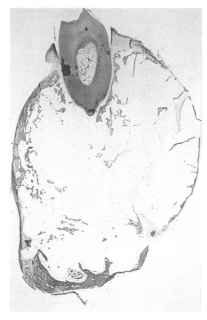

Fig. 11.37 Odontogenic myxoma. This cross-section of the mandible through a myxoma shows extensive bony resorption and gross expansion. The pale-staining myxoid lesion gives the tumour an empty appearance.

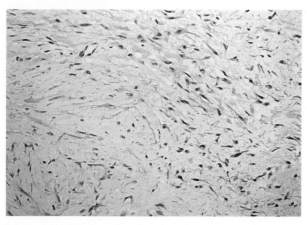

Fig. 11.38 Odontogenic myxoma. High-power view showing the typical appearance of sparse fibroblasts lying in a myxoid of ground substance-rich matrix.

> **Box 11.9 Odontogenic myxoma: key features**
> - Neoplasm of odontogenic myxoid fibrous tissue
> - Usually seen in young adults
> - Benign but prone to recurrence
> - Forms a multilocular, or honeycomb or soap-bubble radiolucency
> - Most common site is posterior mandible
> - Resembles normal dental follicle histologically
> - Treated by excision

hyaluronic acid and chondroitin sulphate, as in normal tissue, but excessive in amount. A few collagen fibres may also form, and there may be small, scattered epithelial rests. The margins of the tumour are ill-defined, and peripheral bone is progressively resorbed.

Myxomas are benign, but grow by secretion of the ground substance by the fibroblasts rather than cell proliferation. The gelatinous consistency allows the tumour tissue to permeate widely between medullary bone trabeculae without a clear margin, making removal very difficult. Excision with a margin of normal bone and removal of associated teeth is required but, in spite of vigorous treatment, some tumours recur.

Key features are summarised in Box 11.9.

Radiology PMID: 9482003

Review PMID: 10587272

Treatment PMID: 19027311

Normal dental follicle

The normal dental follicle resembles odontogenic myxoma histologically and sometimes shows enlargement, often on impacted unerupted teeth ('hyperplastic follicle'). If removed on suspicion of a dentigerous cyst or other odontogenic tumour, it can be mistaken for myxoma if the pathologist is not aware of the clinical presentation. The shape and location are diagnostic and should prevent misdiagnosis and overtreatment.

Misdiagnosis risk PMID: 10587272

CEMENTOBLASTOMA

→ Summary charts 11.1 and 12.1 pp. 185, 202

Cementoblastoma is a benign neoplasm of cementoblasts that forms a mass of cementum on a tooth root.

Some authorities, considering cementoblasts to be no more than osteoblasts, prefer to classify this lesion as an osteoblastoma, a neoplasm of osteoblasts normally found in long bones and vertebral column. However, cementoblasts are unequivocally odontogenic, and the presentation and behaviour of cementoblastoma is distinct from osteoblastoma, even though the histopathology is almost identical.

Clinically, cementoblastomas mainly affect young adults, particularly males, typically younger than 25 years. They are slow growing, sometimes painful and expand the jaw or are chance radiographic findings. The lower first permanent molar is the tooth that is almost always affected.

Radiographically, there is a radiopaque mass, with a thin radiolucent margin, attached to the root of a tooth

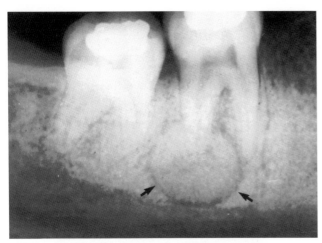

Fig. 11.39   Periapical radiograph showing the typical appearances of a cementoblastoma. A radiopaque mass with a radiolucent rim is attached to the root apex. *(By kind permission of Mr E Whaites.)*

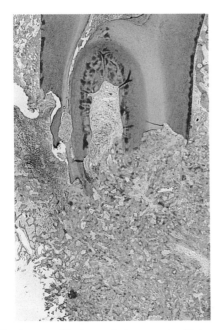

Fig. 11.40   Cementoblastoma. A dense mass of interconnected trabeculae of osteoid is fused to the resorbed roots of the first permanent molar.

(Fig. 11.39). The mass may be rounded or irregular in shape and mottled in texture. Resorption of related roots is common, but the tooth remains vital.

Pathology

The mass consists of cementum fused to a resorbed tooth root. The cementum often has many reversal lines, resembling Paget's disease centrally and a radiating structure of unmineralised matrix at the periphery. The cementoblasts are larger and more darkly stained than normal osteoblasts, and often several cell layers lie on the surface of the matrix. Outside the actively growing rim is a thin fibrous capsule (Figs 11.40 and 11.41).

Cementoblastomas are benign and treated by extraction of the tooth and enucleation and curettage of the bony

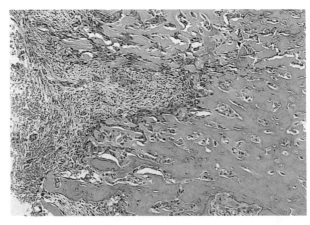

Fig. 11.41   Cementoblastoma. At high power at the periphery of the lesion there are seams of osteoid radiating from the centre of the lesion (to the right) with a thick layer of atypical cementoblasts on their surface. The capsule of the lesion is to the left.

Box 11.10   Cementoblastoma: key features

- Benign neoplasm of cementoblasts
- Usually seen in young adults
- Most commonly at the apex of a vital lower first molar
- Radiopaque with a narrow lucent rim
- Treated by enucleation

---

cavity. Recurrence is unusual, but incomplete removal leads to regrowth.

Key features are summarised in Box 11.10.

Review PMID: 11925541

'Cementomas'

Some sources refer to a group of lesions called *cementomas*. This historic designation used to be applied to all localised cementum lesions, but it is no longer used because the causes have become better characterised and require different treatments. Current terms for 'cementomas' are shown in Box 11.11.

Box 11.11   Localised lesions of cementum

- Cementoblastoma
- Osseous dysplasia
  - Periapical form
  - Focal form
  - Florid form
- Cemento-ossifying fibroma
- Hypercementosis
  - Paget's disease
  - Inflammatory hypercementosis

FIBROOSSEOUS ODONTOGENIC LESIONS

As noted later, fibro-osseous lesions as a group are defined histologically and can be neoplasms, dysplasias, odontogenic or non-odontogenic lesions. Fibrous dysplasia is discussed in Chapter 13, others in Chapter 12 and the odontogenic lesions later in this chapter.

CEMENTO-OSSIFYING FIBROMA

→ Summary charts 11.1 and 12.1 pp. 185, 202

The name cemento-osseous fibroma has recently been reinstated for this lesion to emphasise its odontogenic nature. In the past is has been called a type of ossifying fibroma, but the presentation and restriction to the jaws confirm the odontogenic origin. These lesions are presumed to originate from periodontal ligament or lamina dura bone of the socket, part of which is odontogenic in origin. The name *cemento-ossifying fibroma* also has the advantage of avoiding confusion with the ossifying fibromas of the facial skeleton (Ch. 12).

Cemento-ossifying fibroma

Cemento-ossifying fibromas are uncommon benign neoplasms, arise exclusively in the jaws and typically cause a painless swelling in the mandibular premolar or molar region. Patients are usually between 20 and 40 years of age on diagnosis, but the range is wide. Females are affected several times more frequently than males.

Like other fibro-osseous lesions, the cemento-ossifying fibroma starts as a small radiolucency and expands slowly. Calcification develops centrally while the lesion enlarges. Most become densely calcified given time and then appear largely radiopaque. At all stages, the lesion has a sharply defined margin, often with a thin radiolucent rim surrounded by a narrow zone of cortication. This circumscription is a key diagnostic feature and can be detected both radiographically (Figs 11.42 and 11.43) and histologically (Figs 11.44 and 11.45). Roots of related teeth can be fused to the lesion or displaced.

Microscopy

Being a fibro-osseous lesion, it has histological similarity to fibrous dysplasia and cemento-osseous dysplasias, and it cannot always be differentiated from them on the basis of its microscopic appearances alone. One key distinguishing feature is the well-demarcated periphery, sometimes with a fibrous capsule between the lesion and surrounding bone. Clinical and radiographic findings are required for definitive diagnosis.

The histological appearances vary widely and range from predominantly fibrous tumours to densely calcified masses depending on size and duration.

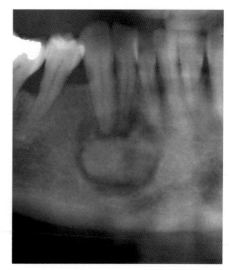

Fig. 11.43 Cemento-ossifying fibroma. This example is more densely mineralised, and the peripheral radiolucent rim is readily apparent.

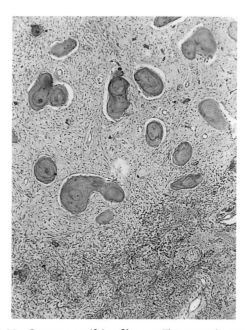

Fig. 11.44 Cemento-ossifying fibroma. This example contains densely mineralised and darkly staining islands of cementum-like tissue lying in cellular fibrous tissue. Toward the actively growing periphery of the lesion (*lower part*) the fibrous tissue is more cellular and is forming woven bone.

Both trabeculae of woven bone with osteoblastic rimming and dense rounded islands of acellular bone are seen, usually a mixture of both (see Fig. 11.44). Foci of bone gradually grow, fuse and, ultimately, form a dense mass (Fig. 11.45).

Management

Cemento-ossifying fibromas can usually be readily enucleated, separating from bone in the plane of their capsule. Occasionally, large tumours that have distorted the jaw require local resection and bone grafting. Recurrence is rare. Densely mineralised lesions are relatively avascular and can become a focus for chronic osteomyelitis following dental extraction.

Review PMID: 3864113

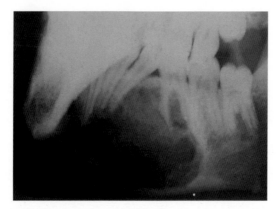

Fig. 11.42 Cemento-ossifying fibroma. The tumour forms a characteristic rounded well-circumscribed lesion radiographically. This example is cloudily radiolucent and slow-growing, as can be seen by the displacement of the teeth.

Juvenile ossifying fibroma

It is controversial whether this is just a histological variant of cemento-ossifying fibroma reflecting diagnosis at a younger age or is a distinct entity. It is found in children aged 8–15 years and histologically appears worrying, resembling osteosarcoma. This misdiagnosis can be avoided by noting the radiological circumscription.

The loose, fibroblastic stroma contains very fine, lace-like trabeculae of immature osteoid entrapping plump osteoblasts. Mitoses may be seen, and focal collections of giant cells are common.

The juvenile type grows rapidly, but it responds to enucleation and curettage despite the worrying presentation.

Juvenile trabecular type PMID: 23052375

Multiple and syndromic cemento-osseous fibromas

Patients with presentation in childhood, multiple cemento-osseous fibromas, or a family history of similar lesions in relatives should be questioned about the signs shown in Table 11.1 because there are syndromic presentations

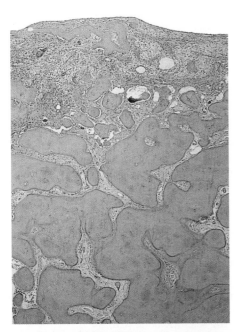

Fig. 11.45 Cemento-ossifying fibroma. In this mature lesion, there are large coalescing islands of dense bone and little fibrous tissue. Note the well-demarcated periphery of fibrous tissue which has shelled away from the adjacent bone during removal.

that have significant implications for the patient or their family.

Malignant neoplasms of parathyroid gland and the possibility of renal disease are the main significant risks in the hyperparathyroidism jaw tumour syndrome. Jaw lesions in hyperparathyroidism might be expected to be brown tumours as a result of high parathormone levels (Ch. 13), but in this syndrome the jaw lesions are fibro-osseous, not giant cell lesions. The cemento-ossifying fibromas and hyperparathyroidism can arise in different relatives. Treatment of the cemento-ossifying fibromas is as for the non-syndromic type.

HRPT2 case report PMID: 16448924

CEMENTO-OSSEOUS DYSPLASIAS

These poorly understood diseases are non-neoplastic disturbances of growth and remodelling of bone and cementum. They are, by far, the most common fibro-osseous diseases of the jaws and are common enough to be seen from time to time in general dental practice. It is unclear whether the various subtypes are all truly related. They have similar histological and radiological features and differ mainly in their extent and radiographic appearances.

All types have a strong predilection for females, accounting for more than 90% of cases, particularly those of African descent. Patients tend to be seen between 30 and 50 years, but probably after many years of asymptomatic disease.

Previously these diseases have been known as *osseous dysplasias*. However, because they affect only the alveolar bone and appear odontogenic, the name *cemento-osseous dysplasia* has been reinstated. This avoids confusion with several inherited osseous dysplasia syndromes of long bones.

Periapical cemental dysplasia

→ Summary chart 13.1 p. 222

In the periapical form, several adjacent teeth are affected, usually lower incisors.

The condition is asymptomatic and often a chance radiographic finding of rounded radiolucent areas related to the apices of the teeth. These simulate periapical granulomas but the related teeth are vital. During a period of years the separate lesions enlarge, may fuse and develop internal calcification. Mineralisation starts centrally and gives each lesion a target-like appearance radiographically. Eventually the lesions cease to enlarge, rarely exceeding 8–10 mm, and become densely radiopaque (Fig. 11.46). All stages of development may be seen at the same time in different lesions in the same patient. The teeth remain vital throughout.

Natural history PMID: 25425097

Table 11.1 Syndromes with cemento-ossifying fibromas

Syndrome	Cause and inheritance	Additional features
Hyperparathyroidism jaw tumour syndrome	Mutation in the *CDC73* gene (also known as *HRPT2* gene) encoding parafibromin, a tumour suppressor gene in the WNT signalling pathway. Inherited as an autosomal dominant but with very variable phenotype and expressivity	Hyperparathyroidism caused by parathyroid adenomas or carcinomas, renal cysts, renal tumours and uterine tumours. Cemento-ossifying fibromas in both mandible and maxilla, often multiple
Gnathodiaphyseal dysplasia	Mutation in the ANO5 gene, which encodes a transmembrane ion channel, inherited as an autosomal dominant	Presents in infants or children. Frequent bone fractures with normal healing, bowing and cortical thickening of the long bones
Familial ossifying fibroma	Unknown	Jaw lesions only. It is possible some of these cases are mildly affected patients with the two other syndromes in this table.

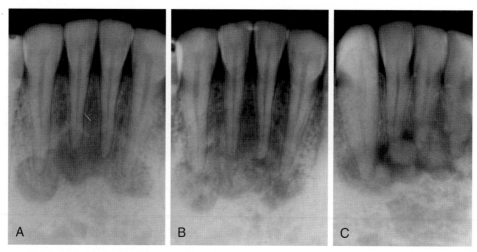

Fig. 11.46 Periapical cemento-osseous dysplasia. Three films taken over a period of years showing, (A) the early radiolucent stage resembling periapical granulomas, (B) intermediate stage with patchy mineralisation and (C) the late stage with well-defined masses of cementum in the centre of lesions. *(By kind permission of Mr EJ Whaites.)*

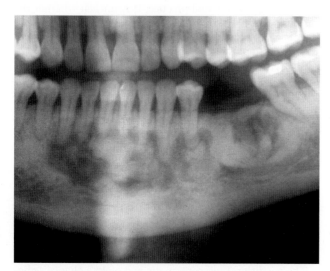

Fig. 11.47 Florid cemento-osseous dysplasia. Section of a panoramic tomogram showing the typical appearances of multiple irregular radiopaque masses centred on the roots of the teeth. The periphery of each is radiolucent, and the surrounding bone shows some sclerosis. Similar lesions were present in the contralateral molar region and on some maxillary teeth.

Florid cemento-osseous dysplasia

→ Summary chart 13.1 p. 222

In the florid form, multiple teeth are affected in more than one quadrant. The affected areas are frequently symmetrically distributed and may involve all teeth in all four quadrants, although the mandibular teeth are more commonly and more severely affected in most cases.

Individual lesions develop around the root apices exactly as in the periapical form but become larger and occasionally expand the jaw. The target-like appearance with central sclerosis resembling cementum on the root apex, surrounded by a radiolucent trim with a further outer zone of sclerosis in the surrounding bone is characteristic. Eventually dense radiopaque, somewhat irregular masses of sclerotic bone without a radiolucent border develop, producing a radiographic appearance similar to chronic osteomyelitis (Fig. 11.47). As in the periapical form, tooth vitality is not affected.

The florid form becomes the most sclerotic and is particularly liable to become infected after extraction (Ch. 8).

Some patients also develop solitary bone cysts in association with the lesions.

Radiology PMID: 9927089

Review PMID: 9394387 and 9377196

With solitary bone cyst PMID: 16182928

With expansion PMID: 21237426

Focal cemento-osseous dysplasia

→ Summary chart 13.1 p. 222

This term is given to changes similar to florid osseous dysplasia but forming a single lesion on one tooth. The lesion resembles a cemento-osseous fibroma radiographically, but shows the maturation sequence typical of this group of lesions. Lesions are usually in the posterior mandible.

Review PMID: 7838469

Microscopy

It must be emphasised that biopsy should **not** be performed for diagnosis. The diagnosis should be made radiographically, and biopsy avoided because it risks introducing infection into the sclerotic bone (Ch. 8).

All types are fibro-osseous in nature with cellular fibrous tissue containing woven bone trabeculae and islands of dense cementum-like bone. Progressive calcification leads to the formation of a solid, bony mass with prominent resting and reversal lines (Fig. 11.48).

Management of cemento-osseous dysplasias

Osteomyelitis starting in these lesions following extraction must be avoided because the widespread sclerosis of the late stages makes the infection difficult to treat. Wide excision may then be required to allow resolution. Treatment is otherwise not indicated except, rarely, for cosmetic reasons if there is expansion or if solitary bone cysts develop.

Familial gigantiform cementoma

This extremely rare autosomal dominant condition causes extremely large and disfiguring lesions, usually in all

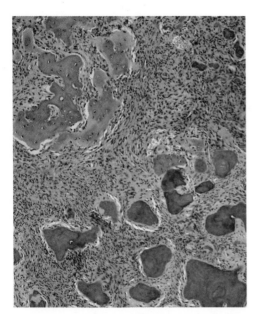

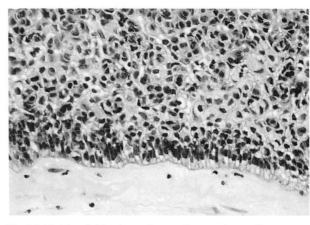

Fig. 11.49 **Ameloblastic carcinoma.** Very rarely a malignant variant of the ameloblastoma is encountered. Histologically, they may be indistinguishable from other carcinomas but, in some cases, as here, a peripheral layer of palisaded ameloblast-like cells remains, indicating the tumour's odontogenic nature.

Fig. 11.48 **Cemento-osseous dysplasia.** All three types have the same histological appearances, a very cellular fibrous tissue containing trabeculae of woven and sclerotic bone and islands of dense basophilic cementum-like bone. In early lesions the fibrous component predominates; late lesions become densely mineralised and sclerotic.

quadrants and presenting in childhood. In at least some cases, the origin appears to be at the tooth roots. Lesions grow progressively and recur after incomplete removal, so that it is unclear whether the condition is one of multiple cemento-ossifying fibromas or a type of cemento-osseous dysplasia.

The term *gigantiform cementoma* must not be used for florid cemento-osseous dysplasia with expansion, and is best reserved for the inherited condition in which the multiple tumours reach 10 or 20 cm in diameter. Conventional ossifying fibromas can be multiple and reach a large size, but not all such cases are gigantiform cementoma.

Cases and review PMID: 11312460

MALIGNANT ODONTOGENIC TUMOURS

Malignant odontogenic tumours are very rare, and there are many histological types. A malignant equivalent exists of most of the odontogenic tumours except adenomatoid odontogenic tumour and odontome.

The malignant tumours, either carcinomas or sarcomas, can present with typical signs of malignancy, such as progressive growth of a swelling of the jaw, pain, ulceration, loosening of teeth, nerve signs and invasion beyond bone into soft tissues. However, they are not necessarily clinically evident as malignant, and sometimes the diagnosis is not suspected until a biopsy is examined. The main significance is to be aware of their existence and be alert for minor features of malignancy in the clinical and radiographic appearance of jaw tumours: nerve signs, an indistinct moth-eaten outline and tooth root resorption.

Most arise in the posterior jaws, more frequently in the mandible. All are more common in the elderly.

Malignant neoplasms in the jaws are much more likely to be metastatic than odontogenic (Ch. 12). Metastases tend

to develop in the bone marrow below the inferior dental canal in the mandible. The malignant odontogenic tumours usually develop in the alveolar bone or retromolar region.

> **Key learning point:** Malignant neoplasms in the jaws are usually metastatic

Ameloblastic carcinoma is a carcinoma that resembles an ameloblastoma histologically, with palisaded basal cells (Fig. 11.49).

Primary intraosseous carcinoma is a carcinoma arising in the jaws with no resemblance to a specific odontogenic tumour. Almost all are squamous carcinomas, and approximately 40% appear to arise in odontogenic cysts, radicular, dentigerous or odontogenic keratocyst (Fig. 11.50). Sclerosing odontogenic carcinoma is a primary intraosseous carcinoma that induces a dense collagenous stroma (Fig. 11.51).

Clear cell odontogenic carcinoma is a carcinoma comprising sheets and islands of cells with clear cytoplasm (Figs 11.52 and 11.53).

Ghost cell odontogenic carcinoma is a carcinoma containing scattered islands of ghost cells. It is the malignant counterpart of dentinogenic ghost cell tumour.

Ameloblastic fibrosarcoma is the rare malignant counterpart of ameloblastic fibroma. It is invasive and destructive but has little tendency to metastasise. As many as half of cases seem to develop in ameloblastic fibromas that have been repeatedly inadequately treated. In these sarcomas the epithelial component remains benign, but the dental-papilla like component becomes very cellular and atypical (Fig. 11.54). Those that contain mineralisation are known as *ameloblastic fibro-dentinosarcoma* or *odontosarcoma*, but behave similarly.

Review all types PMID: 10587275

Clear cell carcinoma cases PMID: 26232924

Clear cell carcinoma translocation PMID: 23715163

Arising in cysts PMID: 21689161

Odontogenic sarcomas PMID: 10587276

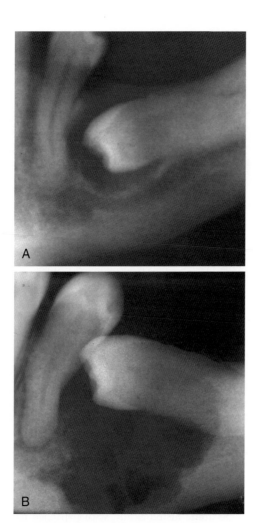

Fig. 11.50 **A primary odontogenic carcinoma** arising in a cyst or enlarged follicle. A. initially the radiological appearance is almost benign, but with subtle erosion of the cortication around the cyst. B. Two years later the carcinoma has enlarged to destroy surrounding bone and caused a pathological fracture.

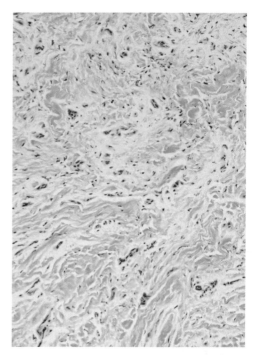

Fig. 11.51 **Sclerosing odontogenic carcinoma.** This type comprises a very dense collagenous stroma in which the small strands and islands of malignant epithelium are difficult to discern.

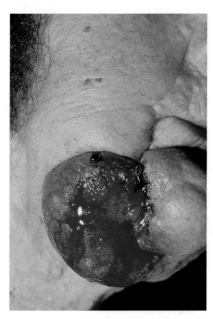

Fig. 11.52 **Clear cell odontogenic carcinoma.** This neglected tumour has fungated through the cheek.

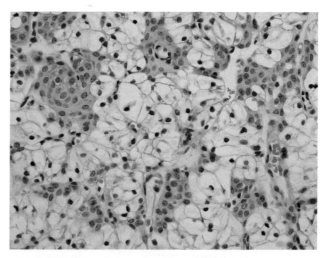

Fig. 11.53 **Clear cell odontogenic carcinoma.** This rare epithelial odontogenic tumour contains cells with vacuolated clear cytoplasm.

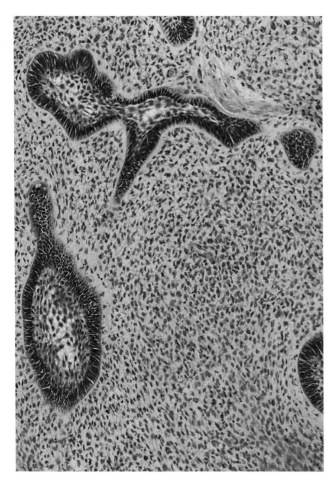

Fig. 11.54   Ameloblastic fibrosarcoma. The tumour has strands and islands of epithelium with ameloblasts and stellate reticulum, as seen in ameloblastic fibroma, but the dental papilla-like mesenchymal tissue in the background is malignant, showing hypercellularity, enlarged cells and, seen only at higher power, frequent mitoses.

Summary chart 11.1   Differential diagnosis and management of sharply defined mixed radiolucencies in the jaws.

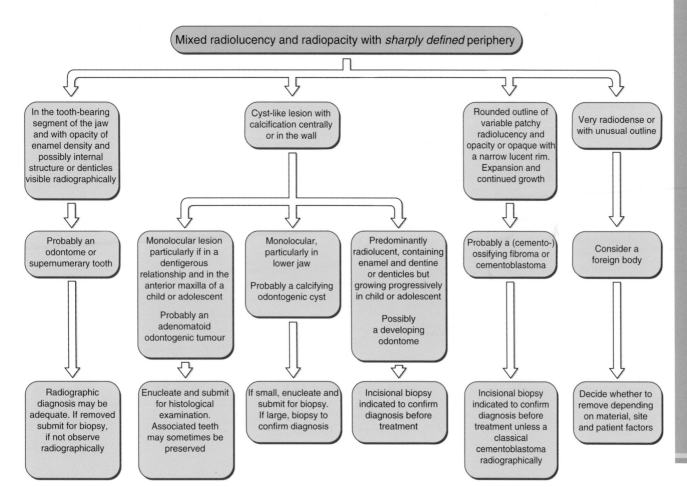

Appendix 11.1

World Health Organization classification of odontogenic and maxillofacial bone tumours 2017*

Name	Growth pattern†	Relative incidence‡	Notes
Odontogenic carcinomas			
Ameloblastic carcinoma	MN		
Primary intraosseous carcinoma NOS	MN		Includes those arising in cysts
Sclerosing odontogenic carcinoma	MN		New entity in this classification
Clear cell odontogenic carcinoma	MN	All are very rare	
Ghost cell odontogenic carcinoma	MN		
Odontogenic carcinosarcoma	MN		Entity reinstated from penultimate classification
Odontogenic sarcomas	MN		
Benign epithelial odontogenic tumours			
Ameloblastomas			
Ameloblastoma	BN	Common	Previously called solid/multicystic type
Ameloblastoma, unicystic type	BN	Common	No longer includes the 'mural' type
Ameloblastoma peripheral/ extraosseous type	BN	Rare	
Metastasizing ameloblastoma	BN	Very rare	Has been moved from the malignant category
Squamous odontogenic tumour	BN	Rare	
Calcifying epithelial odontogenic tumour	BN	Rare	
Adenomatoid odontogenic tumour	H	Common	
Benign mixed epithelial and mesenchymal odontogenic tumours			
Ameloblastic fibroma	BN	Rare	
Primordial odontogenic tumour	?BN	Very rare	New entity in this classification
Odontome (developing/compound and complex)	H	Common	Includes ameloblastic fibrodentinoma and fibro-odontome
Dentinogenic ghost cell tumour	BN	Very rare	
Benign mesenchymal odontogenic tumours			
Odontogenic fibroma	BN	Rare	
Odontogenic myxoma / myxofibroma	BN	Common	
Cementoblastoma	BN	Rare	
Cemento-ossifying fibroma	BN	Common	Reinstated as an odontogenic tumour
Odontogenic Cysts			See Ch. 10
Fibro- and chondro-osseous lesions			
Cemento-ossifying fibroma	BN	Rare	See Chs 11 and 12
Fibrous dysplasia	D	Rare	See Ch. 13
Cemento-osseous dysplasia	D	Very common	
Osteochondroma	BN	Very rare	See Ch. 12
Giant cell lesions and simple bone cyst			
Central giant cell granuloma	U	Common	See Ch. 12
Peripheral giant cell granuloma	R	Common	Giant cell epulis, see Ch. 24
Cherubism	D	Rare	See Ch. 13
Aneurysmal bone cyst	BN & D	Rare	See Ch. 13
Simple bone cyst	U	Rare	See Ch. 13

*The classification has been simplified since last published in 2005. The keratocystic odontogenic tumour has reverted to its previous name of odontogenic keratocyst. Bone and cartilaginous tumours are omitted for clarity, see chapters 12 and 13.

†MN malignant neoplasm; BN benign neoplasm; H hamartoma; D Dysplasia. B Borderline – benign but can infiltrate locally, R reactive, U unknown

‡Refers to incidence in jaws and is relative, overall, all these tumours are rare.

Non-odontogenic tumours of the jaws

12

Tumours of the jaws are conventionally divided into odontogenic, as in the previous chapter, and non-odontogenic types. Sometimes this artificially separates clinically, radiologically or histologically similar lesions, as seen with ossifying fibromas. Other conditions including dysplasias can also cause swellings and destructive jaw lesions. Only a few are more common in the jaws than in other bones, and only the more important examples (Box 12.1) are considered here.

EXOSTOSES AND TORI

These localised swellings of bone are thought to be developmental and are very common. They are extensions of the normal bone structure, with a surface cortical compact bone layer and, if large, a core of normal medullary bone. No clear genetic inheritance has been shown, although there is a genetic contribution to developing a torus palatinus.

A *torus mandibularis* develops on the lingual aspect of the mandible above the mylohyoid muscle and floor of mouth mucosa, usually lingual to the canine and premolars (Fig. 12.1). When small, they are smooth, but larger examples have a lobular shape and can also form a row of nodules extending back to the third molars. Mandibular tori are almost always symmetrical.

Torus palatinus commonly forms toward the posterior of the midline of the hard palate (Fig. 12.2). The swelling is rounded and symmetrical, sometimes with a midline groove or lobular surface if large. It is not usually noticed until middle age.

Other small exostoses are occasionally seen, usually on the surface of the alveolar processes of the maxilla buccally (Fig. 12.3). Sometimes these are multiple and symmetrical, forming a row of nodules.

Until recently, tori have been considered insignificant, but their thin mucosal covering is prone to damage. Their prophylactic removal has been suggested to prevent medication-related osteonecrosis (Ch. 8), which develops more commonly in areas of mucosal trauma. This would only seem justified for the largest and most trauma-prone examples.

OSTEOCHONDROMA (CARTILAGE-CAPPED OSTEOMA)

These are small columns of bone with a cartilaginous cap at the outer growing end. They form a hard bony protuberance, usually from the anteromedial aspect of the condyle that limits mouth opening or causes displacement. If located

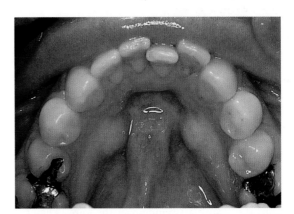

Fig. 12.1 Mandibular tori. The typical appearance of bilateral tori lingual to the lower premolars.

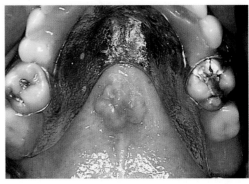

Fig. 12.2 Torus palatinus. Palatal tori range from small smooth elevations to lobular swellings such as this. The bone is covered by only a thin mucosa which is prone to trauma.

Box 12.1 Non-odontogenic tumours of bone.

- Non-neoplastic
  - Exostoses and tori*
  - Osteochondroma
  - Central giant cell granuloma*
- Histiocytoses
  - Langerhans cell histiocytosis*
- Primary: benign neoplasms
  - Osteoma
  - Ossifying fibroma*
  - Haemangioma
  - Melanotic neuroectodermal tumour*
- Primary: malignant neoplasms
  - Osteosarcoma
  - Chondrosarcoma
  - Ewing's sarcoma
  - Multifocal or potentially multifocal: myeloma
- Secondary: metastatic malignant neoplasms
  - Carcinoma

Those marked * are more common in the jaws than in other bones.

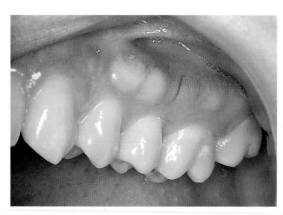

Fig. 12.3 Exostoses. Bony exostoses, aside from tori, are found most frequently buccally on the alveolar bone and are often symmetrically arranged.

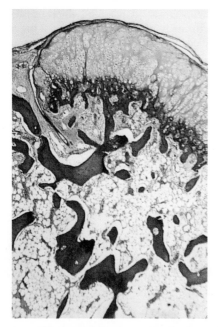

Fig. 12.4 Osteochondroma. There is a superficial cap of hyaline cartilage which undergoes endochondral ossification to form normal trabeculae of lamellar bone. The marrow spaces contain normal marrow continuous with those in the underlying bone.

laterally, they cause a swelling over the joint. They can be detected at almost any age, unlike the long bone equivalent that is usually found in children and young adults.

Osteochondroma is characteristic radiologically and may be diagnosed with reasonable certainty on cone beam computed tomography, although the cartilaginous cap will not be visible.

Pathology

Diagnosis is confirmed after surgical removal. The lesion is subperiosteal and has a cap of hyaline cartilage or fibrocartilage similar to the condyle, showing normal endochondral ossification with vertical rows of aligned cartilage cells (Fig. 12.4). With time the mass progressively ossifies.

In the jaw, these benign bony growths cease to grow after skeletal maturation. Removal is therefore curative. In other parts of the skeleton, they are considered neoplastic.

Case series PMID: 20346630

Case report PMID: 3159417

Box 12.2 Differential diagnosis of giant cell lesions of the jaws

- *Central giant cell granuloma.* Almost only develops in the jaws, usually solitary. No serological or radiographic features of hyperparathyroidism (Ch. 13)*
- *Brown tumour of hyperparathyroidism.* Serum calcium levels and parathormone levels are raised (Ch. 13)
- *Cherubism.* Lesions are multiple, symmetrical, near the angles of the mandible, family history usually present, patients have mutations in the SH3BP2 gene (Ch. 13)
- *Aneurysmal eurysmal bone cysts* may contain many giant cells but consist predominantly of multiple blood-filled spaces, some lesions have a characteristic t(16;17)(q22;p13) translocation (Ch. 13). May arise in conjunction with fibro-osseous lesions.

Giant cell tumour is an intermediate (destructive but rarely metastasising) neoplasm of long bones, with a characteristic H3F3A mutation in the tumour. These are very rare in the jaws, if they occur at all, and must not be confused with giant cell granuloma.

CENTRAL GIANT CELL GRANULOMA

→ Summary chart 10.2 p. 164

The central giant cell granuloma is a localised tumour of fibrous tissue containing numerous osteoclasts. It is one of a group of histologically similar conditions called the giant cell lesions (Box 12.2), the other types of which are discussed in other chapters. The more common giant cell lesions of the jaws are, in order of reducing frequency, central giant cell granuloma, aneurysmal bone cyst and hyperparathyroidism.

In small biopsy samples it may be impossible to differentiate these giant cell–rich lesions, and radiological features, blood chemistry, and sometimes genetics are necessary to make a definitive diagnosis.

Peripheral giant cell granuloma is an unrelated gingival hyperplastic lesion better called *giant cell epulis* to avoid confusion (Ch. 24).

Giant cell granuloma is seen in females twice as frequently as males and usually in people younger than 30 years, although there is a broad age range. Two-thirds of lesions develop in the mandible, anterior to the first molars, where the teeth have had deciduous predecessors. There is frequently only a painless swelling, but growth is sometimes rapid, and the mass can, rarely, erode through the bone, particularly of the alveolar ridge, to produce a purplish soft tissue swelling (Fig. 12.5). Lesions are typically several centimetres across.

Radiographs show a rounded cyst-like radiolucent area, often faintly loculated or with a soap-bubble or honeycomb appearance (Fig. 12.6). Roots of teeth can be displaced or occasionally resorbed.

Pathology

The pathogenesis is unknown. Historically, it was considered a process of frustrated repair following trauma and, more recently, hyperplastic, reactive or possibly neoplastic. No genetic cause has been identified.

A giant cell granuloma is a lobulated mass of proliferating vascular connective tissue packed with giant cells (osteoclasts; Figs 12.7 and 12.8). The giant cells are arranged

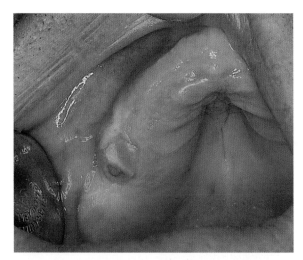

Fig. 12.5   Giant cell granuloma. This maxillary lesion has perforated the cortex and formed an ulcerated bluish soft-tissue mass on the alveolar ridge. The underlying alveolar bone is considerably expanded.

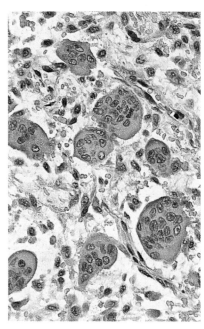

Fig. 12.8   Giant cell granuloma. High power showing the osteoclast-like giant cells with numerous, evenly dispersed nuclei.

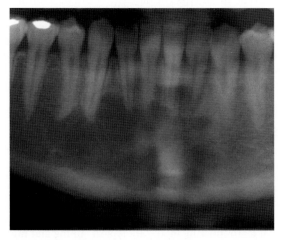

Fig. 12.6   Giant cell granuloma. Characteristic radiographic appearance of a radiolucency with scalloped margins and apparently multilocular.

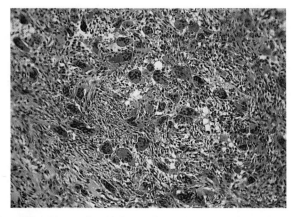

Fig. 12.7   Giant cell granuloma. This tissue is vascular and contains much extravasated blood, around which giant cells are clustered.

in clusters around areas of haemorrhage and deposits of haemosiderin from breakdown of erythrocytes. The lobules are separated by fibrous tissue septa, and sometimes a thin layer of osteoid or bone forms in them, giving the lesion its characteristic faint honeycomb or multilocular appearance radiographically. It seems likely that the fibroblasts are the underlying abnormality, and that the giant cells form in response to cytokines or other signals produced by the fibroblasts or blood vessels. Although the histological appearances are very similar to the brown tumour of hyperparathyroidism, there is no association with hyperparathyroidism.

Management

Many giant cell granulomas grow slowly, and some have even been shown to resolve spontaneously. However, the majority enlarge and require removal by curettage. Approximately 15% of lesions recur, but a second curettage is usually curative.

Some granulomas enlarge rapidly, perforate the cortex and resorb tooth roots. Such behaviour indicates a higher risk of recurrence, and the surgeon may elect to excise the lesion with surrounding bone, particularly in the maxilla and facial bones where effective curettage in thin bones is difficult to achieve. Very large lesions may require en bloc resection. In the majority of cases, complete removal is not necessary for effective treatment.

A variety of medical treatments are available that have been shown to partially control growth, and these may be used for particularly rapidly enlarging examples, when patient factors prevent immediate surgery or in children where facial growth might be affected by surgery. Injection of corticosteroids converts the lesions to fibrous tissue, usually in about three doses during several months, and calcitonin, interferon alpha and bisphosphonates all slow growth. However, residual lesion may still require surgery.

Key features are summarised in Box 12.3.

Review PMID: 8426719

Treatment PMID: 17703964

Noonan and other syndromes

Multiple giant cell granulomas occur in Noonan syndrome, the genetic cause of which is known to be mutation of the PTPN11 gene or others in the RAS pathway, inherited in an autosomal dominant pattern. Patients have cardiac abnormalities, short stature and learning difficulties and a characteristic facial appearance. Patients with the giant cell granulomas are a minority of patients who have a variant of the syndrome. Multiple giant cell lesions in the jaws are also seen in cherubism (Ch. 13).

Case and review PMID: 22848035

LANGERHANS CELL HISTIOCYTOSIS

Langerhans cells are dendritic antigen-presenting cells that derive from the bone marrow and migrate to function within epithelia. In this group of conditions they proliferate excessively and localise in bone, organs and skin. Three main forms are recognised, and their features are shown in Table 12.1 but, in practice, this is a continuous spectrum of disease severity and no single classification has yet proved satisfactory.

Table 12.1   Presentations of Langerhans cell histiocytosis

Classification	Presentation	Features
Chronic unifocal form	Solitary eosinophilic granuloma	Adults, usually bones (80%), lymph nodes or lungs affected
Chronic multifocal form	Multifocal eosinophilic granuloma (including Hand–Schuller–Christian disease)	Young adults and adolescents. Single system involvement but multiple lesions, usually in skull, skin, nodes, brain, liver
Acute disseminated form	Letterer–Siwe disease	Young children and infants. Multiple organ systems and bone

Key features of oral lesions are summarised in Box 12.4. The cause is unknown, but evidence is emerging that at least the systemic forms are neoplastic because the cells are clonal and approximately half of cases carry mutations in the BRAF oncogene. However, the localised forms may well be reactive to a viral infection or a result of abnormal immune regulation because they are less likely to recur and occasionally resolve spontaneously.

Oral involvement is present in approximately 10% of both child and adult patients, and the mandible is affected in nearly 75%, either alone or in polyostotic disease. Langerhans cell histiocytosis restricted to the oral mucosa, as opposed to bone, is extremely rare and causes ulcers.

Pathology

There are varying proportions of Langerhans cells and eosinophils, sometimes with other types of granulocytes. The Langerhans cells have pale, vesicular and often lobulated nuclei and weakly eosinophilic cytoplasm (Fig. 12.9). Langerhans cells in all types of the disease can be identified for diagnosis in a biopsy by immunocytochemistry for the CD1a surface marker or the CD207 receptor langerin found in the cell membrane and cytoplasmic granules. Electron microscopy for the Birbeck granules has been superseded by these stains. There may also be necrosis. Biopsy is required for diagnosis.

Solitary or multifocal eosinophilic granuloma

An eosinophilic granuloma of the jaw causes localised bone destruction with swelling and often pain (Fig. 12.10). Lesions are often centred in the alveolar bone and destroy the bone and soft tissue of the periodontium to expose the roots of the teeth. A rounded area of radiolucency with indistinct margins (Figs 12.11 and 12.12) and an appearance of teeth 'floating in air' are typical. Young and middle-aged adults are mainly affected, and the lesion is most frequently in the mandible. When one lesion is found, a search for others should be made.

Chronic multifocal Langerhans cell histiocytosis

In this form, the skull, axial skeleton and femora, and also sometimes the viscera (liver and spleen) or the skin may be involved. When the skull is affected, there are multiple lesions in the jaws and base of skull and a minority of patients are seen with the Hand–Schuller–Christian triad of exophthalmos, diabetes insipidus and lytic skull lesions. Exophthalmos and diabetes result from involvement of orbital tissues and base of skull extending to the pituitary gland. The histological features are the same as eosinophilic granuloma.

Acute disseminated Langerhans cell histiocytosis

This aggressive form of histiocytosis, previously called *Letterer–Siwe syndrome*, affects infants or young children and behaves like a lymphoma of Langerhans cells. Progression to widespread disease, with involvement of skin, viscera

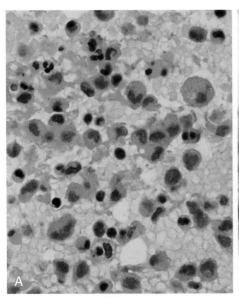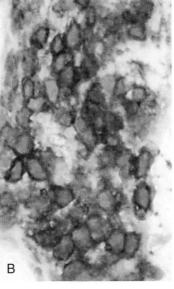

Fig. 12.9 Langerhans cell histiocytosis. High power showing the large round paler-staining Langerhans cells with their characteristic folded, bilobed (coffee bean) nuclei and some eosinophils, smaller and brighter red (*A*). The Langerhans cells are more easily identified by positive brown immunohistochemical staining for their membrane protein CD1a (*B*).

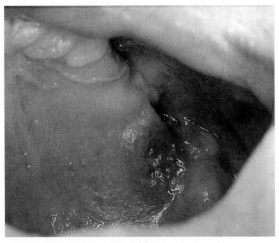

Fig. 12.10 Langerhans cell histiocytosis. This localised lesion (eosinophilic granuloma) has produced an ulcerated mass on the maxillary alveolar ridge. The clinical appearances are non-specific.

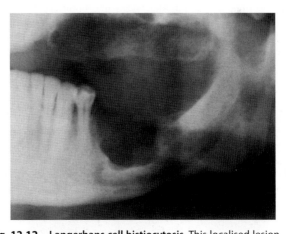

Fig. 12.12 Langerhans cell histiocytosis. This localised lesion (eosinophilic granuloma) shows the characteristic appearance of a well-defined radiolucency scooped out of the alveolar bone. The margin is corticated in places, but less well-defined elsewhere.

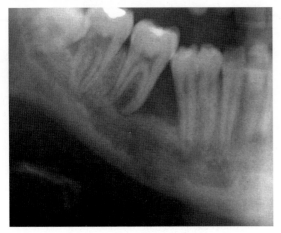

Fig. 12.11 Langerhans cell histiocytosis. Destruction of interdental bone and extension down to a scalloped margin at the lower border of the mandible.

and bones, can be rapidly fatal, despite treatment by irradiation and/or chemotherapy. There is a 50% 5-year survival.

Treatment

Overall, the behaviour of Langerhans cell histiocytosis is unpredictable, but the younger the patient and the greater the number of organ systems affected, the worse the prognosis. All affected patients should be investigated for multifocal disease with a skeletal survey or bone scan.

For eosinophilic granulomas in the jaw, the traditional treatment has been curettage, and the response is usually good. However, spontaneous regression during months or years is reported, and currently more conservative medical treatment with azathioprine or methotrexate is under evaluation. These treatments seem to work well for skin lesions and some jaw lesions and should be first-line treatment. Whether destructive lesions threatening many teeth may require surgical intervention is unclear. Intralesional injection of corticosteroids may be given as adjunctive treatment and may be safe and effective for monostotic disease.

Irradiation may be given if other measures fail or for inaccessible lesions of the skull base. Prolonged follow-up is desirable because of the risk of recurrence and because the apparently single lesion may have been an early manifestation of multifocal disease.

For multisystem disease, a combination of cytotoxic chemotherapy, corticosteroids and irradiation of active bone lesions is required. The poor survival and rapid progression in infants with acute disseminated disease was noted previously. Those surviving long enough may benefit from marrow transplantation.

Oral lesions PMID: 19758405

Treatment PMID: 20188480

OSTEOMAS → Summary chart 12.1 p. 202

Genuine osteomas are benign neoplasms and thus show progressive growth. They must be differentiated from exostoses and tori for this reason. Osteomas are relatively rare in the jaws, but the sinuses are a site of predilection and they occasionally grow in a jaw (Fig. 12.13).

Compact osteomas are a nodule of dense lamellar bone, sometimes in parallel layers like bone cortex rather than in Haversian systems (Fig. 12.14). This dense bone contains occasional vascular spaces and grows very slowly. **Cancellous osteomas** have a peripheral cortical layer and

central zone of medullary bone with marrow spaces (Fig. 12.15). Osteomas are easily excised if they become large enough to cause symptoms or interfere with the fitting of a denture.

Jaw lesions review PMID: 18602294

Gardner's syndrome

Gardner's syndrome is a variant of familial adenomatous polyposis (FAP) caused by mutation in the APC gene and

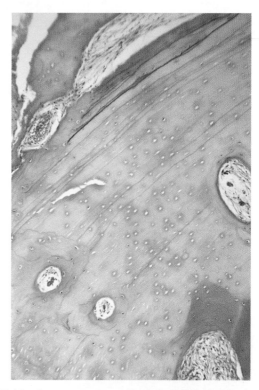

Fig. 12.14 Compact osteoma. Dense bone is laid down in lamellae with occasional vascular spaces, but there is no attempt to form Haversian systems in the compact variant, which resembles cortical bone.

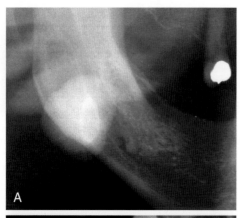

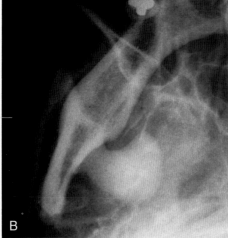

Fig. 12.13 Compact osteoma. A large mass seen on a panoramic film (*A*) is seen to be pedunculated from the medial aspect of the mandible in an axial computed tomography scan (*B*).

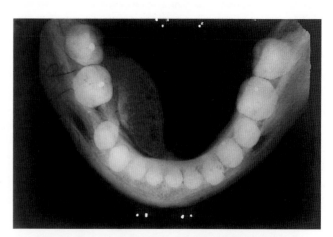

Fig. 12.15 Cancellous osteoma of the mandible. The tumour has arisen from a relatively narrow base lingually to the molars but has been moulded forward during growth by pressure of the tongue. The trabecular pattern of cancellous bone can be seen. A torus mandibularis arises further forward on the jaw, arises from a broad base and is usually bilateral and does not grow progressively.

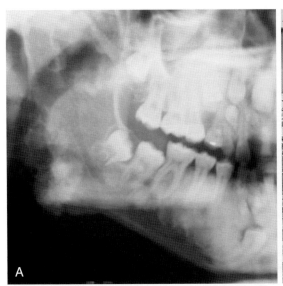
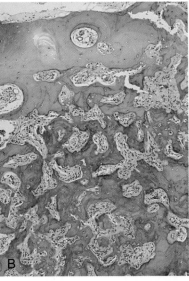

Fig. 12.16 Gardner's syndrome. *A*, Panoramic radiograph showing multiple unerupted supernumerary teeth and sclerotic bone areas in the jaws, the same patient as shown in Fig. 2.39. *B*, Patch of sclerotic bone from the maxilla covered by normal cortex.

inherited as an autosomal dominant trait. The mutation carries a high risk of colon carcinoma. Only a small proportion of those with the mutation have the Gardner variant of the FAP syndrome. This has the additional signs of multiple osteomas of the jaw, fibromas and epidermal cysts, together with a range of other less frequent abnormalities. These extra features are associated with mutations at specific codons in the gene. Dental features include odontomes, supernumerary teeth and sclerotic zones of bone in the jaws, in addition to the typical osteomas.

Osteomas and dental features are visible radiographically before the colonic polyposis becomes evident in the second decade of life. Early recognition may save the life of a patient, particularly in the 30% of patients who have a spontaneous mutation and thus no family history. The dental changes, when present, are easily identified; the jaws, facial bones and skull are the most common site for osteomas. Superficial osteomas cause visible deformity, and the multiple skin cysts and nodules also often affect the face.

Genetic carriers may also have jaw osteomas.

The risk of colonic adenocarcinoma is approximately 10% by age 21 years and 95% by age 50 years, and prophylactic colectomy is indicated.

Review oral features PMID: 17577321

Treatment PMID: 20594634

Genetics supernumerary teeth PMID: 24124058

Web URL 12.1 Syndrome and genetics http://omim.org/ and enter 175100 into search box

OSSIFYING FIBROMAS

→ Summary charts 11.1 and 12.1 pp. 185, 202

The group of ossifying fibromas is somewhat confusing because some types develop only in the jaw and are considered odontogenic tumours (cemento-ossifying fibromas), whereas others develop in facial or long bones and must therefore be non-odontogenic (ossifying fibromas; Table 12.2). All types are also classified as fibro-osseous lesions because of their histological appearances. The psammomatoid type of ossifying fibroma is discussed here and the others with the odontogenic tumours in Chapter 11.

Table 12.2 Types of ossifying and cemento-ossifying fibromas

Type	Origin	Sites
Conventional cemento-ossifying fibroma	Odontogenic	Alveolus and adjacent bone of jaw
Juvenile trabecular cemento-ossifying fibroma	Odontogenic	Alveolus and adjacent bone of jaw
Psammomatoid ossifying fibroma	Non-odontogenic	Facial bones, sinuses, skull and jaws

Psammomatoid ossifying fibroma

This ossifying fibroma has also been called juvenile (active) ossifying fibroma but is now known to develop at all ages, though most present between 15 and 35 years of age. They affect the maxilla, facial bones and base of skull, particularly the ethmoid region, more frequently than the mandible.

Lesions cause asymptomatic expansion of bone, displacing adjacent structures such as sinuses or orbit (Fig. 12.17). Radiological appearance depends on the degree of mineralisation, but most are radiolucent or of even mixed density (Figs 12.18 and 12.19).

Histologically, the lesion consists of a highly cellular fibroblastic tissue containing compact, rounded dense calcifications, larger than, but reminiscent of, the so-called *psammoma bodies* in thyroid carcinomas (Fig. 12.20). These small mineralised balls do not usually fuse together as the lesion matures.

The treatment is enucleation and curettage. There is a risk of recurrence, perhaps because these lesions often arise in thin facial bones that make treatment difficult. However, any recurrence is usually eradicated by a second or third curettage, so that conservative surgery is all that is required.

Review case series PMID: 7823298

Detailed description PMID: 1843064

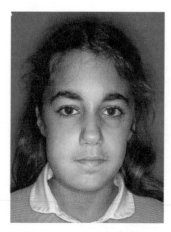

Fig. 12.17 **Psammomatoid ossifying fibroma.** A lesion in the mandible of a 12-year-old girl producing asymmetry by expansion of the mandibular ramus. *(Fig. 8 from Papadaki, M., Troulis, M.J., and Kaban, L.B. 2005. Advances in diagnosis and management of fibro-osseous lesions. Oral Maxillofac Surg Clin North Am 17(4):415-434.)*

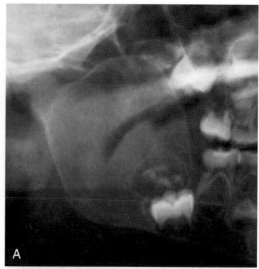

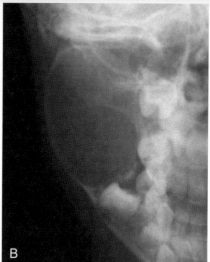

Fig. 12.19 **Psammomatoid ossifying fibroma.** This example in the mandible shows a typically very large expansile lesion (A). In this young child the lesion is in an early phase and no internal mineralisation is evident radiographically. The postero-anterior (PA) jaws projection shows marked expansion of the ramus lingually and buccally (B).

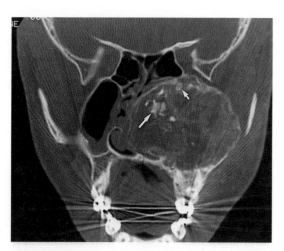

Fig. 12.18 **Psammomatoid ossifying fibroma.** Computed tomography showing a lesion in the typical site involving maxilla, maxillary and ethmoid sinuses and nasal cavity, and expanding the maxilla toward the coronoid process. This example has internal mineralisation visible (*arrowed*). *(From Wenig, B.M., Mafee, M.F., Ghosh, L., 1998. Fibro-osseous, osseous, and cartilaginous lesions of the orbit and paraorbital region. Correlative clinicopathologic and radiographic features, including the diagnostic role of CT and MR imaging. Radiol. Clin. North Am. 36, 1241-1259, xii.)*

HAEMANGIOMA OF BONE

Intraosseous haemangiomas are rare, and it is unclear whether they are hamartomas or benign neoplasms, but they tend to present in patients younger than 30 years of age, and more frequently in females. Three-quarters of lesions arise in the mandible.

Clinically, haemangiomas in bone are usually asymptomatic and are often chance radiographic findings. However, some cause progressive painless swellings which, when the overlying cortex is resorbed, may form a pulsatile bluish soft tissue swelling. Teeth may be loosened, and there may be bleeding, particularly from any involved gingival margins.

Radiographically, the features of haemangioma are extremely varied. They range from a sharply defined cyst-like appearance to poorly defined lobulated radiolucencies or even a soap-bubble appearance (Fig. 12.21). A serpiginous outline is particularly suggestive.

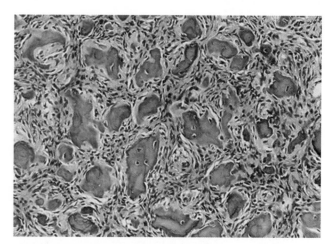

Fig. 12.20 **Psammomatoid ossifying fibroma,** comprising small darkly stained mineralised nodules of bone in a cellular fibrous tissue. Whether mineralisation is psammomatoid or not can be detected histologically but not radiographically.

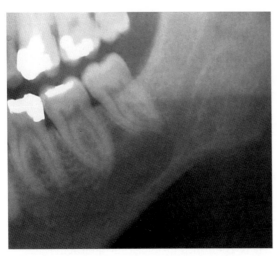

Fig. 12.21   Haemangioma of bone. This well-circumscribed haemangioma below the second and third molars was thought to be a solitary bone cyst. Clues as to its real nature are few. It is not as radiolucent as a cyst, and it communicates with the inferior dental canal, where its feeder vessels originate. Biopsy was associated with considerable bleeding.

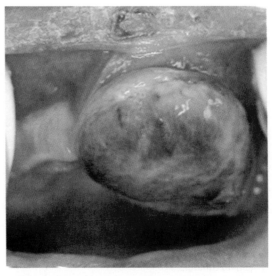

Fig. 12.23   Melanotic neuroectodermal tumour of infancy. This example has become ulcerated, and the dark pigment can be seen as speckles in the tissue. *(Fig. 9.36 from Woo, S.B., 2012. Oral pathology: a comprehensive atlas and text. Saunders, Philadelphia, p. 215.)*

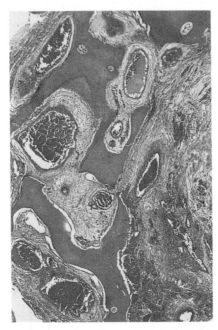

Fig. 12.22   Haemangioma of bone. The marrow spaces contain very large blood-filled sinuses with thin walls; the lesion is poorly localised and permeates between the bony trabeculae.

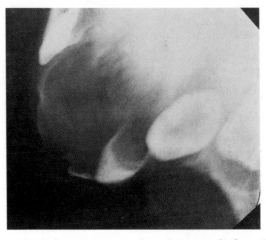

Fig. 12.24   Melanotic neuroectodermal tumour of infancy. The anterior maxilla of this neonate contains an expansile radiolucency that has displaced tooth germs and eroded the alveolar bone.

Pathology

Haemangiomas of bone are essentially similar to those in soft tissues (Ch. 25). They are usually cavernous, with low flow and pressure (Fig. 12.22), but there is also an arteriovenous type (fast-flow angioma) which has large feeder arteries, tends to expand rapidly and is likely to bleed severely if opened.

Intrabony vascular malformations PMID: 25703595

Management

A haemangioma may not be suspected if its vascularity is not obvious. Opening it or extracting a related tooth may therefore release torrents of blood, occasionally with fatal results.

If there are identifiable feeder vessels, selective arterial embolisation can be performed either as a treatment or to reduce size and blood flow before surgery. However, the complexity of the arterial tree in the head and neck makes this a skilled procedure and often only partial embolisation can be achieved. Surgery after embolisation is considerably safer. For the largest haemangiomas, a wide en bloc resection may be the only practical treatment.

MELANOTIC NEUROECTODERMAL TUMOUR OF INFANCY

→ Summary chart 26.1 p. 390

This rare benign but destructive neoplasm arises from the neural crest and affects children in the first few months of life. Two-thirds of lesions arise in the maxilla, usually anteriorly, with occasional examples in the mandible, skull or brain. It is usually painless and expands slowly forming a bluish-black pigmented mass (Fig. 12.23).

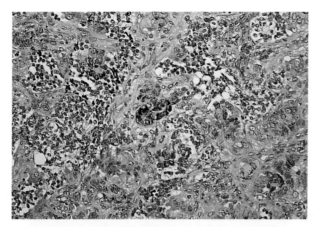

Fig. 12.25 **Melanotic neuroectodermal tumour of infancy.** Pale pink-staining epithelial cells, some of which are pigmented (centrally), arranged in clusters and surrounded by small, round, darkly staining tumour cells.

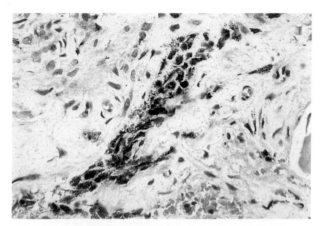

Fig. 12.26 **Melanotic neuroectodermal tumour of infancy.** Higher power showing the melanin pigment granules within a strand of epithelium.

Radiographically, there is an area of bone destruction, frequently with ragged margins, and displacement of the developing teeth (Fig. 12.24) that can simulate a malignant neoplasm.

Pathology

Microscopy reveals that the tumour has two components and a very striking appearance. The first is melanin-containing epithelium, comprising cuboidal epithelial cells forming islands and lining slit-like spaces (Figs 12.25 and 12.26). The second is a population of small darkly stained cells with round nuclei and little cytoplasm. These grow either in the centre of the small epithelial lined cysts or in clusters in the fibrous tissue that supports both components. Some degree of atypia and infrequent mitotic figures are often seen. The round cells resemble neuroblasts and secrete vanillylmandelic acid (VMA), which can be detected in the urine. This is a metabolic degradation product of the epinephrine pathway produced by many neuroendocrine tumours.

Frequent mitotic figures and loss of differentiation of the melanocyte-like cells suggest more aggressive behaviour.

Case series PMID: 12142876

Management

A destructive maxillary tumour in the maxilla in an infant, together with submucosal pigmentation and high levels of urinary vanillylmandelic acid, are distinctive, and to provide treatment rapidly and avoid further destruction, the diagnosis may be confirmed histologically after removal.

Surgery is the treatment of choice, but the extent of the resection is controversial and can range from local excision and curettage to total maxillectomy. The tumour is non-encapsulated but usually separates easily from the bone at operation. Conservative surgery is usually curative but, even when excision is incomplete, recurrence is rare.

Serum levels of epinephrine, norepinephrine and urinary VMA return to normal after treatment and may be monitored for evidence of recurrence. As many as 15% may recur and a very few have metastasised and disseminated widely and these malignant examples cannot be predicted in advance. Histology is an unreliable guide to behaviour, as even those tumours that show histologically malignant features may do well.

Key features are summarised in Box 12.5.

Surgical management PMID: 19070747

MALIGNANT NEOPLASMS OF BONE

OSTEOSARCOMA

➔ Summary chart 13.1 p. 222

Osteosarcoma is defined as a malignant neoplasm that forms bone or osteoid. Most osteosarcomas arise in long bones of children and adolescents, are highly malignant, metastasise early to lung and are frequently fatal. In contrast, osteosarcomas of the jaws tend to arise between 30–50 years of age, seem to grow more slowly and have a much better prognosis.

Only about 5% of osteosarcomas arise in the jaws; males are slightly more frequently affected, and the body of the mandible is a common site.

There is typically a firm swelling that grows noticeably in a few months and becomes painful (Fig. 12.27). Teeth may be loosened, and there may be paraesthesia or loss of sensation in the mental nerve area.

Radiographically, appearances are variable but irregular bone destruction with a poorly defined moth-eaten margin is usual. Bone formation within osteosarcomas varies in extent, but when the sarcoma extends beyond bone into soft tissue, even small amounts of bone can be seen clearly and aid diagnosis (see Fig. 12.27). Rapid enlargement pushes the periosteum away from the bone and triggers formation of a periosteal new bone layer over the tumour, giving rise to a sun-ray appearance and Codman's triangles at the margin. Although characteristic, this reflects rapid growth and is not specific to osteosarcoma. Widening of the periodontal ligament is sometimes an early feature.

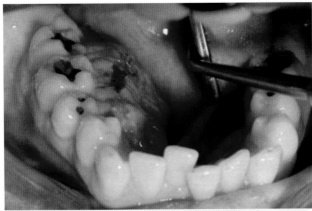

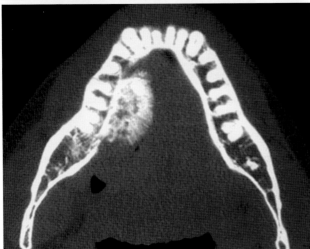

Fig. 12.27 **Osteosarcoma of the jaw.** *Upper panel*, a bony hard expansion of the alveolus. *Lower image*, computed tomography showing the original outline of the mandible to be intact, but the expanded tissue contains bone and has a radiating 'sun ray' appearance. *(Figure from Fernandes, R., et al., 2007. Osteogenic sarcoma of the jaw: a 10-year experience. J. Oral Maxillofac. Surg. 65 (7), 1286-1291.)*

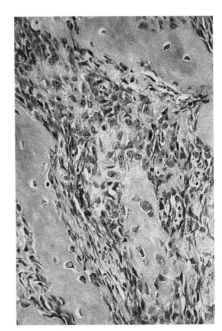

Fig. 12.28 **Osteosarcoma.** Trabeculae of abnormal woven bone surrounded by atypical cells in which mitoses are frequent and pleomorphism is conspicuous.

Box 12.6 Osteosarcoma of the jaws: key features

- Rare
- Patient mean age is approximately 35 years
- Usually affects the mandible
- Radiographically, bone formation is seen in a soft tissue mass
- Treated by radical surgery, sometimes with additional chemotherapy
- Better prognosis than osteosarcoma of the long bones, infrequent metastasis
- Occasionally follows irradiation

Pathology

The cause of osteosarcoma is unknown, though causative mutations in the retinoblastoma gene RB1 and p53 are recognised in long bone lesions.

The mass comprises disorganised neoplastic osteoblasts that vary in size and shape, from spindle cells to angular or large and hyperchromatic (Fig. 12.28). Bone formation is not necessarily prominent, and a search must be made for the diagnostic zones of osteoid and disorganised woven bone. Mitoses may be seen, particularly in the more highly cellular areas. Cartilage and clusters of osteoclasts may also be found. The variable appearance and sparse osteoid in some lesions make diagnosis difficult in a small biopsy.

Longstanding Paget's disease predisposes to osteosarcoma, but because the jaws are rarely affected by Paget's disease, this is not a significant risk factor. However, osteosarcoma may develop in skull and facial bones affected by Paget's disease, and also occasionally many years after head and neck irradiation for another cancer.

Key features are summarised in Box 12.6.

Case series PMID: 10982954

Management

Treatment is by radical surgery, a wide en bloc resection including any soft tissue extension, usually a minimum of a hemimandibulectomy or a total maxillectomy. In recent years it has been common to add radiotherapy and/or chemotherapy as would be provided for long bone sarcoma. However, distant metastasis from jaw lesions is much less frequent than from long bone sarcomas and the additional benefit is marginal. The prognosis depends mainly on the extent of the tumour and deteriorates with spread to the soft tissues, to lymph nodes (in about 10% of cases) or to the base of the skull. In approximately 50%, there is local recurrence within a year of treatment. The 5-year survival rate may range from 70% for tumours less than 5 cm in diameter to zero for tumours greater than 15 cm, and death usually follows local recurrence rather than distant metastasis.

Treatment PMID: 24246156 and 12237918

CHONDROSARCOMA

→ Summary chart 13.1 p. 222

Malignant neoplasms that form cartilage are chondrosarcomas. Those that form both cartilage and osteoid or bone are considered osteosarcomas. Chondrosarcomas of the jaws behave in a similar fashion to those in the commoner sites in the vertebrae, ribs and skull.

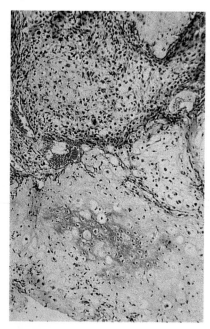

Fig. 12.29   Chondrosarcoma. Lobules of abnormal hyaline cartilage are formed in a disorganised fashion by sheets of malignant cells.

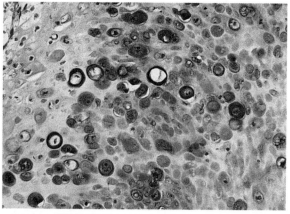

Fig. 12.30   Chondrosarcoma. High power of cartilage in a chondrosarcoma showing the abnormal chondrocytes and disorganised mineralisation.

Chondrosarcomas of the jaws are even rarer than osteosarcomas and affect adults at an average age of approximately 45 years. The anterior maxilla is the site in 60% of cases. A painless swelling or loosening of teeth associated with a radiolucent area are typical. The radiolucency can be well or poorly circumscribed, or may appear multilocular. Calcifications are frequently present and may be widespread and dense.

Pathology

Chondrosarcomas are graded on the basis of how well the cartilage is differentiated and how pleomorphic and mitotically active the cells are. Jaw osteosarcomas are usually at the low-grade end of the spectrum. The cartilage is comparatively well formed, with mild atypia in chondrocytes and only an occasional mitosis (Figs 12.29 and 12.30).

Chondrosarcomas must be widely excised as early as possible as radiotherapy and chemotherapy have no effect on low-grade tumours. Greater margins are required with

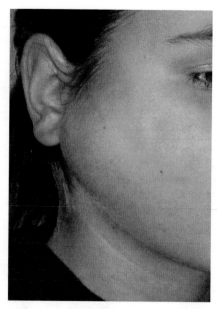

Fig. 12.31   Rapidly enlarging swelling of the ramus caused by Ewing's sarcoma in a patient aged 12 years.

increasing grade, from 1–3 cm. Survival is good, with a 75% 5-year survival. Death usually follows repeated recurrence, and extension to the skull. Metastasis is unusual.

Mesenchymal chondrosarcoma is a rare but highly malignant variant. It is a highly cellular tumour in which there are only small foci of tissue recognisable as poorly formed cartilage. The jaws are common sites, and patients are usually younger than for other chondrosarcomas, in their second or third decade.

Case series PMID: 3131505

All cartilaginous lesions PMID: 20614285

Mesenchymal chondrosarcoma PMID: 17681487

EWING'S SARCOMA

Ewing's sarcoma of bone and its near relative, the primitive neuroectodermal tumour of soft tissue, are members of a group of malignant neoplasms that are essentially undifferentiated but show some neural features.

Ewing's sarcoma is rare overall, and only 1% or so of these already rare lesions arise in the jaws. It has a predilection for the body of the mandible in children or young adults, aged 10–20 years. Typical symptoms are bone swelling and often pain, progressing over a period of months to perforate the cortex and form a soft tissue mass (Fig. 12.31). Teeth may loosen, and the overlying mucosa ulcerate. Fever, leukocytosis, a raised erythrocyte sedimentation rate (ESR) and anaemia may be associated and indicate a poor prognosis.

Radiographically there is a very poorly defined radiolucency that can be difficult to see in its early stages on plain radiographs or panoramic views but later may produce a prominent 'onion-skin' periosteal reactive bone visible on CT or cone beam CT (Fig. 12.32).

Genetics

Ewing's sarcoma is caused by one of several similar characteristic reciprocal translocations. In 85% this is a t(11;22) translocation that fuses two genes (Ewing's sarcoma gene

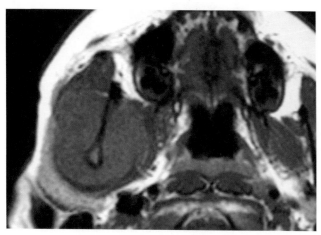

Fig. 12.32 **Axial magnetic resonance imaging scan of Ewing's sarcoma in the mandibular ramus.** The features are not specific but indicate a rapidly growing lesion because the cortex of the ramus is still visible in the centre of the large round tumour mass.

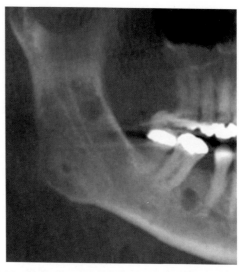

Fig. 12.33 **Multiple myeloma.** There are multiple small relatively well-defined radiolucencies in the ramus, alveolus, body and near the angle. *(By kind permission of Mrs J Brown.)*

EWSR1 and *Fli1*) that then produce an abnormal transcription factor responsible for transforming the cells. Other causative translocations are recognised and are useful diagnostic tests routinely performed on biopsy samples.

Pathology

Ewing's sarcoma cells resemble lymphocytes but are approximately twice their size. They have a darkly staining nucleus and a rim of cytoplasm, which is typically vacuolated and stains for glycogen. The cells form diffuse sheets or loose lobules, separated by septa. Distant spread is usually to the lungs and other bones rather than lymph nodes.

The initial treatment is chemotherapy followed by wide excision and radiotherapy. Chemotherapy improves the survival but, unfortunately, increases the risk of lymphoid tumours in later life. If the disease is localised, 70% of patients will survive 5 years, but the survival in those with disseminated disease is less than 20%. Jaw lesions appear to have a better prognosis than long bone lesions, probably because they are diagnosed at a smaller size; this is the main prognostic indicator.

Case series PMID: 21107767

MYELOMA

Multiple myeloma is a malignant neoplasm of plasma cells. The malignant plasma cells localise in the bone marrow, multiply to displace the normal marrow and cause multiple foci of bone destruction. Myeloma is a systemic disease from the outset. It is rare for a jaw lesion to cause the initial symptoms, but the skull is a common site of involvement and a third of patients may have a focus in the jaws. Myeloma is usually diagnosed in patients older than 60 years.

Clinically, myeloma lesions may be asymptomatic or cause bone pain and tenderness, weakening of bones and pathological fracture. The malignant plasma cells secrete immunoglobulin in great quantities causing a markedly raised ESR. The excess immunoglobulin is detectable by serum electrophoresis for diagnosis.

Radiologically myeloma lesions are radiolucencies, traditionally multiple 'punched out' radiolucencies in the vault of the skull. Presentation with jaw lesions is uncommon, but multiple small foci of bone destruction is a common presentation in those under treatment or in relapse (Fig. 12.33).

Genetics

Myeloma arises by one of several mechanisms involving chromosomal translocations. These bring together one of a variety of oncogenes, often the cell cycle regulator cyclin D1, with genes for immunoglobulins, both transforming the cell and inducing the excessive immunoglobulin synthesis. Myeloma arises from a single cell, and so all the malignant plasma cells are monoclonal; they all secrete antibody of the same immunoglobulin (Ig) class and antigen specificity.

Pathology

Myeloma lesions are masses of neoplastic plasma cells that may be well or poorly differentiated. Because the cells are monoclonal, they secrete only one type of immunoglobulin light chain, either kappa or lambda, and this is helpful in diagnosis (Fig. 12.34). Diagnosis can also be aided by serum electrophoresis showing a monoclonal band. Light chain overproduction is usual and leads to Bence-Jones proteinuria and often amyloidosis.

General review PMID: 23803862

Treatment

Myeloma is considered incurable, but treatment has developed to the stage that life can be extended for many years. Initially, most patients will be treated with combination chemotherapy including steroids and a thalidomide analogue and the proteasome inhibitor bortezomib, and there is frequently a good initial response. Remission is maintained and prolonged with a progression of drug regimens selected to match disease progression and avoid adverse effects.

If patients are fit enough, autologous stem cell transplants provide the best survival. During remission, the patient's own stem cells are harvested, either from blood or bone marrow, and reintroduced after high-dose chemotherapy. Localised lesions may be treated with radiotherapy or occasionally surgery if they threaten adjacent important structures or fracture. When bone metastases are widespread or symptomatic, they may be treated with bisphosphonates to

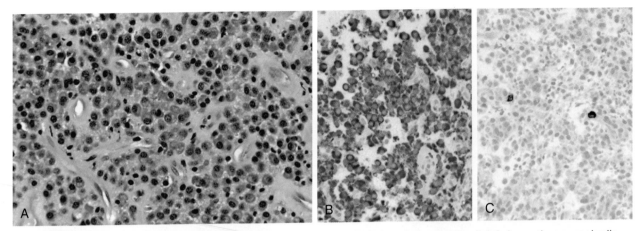

Fig. 12.34 **Multiple myeloma.** A. the tissues are infiltrated by a uniform population of plasma cells, slightly larger than normal cells. Myeloma is confirmed by immunohistochemistry for immunoglobulin light chains in the right panels. B. staining for kappa light chain and, (C), lambda light chain; brown stain is positive (see also Fig. 1.8 for method). It can be seen that almost all the plasma cells are secreting kappa light chain containing antibody, whereas only an occasional cell (probably inflammatory plasma cells not part of the myeloma) contain lambda light chain. The plasma cell population is therefore clonal and neoplastic.

Box 12.7   Multiple myeloma: key features

- Myeloma is a disseminated malignant neoplasm of plasma cells
- Radiographically, punched-out lesions appear particularly in the skull
- Similar lesions may appear in the jaws
- Monoclonal immunoglobulin (usually immunoglobulin G) produced
- Anaemia, purpura or immunodeficiency may be associated
- Excess immunoglobulin light chain production can lead to amyloidosis
- Many implications for dental treatment

Box 12.8   The most common primary sites for malignant neoplasms that metastasise to the jaws

- Breast
- Bronchus
- Prostate
- Thyroid
- Kidney

SOLITARY PLASMACYTOMA

A plasmacytoma is a solitary neoplasm of plasma cells that can be thought of as a localised form of myeloma. Approximately 80% of these rare tumours form in the soft tissues of the head and neck region, often in the nose and sinuses. Multiple myeloma develops in as many as 50% of patients within 2 years, demonstrating a link between these conditions and suggesting that plasmacytoma is often the initial and presenting lesion of myeloma.

Solitary plasmacytoma occasionally affects the jaws and nasal cavity, and the signs and symptoms are as for a deposit of multiple myeloma. Treatment is by radiotherapy. More than 65% of patients survive for 10 or more years, but multiple myeloma develop in the majority eventually, sometimes many years later.

Histologically, the appearances of plasmacytoma and multiple myeloma are the same (see Figs 12.33 and 12.34).

LYMPHOMAS

As discussed later, lymphomas of the oral soft tissues are uncommon except in association with HIV infection and are more likely to present as enlarged cervical lymph nodes (Ch. 27) or parotid gland swelling, the latter in Sjögren's syndrome (Ch. 22).

METASTASES TO THE JAWS

→ Summary chart 13.1 p. 222

Blood-borne metastasis to bone is almost always from a carcinoma, usually an adenocarcinoma (Box 12.8).

reduce bone resorption, reduce bone pain and hypercalcaemia and prevent fractures and collapse of vertebrae. Median survival for patients recently diagnosed is 8 years, and 15 years is currently the likely maximum.

Dental aspects

A myeloma deposit in the jaws or amyloid deposition in the oral soft tissues can be the first manifestation of the disease.

Complications of disease and its treatment affect delivery of dental treatment. Bone marrow replacement causes thrombocytopenia, anaemia, bleeding and purpura. Immunosuppression from steroids and loss of normal lymphocytes cause immunosuppression and opportunistic infections arise. Antibiotic prophylaxis may be required for surgery depending on stage of disease. High-potency bisphosphonates given intravenously include pamidronate and zoledronic acid, and this treatment carries a risk of medication-induced osteonecrosis (see Ch. 8).

Key features are summarised in Box 12.7.

Oral presentations PMID: 24048519

Amyloidosis

Amyloidosis is a complication of myeloma resulting from deposition of excess secreted Ig light chains in the tissues; this is discussed in Chapter 17.

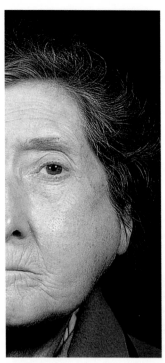

Fig. 12.35 Metastatic carcinoma of the mandible. Swelling developed in the ramus quite suddenly in this apparently fit patient. Investigations showed a deposit of poorly differentiated carcinoma in the jaw and signs of a bronchial carcinoma.

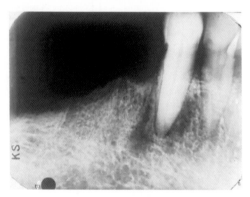

Fig. 12.36 Metastatic bronchogenic carcinoma. This small metastasis in the alveolar bone has produced a poorly demarcated, patchy radiolucency and destroyed the lamina dura around a root apex. Such small lesions could easily be mistaken for periapical granulomas radiographically, but have ragged margins.

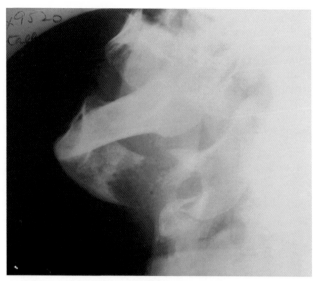

Fig. 12.37 Metastatic carcinoma in the mandible. A large and poorly defined radiolucent metastasis has destroyed most of the posterior body of the mandible, resulting in a pathological fracture.

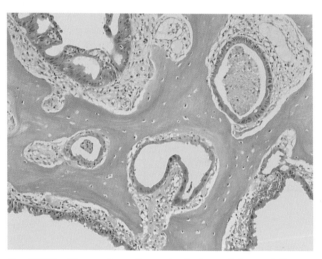

Fig. 12.38 Metastatic carcinoma in the jaw. All the medullary spaces contain adenocarcinoma, forming glands and duct-like spaces.

Metastasis to bone affects those bones with the greatest medullary volume, the spine, pelvis, ribs and femur. Jaw metastases are relatively unusual and almost always signify late-stage disease and widespread bony and other metastases. It is rare that a metastasis to the jaw is the first sign leading to diagnosis of the primary malignancy.

Jaw metastases are much more common than primary malignant neoplasms of bone.

Patients are usually middle-aged or elderly, reflecting the age distribution of carcinoma at the primary sites. The vast majority of metastases are in the mandible. Common symptoms are pain or swelling of the jaw (Fig. 12.35), trismus and paraesthesia or anaesthesia of the lip. A non-healing tooth socket is an important presentation for dentists.

There is typically an area of radiolucency with a hazy outline (Figs 12.36 and 12.37). This sometimes simulates an infected cyst or may be quite irregular and simulate osteomyelitis. One key feature is that metastases seed in the marrow spaces and, in the mandible, most of the marrow lies below the inferior dental canal. This localisation helps distinguish potential metastases from lesions associated with the teeth. However, it is important to be alert for metastases mimicking infection or dental disease if the radiographic features are unusual or treatment is ineffective. Sometimes the entire mandible may have a moth-eaten appearance from complete replacement of the medulla, usually by lymphoma. Bone sclerosis is a typical result of prostatic carcinoma metastasis.

Pathology

Diagnosis requires biopsy unless extensive bony metastases are already known. In such circumstances a biopsy is confirmatory but will not alter the treatment. In new lesions, biopsy is required and the histological appearances will be those of the primary carcinomas. The malignant tissue infiltrates adjacent marrow spaces and induces osteoclastic bone resorption (Fig. 12.38).

When a new metastasis is found, others are probably present elsewhere and a skeletal survey, bone scan, positron emission tomography scan or other survey technique will show the extent of the disease. Few patients survive more than a few months after diagnosis of a jaw metastasis and patients are treated palliatively. For the few carcinomas that respond to hormonal treatment, such as prostate or breast, this may induce a relatively long remission. Palliative radiotherapy may sometimes make the lesion in the jaw regress for a time and lessen pain.

Case series PMID: 17138711 and 25409855

Summary Chart 12.1   Differential diagnosis of a well-defined radiopaque lesion in the jaws or soft tissues.

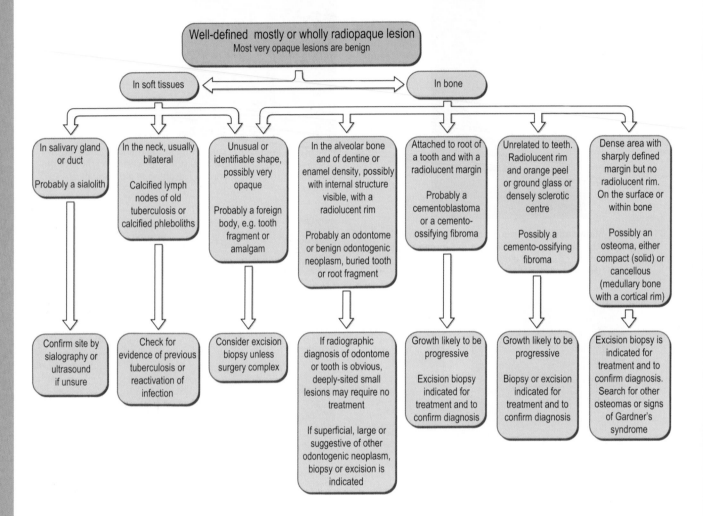

Summary Chart 12.2 Differential diagnosis of an ill-defined or diffuse radiographic lesion in the jaws.

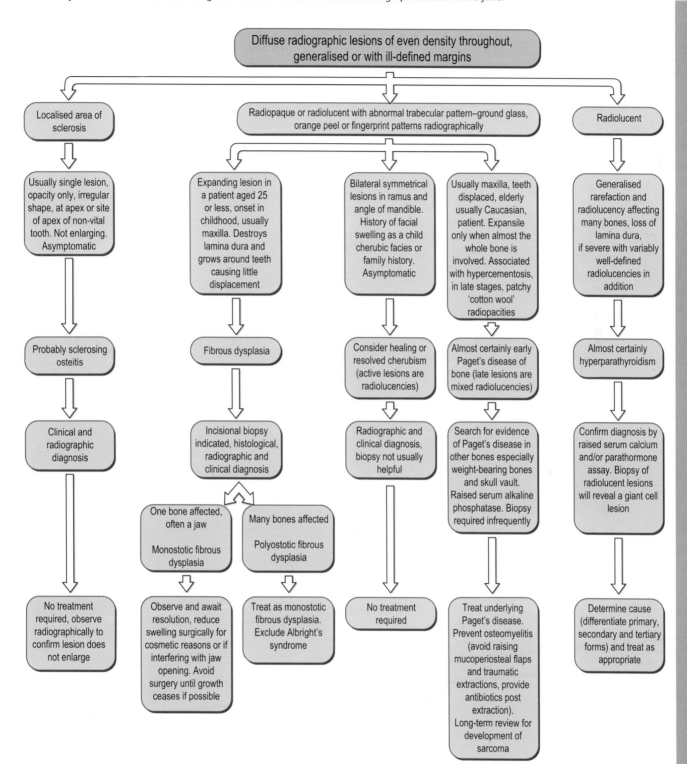

Genetic, metabolic and other non-neoplastic bone diseases

13

Bone diseases of dental significance are summarised in Box 13.1.

GENETIC DISEASES OF BONE

Osteogenesis imperfecta

Osteogenesis imperfecta is a group of genetic conditions in which the bones have reduced bone density and fracture

---

Box 13.1   Bone diseases of dental significance

- Osteogenesis imperfecta – associated dentinogenesis imperfecta
- Osteopetrosis – anaemia and risk of osteomyelitis
- Cleidocranial dysplasia – multiple unerupted teeth
- Cherubism – cyst-like giant cell lesions
- Rickets – hypocalcification of teeth in severe cases
- Scurvy – purpura, swollen, bleeding gingivae
- Hyperparathyroidism – 'cyst-like' giant cell lesions
- Paget's disease – overgrowth of maxilla sometimes
- Fibrous dysplasia – typically, hard swelling of maxilla
- Solitary bone 'cyst' – cyst-like radiolucency
- Aneurysmal bone 'cyst' – cyst-like radiolucency
- Gardner's syndrome – risk of colon carcinoma

---

easily. The term *brittle bone disease* is usually taken to mean this genetic condition but has also been applied to osteoporosis.

Pathology

Most types are inherited as an autosomal dominant trait, and the more common causal genes are the COL1A1 and COL1A2 procollagen genes. Procollagen fails to form a normal alpha helix, polymerise into normal type 1 collagen in the bone matrix and the collagen cannot mineralise. Without appropriate matrix, osteoblasts are unable to form normal amounts of bone, leading to fractures. However, there is remarkable molecular and clinical diversity, and the classification now extends to a proposed 17 types, based on inheritance pattern, genes affected and severity of the clinical phenotype. Even within one type there is variability of the effects. No gene is known for some types (Table 13.1). All types together affect approximately 1 in every 20,000 live births.

The bones are thin and lack the usual cortex of compact bone (Fig. 13.1), but development of epiphyseal cartilages is unimpaired so that bones in most types can grow to their normal length. Nevertheless, they may become grossly distorted by multiple fractures and result in dwarfism. The most severe cases (type II) usually die at birth or soon after; mild cases (type V) may have little disability. In the more common form (type I), the many fractures can cause severe

Table 13.1   Types of osteogenesis imperfecta

Type	Inheritance	Phenotype	Gene	Hereditary opalescent teeth
I	AD	Mild	COL1A1	rare
	X-linked	Mild	PLS3	rare
II	AD	Severe, ultimately lethal	COL1A1 or COL1A2	no
III	AD	Progressive deformity	COL1A1 or COL1A2	frequent
IV	AD	Moderate	COL1A1 or COL1A2	frequent
V	AD	Moderate, hypertrophic callus and ossification of the interosseous membrane	IFITM5	no*
VI	AR	Moderate to severe	SERPINF1	no
VII	AR	Severe to lethal	CRTAP	no
VIII	AR	Severe to lethal	LEPRE1	no
IX	AR	Severe to lethal	PPIB	no
X	AR	Severe	SERPINH1	rare
XI	AR	Progressive deformity, contractures	FKBP10	no
XII	AR	Moderate	SP7	no
XIII	AR	Severe	BMP1	no
XIV	AR	Variable severity	TMEM38B	no
XV	AR	Variable severity	WNT1	no
	AD	Early-onset osteoporosis	WNT1	no

AD, autosomal dominant; *AR*, autosomal recessive.
*Type V has no dentinogenesis imperfecta but does show hypodontia and short roots in some families.

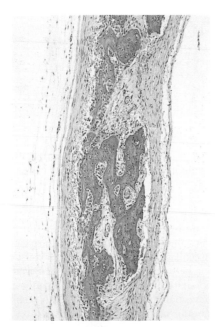

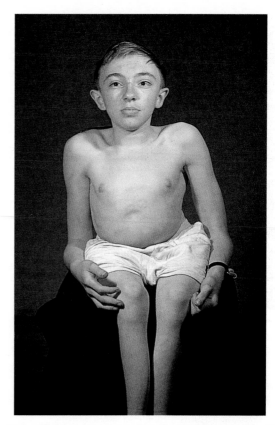

Fig. 13.1 Osteogenesis imperfecta. A section from the vault of the skull of a stillborn infant with type II disease; the most severe form of osteogenesis imperfecta shows that the bone is small in amount, primitive (woven) in character and shows no attempt at differentiation into cortical plates and medullary space.

Fig. 13.3 Clinical appearance of a severely affected child with osteogenesis imperfecta type III in which there is progressive deformity.

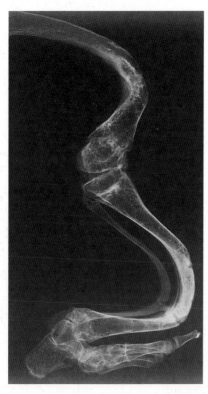

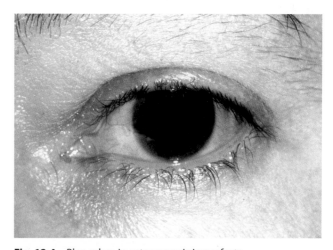

Fig. 13.4 Blue sclera in osteogenesis imperfecta.

Natural history and types PMID: 24754836

Types and genetics PMID: 24715559

Fig. 13.2 Osteogenesis imperfecta. Leg of an infant with a severe type of osteogenesis imperfecta showing severe bending as a result of multiple fractures under body weight.

deformity (Figs 13.2 and 13.3). The sclera of the eyes may also appear blue because their thinness allows the pigment layer to show through (Fig. 13.4). Deafness also develops.

In addition to fractures, patients with the milder types also tend to suffer from back and joint pain usually due to osteoarthritis. Approximately 60% have joint hypermobility, but otherwise, the majority have good health.

Dental effects

Because collagen type 1 is a major matrix protein of dentine too, some patients have abnormal teeth. It is difficult to be certain about the exact relationship between the two conditions because some types are described in few families, and often there has only been clinical examination and no examination of extracted teeth. Types III and IV account for most cases with abnormal teeth. The effects on teeth are described in Chapter 2 and appear identical to those in dentinogenesis imperfecta, though these result

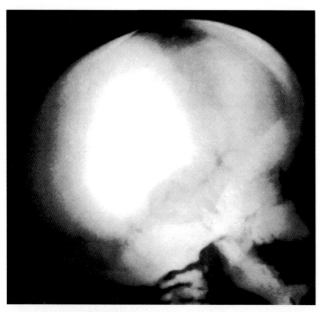

Fig. 13.5   Osteopetrosis. In contrast to osteogenesis imperfecta, the bone is excessively thick and dense as a result of defective resorption.

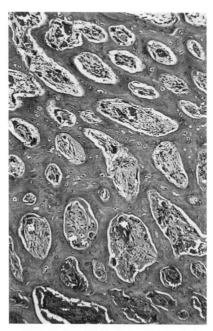

Fig. 13.6   Osteopetrosis. Almost solid bone with only small medullary spaces.

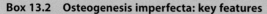

Box 13.2   Osteogenesis imperfecta: key features
• Thin fragile bones
• Usually an autosomal dominant trait
• Multiple fractures typically lead to gross deformities
• Teeth affected, especially in types III and IV
• Jaw fractures are uncommon

Box 13.3   Osteopetrosis: key features
• Rare genetic defect of osteoclastic activity
• Bones lack medullary cavities but are fragile
• Anaemia is common
• Osteomyelitis a recognised complication
• Delayed tooth eruption

from mutations in different genes. The dental changes in osteogenesis imperfecta are currently called 'osteogenesis imperfecta with hereditary opalescent teeth', whereas those affecting the teeth alone caused by other mutations are called 'dentinogenesis imperfecta'.

Dental effects PMID: 7285471 and 24700690

Management

Treatment with a bisphosphonate may be given to prevent resorption of what bone does form and this carries a risk of future osteonecrosis. No other treatment is effective, except to protect the child from even minor injuries and to minimise deformity by attending to fractures. Care must be taken during dental extractions, but fractures of the jaws are uncommon. Implants appear to osseointegrate in the few cases reported, enabling treatment of late dental effects.

Key features are summarised in Box 13.2.

Gnathodiaphyseal dysplasia

This recently described and very rare autosomal dominant condition was previously thought to be a variant of osteogenesis imperfecta with frequent fractures but normal healing. Its other features include bowing and cortical thickening of the long bones and multiple ossifying fibromas of the jaws. The teeth are normal (Ch.11).

Osteopetrosis: marble bone disease

Osteopetrosis is a rare genetic disease in which the bones become solidified and dense (Fig. 13.5) but brittle, as a

result of a variety of mutations in proteins that inactivate osteoclasts, preventing normal bone remodelling. There are several types of variable severity and inheritance pattern, and the disease can present in children or adults.

Medullary spaces are minute (Fig. 13.6), and the epiphyseal ends of the bones are club-shaped. Because of the deficiency of marrow space, the liver and spleen take on blood-cell formation, but anaemia is common, and defective white cells can lead to abnormal susceptibility to infection.

General review PMID: 23877423

Dental aspects

There may be compression of cranial nerve canals so that trigeminal or facial nerve neuropathies result. Despite its density, bone can be brittle so that the jaw may fracture during extractions. The reduced vascularity and sclerosis predispose to osteomyelitis, and prevention of dental infections is important. There is no effective treatment apart from marrow transplantation, and then only rarely. The dense bone delays tooth eruption.

Key features are summarised in Box 13.3.

Dental changes PMID: 4505753

Achondroplasia

Achondroplasia is the most common type of genetic skeletal disorder and manifests itself as 'disproportionate dwarfism', short-limbed individuals with normal trunk and head. The

Box 13.4   Achondroplasia: key features

- A common type of genetically determined restricted growth
- Failure of proliferation of cartilage in epiphyses and base of skull
- Short limbs but normal-sized skull
- Middle third of face retrusive due to reduced growth of skull base
- Malocclusion may need correction

cause is a homozygous mutation in the fibroblast growth factor receptor 3 gene, that prevents bone forming from cartilage at the epiphyses and base of the skull. Inheritance is autosomal dominant, but homozygous mutation is lethal.

Dental aspects

The head is of normal size with a high forehead, but reduced growth at the base of the skull causes the middle third of the face to be retrusive. The mandible is often protrusive, and there is usually severe malocclusion and sometimes posterior open bite. Associated macroglossia has been described.

Key features are summarised in Box 13.4.

Case and review: PMCID: PMC3804960

Cleidocranial dysplasia

In this rare familial disorder, there is a mutation in the *RUNX2* gene that controls osteoblast and chondroblast differentiation. There is defective formation of the clavicles, delayed closure of fontanelles and sometimes retrusion of the maxilla and a range of other features, many affecting the skull. Partial or complete absence of clavicles allows the patient to bring the shoulders together in front of the chest (Fig. 13.7).

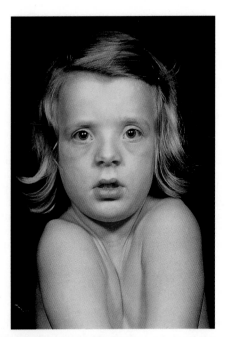

Fig. 13.7   Cleidocranial dysplasia. Defective development of the clavicles allows this abnormal mobility of the shoulders. Other members of the family were also affected.

Dental aspects

Cleidocranial dysplasia is one of the few identifiable causes of delayed eruption of the permanent dentition. Many permanent teeth may remain embedded in the jaw (Fig. 13.8) and frequently give rise to dentigerous cysts (see Ch. 10). The deciduous teeth are retained. The *RUNX2* gene that is mutated in this condition normally controls alveolar bone remodelling, tooth and periodontal ligament development, all required for tooth eruption.

Key features are summarised in Box 13.5.

Case series and review PMID: 22023169

Box 13.5   Cleidocranial dysplasia: key features

- Absent clavicles, delayed closure of fontanelles
- Many or most permanent teeth typically remain embedded in the jaw
- Delayed eruption then prolonged retention of deciduous teeth
- Many supernumerary unerupted teeth also present
- Long-term risk of developing dentigerous cysts
- Sinuses reduced in size
- High arched palate and sometimes cleft palate
- Large skull with frontal bossing
- Ocular hypertelorism
- Short stature

Cherubism

→ Summary chart 10.2 p. 164

Cherubism causes multiple multilocular bone lesions in the mandible and maxilla that develop in early childhood, enlarge and then regress over many years. Cherubism is caused by one of several mutations in the SH3BP2 gene that encodes a signalling protein. It is inherited as an autosomal dominant trait.

Although a dominant condition, there may be no family history because of variable expressivity and penetrance. As a result of weaker penetrance of the trait in females, the disease is approximately twice as frequently clinically evident in males. Non-familial cases may also be new mutations. Usually, only isolated cases are encountered, but a family with no fewer than 20 affected members has been reported. Cherubism is not a familial form of fibrous dysplasia.

The onset is typically between the ages of 6 months and 7 years, but rarely is delayed until late teenage or after puberty. Typically, symmetrical swellings are noticed at the age of 2–4 years in the region of the angles of the mandibles and, in severe cases, in the maxillae. The symmetrical mandibular swellings give the face an excessively chubby appearance (Fig. 13.9). The alveolar ridges are expanded, and the mandibular swellings may sometimes be so gross lingually as to interfere with speech, swallowing or even breathing, but the rapidity and extent of growth is very variable. Teeth are frequently displaced and loosened.

Maxillary involvement is usually associated with widespread mandibular disease and is uncommon. Extensive maxillary lesions cause the eyes to appear to be turned heavenward; this, together with the plumpness of the face, is the reason for these patients being likened to cherubs. The appearance of the eyes is due to such factors as the maxillary masses pushing the floors of the orbits and eyes

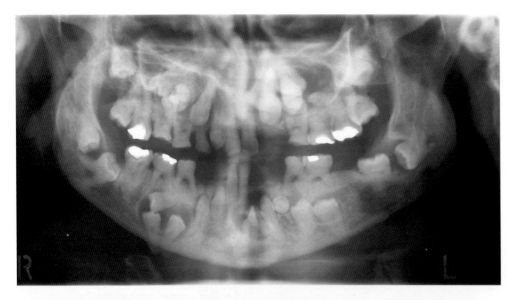

Fig. 13.8 Cleidocranial dysplasia. There are many additional teeth but widespread failure of eruption and possibly development of dentigerous cysts.

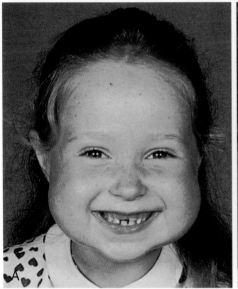

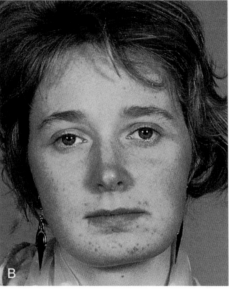

Fig. 13.9 Cherubism. The typical expansion of the mandibular rami in a child have regressed 10 years later. *(From Cawson, R.A., Binnie, W.H., Barrett, A.W., et al., 2001. Oral disease. Third ed. Mosby, St. Louis.)*

upward and exposing the sclera below the pupils. Expansion of the maxillae may also cause stretching of the skin and some retraction of the lower lids.

There is frequently cervical lymphadenopathy. This is typically seen in the early stages and may completely subside by puberty.

Radiographic changes may be seen considerably earlier than clinical signs and are usually more extensive than the clinical swelling would suggest. The body and ramus of the mandible are particularly involved by large radiolucent lesions with fine bony septa producing a multilocular appearance (Fig. 13.10). Lesions often destroy the involved tooth germs, leading to missing teeth. Maxillary involvement is shown by diffuse rarefaction of the bone and extension to obliterate the sinuses. Extent is most clearly visualised by computed tomography scanning.

Growth is rapid for a few years and then slows down until puberty is reached. There is then slow regression until, by adulthood, normal facial contour is typically completely restored, although bone defects may persist radiographically. Severely affected patients may suffer permanent deformity, particularly if bony support for the eye has been destroyed.

General review PMID: 22640403

Pathology

The jaw lesions consist of loose fibrous tissue containing clusters of multinucleate giant cells (Fig. 13.11), overall resembling giant cell granulomas or hyperparathyroidism. With the passage of time, giant cells become fewer and there is bony repair of the defect (Fig. 13.12).

Management

Because of natural regression of the disease, treatment can usually be avoided. If disfigurement is severe, the lesions respond to curettage or to paring down of excessive tissue. Treatment in the early stages is likely to lead to recurrence.

Key features are summarised in Box 13.6.

Natural history PMID: 11113824

Hypophosphatasia

Hypophosphatasia is an uncommon recessive genetic disorder caused by lack of the enzyme alkaline phosphatase. There are several types of variable severity, milder forms presenting at an older age. The early-onset type causes rickets-like skeletal disease with defective mineralisation. Teeth lack cementum and therefore periodontal attachment

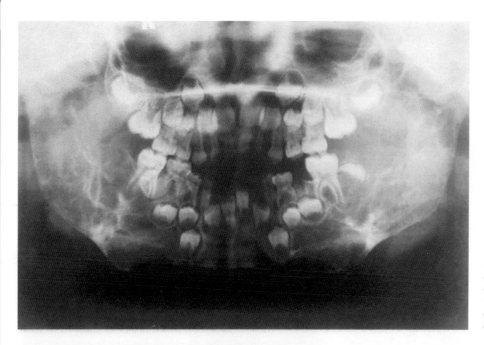

Fig. 13.10 Cherubism. Both rami, much of the body of the mandible and the posterior maxillae are expanded by multilocular radiolucent lesions that have displaced and destroyed developing teeth.

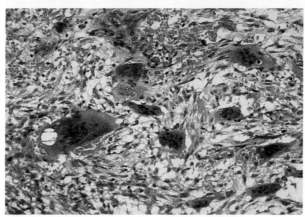

Fig. 13.11 Cherubism. An early lesion showing multinucleate giant cells lying in haemorrhagic oedematous fibrous tissue. The appearances are indistinguishable histologically from giant cell granuloma.

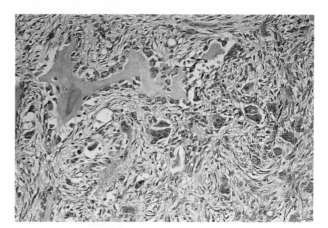

Fig. 13.12 Cherubism. In a late lesion, there is formation of woven bone by the fibrous tissue and giant cells are less numerous. Eventually bone remodelling will restore the contour and quality of the bone.

Box 13.6 Cherubism: key features

- Inherited as autosomal dominant trait
- Jaw swellings appear in infancy
- Angle regions of mandible affected symmetrically giving typical chubby face
- Symmetrical involvement of maxillae in more severe cases
- Radiographically, lesions appear as multilocular cysts
- Histologically, lesions consist of giant cells in vascular connective tissue
- Lesions regress with skeletal maturation
- Normal facial contour restored unless severely affected

---

to bone, causing premature loss. This is sometimes the only sign of the disease (see Fig. 2.37). Diagnosis is made by the low levels of plasma alkaline phosphatase and raised urinary phosphoethanolamine. Late-onset hypophosphatasia presents with bone fractures. See also Chapter 2.

Dental effects PMID: 19232125

Sickle cell anaemia and thalassaemia major

Both these haemoglobinopathies can cause bone changes, but only in the most severely affected. Thalassaemia is the more likely to do so. In thalassaemia, the bone marrow becomes hyperplastic, responding to chronic hypoxia, expanding the marrow spaces in all bones. Trabecular bone becomes less dense, and there is painless expansion of bones, with eventual obliteration of the maxillary sinuses. Bones are thus larger but osteoporotic. Skull radiographs may show a 'hair-on-end' appearance caused by periosteal growth expanding the bone, large maxilla and a thin cortex in all bones. The teeth may be displaced, causing malocclusion.

In sickle cell anaemia, the changes are less marked, but in addition the abnormal erythrocytes sludge in vessels under low oxygen tension, block them and cause painful infarcts in the bones. Symptomatically and radiographically, infarcts can mimic osteomyelitis. Bone infarcts may appear relatively radiolucent at first, but become sclerotic.

Gigantism and acromegaly

Overproduction of pituitary growth hormone, usually by an adenoma, before the epiphyses fuse, gives rise to gigantism with overgrowth of the whole skeleton. After fusion of the epiphyses, overproduction of growth hormone gives rise to acromegaly. The main features are continued growth at the mandibular condyle, causing gross prognathism, macroglossia, thickening of the facial soft tissues and overgrowth of the hands and feet (see Ch. 36).

METABOLIC BONE DISEASE

Rickets

Rickets in developing countries is usually due to deficiency of dietary calcium, whereas in developed countries it is rare and caused by deficiency of vitamin D, either in the diet or through lack of exposure to sunlight (Ch. 35). Rickets causes defective calcification and development of the skeleton. Similar changes may also result from excess mineral excretion in chronic renal diseases (renal rickets) including renal tubular acidosis, hypophosphatemic rickets and defects in vitamin D metabolism in the kidney.

The onset of rickets is usually in infancy. The main defects are broadening of the growing ends of bones and prominent costochondral junctions due to the epiphyseal defects (Figs 13.13 and 13.14). The weakened bones bend readily. Typical changes in the skull are wide fontanelles, bossing of the frontal and parietal eminences and thinning of the back of the skull.

Treatment of rickets is with vitamin D.

Dental aspects

Teeth have priority over the skeleton for minerals, and dental defects rarely result from rickets except in the most severe cases. Hypocalcification of dentine, with a wide band of predentine and excessive interglobular spaces, may be seen in unusually severe rickets. Eruption of teeth may also be delayed in such cases. Rachitic children are not abnormally susceptible to dental caries.

Dental effects PMID: 23939820

Vitamin D–resistant rickets

This condition caused by genetic failure of reabsorption of phosphate in the kidney is associated with characteristic dental defects and is discussed in Chapter 2.

Hyperparathyroidism

→ Summary charts 10.2 and 12.2 pp. 164, 203

Overproduction of parathormone (PTH) mobilises calcium from the skeleton and raises the plasma calcium level. In primary hyperparathyroidism the cause is usually an adenoma of the parathyroid glands, uncommonly hyperplasia of the gland and rarely a parathyroid carcinoma. Mostly elderly women are affected. This is less common than secondary hyperparathyroidism, in which PTH secretion is maintained by low calcium levels, usually caused by vitamin D deficiency or chronic renal failure (because the kidney enzymatically activates vitamin D). The major symptoms of all types result from renal damage which leads to hypertension or cardiovascular disease.

Bone disease is rarely seen now because of early treatment, but identical features can follow primary and secondary disease. Radiographically there are diffuse changes:

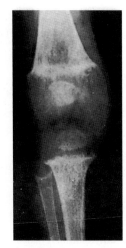

Fig. 13.13 Rickets. Overgrowth of cartilage (as shown in the section in Fig. 13.14) causes the epiphyseal plate to be broad, thick and irregular, and the ends of the bone become splayed. The growing end of the bone is ill-defined and calcification defective.

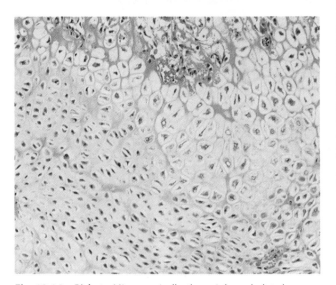

Fig. 13.14 Rickets. Microscopically, the epiphyseal plate has become disorganised with loss of the well-drilled lines of chondrocytes. There is also fibrous proliferation, but no calcification.

thinning of bone trabeculae, subperiosteal resorption of the bone of the fingers and resorption of the terminal phalangeal tufts. Dental radiographs may reveal reduced bone density, loss of trabecular pattern and definition of the lamina dura around the teeth. In severe disease these changes are more marked, and in addition the patient may develop one or more brown tumours. These cyst-like radiolucencies may appear unilocular or multilocular (Figs 13.15–13.17) and are more likely to be seen in secondary disease because of its long-term course. Bony changes can cause pathological fractures but reverse with treatment (Figs 13.18 and 13.19). A second effect seen in hyperparathyroidism secondary to renal disease is diffuse mandibular enlargement.

Hyperparathyroidism is also present in 95% of patients with type 1 multiple endocrine neoplasia (MEN 1) syndrome (Ch. 36).

Teeth primary hyperparathyroidism PMID: 13912943

Diffuse mandibular enlargement PMID: 22676829

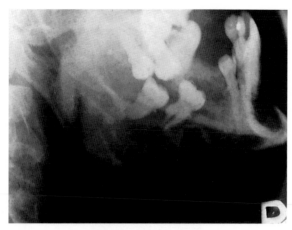

Fig. 13.15 Hyperparathyroidism. A patient of 51 years with hyperparathyroidism as a result of a parathyroid adenoma. There is an area of bone destruction simulating a multilocular cyst. The radiograph quality is low because of the loss of bone mineral.

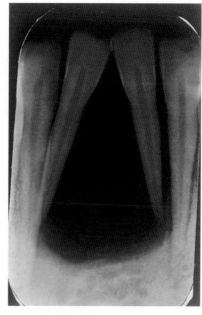

Fig. 13.17 Hyperparathyroidism. In this patient with hyperparathyroidism as a result of rejection of a kidney graft, there is a well-defined area of bone loss caused by a brown tumour.

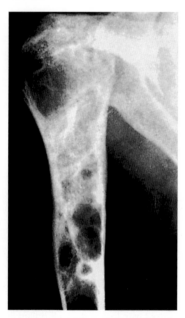

Fig. 13.16 Hyperparathyroidism. Osteitis fibrosa cystica in the humerus of the same patient with a parathyroid adenoma.

Pathology

Histologically, the brown tumour comprises foci of osteoclasts in a highly vascular stroma (Fig. 13.20). There is extensive internal haemorrhage. Breakdown of erythrocytes produces haemosiderin pigment and colours the lesion brown, hence its name. The histological appearances are indistinguishable from a giant cell granuloma of the jaws (see Ch. 12)

Diagnosis cannot, therefore, depend on histology alone, and radiographs and blood chemistry are essential whenever histology reveals a giant cell lesion (Box 13.7), with a search for involvement of other bones if test results suggest hyperparathyroidism.

The increased excretion of calcium leads ultimately to renal stone formation and renal damage. Other clinical features also result from the hypercalcaemia. The severe complications make early diagnosis of this disease particularly important.

Brown tumours in jaws PMID: 16798410

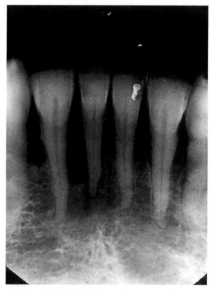

Fig. 13.18 Hyperparathyroidism. A periapical view reveals the relative radiolucency of the bone. There is loss of lamina dura around the roots, loss of trabeculae centrally and coarsening of the trabecular pattern elsewhere.

Management

In primary hyperparathyroidism, surgical removal of the causative adenoma is curative. A sestamibi scan (a form of technetium 99 scan) can often identify the hyperactive gland. For secondary hyperparathyroidism, treatment depends on the success of management of the renal failure. Bone lesions may respond to oral administration of vitamin D, whose metabolism is abnormal as a result of the renal disease. Surgery may also become necessary in late-stage renal failure to remove parathyroid glands that secrete excessively in response to the low serum calcium, so-called *tertiary hyperparathyroidism*.

Key features are summarised in Box 13.8.

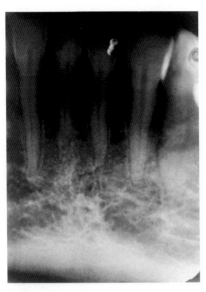

Fig. 13.19 Hyperparathyroidism. The same patient after treatment shows improved bone density and reformation of the lamina dura and cortex.

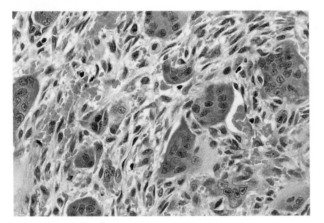

Fig. 13.20 Hyperparathyroidism. Multinucleate osteoclast-like giant cells are lying in a haemorrhagic fibrous tissue. The appearances are indistinguishable from giant cell granuloma histologically.

OTHER BONE DISEASES

Paget's disease of bone* (osteitis deformans) → Summary chart 13.1 p. 222

Paget's disease is a disturbance of bone turnover that causes irregular resorption, softening and sclerosis of bones. Paget's disease affects the elderly, with onset older than the age of 45 years. Anglo-Saxon races have the highest incidence, and in Britain, as many as 3% of people older than 40 years may have radiographic signs. Men are more frequently affected than women.

The possibility that Paget's disease is caused by a virus, possibly measles or a canine virus, is now considered less likely than genetic causes. However, there must be

---

*Sir James Paget (1814–1899), pioneer surgical pathologist, described several diseases that bear his name: Paget's disease of the nipple (intraductal breast carcinoma involving the nipple), extramammary Paget's disease, Paget's abscess and Paget's disease of bone. In general usage, the additional 'of bone' is understood when Paget's disease is referred to, but may need to be specified to avoid confusion.

Box 13.7 Biochemical findings in primary hyperparathyroidism

- Raised plasma calcium
- Low serum phosphorus
- Raised plasma parathyroid hormone levels
- Raised serum alkaline phosphatase

Box 13.8 Hyperparathyroidism: key features

- Overproduction of parathyroid hormone due to hyperplasia or adenoma of parathyroid glands
- Calcium mobilised from bone to serum, then lost in urine
- Common effects are malaise, hypertension or peptic ulcer and kidney stones
- Significant bone disease now uncommon
- Generalised rarefaction of bone, loss of density and lamina dura
- Brown tumours in the jaw appear radiographically as multilocular cyst-like areas
- Histologically, brown tumours are indistinguishable from giant cell granulomas
- Diagnosis confirmed by raised parathyroid hormone level (and serum calcium)

environmental factors because the incidence and severity have decreased dramatically in the UK during the last 50 years. This, together with effective treatment, has made clinically evident disease uncommon.

Several genes are recognised to be associated with different disease types, but the main candidates are the SQSTM1 and RANK genes, both of which are important for osteoclast function. As many as 30% of cases have a genetic background, and mutations can be detected in diseased bone, but not always in the rest of the body.

The bones most frequently affected are the sacrum, spine, skull, femora and pelvis. The disease may be widespread and is usually symmetrical, but sometimes a single bone is affected. In a severely affected patient, the main features are an enlarged head, thickening of long bones, which bend under stress, and tenderness or aching bone pain which can be severe.

Paget's disease is now largely effectively treated by bisphosphonates, either orally or given as intravenous infusion during active disease. Calcitonin can also be used to inactivate osteoclasts but is no longer used for long-term treatment because there is a risk for cancer of various types, although the risk is low. It is reserved for disease not responding to bisphosphonates and limited to 3 months of treatment. Calcium and vitamin D supplementation are also required.

General review PMID: 25585180

Pathology

Resorption, softening and then sclerosis of bones develop in sequence. A focus of diseased bone gradually enlarges, spreading along a bone like a wave, leaving an enlarging central zone of the bone sclerotic and distorted. Bone resorption and replacement becomes rapid, irregular, exaggerated and purposeless, and the ultimate result is diffuse thickening of affected bones. Closely adjacent parts of the bone may show different stages of the disease; a common result is therefore patchy areas of osteoporosis and of sclerosis (Figs 13.21 and 13.22).

Repeated bone resorption and deposition is marked histologically by blue-staining resting and reversal lines. Their irregular pattern characteristically produces a jigsaw puzzle ('mosaic') appearance in the bone (Figs 13.23 and 13.24). Both osteoclasts and osteoblasts are more prominent than in normal bone, and the osteoclasts are abnormally large and with more nuclei than normal. In the late stages, affected bones are thick, the cortex and medulla are obliterated and the whole bone is spongy in texture. There is also fibrosis of the marrow spaces and increased vascularity with large vessels. These shunt the majority of the blood flow direct from the arterial to venous circulation, reducing the perfusion of bone and peripheral resistance. This places a strain on the heart and may lead to eventual high-output cardiac failure.

Serum calcium and phosphorus levels are usually normal, but the alkaline phosphatase level is particularly high and may reach 700 IU/L. This is the primary diagnostic test for Paget's disease, and with typical radiological appearances, no biopsy is necessary.

The development of osteosarcoma is a recognised but rare complication of Paget's disease that carries a very poor prognosis. Osteosarcoma developing in the jaws is extremely rare in comparison with other bones but does develop occasionally.

Many patients live to an advanced age in spite of their disabilities.

Pathology review PMID: 24043712

Dental aspects

The skull is the most frequently affected bone in the head and neck. The softened skull vault deforms under the weight of the brain and sags down around the sides to produce the radiological sign of tam o'shanter skull, said to resemble the Scottish hat of the same name. Involvement of the skull base narrows foramina and in severe cases leads to cranial nerve deficits, commonly deafness.

Approximately 20% of patients used to have jaw involvement, but reducing severity during the last decades seems to have reduced the incidence in the jaws. When they are affected, the maxilla is considerably more frequently and severely affected than the mandible (see Fig. 13.21). The alveolar process becomes symmetrically and grossly enlarged (Figs 13.25 and 13.26). The sinuses are obliterated in severe cases, and the nasal airway can be reduced in size. Outward

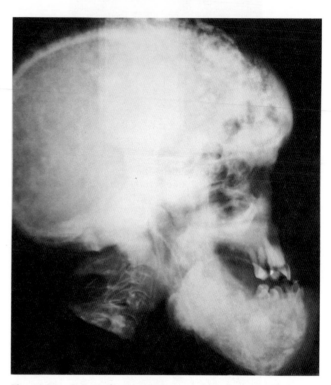

Fig. 13.22   Paget's disease. A very severely affected individual with extensive sclerosis and enlargement of all skull bones and jaws including, unusually, the mandible.

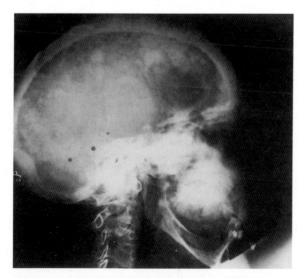

Fig. 13.21   Paget's disease of the skull and maxilla. The thickening of the bone and the irregular areas of sclerosis and resorption, which give it a fluffy appearance, are in striking contrast to the unaffected mandible.

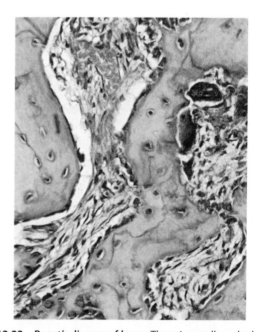

Fig. 13.23   Paget's disease of bone. There is a well-marked irregular ('mosaic') pattern of reversal lines due to repeated alternation of resorption and apposition. The marrow has been replaced by fibrous tissue; many osteoblasts and osteoclasts line the surface of the bone.

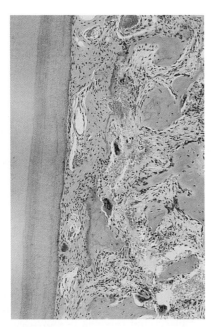

Fig. 13.24 Paget's disease affecting the jaw results in destruction of the lamina dura surrounding the teeth and, at a later stage, causes hypercementosis (see Fig. 6.16) and sometimes ankylosis.

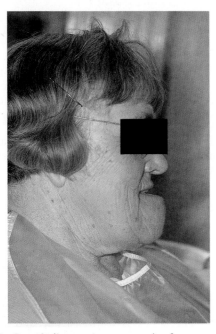

Fig. 13.26 Paget's disease. A rare example of severe mandibular involvement.

expansion of the alveolus carries the teeth with it so that spacing develops and dentures no longer fit. When the maxilla and base of skull are greatly enlarged, the orbits are pushed laterally, and hypertelorism and the additional facial height contribute to the appearance known as 'leontiasis ossea', a deformity somewhat incongruously likened to the appearance of a lion's face and now of only historical interest.

There may also be gross and irregular hypercementosis of teeth that can extend through the apex into the pulp. The lamina dura around the teeth is lost, and teeth may become ankylosed if the hypercementosis becomes fused to sclerotic areas of the bone. Attempts to extract affected teeth may succeed only by tearing away a large mass of bone. Severe bleeding from the vascular bone may follow. In the longer

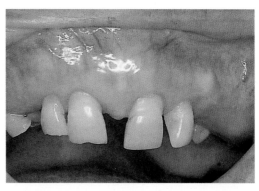

Fig. 13.25 Paget's disease of bone. Characteristic features of the involved maxilla are the broadening and deepening of the alveolar process, generalised bone enlargement and spacing of the teeth.

Box 13.9 Paget's disease: key features

- Persons past middle age affected
- Thickening but weakness of long bones and bone pain are typical of severe disease
- Often a radiographic finding. Less common as clinical disease
- Enlargement of skull
- Maxilla occasionally, but mandible rarely affected
- Teeth may show gross irregular hypercementosis
- Radiographically, patchy sclerosis and resorption give a cotton-wool appearance
- Histologically, irregular resorption and apposition leaves jigsaw puzzle ('mosaic') pattern of reversal lines
- Serum alkaline phosphatase markedly raised

term the dense cemental and bone sclerosis are prone to osteomyelitis and heal slowly. Antibiotic cover is necessary for extractions if the alveolus is sclerotic, and biopsy of involved jaws for diagnosis should be avoided.

The main radiographic features are lower density of the bone in the early stages and sclerosis in the later stages. Changes are patchily distributed, and loss of normal trabeculation and patchy sclerosis cause the characteristic 'cotton-wool' appearance.

Prolonged bisphosphonate treatment gives patients with Paget's disease a risk of osteonecrosis (Ch. 8).

In the diagnosis of Paget's disease in the jaws, alternatives to consider are fibro-osseous lesions, particularly florid cemento-osseous dysplasia (see Ch. 11). The patchy radiolucent and sclerotic appearances are very similar, but cemento-osseous dysplasia always starts in the alveolar processes of the jaws and is much more common in the mandible.

Key features are summarised in Box 13.9.

Dental relevance PMID: 6459433

FIBRO-OSSEOUS LESIONS

A fibro-osseous lesion is one in which bone is replaced by cellular fibrous tissue, which grows and then gradually matures back to bone. The degree of maturation varies between diseases and takes many months or years. Sometimes the maturation never proceeds beyond woven bone, or the woven bone may mature further to disorganised

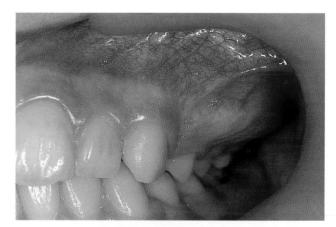

Fig. 13.27   Fibrous dysplasia. Typical presentation with a poorly defined, rounded expansion of the maxilla with no displacement of teeth and intact overlying mucosa.

lamellar bone or very dense sclerotic amorphous mineralisation.

The concept of fibro-osseous lesions is somewhat difficult because they are defined only by their histological appearances. This is not very helpful in diagnosis, particularly when biopsy should be avoided in the commonest disease of the group in the jaws. Because of their histological similarities, the diagnosis depends greatly on the clinical and radiographic findings. The presentation and behaviour of the different diseases are strikingly different. Fibro-osseous lesions are listed in Box 13.10.

Review all types PMID: 25409854

Fibrous dysplasia and Albright's syndrome → Summary chart 12.2 p. 203

Fibrous dysplasia is a growth disturbance of bone caused by mutation in the *GNAS1* gene. This gene encodes a G protein signalling molecule, and the mutation inactivates the G protein, allowing cyclic AMP to levels to rise, activating the affected cell.

The mutation is not inherited but occurs in a stem cell in the very early embryo, as early as a week or two after fertilisation, before placenta and embryonic tissues have started to form. The clone of cells carrying the mutation develops normally, and its daughter cells become distributed and incorporated into different tissues so that any patient is a mosaic for the mutation. Mutation at this very early stage means that the mutated cells can be mesodermal, endodermal or ectodermal and could give rise to almost any tissue. If the mutation arises later in development after tissues have started to develop, then the affected daughter cells will be limited to one tissue. The extent of the mosaicism, that is, the number of cells affected by the mutation, defines the clinical presentation.

There is no family history for any of the following presentations because this is a somatic mutation.

General review PMID: 17982387

Monostotic fibrous dysplasia

Monostotic fibrous dysplasia causes enlargement of one bone or part of one bone. This typically starts in childhood but usually stops growing in early adulthood. The jaws are the most frequent sites in the head and neck region and a common site overall, followed by skull bones, ribs and femur. Males and females are almost equally frequently affected. It is the commonest presentation of fibrous dysplasia, six times commoner than the polyostotic form.

In monostotic disease the *GNAS1* mutation arises late in development, so that the clone of affected cells is present in only one bone, forming both the osteoblasts and the fibrous tissue in the marrow spaces. In the affected region, the activated fibroblasts and osteoblasts grow excessively, but they remain under some degree of growth control, and the increased growth usually develops at a time when the bone would normally be growing and ceases at around the time the bone would normally be mature.

When the jaws are involved, a painless, smoothly rounded swelling, usually of the maxilla, is typical (Fig. 13.27). This is often centred around the zygomatic region or more posteriorly. Initially, the teeth are aligned but, if the mass becomes large, it will displace teeth. Patients with fibrous dysplasia may have missing teeth and enamel hypoplasia, but the dental defects are mild and poorly described. Lesions affecting the maxilla may spread to involve contiguous skull bones causing deformity of the orbit, base of skull and cranial nerve lesions (craniofacial fibrous dysplasia). The swelling usually grows very slowly, but with occasional rapid growth spurts.

Radiographically, the features reflect the structure of the abnormal bone described later in this chapter, and this varies depending on the stage of the process. Early lesions are patchy radiolucencies but develop into weak radiopacities, with a ground glass or fine orange-peel texture while the lesion mineralises. The degree of radiopacity increases, and late lesions are sclerotic and lack the trabecular pattern of normal bone. A fingerprint pattern of coarse trabeculae may be seen in very old lesions. The cortex and lamina dura are affected by the process, and their definition is lost radiographically. The cortex is expanded but thin and barely discernable during growth (Fig. 13.28). Two key diagnostic features are that the margins merge imperceptibly with the surrounding normal bone and that there is always expansion of the bone (Fig. 13.29).

Pathology

The microscopic appearances vary with stage. In the early radiolucent phase there is loose cellular fibrous tissue that forms slender trabeculae of woven bone. These link together in complex and variable shapes. At the margin there is a gradual imperceptible merging into surrounding normal bone (Figs 13.30 and 13.31). During this phase the bone enlarges and radiographically has a featureless ground glass appearance with no cortex or lamina dura.

After several years, while skeletal growth slows, the bone gradually starts to mature, though abnormally. The woven bone trabeculae are larger and more heavily mineralised but

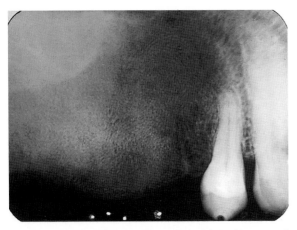

Fig. 13.28 Fibrous dysplasia. This well-established lesion with a rounded swelling merges imperceptibly with normal bone surrounding the canine. There is loss of lamina dura and cortex in the affected area, and the fine trabecular pattern produces an orange-peel or thumb-print appearance.

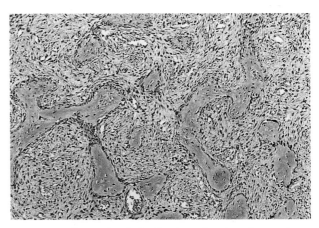

Fig. 13.30 Fibrous dysplasia. Slender trabeculae of woven bone, said to resemble Chinese characters in shape, lying in a very cellular fibrous tissue. With maturation there is progressively more bone formation.

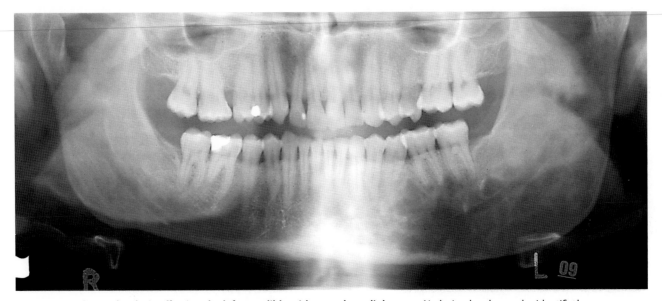

Fig. 13.29 Fibrous dysplasia affecting the left mandible with a patchy radiolucency. No lesion border can be identified.

only develop a minimal peripheral osteoblast layer and a little thin lamellar bone. Radiographically, the bone is visible as the coarse trabecular pattern of the orange peel appearance. In addition, there may be islands of very dense heavily mineralised bone, but these are not cementum as sometimes claimed. Occasional loose foci of giant cells can also be seen, but these are not a major feature as they are in giant cell lesions. Gradually a partial cortex reforms and growth ceases.

The bone remains mostly woven in type for many years but eventually develops partially into lamellar bone and slowly remodels. By middle age, only subtle radiographic features remain.

Biopsy is required to confirm a fibro-osseous lesion, but cannot distinguish fibrous dysplasia from other fibro-osseous lesions with certainty. Identification of the *GNAS1* mutation by DNA sequencing of cells from the lesion is diagnostic. However, the combination of a fibro-osseous lesion on biopsy, radiological features and the clinical presentation are usually conclusive. The vascular soft bone may bleed significantly on biopsy.

Very occasionally lesions can reactivate and grow in later life, but the reasons are unknown.

Jaw lesions PMID: 4513065 and 25409854

Craniofacial involvement PMID: 22771278

Treatment

The disease is self-limiting, but lesions become quiescent rather than resolve. The lesion is not well demarcated and cannot be excised. Disfiguring lesions may be pared down to a normal contour, but this should be delayed until the process has become inactive, usually just after the end of the second decade, slightly earlier in females. Surgery to active or recently active lesions risks reactivation and rapid growth. However, extraction of teeth from affected bone does not increase bone growth, fractures heal normally and implants can be placed.

The late sclerotic bone is prone to osteomyelitis, and the long-term success of implants is unclear, in part because they lack the support of an organised cortical bone layer.

During growth the bone may be painful, and in rapidly enlarging lesions treatment with bisphosphonates reduces pain and may be used to limit growth, but is rarely used for jaw lesions.

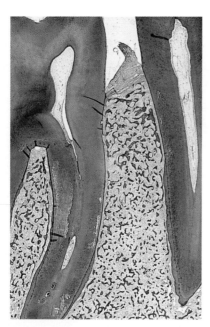

Fig. 13.31   Fibrous dysplasia. There is loss of lamina dura around the teeth and its replacement by lesional bone. These numerous small trabeculae give rise to the ground-glass and orange-peel appearances radiographically.

There is a small risk of sarcomatous change in later life. This complication is more frequent in craniofacial bones but not the jaws and affects less than 1% of patients. Osteosarcoma is the usual type of sarcoma to develop.

Key features are summarised in Box 13.11.

Ref treatment and dental treatment PMCID: PMC3359960

Polyostotic fibrous dysplasia

Polyostotic fibrous dysplasia is rare and, unlike the monostotic form, females are affected three times more frequently than males and onset is at a slightly younger age.

Polyostotic fibrous dysplasia involves the head and neck region in as many as 50% of cases. A jaw lesion may then be the most conspicuous feature and polyostotic disease may not be suspected initially. Thus, all patients with an apparently solitary jaw lesion should be screened for involvement of other bones and for the features of Albright's syndrome.

Long bone involvement causes most problems, with bowing of weight bearing bones, bone pain and pathological fractures.

Histologically and radiographically, the individual lesions are indistinguishable from the monostotic form.

Albright's syndrome

Albright's syndrome (also known as *McCune-Albright syndrome*) comprises polyostotic fibrous dysplasia, skin pigmentation and endocrine abnormalities. Most patients are girls aged less than 10 years at onset.

The bone lesions are more numerous than in nonsyndromic polyostotic fibrous dysplasia, and more than three-quarters of cases have one or both jaws involved and nearly all have skull involvement. Skin pigmentation consists of brownish macules with irregular outlines that frequently overlie affected bones and appear especially on the back of the neck, trunk, buttocks or thighs, and only very occasionally on the oral mucosa. These are caused by

---

melanocytes carrying the GNAS1 mutation, which activates melanin synthesis.

Endocrine dysfunction is usually manifest as precocious puberty, but other thyroid, pituitary and adrenal anomalies may develop. Hypothyroidism, Cushing's syndrome and acromegaly can all be found. Malignant neoplasms in the affected organs are very rare; only the bone lesions have a significant risk. The risk is higher in Albright's syndrome than in the monostotic form, but is still very low.

Histologically and radiographically, the individual bone lesions are indistinguishable from the monostotic form.

Review PMID: 22640971

Osseous dysplasias

Osseous dysplasias (cemento-osseous dysplasias) are growth disturbances of alveolar bone and cementum. They are fibro-osseous in nature but are discussed in Chapter 11 because they are odontogenic.

BONE 'CYSTS'

This group of lesions produces well-defined radiolucencies in the jaws and other bones that appear cyst-like, but they lack an epithelial lining. When these lesions are detected radiologically, they are often thought to be cysts and are not recognised until opened for biopsy. Whether the lack of an epithelial lining makes these lesions pseudocysts as opposed to cysts is a common but futile discussion because it depends on which definition of cyst is accepted.

Solitary bone cyst

→ Summary charts 10.1 and 10.2 pp. 163, 164

Solitary bone cysts are cavities in bones, either filled with fluid or apparently empty.

Solitary bone cysts are almost always single lesions and are found mostly in teenagers and those younger than 25 years. They are most common in long bones, usually the femur or humerus. When the jaws are affected, cavities are found almost exclusively in the mandible and in the alveolus and body rather than the ramus. Males and females are equally affected by jaw lesions.

Most jaw solitary bone cysts are asymptomatic and are often chance radiographic findings. Approximately one-quarter of patients have a painless swelling. The vitality of adjacent teeth is not affected despite their apices extending into the cavity. The apices are sometimes slightly resorbed.

Radiographically, the cavities form rounded, radiolucent areas that tend to be less sharply defined than odontogenic cysts and have two unusual features. First, the area of radiolucency is typically much larger than the size of any swelling suggests. Second, the cavity often arches up between the roots of the teeth and may as a consequence be seen first on a bitewing radiograph (Figs 13.32 and 13.33). Cavities usually appear unilocular but larger examples as large as 10 centimetres across may appear multilocular.

Pathology

Solitary bone cysts are of unknown cause. There is little or no evidence to support the old theory that they result from injury to, and haemorrhage within, the bone followed by defective repair. A common form of treatment is to open solitary bone cysts to allow bleeding into the cavity. Normal healing then follows.

The cavity has a smooth bony wall. There may be a thin connective tissue lining or only a few red cells, blood pigment or giant cells adhering to the bone surface (Fig. 13.34). There are often no cyst contents, but there may sometimes be a little fluid and some fibrin. There is no epithelial lining.

Key features of solitary bone cysts are summarised in Box 13.12.

Review possible causes PMID: 18940504

Jaw lesion radiology PMID: 9503460

> **Box 13.12 Solitary bone cysts: key features**
> - Often chance radiographic findings
> - Rarely expand the jaw
> - Are of unknown aetiology
> - Have no epithelial lining. Appear empty at operation or contain pale fluid
> - Diagnosis suggested by radiographic features (especially extension between tooth roots) and findings at operation
> - Histology confirms the lack of epithelial lining
> - Resolve after surgical opening and closure, or occasionally spontaneously

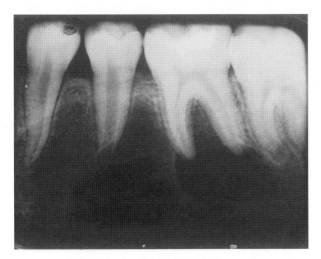

Fig. 13.32   Solitary bone cyst. Typical appearance showing a moderately well-defined but non-corticated radiolucency extending up between the roots of the teeth.

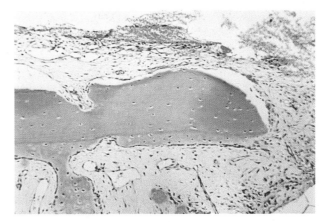

Fig. 13.34   Solitary bone cyst. The scanty cyst lining comprises bone and a thin layer of fibrous tissue. Epithelium is not present, and in some cases even the fibrous lining is lacking.

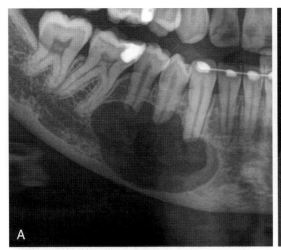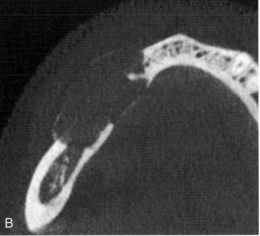

Fig. 13.33   Solitary bone cyst. Panoramic radiograph (**A**) showing a rounded expansile radiolucent lesion with a tendency to dip up between the roots of the teeth. This example shows minor root resorption; most cause none. In axial computed tomography (**B**), the minimal lingual expansion and limited buccal expansion can be seen, outlined by a thin periosteal new bone layer. *(By kind permission of Dr D Baumhoer.)*

Management

When radiological features are typical, there may be no need for intervention, and some lesions resolve spontaneously. Biopsy plays no role in diagnosis because there is minimal tissue to sample, but opening the cyst will reveal the characteristic empty cavity, and the usual treatment is light curettage to remove a sample for histological examination and trigger bleeding and subsequent healing. Recurrence is minimal.

Cysts similar to solitary bone cysts may develop in florid cemento-osseous dysplasia. These cause more expansion than typical solitary bone cysts and do have a low recurrence rate.

Aneurysmal bone 'cyst'

→ Summary chart 10.2 pp. 163, 164

There are two types of aneurysmal bone cyst, primary and secondary. Both replace and expand bone with a vascular soft tissue containing numerous giant cells. Primary aneurysmal bone cysts have recently been discovered to be clonal and are now considered to be benign neoplasms of bone rather than vascular malformations. They are much more common in long bones; jaw lesions account for only 1%–2% of the total. The usual site is posterior body and ramus, sparing the condyle.

Secondary aneurysmal bone cysts lack the genetic translocations of primary examples and develop in association with other pre-existing bone lesions. In the jaws, the most common lesions to be associated with secondary aneurysmal bone cyst formation are fibrous dysplasia and giant cell granuloma. Secondary cysts are usually less expansile than primary and more easily treated without recurrence.

Most patients are between 10 and 20 years of age, and there appears to be no strong predilection for either sex. The main manifestation is usually a rapidly growing painless swelling. The name *aneurysmal* is given to indicate the ballooning expansion that is characteristic, similar to the shape of a dilated vascular aneurysm.

Radiographically, the radiolucent cavity may appear multilocular or be divided by faint septa (Fig. 13.35). Adjacent teeth are displaced, occasionally resorbed but vital. Extensive 'blow out' periosteal expansion with a thin cortex is usual, rather than cortical perforation.

There is a relationship between giant cell granuloma and aneurysmal bone cyst that extends beyond the secondary development of the cyst. USP6 rearrangements have been found in some, but not all, giant cell granulomas, suggesting that they may be a solid type of aneurysmal bone cyst.

Key features of aneurysmal bone cysts are summarised in Box 13.13.

Causes PMID: 15509545

Pathology

Primary aneurysmal bone cysts have a clonal chromosomal translocation. Several are described involving different chromosomes, but all activate the *USP6* gene. How *USP6* upregulation produces the lesion is unclear, possibly by triggering bone resorption and inflammation. Only the fibrous cells in the lesions carry the translocation.

Histologically, there is a highly cellular mass of blood-filled spaces without an endothelial lining. When seen at operation, the appearance has been likened to a blood-filled sponge (Fig. 13.36). The spaces are separated by fibrous septa formed by the causative fibroblasts. However, the histology is dominated by other cell types without the genetic

---

Box 13.13   Aneurysmal bone cyst: key features

- Primary examples are benign neoplasms
- Secondary lesions arise with fibro-osseous and other lesions, and are not neoplasms
- Rare in the jaws
- Jaw lesions are usually in the mandibular ramus and angle
- Affects patients usually between 10 and 20 years
- Form very expansile soap-bubble radiolucencies
- Radiologically resemble ameloblastoma or giant cell granuloma
- Histologically, consist of a mass of blood-filled spaces with scattered giant cells
- Are treated by curettage but sometimes recur

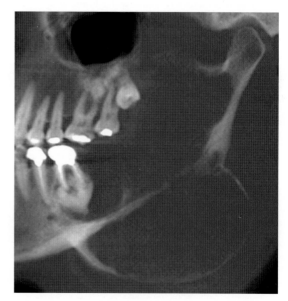

Fig. 13.35   Aneurysmal bone cyst. Part of a panoramic radiograph showing the typically very expansile radiolucency with faint internal septa. The patient also has florid cemento-osseous dysplasia, suggesting that this is a secondary aneurysmal bone cyst.

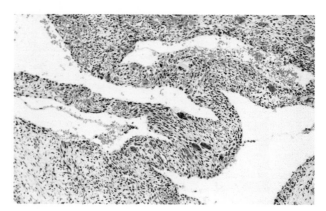

Fig. 13.36   Aneurysmal bone cyst. Cyst wall composed of loose fibrous tissue containing occasional giant cells and large blood-filled spaces.

changes: osteoclast-type giant cells and osteoblasts that form osteoid and woven bone. These other cells cluster in the fibrous tissue and are presumably attracted by cytokines, haemorrhage or inflammation.

Biopsy is necessary for diagnosis. Detecting the genetic changes is not usually necessary for diagnosis but may be helpful in difficult cases or to differentiate aneurysmal bone cyst from giant cell granuloma, or primary from secondary lesions.

Treatment consists of thorough curettage, which may need to be repeated because the lesion recurs in approximately 20% of cases. Very large examples may require extensive resection. For secondary cysts, the associated lesion also needs to be treated.

Case series PMID: 24931106 and 19233862

Osteoporotic bone marrow defect

This is an anatomical variant rather than a lesion and is included here because it may be misdiagnosed radiographically for solitary bone cyst (Fig. 13.37).

The defect is simply a very large marrow space filled with haemopoietic or fatty marrow. The common site is the posterior body of mandible, and there are no symptoms. No treatment is required, but large and radiographically well-defined examples are often submitted to biopsy assuming the changes to be pathological.

Cases and review PMID: 4528570

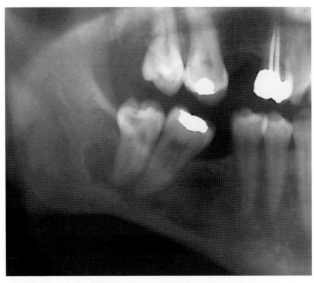

Fig. 13.37 Osteoporotic bone marrow defect affecting a typical site. Large lesions with well-defined borders such as this are often subjected to unnecessary biopsy.

Summary chart 13.1 Mixed patchy radiolucent and radiopaque lesion with poorly defined margin.

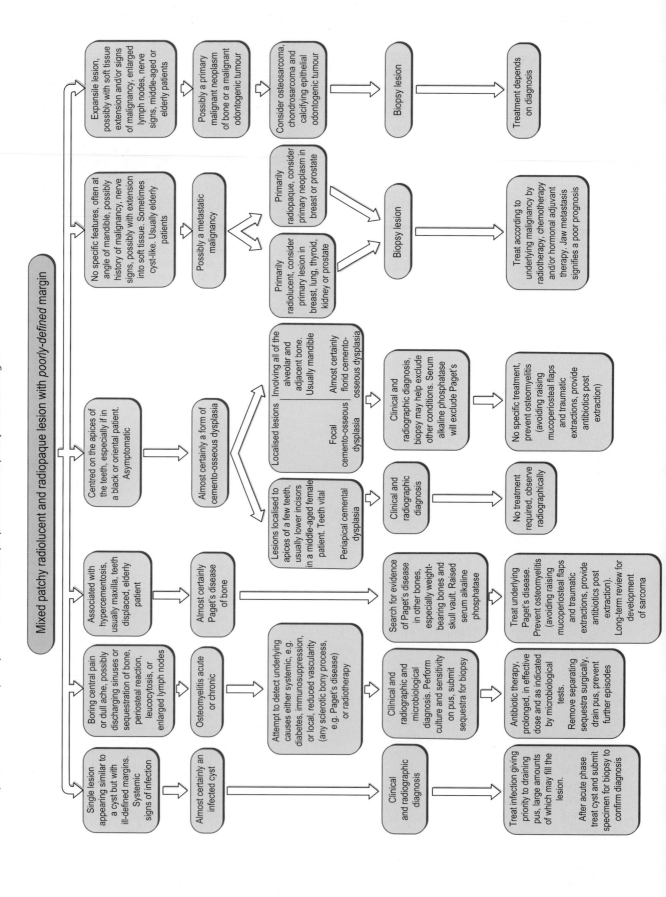

Disorders of the temporomandibular joints and trismus

14

Temporomandibular joint (TMJ) disorders can cause various combinations of limitation of movement of the jaw, pain, locking or clicking sounds. Pain, in particular, is a frequent cause of limitation of movement. These complaints are rarely due to organic disease of the joint, but diagnosis requires organic disease to be excluded. Important causes of limitation of mandibular movement are summarised in Boxes 14.1 and 14.2.

Trismus is correctly defined as inability to open the mouth due to muscle spasm, but the term is usually used for limited movement of the jaw from any cause and usually refers to temporary limitation of movement. The term *ankylosis* means reduced movement due to causes within the joint, usually bony or fibrous union as a result of infection or trauma (see Box 14.2). Inability to open the mouth

fully is usually temporary, and causes are summarised in the following sections.

TEMPORARY LIMITATION OF MOVEMENT (TRISMUS)

Temporomandibular pain dysfunction syndrome

Pain dysfunction syndrome is by far the most common cause of temporary limitation of movement of the temporomandibular joint, as discussed later in this chapter.

Infection and inflammation in or near the joint

Any infection or inflammation involving the muscles of mastication will lead to trismus, either by making opening painful or because oedema or swelling prevent movement. The main causes are surgical extraction of third molars, acute pericoronitis and infections of dental origin in fascial spaces (Ch. 9).

Submasseteric abscess results in profound trismus. Mumps makes eating painful and limits movement because the parotid is compressed by the mandibular ramus on opening. Rare causes include suppurative arthritis, osteomyelitis, cellulitis and suppurative parotitis.

Mandibular block injections may cause inflammation and oedema in medial pterygoid muscle, usually through bleeding. Needle-track infections are now only of historic interest since single-use sterile needles have been used.

Injuries

Unilateral condylar neck fracture usually produces only a mild limitation of opening with deviation of the jaw to the affected side, but closing into intercuspal occlusion may be difficult. Bilateral displaced condylar fractures cause an anterior open bite with limited movement. A major 'guardsman's fracture' with damage to the fossa causes severe restriction of all movements. Less severe injuries frequently result in an effusion into the temporomandibular joint; both wide opening and complete closure are then prevented during the acute phase.

Bleeding into the joint space after a condylar fracture fills the joint with blood clot and organisation can lead to bone formation in the clot, either in one compartment of the joint or both, the latter resulting in bony ankylosis. Early mobilisation of condylar fractures prevents this complication.

Any unstable mandibular fracture causes protective muscle spasm and limitation of movement. Patients suffering from displaced Le Fort II or III fractures often complain of limited opening whereas, in reality, they are half open

---

Box 14.1   Causes of limitation of mandibular movement

Pericapsular and remote causes

- Infection and inflammation in adjacent tissues
- Injury, condylar neck or zygoma fracture
- Irradiation and other causes of fibrosis
- Fibrous ankylosis in the periarticular tissues
- Oral submucous fibrosis
- Systemic sclerosis

Intracapsular causes

- Traumatic arthritis and disk damage
- Infective arthritis
- Rheumatoid and osteoarthritis
- Intracapsular condylar fracture
- Neoplasms of the joint
- Loose bodies in joint
- Intracapsular fibrous ankylosis, caused by any of the above

Muscular

- Temporomandibular joint pain-dysfunction syndrome
- Myalgia caused by bruxism
- Cranial arteritis
- Tetanus and tetany
- Haematoma from ID block

Other

- Drugs
- Dislocation
- Craniofacial anomalies involving the joint

with the jaws wedged apart by the displaced middle third. Reduction of the fracture allows closure.

Drugs

Tardive dyskinesia is an adverse effect of long-term treatment with drugs, causing uncontrollable repetitive involuntary movements. These often affect the face and muscles of mastication and produce trismus. The antiemetic metoclopromide and antipsychotics including butyrophenones and phenothiazines are causes. These effects may reverse on drug withdrawal, if that is possible, but may also persist long after cessation of treatment.

Tardive dyskinesia PMID: 25556809

PERSISTENT LIMITATION OF MOVEMENT: EXTRACAPSULAR CAUSES

Extracapsular causes of persistent limitation of opening are caused by some degree of mechanical interference to mandibular movement (see Box 14.2).

Irradiation

Radiation-induced trismus is a common effect of head and neck radiotherapy and results primarily from damage to the muscles of mastication, particularly the pterygoid muscles. The severity is proportional to the dose, and the cause is inflammation followed by fibrosis. The effect is long term, developing during months and years, and is slowly progressive. Irradiation of the joint itself does not appear to be as significant.

Modern intensity modulated radiotherapy allows accurate localisation of radiotherapy, and this effect is likely to be less common in future. However, it is impossible to deliver

---

curative doses to tumours of the posterior oral cavity, maxilla, pharynx and salivary glands without involving the masticatory muscles, and as many as half of patients suffer this adverse effect.

Jaw exercises and stretching are ineffective once the process is established but are prescribed prophylactically. Stretching is painful, and dedication is required to achieve a good result. Stretching devices (Fig. 14.1) or a trismus screw may aid the process. Otherwise, surgical treatment is difficult and may involve division of muscle attachments from the jaw or section of the angle or body of the mandible to produce a false joint. Bone surgery is complicated by the risk of osteoradionecrosis and infection (see Ch. 8).

Treatment in cancer patients PMID: 26876238

Oral submucous fibrosis

Oral submucous fibrosis, caused by betel nut habit, causes limitation of opening and predisposes to oral carcinoma. Fibrosis of the buccal mucosa, soft palate and the pillars of the fauces render the mucosa firm and hard and prevents opening. Fibrosis extends deeply into muscles of mastication and is progressive. Ultimately, opening the mouth may be completely impossible, and tube feeding may become necessary. There is no effective treatment. This condition is considered in detail in Chapter 19.

Systemic sclerosis (scleroderma)

Systemic sclerosis is an uncommon connective tissue disease characterised by widespread subcutaneous and submucous fibrosis. Although the most obvious feature is the progressive stiffening of the skin, the gastrointestinal tract, lungs, heart and kidneys can also be affected.

Clinically, women between the ages of 30 and 50 years are predominantly affected. Raynaud's phenomenon is the most common early manifestation, often associated with arthralgia.

The skin becomes thinned, stiff, smooth, tethered, pigmented and marked by telangiectases. A hallmark of the disease is involvement of the hands causing such changes as atrophy of, or ischaemic damage to, the tips of the fingers. Contractures prevent straightening of the fingers (Fig. 1.3).

The head and neck region is involved in more than three-quarters of patients and, in a minority, symptoms start there. Narrowing of the eyes and taut, mask-like limitation

---

> **Box 14.2   Extracapsular causes of limitation of temporomandibular joint movement ('false ankylosis')**
>
> **Mechanical interference with jaw movement**
> - Trauma: depressed fracture of the zygomatic bone or arch
> - Hyperplasia: developmental overgrowth of the coronoid process
> - Neoplasms: osteochondroma, osteoma of the coronoid process
> - Irradiation fibrosis
> - Miscellaneous:
>   - myositis ossificans in masticatory muscles
>   - taut skin in systemic sclerosis
>   - taut mucosa in oral submucous fibrosis
>   - congenital anomalies of the jaw or face
>
> **Capsular causes**
> - Trauma: periarticular fibrosis from wounds or burns
>   - Posterior or superior dislocation
>   - Longstanding anterior dislocation
> - Infection: fibrosis from chronic periarticular suppuration
> - Joint capsule fibrosis
>   - Irradiation
>   - Post-surgical scarring

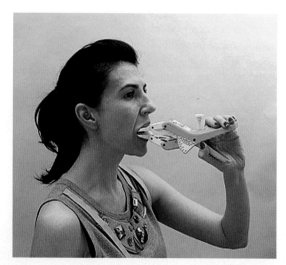

Fig. 14.1 A muscle and fibrosis stretching device for trismus.

of movement can give rise to a characteristic appearance (Mona Lisa face). The lips may be constricted (fish mouth) or become pursed with radiating furrows. Occasionally, involvement of the periarticular tissues of the temporomandibular joint together with the microstomia may greatly limit opening of the mouth (Fig. 14.2). Involvement of the oral submucosa may cause the tongue to become stiff and narrowed (chicken tongue). Oesophageal stiffness causes dysphagia and allows gastric reflux.

Systemic sclerosis has autoimmune and environmental causes, and probably a genetic predisposition. Autoantibodies are found against centromeres, topoisomerase (anti Scl70) and RNA polymerase, but the cause of the fibrosis appears to be T lymphocytes secreting transforming growth factor beta, to which the patient's fibroblasts are particularly sensitive. The initial trigger remains unknown.

Widening of the periodontal ligament space is another abnormality characteristic of systemic sclerosis but is seen in fewer than 10% of cases. The mandibular angle and ramus shows an unusual pattern of resorption in 15% of patients, and more rarely, there is gross extensive resorption of the jaw with a risk of pathological fracture. Tooth root resorption is also reported but appears rare. Sjögren's syndrome also develops in a significant minority.

Histologically, there is great thickening of the subepithelial connective tissue, degeneration of muscle fibres and atrophy of minor glands. The collagen fibres are swollen and eosinophilic. There are scattered infiltrates of chronic inflammatory cells around vessels, and arterioles typically show thickening of their walls.

Features of systemic sclerosis relevant to dentistry are shown in Box 14.3.

General review PMID: 23806160

Oral features PMID: 6584594

Jaw radiology PMID: 9084272

Complications and prognosis

Skin disease alone, although debilitating, is rarely fatal. The main disabilities are dysphagia and pulmonary, cardiac or renal involvement. Pulmonary involvement leads to impaired respiratory exchange and, eventually, dyspnoea and pulmonary hypertension. Cardiac disease can result from the latter or myocardial fibrosis. Renal disease secondary to vascular disease is typically a late effect; it leads to hypertension and is an important cause of death. The overall 10-year survival rate is 70%, but much reduced with visceral involvement.

No specific treatment is available. Immunosuppressive drugs are ineffective. Penicillamine may be given to depress fibrous proliferation but can cause loss of taste, oral ulceration, lichenoid reactions and other complications.

CREST syndrome

CREST syndrome is the combination of Calcinosis, Raynaud's phenomenon Esophageal dysfunction, Sclerodactyly and Telangiectasia and can be thought of as a limited cutaneous form of scleroderma with a better prognosis. It affects elderly females. Calcinosis is seen as calcified skin nodules a few millimetres in diameter; telangiectasia can result in prolonged bleeding. The remaining features are as seen in systemic sclerosis.

Oral features PMID: 8217427

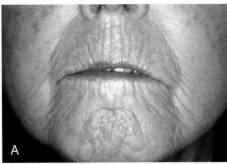
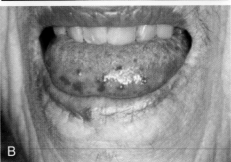

Fig. 14.2 Systemic sclerosis. Fibrosis of perioral skin with furrowing (A) and telangiectases of lips and tongue (B). *(From Varga, J., 2015. Systemic sclerosis (scleroderma). In: Goldman, L., Schafer, A.I. Goldman-Cecil medicine, twenty-fifth ed. Elsevier Saunders, New York, pp. 1777–1785.e2.)*

Box 14.3 Dental relevance of systemic sclerosis

- Limitation of opening
- Limited oral access from microstomia
- Prominent gingival recession in a minority
- Coup de sabre linear scars of face and tongue
- Firm whitish-yellow fibrotic mucosal plaques, very rarely
- Widening of periodontal ligament radiographically in 7% cases
- Dental erosion from gastric reflux
- Mandibular resorption at angle and ramus
- Dry mouth
- Risk of Sjögren's syndrome (Ch. 22)
- Dentally relevant effects of drug treatment may include
  - Nifedipine given for Raynaud's phenomenon
  - Immunosuppression from ciclosporin, methotrexate or steroids
  - Lichenoid reactions to angiotensin-converting enzyme inhibitors for hypertension or penicillamine
  - And others depending on specific presentation

Morphoea

Morphoea, or localised scleroderma, is considered a very localised form of limited skin involvement producing scar-like fibrosis, as oval patches or sometimes linear deep scars with a characteristic *scleroderma en coup de sabre* ('sabre cut') morphology (see Fig. 14.3). This latter type often affects the forehead or scalp, with hair loss, deep contraction and resorption of underlying bone (Fig. 14.4), and it occasionally affects the tongue. Childhood morphoea is a possible cause of facial hemiatrophy.

Morphoea review PMID: 24048434

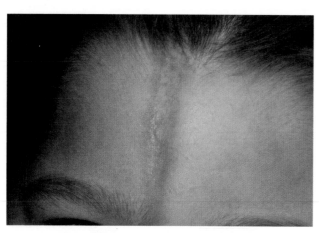

Fig. 14.3   Scleroderma en coup de sabre. Linear atrophy and fibrosis across the forehead. *(From Paller, A.S., Mancini, A.J., 2016. Collagen vascular disorders. In: Paller, A.S., Mancini, A.J. 2016. Hurwitz clinical pediatric dermatology, fifth ed. Elsevier, Philadelphia, pp. 509–539.e8.)*

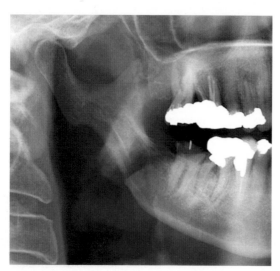

Fig. 14.4   Scleroderma. Resorption of the posterolateral ramus is characteristic but seen only in severe cases. *(By kind permission of Dr M Payne.)*

PERSISTENT LIMITATION OF MOVEMENT: INTRACAPSULAR CAUSES

Almost all intracapsular causes of limited opening are caused by ankylosis, due to fibrous or bony union of the condyle and temporal bone. Causes of ankylosis are shown in Box 14.4. A few, such as neoplasms of the joint itself or synovial chondromatosis, produce mechanical interference without ankylosis.

Treatment of ankylosis

Ankylosis is treated in a similar fashion regardless of which of the following causes is responsible, and relatively aggressive surgical intervention is necessary. All the fibrous or bony tissue causing ankylosis is removed, and interposition of a temporalis muscle flap or other implant material prevents healing across the defect. In the growing patient, joint reconstruction using a free costochondral bone graft gives better results because, in many cases, the graft will grow with the patient, preventing subsequent facial deformity. Early mobilisation with aggressive physiotherapy is required to prevent the ankylosis reforming.

> **Box 14.4   Important causes of ankylosis ('true' or intracapsular ankylosis)**
>
> **Trauma**
> - Intracapsular fracture of the condyle
> - Penetrating wounds
> - Forceps delivery at birth
>
> **Infection**
> - Otitis media/mastoiditis
> - Osteomyelitis of the jaws
> - Haematogenous – pyogenic arthritis
>
> **Arthritides**
> - Systemic juvenile arthritis
> - Psoriatic arthropathy
> - Osteoarthritis (rarely)
> - Rheumatoid arthritis (rarely)
>
> **Neoplasms of the joint**
> - Chondroma
> - Osteochondroma
> - Osteoma
>
> **Miscellaneous**
> - Synovial chondromatosis

Arthritis

The main causes are:

Traumatic arthritis. Follows dislocation or fracture. Surprisingly, undisplaced fractures of the neck of the condyle can remain unnoticed for many weeks until pain of arthritis develops.

Infection and inflammation. Acute pyogenic arthritis is exceedingly rare but exceedingly painful.

Rheumatoid and other arthritides. These are discussed below.

Rheumatoid arthritis

Rheumatoid arthritis is an autoimmune disease of unknown cause, but with a strong genetic background, that affects approximately 2% of the population. The disease target is the synovial membrane, which is infiltrated by inflammatory cells, enlarges and grows across the joint surface causing resorption and joint destruction.

Deposition of immune complexes of immunoglobulin M complement-activating autoantibody against immunoglobulin receptor (rheumatoid factor) may be an initiating factor, but the disease is self-perpetuating as a result of systemic immune activation.

The main features are chronic inflammation of many joints, pain and progressive limitation of movement of small joints. Rheumatoid arthritis is the only important inflammatory disease of the temporomandibular joints, but is rarely symptomatic in this joint.

General review PMID: 22150039

Clinical features

Women are affected, particularly in the third and fourth decades. The smaller joints are mainly affected (particularly those of the hands), and the distribution tends to be symmetrical. Extra-articular manifestations include vasculitis and involvement of almost any organ system. Loss of

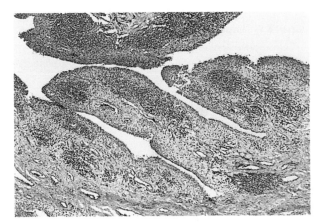

Fig. 14.5 **Rheumatoid arthritis.** Inflamed villi of pannus growing across the surface of a temporomandibular joint severely affected by rheumatoid arthritis. The condylar surface is destroyed.

weight, malaise and depression are common as secondary effects

The temporomandibular joints are never involved alone, and temporomandibular joint involvement is usually a late sign. Although three-quarters of patients have clinical or radiological abnormalities of the temporomandibular joints, pain and swelling are not features. When there are symptoms of temporomandibular joint involvement, they are crepitus and limitation of movement with pain on clenching or chewing, rather than opening and closing. The shape of the condyle is flattened at first. In severely involved joints, the shape of both condyle and glenoid fossa can be lost, predisposing to dislocation.

Radiography shows flattening of the condyles with loss of contour and irregularity of the articular surface as typical findings. The joint space may be widened by exudate in the acute phases but later narrowed. The underlying bone is often osteoporotic, and the margins of the condyles become irregular.

Biopsy is not used for diagnosis because joint involvement is always seen in established cases. If examined histologically, there is proliferation of the synovial lining cells and infiltration of the synovium by dense collections of lymphocytes and plasma cells (Fig. 14.5). The synovial fluid contains neutrophils and fibrinous exudate from the hyperaemic vessels in the synovial membrane. A vascular, inflamed mass of granulation tissue (pannus) spreads over the surfaces of the articular cartilages from their margins and is followed by death of chondrocytes and loss of intercellular matrix. Fibrous adhesions form between the joint surfaces and the meniscus. The meniscus may eventually be destroyed, and inflammatory changes in the ligaments and tendons can then lead to fibrous or bony ankylosis, though this very rare. Collapse of the joint is a more likely outcome in severe disease, with development of an anterior open bite as a consequence.

TMJ radiology PMID: 8734713 and 11426029

Management

Diagnosis is based on the clinical, radiographic and autoantibody findings. Patients may be taking a range of medications including non-steroidal anti-inflammatory drugs, penicillamine, antimalarial drugs and colloidal gold injections, methotrexate, azathioprine, ciclosporin and infliximab or golimumab (anti-tumor necrosis factor α monoclonal antibodies). Many of these drugs have oral adverse effects

(Box 14.6). Low-dose methotrexate is a popular maintenance treatment for severe disease in remission.

If joint symptoms are severe, a corticosteroid injection into the joint space may reduce pain and swelling, but cannot be repeated frequently without inducing bone resorption. There is no effect of steroids on disease progression and no evidence that they can allow normal condylar growth in juvenile rheumatoid arthritis.

Joint surgery is rarely performed, but if required, a functional joint may be restored with various implant materials or a custom-made artificial joint. Replacement joints tend to be reserved for patients with mandibular growth disturbance as a result of juvenile rheumatoid arthritis, as part of an orthognathic treatment plan to advance the hypoplastic mandible.

Dental aspects

Generally speaking, although rheumatoid arthritis is a common disease, specific treatment of TMJ symptoms is unlikely to be necessary. The mainstay of treatment is the use of non-steroidal anti-inflammatory drugs, but any gross abnormalities of occlusion, such as overclosure, should be corrected to reduce abnormal movement at the temporomandibular joints. Sjögren's syndrome is associated in approximately 15%. Important features of rheumatoid arthritis are summarised in Box 14.6.

Dental care PMID: 18820621 and 27857093

Osteoarthritis

Osteoarthritis is a disorder of cartilaginous repair. Joints are more susceptible than normal to daily wear, so that large weight-bearing joints are the most frequently affected. Alterations in cartilage matrix appear to be the cause and are linked to several gene defects. Erosion of cartilage causes resorption of the underlying bone, which distorts, collapses and becomes sclerotic in response. New bone grows at the edge of the joint (osteophytes), limiting movement, and the capsule and ligaments are thickened. Inflammation is mild.

In diseases in which joint movement is abnormal or a joint is malformed, osteoarthritis may develop as a secondary complication, for instance in congenital hip disease or Ehlers-Danlos syndrome. Trauma and diabetes also predispose.

Osteoarthritis is very common. Severe disease affects 2% of the population, but by the age of 70 years, three-quarters of individuals have some radiographic features. Presentation is usually in middle age or the elderly because it takes many years of cumulative damage for the effects to become significant. Stress, particularly on weight-bearing joints, is the

Box 14.6 Rheumatoid arthritis: dental implications

- Difficulty with oral hygiene, reduced manual dexterity and limited range of movement
- Oral access reduced by limited opening
- Difficulty lying in dental chair
- Anaemia
- Sjögren's syndrome in about 15%
- Mild bleeding risk from thrombocytopenia
- Cervical lymph nodes may be enlarged during active disease
- Risk of atlantoaxial subluxation if cervical spine involved
- Adverse effects of drug treatment
  - Lichenoid reactions from gold, antimalarials and penicillamine
  - Immunosuppression from ciclosporin, methotrexate and infliximab
  - Candidosis from immunosuppression and anaemia
  - Oral ulceration from methotrexate
  - Anaemia from non-steroidal anti-inflammatory drugs
  - Interactions with drugs prescribed for dentistry

Box 14.7 Important features of osteoarthritis

- Onset mainly older than 60 years
- Slow development of pain and wear of weight-bearing joints
- Usually one or a few joints involved
- Heberden's nodes
- Palpable coarse crepitus of affected joints
- Bony swelling and deformity
- Secondary muscle weakness and wasting
- Little or no inflammation and no systemic effects

Box 14.8 Dental implications of osteoarthritis

- Pain on movement restricts access to care
- Difficulty with oral hygiene, reduced manual dexterity and limited range of movement
- Difficulty lying in dental chair
- Joint replacements do NOT require antibiotic prophylaxis unless there are specific patient indications. Prophylaxis may be *considered* in diabetics, the immunosuppressed or those with previous joint infection
- Adverse effects of drug treatment
  - Anaemia from non-steroidal anti-inflammatory drugs
  - Bleeding tendency in those on aspirin

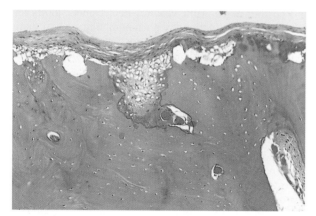

Fig. 14.6 Osteoarthritis. The fibrocartilage layer is split, and the underlying bone shows resorption and repair centrally.

injections have been tried, but in general the more conservative the approach, the better.

Important features of osteoarthritis are summarised in Box 14.7.

Natural history joint damage PMID: 7621016

Dental aspects

Although the temporomandibular joint rarely causes problems, the disease has significant dental implications as shown in Box 14.8.

Dental care PMID: 18511715

Other types of arthritis

Many other types of arthritis can affect the temporomandibular joints but rarely do so. They include psoriatic arthritis, the juvenile arthritides, gout, ankylosing spondylitis, Lyme disease and reactive arthropathy. Psoriatic arthropathy can cause ankylosis of the temporomandibular joint. Juvenile arthritis can be severe and disabling, and destruction of the condylar head leads to severely limited opening and secondary micrognathia.

Condylar hyperplasia

Condylar hyperplasia is a rare, usually unilateral, overgrowth of the mandibular condyle. It causes facial asymmetry, deviation of the jaw to the unaffected side on opening and a crossbite. The condition usually manifests itself after puberty and is slowly progressive. Pain in the affected joint is variable. If the condition is still active at the time of diagnosis, an intracapsular condylectomy should be performed to remove the active growth centre in the condylar surface. If the disease has stabilised – usually at the end of puberty or shortly afterward – corrective osteotomies may

main cause of pain, but frequently joints with radiographic signs of osteoarthritis are painless (Fig. 14.6). A characteristic feature is the presence of Heberden's nodes (bony swellings) of the terminal interphalangeal joints. Affected joints are swollen and warm when the disease is active and produce crepitus on movement.

Osteoarthritis of the temporomandibular joint is occasionally seen by chance in radiographs, but is not a cause of significant symptoms. The unusual structure of the joint, with a fibrocartilage disk rather than hyaline cartilage, and the lack of weight bearing seem to protect it. The disk suffers the worst damage. Any significant limitation of movement is likely to be from osteophytes around the joint or fragments of osteophytes that have fractured and become loose bodies in the joint.

In the rare event that a patient has severe pain and joint deformity associated with osteoarthritis of the temporomandibular joint, any factor contributing to stress on the joint should be relieved. Treatment is symptomatic, and topical agents and anti-inflammatory analgesics are the main line of treatment. Corticosteroid or hyaluronate

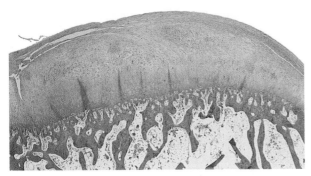

Fig. 14.7   Condylar hyperplasia. The condyle retains an immature structure with a thick cartilage layer, calcification and new bone formation, reflecting the continued growth.

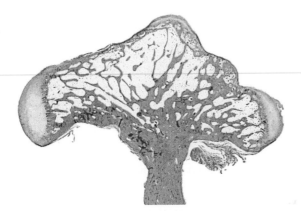

Fig. 14.8   Osteochondroma of the condyle. Two cartilage-capped exostoses arising near the condyle have grown progressively sideways to form a distorted condylar head several centimetres across.

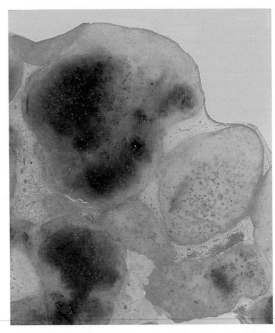

Fig. 14.9   Synovial chondromatosis of the temporomandibular joint. Multiple rounded nodules of benign cartilage growing in the joint capsule.

be needed to restore the occlusion and facial symmetry (Fig. 14.7). This may be complex. The mandible grows down and forward, tilting the occlusal plane and allowing the maxillary alveolus and teeth to grow down into the space.

Coronoid hyperplasia can also occur, but is rarer and usually bilateral.

Review and treatment PMID: 25483450

Tissue changes PMID: 3461098

Neoplasms

Osteochondroma (Fig. 14.8) is probably the most common tumour of the condyle or coronoid process, but even that is very rare. Osteoma and chondroma and their malignant counterparts may develop and are treated in the same way as elsewhere in the skeleton (see Ch. 12).

Synovial chondromatosis and loose bodies in the temporomandibular joints

Loose bodies (or 'joint mice') are fragments of bone or cartilage floating free in the joint space. Compared with other joints, they are rare in the temporomandibular joints where the main causes are synovial chondromatosis and osteochondritis dissecans.

In **synovial chondromatosis** multiple nodules of cartilage develop in the synovial membrane, each as large as approximately 1 mm in diameter. The nodules become separated and fall into the joint space to cause locking, deviation to

the affected side on opening, and crepitus, followed eventually by pain and swelling when the joint is damaged. Synovial chondromatosis is rare and probably a benign neoplasm, but it can erode into the cranial cavity from the joint by pressure effect.

The nodules are seen best on magnetic resonance image scanning because they may not be mineralised. More than 100 may be present in the joint capsule.

Histologically, the nodules of cartilage are benign (Fig. 14.9) and may calcify but can resemble chondrosarcoma. Diagnosis is by imaging, and the diagnosis is confirmed after surgical removal of the loose bodies and the whole of the affected synovium. Endoscopic removal is possible, but incomplete excision can be followed by recurrence.

Osteochondritis dissecans is even rarer and results from trauma or loss of blood supply to the bone below the articular surface, always in the condyle. The bone becomes necrotic, and pieces of the overlying fibrocartilage layer separate to form loose bodies. Diagnosis is by imaging, and the patient has discomfort and episodes of locking. Conservative management may be successful in the young, but surgical removal of the loose body may be required.

Synovial chondromatosis series PMID: 16003619

Osteochondritis dissecans PMID: 16997094

LIMITATION OF MOVEMENT: MUSCLE CAUSES

Temporomandibular pain dysfunction 'syndrome'

This is one of the most controversial areas in dentistry and cause and optimum treatment are unclear. Many interventions appear effective, and the condition is very common, probably the most common cause of trismus and limited jaw movement.

The differing views of this condition are reflected in its many names. In the UK the terms *temporomandibular pain dysfunction syndrome*, *facial arthromyalgia* or *myofascial pain* are used. In the United States, the more generic *temporomandibular disorders* indicates that this is a group of related presentations, but this term includes organic joint disease. None of the names is satisfactory; they emphasise the joint when it is not the primary cause of the condition.

Presentation

Pain dysfunction syndrome comprises a collection of symptoms of pain and tenderness in the muscles of mastication and in or around the joint, limitation of movement and clicking or other sounds from the joint. Onset is occasionally ascribed to violent yawning, laughing or trauma but is usually insidious.

It is estimated that 25% of the population may suffer the symptoms at some time in their life and half may show signs, although this is perhaps a reflection of the poor specificity of the diagnostic criteria. Although the symptoms are common, treatment is much more likely to be sought by young or youngish women. The condition is often considered of low significance and difficult to treat, but it can cause significant discomfort, stress and depression and have a major impact on quality of life. The symptoms and signs wax and wane, sometimes with almost acute severity. They are:

Muscle and joint tenderness felt during jaw movement or mastication, and on palpation. The joint pain may be referred from the muscles or associated with their tendons rather than originating in the joint. The pain is not severe, more an ache or tenderness and often poorly localised by the patient. Muscle symptoms are usually worse on one side or completely unilateral. Pain is classically preauricular.

Limitation of mandibular movement characterised by reduced opening and lateral excursion, associated with pain, making mastication difficult. The mandible deviates to the side of the pain, reflecting muscle spasm. Trismus may be complete in severe phases.

Joint noises are usually clicks or crepitus on movement. The noises can be impressive and surprise the patient, but are not painful. They indicate poor coordination of movement of the disk and mandible. Clicks are very common and do not alone indicate pain dysfunction syndrome.

A series of secondary symptoms have an unclear relationship to the central disorder:

Bruxism is most closely associated and is an understandable cause of muscle spasm (see Ch. 6). Patients who brux at night wake with worse limitation of movement and pain that slowly reduces during the day. Other parafunctional activity or jaw posturing is also sometimes associated.

Headache may be misinterpreted temporalis pain, referred pain or relate to stress, possibly causing or possibly a result of the disorder. Migraine is also associated in an ill-defined way.

Locking of the joint. This does not necessarily indicate organic disease in the joint, but rather uncoordinated movements of the condyle, disk and muscles. Most locking is in an open position. Closed lock is rarer and more likely to indicate a joint derangement.

Ear pain is probably referred pain from the joint and does not indicate damage to the ear itself. Tinnitus can also be associated.

Features are summarised in Box 14.9.

Box 14.9   Typical features of pain dysfunction syndrome

- Female to male preponderance of nearly 4 to 1
- Most patients are between 16 and 40 years
- Onset is usually gradual
- Pain usually one-sided, rarely severe
- Typically, a dull ache is made worse by mastication
- Pain typically felt in front of the ear
- Frequently also limitation of opening
- Clicking or crepitus in the joint
- Ultimately self-limiting
- Causes no long-term damage to joint

Aetiology

The aetiology is unknown and probably multifactorial. Psychosocial factors seem to play a significant role. Some authorities consider the problem to be within the spectrum of chronic facial pain, sharing psychological aetiological factors with burning mouth and atypical facial pain, but this only partly explains the condition and probably not in all patients. Stress and anxiety are well-recognised causes of clenching and bruxing, with constant contraction of facial and masticatory muscles. More than half of patients recognise a stressful life event preceding their symptoms, and many have other stress-associated disorders such as stress headache, irritable bowel or chronic fatigue.

The joint is almost always normal, and it is unclear whether any derangements of the meniscus are primary or secondary changes in the small proportion of patients who have them. If the joint is abnormal, it should be treated as joint disease and not temporomandibular pain dysfunction.

Previous suggestions that the occlusion is a primary cause have not been validated in studies. However, there is clearly some poorly understood relationship between the patterns of movement of the jaw, muscle tenderness and the effect the occlusion exerts on them, as demonstrated by the diagnostic value of splints. Abnormal neuromuscular coordination, causing areas of spasm of the masticatory muscles, appears to be a likely main cause.

Investigation

In view of the absence of objective signs, diagnosis is largely by exclusion. The pain character and distribution are typical and the main function of the history and examination are to exclude organic disease. As in all cases of pain in the region of the jaws, referred pain from the teeth should be carefully excluded.

The muscles should be palpated to identify tender areas that can be confirmed by the patient as the correct source when the pain is poorly localised. Check the movements of the mandible to identify postural positions, limitation of movement and asymmetry.

The temporomandibular joint should be palpated for tenderness or swelling which, if present, suggest organic disease. Crepitus may be felt but is not specific and is not necessarily a sign of significant joint disease.

Radiographs of the joints may be taken to make sure that movements are not excessive in either direction and are equal on both sides. However, the main value of radiographs is to exclude such changes as fluid accumulation (widening of the joint space) or damage or deformity of the joint surfaces, indicating organic disease.

Palpation of the temporal artery will aid exclusion of giant cell arteritis.

Management

Temporomandibular pain dysfunction is ultimately self-limiting and does not progress to permanent damage or degenerative arthritis later in life. No irreversible treatment should be undertaken. Surgery, orthodontics and occlusal adjustment in particular are to be avoided.

There is a strong placebo effect in any form of treatment and reversible treatments, usually in combination, will usually reduce trismus and pain. Possible interventions include exercises and stretching, massage, physiotherapy, soft diet, application of heat to muscles, ultrasound therapy, cognitive behavioural therapy, hypnosis, relaxation and many more. Dividing patients into those who have primarily muscle or joint symptoms for different types of treatment seems logical but is not always easy to do.

The provision of various types of splint has long been a popular dental intervention. There are many types, but specific indications for particular types remain largely without an evidence base. Splints perform two roles, diagnostic and therapeutic. They are perhaps most useful for diagnosis, interfering with the neuromuscular control of jaw movement and breaking learned habits so that a short period of wear may quickly change the pain and joint symptoms to confirm the diagnosis (whether improving or occasionally worsening them). Soft vacuum-formed splints are easily provided for night wear to reduce bruxism, but only last a short time between the teeth of a dedicated bruxist. Hard splints are more complex to make and may either permit movement in all directions – removing the occlusal guidance of jaw movement – or attempt to guide the jaw to some artificial 'correct' posture. Partial coverage splints and flat anterior bite planes risk allowing overeruption of the uncovered teeth in only a few weeks, and full coverage splints are generally preferred.

A broad range of analgesics including non-steroidal anti-inflammatory drugs are used but have no proven benefit. Medication targeting stress, anxiety or depression, such as benzodiazepines or tricyclic antidepressants, also provide minimal or no benefit.

Unless joint disease is identified by imaging, arthroscopy should be avoided.

In practice, a combination of education and reassurance, a soft diet and a soft splint worn at night for 3 months, with some simple jaw exercises, is sufficient intervention to allow the patient to manage the condition until it wanes in severity. More severe cases may merit a trial of non-steroidal anti-inflammatory drugs or a brief course of a benzodiazepine when symptoms are severe. Most cases are amenable to management in primary care, but those with clear psychological factors, widespread pain or locking of the joint are best treated in a specialised centre.

Explaining that the condition may recur and relapse during many years is important for patient acceptance of mild symptoms in the long term.

The main principles of management of pain dysfunction syndrome are summarised in Box 14.10.

Review UK perspective PMID: 27024901

Symptoms PMID: 8995904 and 9973710

Association with pain sensitivity PMID: 26928952

Management advice PMID: 24386767

Meta-analysis splint therapy PMID: 22855899

> **Box 14.10 Principles of management of pain dysfunction syndrome**
> - Exclude joint disease
> - Exclude giant cell arteritis (in the elderly)
> - Exclude pain and infection of dental origin
> - Reassurance and education
> - Conservative management – reversible treatments only
> - Soft diet and jaw exercises
> - Consider need for a splint
> - Analgesics or anxiolytics in selected cases

Controversy over US guideline PMID: 20943030

Occlusal adjustment ineffective PMID: 9656902

Psychosocial model PMID: 9610309

Web URL 14.1 UK clinical guideline: https://www.rcseng.ac.uk/dental-faculties/fds and follow menus to publications and guidelines > clinical guidelines

Web URL 14.2 NICE guidance: http://cks.nice.org.uk/ and enter TMJ in search box

Web URL 14.3 US Guidance for the young: http://www.aapd.org/media/policies_guidelines/g_tmd.pdf

Web URL 14.4 Evidence-based diagnosis: http://www.rdc-tmdinternational.org/ and follow menus to TMD assessment/ Diagnosis

Acute temporomandibular pain dysfunction

In patients with an acute onset there is often a clear cause such as trauma or a prolonged period of forced mouth opening, usually for dental surgery. In such cases analgesics, soft diet and reassurance with instructions to avoid yawning or forced opening for 2 months are usually sufficient.

Giant cell arteritis (temporal arteritis)

Giant cell arteritis is an autoimmune inflammatory disease of large arteries, particularly the cranial arteries causing swelling and narrowing of the lumen.

Clinically, women older than 55 years are predominantly affected. The disease may start with malaise, weakness, low-grade fever and loss of weight. Severe throbbing headache is the most common symptom. The temporal artery is the artery most frequently affected and becomes red, tender, firm, swollen, and tortuous on palpation.

In 20% of patients, there is ischaemic pain in the masticatory muscles, that worsens on mastication, sometimes called 'jaw claudication'.[*] This characteristic combination of headache and pain on mastication can be misdiagnosed as temporomandibular joint dysfunction. Ophthalmic artery involvement is found in as many as half of patients and can cause disturbance of vision or sudden blindness. Soft tissue infarcts may result, sometimes in the tongue.

Histologically, the arterial media and intima are oedematous and inflamed and contain macrophages and multinucleate giant cells. Intimal damage leads to formation of thrombi, and the internal elastic lamina becomes disrupted

---

[*]The term is based on the intermittent claudication in the calves on arterial insufficiency, but is something of a misnomer because claudication means limping.

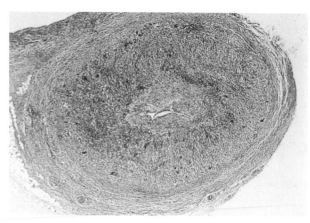

Fig. 14.10 Giant cell (temporal) arteritis. The structure of the artery is disrupted by inflammatory cells, and the lumen is much reduced in size.

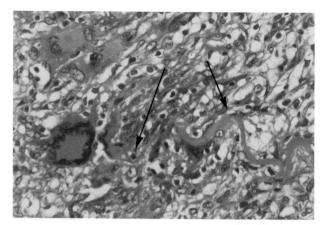

Fig. 14.12 Giant cell (temporal) arteritis. At high power, multinucleate giant cells, lymphocytes and neutrophils may be seen among the remnants of the artery's internal elastic lamina (*arrowed*).

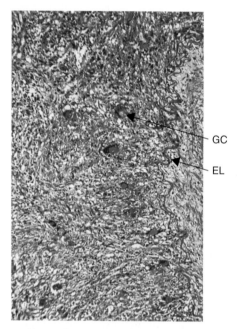

Fig. 14.11 Giant cell (temporal) arteritis. At higher power the internal elastic lamina of the artery may be seen together with giant cells, lymphocytes and neutrophils in the media. *GC*, giant cell; *EL*, elastic lamina.

and eventually destroyed for short lengths of the artery (Figs 14.10–14.12). Healing is by fibrosis and partial recanalisation of the thrombus.

General review PMID: 24461386

Intraoral involvement PMID: 9483933 and 21176820

Management

Biopsy is not required for diagnosis in a typical presentation, and treatment should not be delayed because blindness, which develops in as many as 50% of untreated patients, makes it essential to start treatment early. If a biopsy is required, it must be at least 1 cm and ideally 3 cm long to ensure that it includes the short lengths of affected wall necessary for diagnosis.

Systemic corticosteroids should be given on the basis of inflamed scalp vessels and a high (>70 mm/hour) erythrocyte sedimentation rate (ESR). Corticosteroids are usually quickly effective and should be continued until the ESR falls to normal.

Polymyalgia rheumatica

Half of patients with temporal arteritis have this more extensive condition with weakness, stiffness and pain of the shoulder or pelvic girdles associated with malaise and low fever. The ESR is usually greatly raised.

General review PMID: 23579169

Tetanus and tetany

These are rare causes of masticatory muscle spasm. Lockjaw (trismus) is a classical early sign of tetanus which, although rare, must be excluded because of its high mortality. The trismus is associated with extreme muscle contraction and typically causes spasms of a few minutes at a time. This possibility should be considered whenever a patient develops acute severe limitation of movement of the jaw without local cause, but has had a penetrating wound, particularly a contaminated one, in the previous 4 weeks. Immunisation has almost eradicated the disease in developed countries.

Tetany is most likely to be seen as a result of anxiety and hyperventilation. Tetany is usually associated with typical carpal spasm, and tapping on the facial nerve may trigger spasm of facial muscles (Chvostek's sign).

Tetanus with trismus, case PMID: 26869628

PAIN REFERRED TO THE JOINT

Salivary gland disease, otitis externa, otitis media and mastoiditis are potent causes of pain referred to the temporomandibular joint. Temporomandibular joint dysfunction illustrates referred pain from muscles of mastication, and any disease in these muscles may produce joint pain; indeed joint and ear pain may be referred from almost anywhere in the sensory distribution of the trigeminal nerve. Excluding dental causes for any ear or joint pain is therefore an essential step in diagnosis.

DISLOCATION

The temporomandibular joint may become fixed in the open position by anterior dislocation, when the condyle

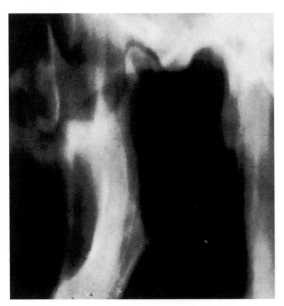

Fig. 14.13 Dislocation of the jaw. Radiography of the temporomandibular joint of the patient seen in Figs 14.14 and 14.15 showed complete dislocation of the condyle in front of the eminentia articularis. *(Figures by courtesy of the late Professor I Curson.)*

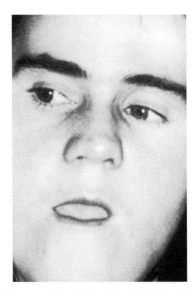

Fig. 14.14 Longstanding dislocation of the jaw. The teeth had been extracted about a month previously; in spite of the patient's inability to close her mouth and the distorted appearance, the dislocation remained unrecognised.

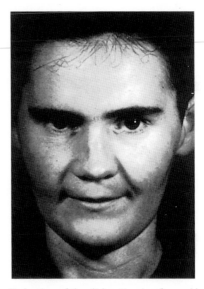

Fig. 14.15 Reduction of the dislocation (performed by open operation because of development of fibrous adhesions) restores the patient's normal appearance and movements of the jaw.

slides over the anterior articular eminence. Causes include forcible opening of the mouth by a blow on the jaw or during dental extractions under general anaesthesia. Epileptic patients sometimes also dislocate during seizures. A minority of patients have a small articular eminence or lax joint capsule and dislocate relatively easily, for instance on yawning. This may be frequent in conditions with generalised 'floppy joints' such as Ehlers–Danlos and Marfan's syndromes.

Dislocation is very painful, and the dislocation should be reduced immediately if possible, but muscle spasm and guarding by the patient tend to maintain the dislocation.

The traditional method to reduce the dislocation is to press downward and backward on or behind the lower posterior teeth with the thumbs while standing behind the patient. This is difficult and sedation may be required. Sudden reflex closing in a conscious patient risks a major bite injury to the thumbs, which must be protected with padding.

Occasionally, the dislocation remains unnoticed and, surprisingly, a patient may tolerate the disability and discomfort for weeks or even months (Figs 14.13–14.15). In these cases, effusion into the joint, following injury, becomes organised to form fibrous adhesions. When this happens, manual reduction may be impossible and open surgical reduction, with division of adhesions, must be carried out.

For recurrent dislocation, augmentation of the eminence by bone graft or down-fracture of the zygomatic arch to enlarge the eminence are overall the most successful procedures

Review PMID: 25483448

Ehlers–Danlos syndrome

Ehlers–Danlos syndrome (see also Ch. 2) is a heritable disease of collagen formation causing, among other features, hyper-extensibility of the skin, lax joint capsules and ligaments, impaired healing and scar formation. Six main types are recognised, all with slightly different combinations of features (see Table 14.1). Not all patients have typical lax skin and joints. Pulp stones seem to affect only some families and are not closely associated with any one type. Short roots and small teeth are also reported. Wrist mobility may impair toothbrushing, leading to poor oral health.

Review oral features PMID: 17052632

Oral and TMJ effects PMID: 15817074

Case, multiple dental defects PMID: 16937863

Table 14.1   Types and features of Ehlers-Danlos syndrome

Type	Inheritance and gene	Features	Dental significance
Classical	Autosomal dominant mutations in collagen V	Skin and joint hypermobility Poor healing	Mitral valve prolapse predisposes to endocarditis Temporomandibular joint (TMJ) dislocation frequent Pulp stones
Hypermobility	Autosomal dominant, possibly mutation in collagen 3	Skin and severe joint hypermobility	TMJ dislocation frequent Early-onset arthritis
Vascular	Autosomal dominant, mutation in collagen 3	Thin skin, arterial and bowel rupture, bruising, joints mostly unaffected	Bleeding risk Marked gingival bleeding on toothbrushing Occasional rapidly progressing periodontitis Poor healing after surgery or trauma TMJ dislocation
Kyphoscoliosis	Autosomal recessive, mutation in PLOD collagen processing enzyme gene	Joint hypermobility, muscle hypotonia, progressive scoliosis from birth	Poor healing
Arthrochalasia	Autosomal dominant, mutations in collagen 1	Severe joint hypermobility	TMJ dislocation
Dermatosparaxis	Autosomal recessive, mutations in collagen 1 processing enzyme gene	Severe skin fragility and sagging skin	Poor healing
Periodontal or type VIII	Genetically heterogeneous	As classical with rapidly progressive periodontitis	Premature loss of permanent teeth and marked alveolar bone resorption

Diseases of the oral mucosa: mucosal infections

15

Few diseases are specific to the oral mucosa. Mucosal changes can be part of an underlying systemic disease, a marker of internal malignancy or of almost no significance. Occasionally mucosal signs indicate potentially life-threatening disease.

The oral mucosa has a limited range of responses to injury. The epithelium may thicken (acanthosis), thin (atrophy), proliferate (hyperplasia), keratinise, separate or break down to form an ulcer. This restricted range of changes means that many oral diseases appear similar. The end result in many diseases is ulceration.

ULCERS

→ Summary charts 15.2, 16.2 and 16.3 pp. 253, 280, 281

Many oral diseases are characterised by ulcers. An ulcer is a break in the continuity of the epithelium, exposing the connective tissue to the oral environment. Ulcers may have sharp well-defined borders or ragged margins, but all are covered by a grey-yellow fibrin slough. The slough has a characteristic appearance, and with experience is readily distinguished from the brighter white colour of keratinisation. Ulcers have a superficial bacterial contamination by oral flora, but the tissue below very rarely becomes infected. The rapid turnover of oral epithelium allows uncomplicated ulcers to heal rapidly.

Important causes are summarised in Table 15.1.

General review diagnosis ulcers PMID: 26650694

HERPESVIRUS DISEASES

The herpesvirus group can cause many oral and head and neck diseases, listed in Table 15.2. All herpesvirus infections are more common in immunosuppression, particularly HIV infection. Infection can then be more severe, persistent or recurrent.

PRIMARY HERPETIC STOMATITIS

→ Summary chart 15.2 p. 253

Primary infection (systemic infection in a non-immune individual) is caused by *Herpes simplex* virus, usually type 1. Herpes viruses have been considered almost ubiquitous. Free virus is transmitted by close living conditions, through saliva in early childhood. In underdeveloped communities, 90% of individuals have been exposed to the virus by adolescence, as demonstrated by antibody levels. In the UK, the proportion of the population who are exposed to the virus before the age of 20 years, and are therefore immune, has reduced to 60%. The consequence is that though the incidence of herpetic stomatitis has declined, but it can now be seen in adolescents or adults, as well as in children.

Clinical features

The great majority of primary infections are subclinical or completely asymptomatic. Only 1% of those infected develop any symptoms, and these are often minimal. Most patients with clinical infection are children aged younger than 6 years.

In clinical disease, vesicles develop on the oral mucosa approximately 1 week after transmission. The hard palate, gingiva and dorsum of the tongue are favoured sites (Figs 15.1–15.3). The vesicles are dome-shaped, tense and filled with clear fluid and increase from 1 mm in diameter to 2–3 mm. There are usually tens or more than 100 tiny vesicles. Rupture of vesicles after a day or two leaves circular, sharply defined, shallow ulcers with yellowish or greyish

Table 15.1	Important causes of oral mucosal ulcers	
	Vesicular and immunobullous diseases	Ulceration without preceding vesiculation
Infectious	Primary herpetic stomatitis	Measles
	Herpes labialis	Glandular fever
	Herpes zoster and chickenpox	Tuberculosis
	Hand-foot-and-mouth disease	Syphilis
	Herpangina	
Non-infectious	Pemphigus vulgaris	Traumatic
	Mucous membrane pemphigoid	Aphthous stomatitis
	Linear IgA disease	Behçet's disease
	Dermatitis herpetiformis	HIV-associated mucosal ulcers
	Bullous erythema multiforme	Lichen planus
		Lupus erythematosus
		Eosinophilic ulceration
		Wegener's granulomatosis
		Some mucosal drug reactions
		Carcinoma (Ch. 20)

Table 15.2 Herpesvirus diseases relevant to dentistry

Human Herpesvirus type	Common name	Diseases	
1	Herpes simplex	Primary herpetic stomatitis Herpes labialis Herpetic whitlow	This chapter
2	Herpes simplex	A rarer cause of oral diseases as type 1, more commonly genital infections of similar type	This chapter
3	Varicella zoster	Chicken pox Shingles (zoster)	This chapter
4	Epstein–Barr virus	Infectious mononucleosis (glandular fever) Hairy leukoplakia Lymphoma Nasopharyngeal carcinoma Hodgkin's disease Mucosal ulcers	Infectious mononucleosis Ch. 31 Hairy leukoplakia Ch. 18
5	Cytomegalovirus	Salivary infection in neonates	This chapter
8	Kaposi sarcoma virus	Kaposi sarcoma Multicentric Castleman's disease	Kaposi sarcoma Ch. 25 Castleman's disease Ch. 31

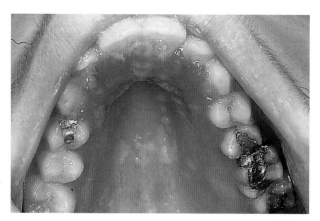

Fig. 15.1 Herpetic stomatitis. Pale vesicles and ulcers are visible on the palate and gingivae, especially anteriorly, and the gingivae are erythematous and swollen.

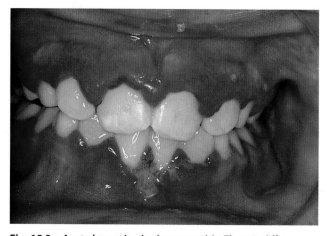

Fig. 15.3 Acute herpetic gingivostomatitis. There is diffuse reddening of the attached gingiva with ulceration in the lower incisor region extending beyond the attached gingiva.

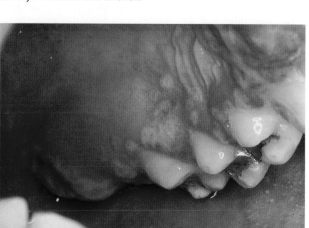

Fig. 15.2 Herpetic stomatitis. A group of recently ruptured vesicles on the hard palate, a characteristic site. The individual lesions are of remarkably uniform size, but several have coalesced to form larger irregular ulcers.

floors and red margins. Initially round, the ulcers enlarge and coalesce to produce more irregular but shallow ulcers. The gingival margins are swollen and red, with or without ulcers.

Symptoms depend on extent of ulceration, but the ulcers are painful and often interfere with eating. There is usually a degree of fever and systemic upset with enlarged cervical lymph nodes. This can be severe, particularly in adults.

Oral lesions usually resolve within a week to 10 days, but malaise can persist so long that an adult may not recover fully for several weeks.

Clinicopathological features PMID: 18197856

Pathology

The DNA virus targets epithelial cells, and replication leads to cell lysis. Clusters of infected cells break down to form the vesicles in the upper epithelium (Fig. 15.4). Virus-damaged epithelial cells with swollen nuclei and marginated chromatin (ballooning degeneration) are seen in the floor of the vesicle and in direct smears from early lesions (Fig. 15.5). Infected cells fuse with normal adjacent cells, spreading the infection and forming multinucleate cells. Later, the full thickness of the epithelium is destroyed to produce a sharply defined ulcer (Fig. 15.6) associated with an inflammatory infiltrate.

Diagnosis

The clinical picture is usually distinctive (Box 15.1). A smear showing virus-damaged cells provides additional

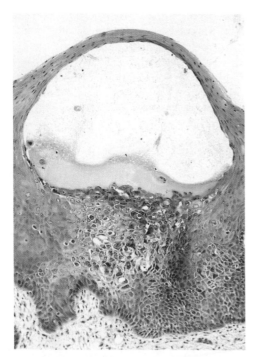

Fig. 15.4 Herpetic vesicle. The vesicle is formed by accumulation of fluid within the prickle cell layer. The virus-infected cells, identifiable by their enlarged nuclei, can be seen in the floor of the vesicle, and a few are floating freely in the vesicle fluid.

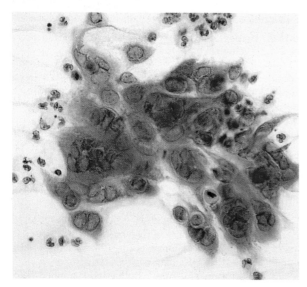

Fig. 15.5 A smear from a herpetic vesicle. The distended degenerating nuclei of the epithelial cells cluster together to give the typical mulberry appearance.

diagnostic evidence. A rising titre of antibodies reaching a peak after 2–3 weeks provides absolute but retrospective confirmation of the diagnosis, as can viral culture of vesicle fluid.

In cases of severe disease, when the patient is immuno-suppressed or complications such as spread to the eye are suspected, rapid definitive diagnosis can be obtained by PCR DNA amplification, ELISA assays or electron microscopy. These virus-specific tests reveal that approximately 15% of cases are caused by the type 2 virus that normally causes genital infection, but the symptoms, signs and treatment are identical.

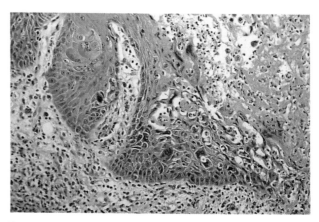

Fig. 15.6 Herpetic ulcer. The vesicle has ruptured to form an ulcer (*right*) and the epithelium at the margin contains enlarged, darkly staining virus-infected cells liberating free virus into the saliva.

Box 15.1 Herpetic stomatitis: key features

- Usually caused by Herpes simplex virus type 1
- Transmitted by close contact
- Usually affects children younger than 6 years
- Vesicles, followed by ulcers, affect any part of the oral mucosa
- Gingiva usually involved
- Lymphadenopathy and fever of variable severity
- Smears from vesicles show ballooning degeneration of viral-damaged cells
- Rising titre of antibodies to HSV confirms the diagnosis
- Supportive treatment important
- Aciclovir very effective if given in first 48 hours

Obtaining a definite diagnosis may not be essential. Hand, foot and mouth disease and herpangina (later in this chapter) produce similar features and, if mild, all are treated only by supportive measures.

Treatment

Patients feel very unwell, and children fail to eat or maintain fluid intake, sleep poorly and are fractious. Addressing these concerns is important for children and stressed parents. Because the disease is ultimately self-limiting, supportive treatment may be all that is required. Bed rest, soft bland diet, drinking through a straw and paracetamol elixir are effective. A sedative antihistamine such as promethazine will aid sleeping. Chlorhexidine mouthwash is sometimes used in an attempt to reduce pain by controlling secondary infection of ulcers. It also helps maintain gingival health while tooth brushing is impossible. The saliva is infectious, and transfer to the eye must be avoided because ocular herpes infections may develop into encephalitis by direct spread along the optic nerves.

Treatment with antiviral drugs is highly effective, but only if administered during the first 48 hours or so after vesicles appear. Aciclovir is a nucleoside analogue that is only phos-phorylated by viral DNA-encoded enzymes in infected cells. The activated drug blocks viral DNA synthesis, preventing viral replication. Aciclovir suspension can be used as a rinse and then swallowed for systemic effect or given in tablet form at 400 mg, five times per day for 5 days in adults and children older than 2 years. Aggressive treatment is essential in the immunosuppressed to prevent infection spreading onto the skin or eye and other complications. Valaciclovir is then preferred for its higher blood level and longer half-life.

Unusually prolonged or severe infections or failure to respond to aciclovir suggest immunodeficiency, and herpetic ulceration persisting for more than a month is an AIDS-defining illness.

Treatment PMID: 17379150

Web URL 15.1 NICE treatment guidance: http://cks.nice.org.uk/herpes-simplex-oral

Latency

Herpes simplex and zoster are neurotropic as well as epitheliotropic viruses. After the immune response develops and mucosal infection subsides, the virus can remain hidden from the immune response in the sensory nerves that supply the site of the primary infection. Virus is transported back along the nerves from the mucosa to the neurone cell bodies in the ganglia where it establishes a lifelong latent infection. During latency there are no symptoms, no virus replication occurs and the patient is not infectious.

Reactivation of the latent infection depends on the host cell, not the virus, and triggers (discussed later in this chapter) switch the virus back into replicative infection, after which it travels back down the neurones to infect the skin or mucosa. Only a small proportion of the latently infected neurones are able to reactivate, so that recurrent lesions are focal. They are almost always on the lip (herpes labialis) but occasionally in the mouth or on the skin. Intraorally the palate is the most frequent site.

Many in the population shed virus intermittently into saliva indicating activation of latent infection. They suffer no symptoms but can transmit the infection.

Persistent infection and infectivity PMID: 17703961

HERPES LABIALIS → Summary chart 15.2 p. 253

Herpes labialis is a secondary infection, that is an infection in an immune individual following reactivation of latent virus. In secondary infection the neutralising antibodies and T-cell responses produced in response to the primary infection are not protective because the virus travels along the nerves inside neurones to the new site.

Reactivation of latent virus to produce a herpes labialis lesion ('cold sore') happens in up to 30% of the population, many more than have ever had a clinically evident primary infection. Recurrent lesions must therefore usually follow a subclinical infection. Triggering factors include the common cold, other febrile infections, exposure to ultraviolet light, menstruation, emotional stress, local trauma, hypothermia, dental treatment and immunosuppression, but often none is identified.

Clinically, changes follow a consistent course with prodromal paraesthesia or burning sensations, then erythema at the site of the attack. Vesicles form after an hour or two, usually in clusters along the mucocutaneous junction of the lips and extending a short distance onto the adjacent skin (Fig. 15.7).

The vesicles enlarge, coalesce and weep exudate. After 2 or 3 days they rupture and crust over, but new vesicles frequently appear for a day or two only to scab over and

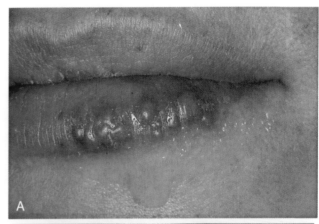

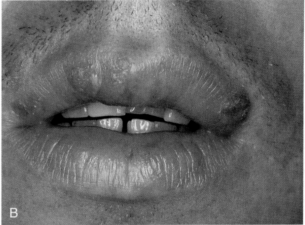

Fig. 15.7 Herpes labialis. (A) Typical vesicles. (B) Crusted ulcers affecting the vermilion borders of the lips.

finally heal, usually without scarring. The whole cycle may take as long as 12 days. In the immunocompromised, lesions are larger, more painful and last longer.

Secondary bacterial infection may induce scarring. Infectious virus is shed from the lesion until it is completely healed, so a dentist with a cold sore should not work.

Recurrent infection can trigger erythema multiforme (Ch. 16).

Treatment

The need for treatment depends on extent. Many stoical patients manage cold sores with over-the-counter preparations of minimal value. Docosanol is a fatty alcohol with a mild effect. In the UK aciclovir, 5% cream, is available without prescription and may be effective if applied before vesicles appear, when premonitory sensations are felt. Penciclovir, on prescription, applied every 2 hours is more effective. These agents must be dabbed and not rubbed onto the lesions to avoid spreading the infectious exudate more widely.

Sunscreen on the lips prevents lesions in those susceptible to ultraviolet light reactivation.

Patients who suffer frequent, multiple or large cold sores may benefit from more aggressive treatment with antiviral drugs. Repeated early high-dose treatment both treats the lesion and reduces the risk of future attacks.

Vaccines are in trial and have greatest potential benefit in the developing world where herpes simplex infections are a common cause of blindness and are common sexually transmitted diseases.

Web URL 15.1 NICE treatment guidance: http://cks.nice.org.uk/herpes-simplex-oral

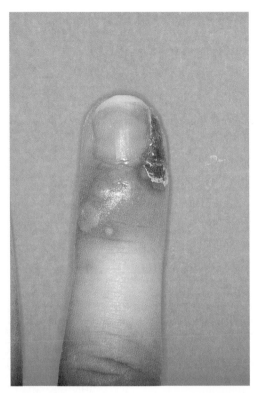

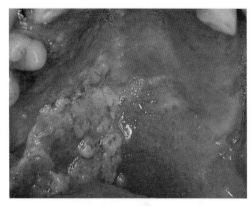

Fig. 15.9   Herpes zoster. A severe attack in an older person shows confluent ulceration on the hard and soft palate on one side.

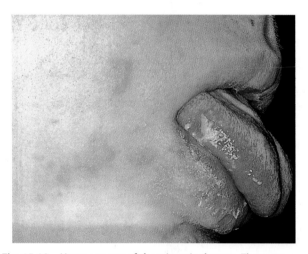

Fig. 15.10   Herpes zoster of the trigeminal nerve. There are vesicles and ulcers on one side of the tongue and facial skin supplied by the first and second divisions. The patient complained only of toothache.

Fig. 15.8   Herpetic whitlow. This is a characteristic non-oral site for primary infection as a result of contact with infected vesicle fluid or saliva. The vesiculation and crusting are identical to those seen in herpes labialis.

Herpetic whitlow

Both primary and secondary herpetic infections are contagious. *Herpetic whitlow* (Fig. 15.8) is a skin infection in a non-immune host after inoculation from another infected site, either another individual or by autoinoculation. Children with a primary infection may transfer the infection by finger sucking. Before gloves became routine in dentistry it was an uncommon occupational hazard for dental surgeons and their assistants.

Antiviral drugs should be prescribed as for a primary infection.

Case and image PMID: 25337767

HERPES ZOSTER OF THE TRIGEMINAL
NERVE → Summary chart 15.2 p. 253

The varicella-zoster virus causes chickenpox in the non-immune, mainly children (later in this chapter), while reactivation of the latent virus in nerves causes zoster (shingles), mainly in the elderly. The mechanism of latency is as described above for herpes simplex, but unlike simplex virus, reactivation is a relatively rare phenomenon, and most patients only ever suffer a single attack of zoster. Although zoster affects as many as one in three adults, the face and mouth are relatively unusual sites.

Clinical features

Zoster usually affects adults of middle age or older. The first signs are pain and irritation or tenderness in the dermatome supplied by the nerve in which the virus has become latent. Unlike simplex infection there is severe neuralgic, often burning, pain initially while the virus replicates in the nerve

and travels to the skin or mucosa. After 2–3 days the pain is felt in the skin and a vesicular rash develops, sharply limited to the dermatome. Facial rash or stomatitis is therefore limited at the midline.

Vesicles are usually numerous and can become confluent and pass through the same sequence of rupture, ulceration, crusting and healing as described for herpes simplex infections over 7–10 days (Figs 15.9 and 15.10). The regional lymph nodes are enlarged and tender. Pain continues until the lesions crust over and start to heal, but secondary infection may cause suppuration and scarring of the skin. Malaise and fever are usually associated.

In its prodromal phase the acute neuralgic pain of trigeminal nerve zoster is a classic mimic of pulpitis, and patients may well present for dental treatment. If no dental cause is evident, this possibility should be considered. This has given rise to the myth that dental extractions can precipitate facial zoster.

Pathology

The varicella-zoster virus produces epithelial lesions similar to those of herpes simplex.

A national programme of vaccination against varicella zoster started in the UK in 2013 for those aged between 70 and 80 years. Vaccination reduces attacks by approximately half and reduces severity in the remaining patients.

Management

Herpes zoster is an uncommon cause of stomatitis, but readily recognisable (Box 15.2) without laboratory investigation, although viral culture and other more rapid tests such as polymerase chain reaction (PCR) are available if required.

Mild attacks may require only analgesia and topical soothing cream. Facial infections are usually treated because of the risk of scarring and higher risk of complications. Oral aciclovir, 5 mg/kg, every 8 hours for 5 days is effective. The dose is doubled in the immunocompromised. The drug must be given at the earliest opportunity for maximum effect, ideally within 72 hours, and complemented with analgesics. Addition of prednisolone speeds recovery and reduces the incidence of post-herpetic neuralgia (Ch. 38). Any patient who is immunosuppressed, suffers complications, has eye involvement or bacterial infection of skin lesions or is very elderly should be managed in a specialist centre. Intravenous aciclovir may be required.

Treatment PMID: 19691461

Web URL 15.2 NICE guidance: http://cks.nice.org.uk/shingles #!scenario:1

Complications

Zoster will occasionally cause tooth devitalisation and even bone necrosis in the affected area, during or after the clinical infection, particularly when the prodromal symptoms included toothache.

Involvement of the tip and lateral tip of the nose indicates involvement of the external nasal branch of the nasociliary nerve, a branch of the ophthalmic division of the trigeminal that also supplies the cornea. This is Hutchinson's sign*, and it indicates a high risk of ocular involvement and need for specialist treatment from the outset.

Zoster in immunosuppression can be a lethal infection if encephalitis develops. Thus, zoster in the very elderly, organ transplant patients, those treated for malignant disease or in HIV infection require aggressive treatment and follow up. Vaccination is not possible in immunosuppression because it uses a live virus.

Post-herpetic neuralgia mainly affects the elderly and is difficult to relieve (Ch. 38).

Case devitalisation teeth PMID: 16054735

Rare oral complications PMID: 20692192

Ramsay Hunt syndrome

Ramsay Hunt** syndrome is reactivated zoster infection in the facial nerve. Virus is latent in the geniculate ganglion, which houses both sensory and motor fibres. On reactivation, patients develop facial paralysis, loss of taste on one side of the anterior tongue and vesicles on the tongue, hard palate and in the external auditory canal. It must be differentiated from Bell's palsy.

Treatment is as for zoster of the trigeminal nerve, but the chances of full recovery are lower than for Bell's palsy.

CYTOMEGALOVIRUS ULCERS

Cytomegalovirus, or herpesvirus type 5, is another almost ubiquitous virus that causes an acute primary disease and can remain latent to cause recurrent infection. Almost all infections are asymptomatic. In those few with clinical disease, primary infection resembles infectious mononucleosis, sometimes with painful swelling and infection of salivary glands.

The main interest is cytomegalovirus ulceration of the oral mucosa in immunodeficiency, particularly in HIV infection. These ulcers show no specific clinical features but are usually large and shallow and solitary. In the immunosuppressed they heal slowly, and biopsy is usually undertaken to identify a cause. The virally infected cells have typical inclusions in their nuclei and can be identified on immunohistochemistry (see Fig. 1.8).

Cytomegalovirus infection is treated with the aciclovir analogue ganciclovir or related drugs.

Review oral signs PMID: 8385303

In immunosuppression PMID: 8705589

HAND-FOOT-AND-MOUTH DISEASE

→ Summary chart 15.2 p. 253

Hand-foot-and-mouth disease is a common viral infection caused by several related strains of enteric viruses, notably coxsackie A16 and enterovirus 71. These are RNA viruses spread by faecal-oral contact and, distantly, related to poliovirus.

The disease is highly infectious and often causes minor epidemics among school children and an occasional parent or teacher, often in the autumn. The incubation period is probably between 3 and 10 days. The disease is unrelated to foot-and-mouth disease of cattle.

Clinical features

This is a mild viral infection characterised by ulceration of the mouth and a vesicular rash on the extremities. Regional lymph nodes are not usually enlarged, and systemic upset is typically mild or absent, but there may be diarrhoea and vomiting. The main features are small, scattered oral ulcers in all areas of the mouth, usually with little pain and an

---

*This is named after the same Sir Jonathan Hutchinson (1828–1913) who described the characteristic incisors of syphilis and who has over a dozen eponymous signs, disease and syndromes named after him.

**There is no hyphen in the name of this disease because it is named after James Ramsay Hunt (1872–1937), not after two people.

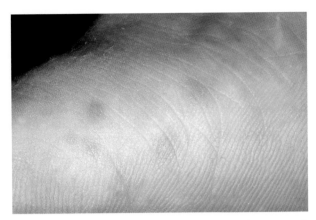

Fig. 15.11 Hand-foot-and-mouth disease. The rash consists of vesicles or bullae on the extremities; in this patient they are relatively inconspicuous.

erythematous background. Unlike herpetic stomatitis, intact vesicles are rarely seen and gingivitis is not a feature.

The rash develops after the oral ulcers and consists of vesicles, sometimes deep-seated, or occasionally bullae, mainly seen on palms and soles and around the base of fingers or toes, but any part of the limbs may be affected (Fig. 15.11). The rash is often the main feature, and such patients are unlikely to be seen by dentists. In some outbreaks, either the mouth or the extremities alone may be affected.

The disease typically resolves within a week. No specific treatment is available or needed, but myocarditis and encephalitis are rare complications.

Key features are summarised in Box 15.3.

Clinical review PMID: 26087425

Oral features PMID: 1061921

More severe variant PMID: 24932735

HERPANGINA

This can be considered related to hand-foot-and-mouth disease, and the features described above also apply. It is slightly less common than hand-foot-and-mouth disease and is caused by enteroviruses, of often the same types, but most often by coxsackie A strains.

The presentation is a similar mild viral disease with a cluster of a few larger ulcers usually limited to the soft palate, tonsils or posterior mouth but no rash. As after hand, foot and mouth disease, occasional complications can occur.

Herpangina review PMID: 20118685

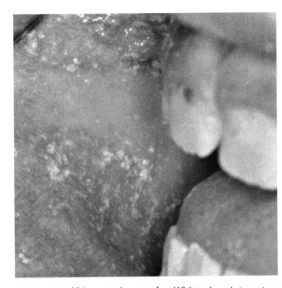

Fig. 15.12 Koplik's spots in measles. White pinpoint spots on an erythematous background, likened to the appearance of grains of salt. *(Fig. 16.7 From Paller, A.S., and Mancini, A.J. 2011. Hurwitz clinical pediatric dermatology: a textbook of skin disorders of childhood and adolescence. Philadelphia: Saunders.)*

MEASLES

Measles, once a common childhood illness, is now rare following introduction of the UK national vaccination scheme, but there are still approximately 2000 cases each year due to poor uptake. Occasional epidemics still occur, but death from measles is now limited to adults, the immunocompromised or those with late complications.

In the prodromal stage of measles, toward the end of a 14-day incubation period, Koplik's spots form on the buccal mucosa and soft palate. These are characteristic pinpoint foci of epithelial necrosis on a red background (Fig. 15.12). Classically, while these break down into ulcers, the patient develops the typical fever and rash starting on the face. However, the spots are very variable, have been reported to be absent in vaccinated children and also to occur late in the disease. Recognising Koplik's spots is therefore very helpful, but the oral lesions require no treatment.

Measles is highly infectious and has many severe complications and in the UK is a notifiable disease. In the developing world and in the immunosuppressed it is potentially fatal and predisposes to noma (page 134).

Case and image PMID: 25754702

Case series, images PMID: 22236551

CHICKEN POX

Chicken pox is caused by infection with varicella-zoster virus in a non-immune host, usually a child younger than 12 years. The UK does not have a universal chicken pox vaccination scheme, and the disease remains endemic. An effective vaccine is available, but use is limited to protecting those at particular risk of complications.

After a 2-week incubation period, there is malaise, nausea, fever, sore throat and the rash appears on the face and trunk producing intensely itchy blisters that break down into ulcers. The oral lesions are identical and usually appear before the rash and appear like herpes simplex vesicles and ulcers except that they tend to occur on the buccal mucosa and palate. There are normally only a few lesions, and numerous ulcers signify a more severe systemic infection.

Treatment is mostly supportive, with aciclovir or related drugs if the diagnosis is made early enough.

Review and cases PMID: 1068230 and 6931841

TUBERCULOSIS

Mucosal infection is described here; tuberculous lymphadenopathy is dealt with in Chapter 31.

The recrudescence of tuberculosis is partly a consequence of the AIDS epidemic, partly explained by multiple drug-resistant mycobacteria and partly due to the reduced effectiveness of the BCG (bacillus Calmette-Guérin) vaccination.

Oral tuberculosis is rare and a complication of active pulmonary disease in which the mucosa is infected from the sputum. Open active tuberculosis is now rare and tends to be seen in elderly men with pulmonary infection and a chronic cough that has progressed unrecognised, those who have neglected treatment or are immunosuppressed. They are likely to show typical signs of pulmonary infection: chest pain, malaise, weight loss and haemoptysis.

The typical lesion is an ulcer on the middorsum of the tongue; the lip or other parts of the mouth are infrequently affected. The ulcer is typically angular or stellate, with overhanging edges and a pale floor, but can be ragged and irregular (Fig. 15.13). It is painless in its early stages, and regional lymph nodes are usually unaffected. A second typical presentation is a non-healing extraction socket.

The diagnosis is rarely suspected before biopsy.

Case series PMID: 22014940

Review PMID: 20486998

Pathology

Typical non-caseating tuberculous granulomas containing occasional Langhans type giant cells are seen in the floor of the ulcers (Fig. 15.14). Mycobacteria are sometimes identifiable in the oral lesion by using special stains but can be demonstrated more easily in the sputum. Chest radiographs usually show advanced infection. In tropical countries and in immunosuppression, similar features arise from fungal or atypical mycobacterial infections.

Management

Diagnosis is confirmed by biopsy, chest radiography and a specimen of sputum. Mycobacterial infection is confirmed by culture or PCR. Interferon gamma release assays used in latent infection are not used to diagnose active infection.

Oral lesions clear up rapidly if vigorous multidrug chemotherapy is given for the pulmonary infection. No local treatment is needed.

SYPHILIS

As a result of contact tracing and early treatment, fewer than 150 cases a year of primary or secondary syphilis were seen in England and Wales in the 1980s. However, since the mid-1990s, the prevalence has risen steadily. There are currently approximately 3000 new cases of syphilis a year in the UK, the highest levels since the 1950s. There are 10,000 a year in the United States, but there is no accurate estimate for Africa where the incidence is highest. This increase is a worldwide trend, and the disease has, for example, become widespread in Eastern Europe.

Most of these increases parallel rates of HIV infection, and most cases are in men who have sex with men. HIV infection predisposes to a fulminant form of the disease and also renders some diagnostic tests based on antibody levels inaccurate.

Oral lesions in each stage of syphilis are clinically quite different from each other. Oral lesions in the UK probably often pass unrecognised outside specialist clinics.

Congenital syphilis

Congenital syphilis arises when an infected mother transmits the infection to her child in utero. After almost vanishing in the developed world, congenital infection is

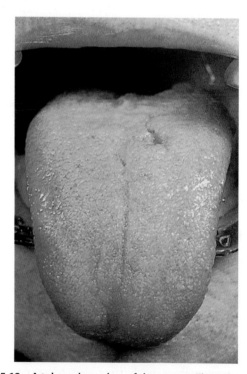

Fig. 15.13   A tuberculous ulcer of the tongue. The rather angular shape and overhanging edges of the ulcer are typical. The patient was a man of 56 with advanced but unrecognised pulmonary tuberculosis.

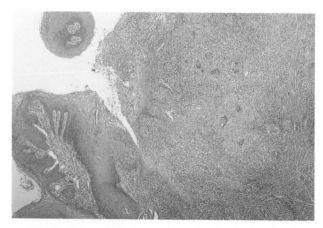

Fig. 15.14   Tuberculous ulcer. At the margin, numerous pale staining granulomas are present in the ulcer bed. The darkly stained multinucleate Langhans giant cells are visible even at this low power.

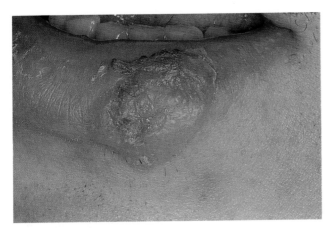

Fig. 15.15　Primary chancre. The lower lip is a typical site for extragenital chancres, but they are rarely seen.

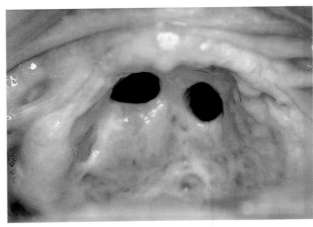

Fig. 15.16　Tertiary syphilis; gummas of the palate. Necrosis in the centre of the palate has caused perforation of the bone and two typical round punched-out holes.

now seen again, even in developed countries, and worldwide it causes the death of half a million infants each year. The widespread infection produces many signs and developmental disturbances, classically diffuse rash, rhinitis, radial scarring around the mouth and periostitis of many bones producing a saddle nose and frontal bossing. The classical triad of interstitial keratitis of the cornea, sensorineural hearing loss and dental anomalies is diagnostic.

Dental anomalies are discussed in Chapter 2.

UK incidence PMID: 26931054

US incidence PMID: 26562206

Primary syphilis

An oral chancre appears 2–8 weeks after infection and may form on the lip, tip of the tongue or, rarely, other oral sites. It consists initially of a firm nodule about a centimetre across (Fig. 15.15). The surface breaks down after a few days, leaving a rounded ulcer with raised indurated edges. Chancres are usually solitary, and multiple lesions suggest immunosuppression. A chancre is typically painless, but regional lymph nodes are enlarged, rubbery and discrete.

A biopsy may only show non-specific inflammation, but sometimes there is conspicuous perivascular infiltration by plasma cells. If infection is suspected, immunohistochemical staining can reveal the treponemal organisms in the epithelium, but the diagnosis is easily missed if not suspected. Diagnosis is best made by serological tests or polymerase chain reaction. Direct examination of smears from oral lesions is not recommended because *Treponema pallidum* cannot be confidently distinguished from other oral commensal spirochaetes.

After 8 or 9 weeks the chancre heals, often without scarring.

Secondary syphilis

The secondary stage develops 1–4 months after infection. It typically causes mild fever with malaise, headache, sore throat and generalised lymphadenopathy, soon followed by a rash and stomatitis.

The rash is variable but typically consists of asymptomatic pinkish ('coppery') macules, symmetrically distributed and starting on the trunk. It may last from a few hours to several weeks, and its presence or history is a useful aid to diagnosis. Oral lesions, which rarely appear without the rash, mainly affect the tonsils, lateral borders of the tongue

and lips. They are usually flat ulcers covered by greyish membrane and may be irregularly linear (snail's track ulcers) or coalesce to form well-defined rounded areas (mucous patches). *Condyloma lata* are raised mucous patches that resemble large flat papillomas.

Discharge from the ulcers contains many spirochaetes, and saliva is highly infectious. Serological reactions (see later in this chapter) are positive and diagnostic at this stage, and biopsy is diagnostic using *T. pallidum*-specific immunohistochemical stains.

Tertiary syphilis

Late-stage syphilis develops in patients approximately 3 or more years after infection in as many as a third of untreated patients but not in those treated effectively. The onset is insidious, and during the latent period the patient may appear well. The late tertiary stage is now very rare. Leukoplakia of the tongue may develop during this late stage (Ch. 19) and other effects of syphilis such as aortitis, tabes or general paralysis of the insane may be associated.

The characteristic oral lesion is the gumma, usually of the palate, tongue or tonsils. This starts as a swelling a few to several centimetres in diameter sometimes with a yellowish centre that undergoes necrosis, leaving a painless indolent deep ulcer. The ulcer is rounded, with soft, punched-out edges. The floor is depressed and pale (wash-leather) in appearance. It eventually heals with severe scarring that may distort the soft palate or tongue, perforate the hard palate (Fig. 15.16) or destroy the uvula.

Microscopically, there is non-specific inflammation with endarteritis and sparse granulomas. However, the appearances can be completely non-specific, and diagnosis depends on laboratory tests.

Review oral lesions PMID: 20596972 and 15953910

Case series PMID: 24045192

Tertiary syphilis cases PMID: 24891485

Management

Management of syphilis in the dental setting is limited to maintaining suspicion to identify cases and screening diagnosis in secondary care. Definitive diagnosis and treatment must be provided by specialists. Clinical diagnosis and biopsy diagnosis with confirmation of *Treponema* by immunohistochemistry is the likely pathway in most cases presenting to dentists as the diagnosis is not usually suspected and a biopsy may well be taken.

When the diagnosis is suspected, specialist testing must be sought as interpretation of the results is complex. The organism cannot be cultured, and serological tests are used. Until recently the specific fluorescent antibody tests and *T. pallidum* haemagglutination or particle agglutination assays were the most specific. Although widely used, the VDRL test is a screening test of low positive predictive value and multiple tests had to be used. Gradually these tests are being replaced by PCR- based rapid molecular assays of very high sensitivity and specificity. Tests indicate the infection, but not the stage.

Benzathine penicillin is the drug of choice, an intramuscular preparation with slow absorption. Syphilis in HIV infection requires more aggressive treatment.

CANDIDOSIS

Candidosis* is caused by several species of candida that are normal commensals in the mouths of a third or more of the normal population, and many more in denture wearers and the elderly. This candida 'carriage' is not associated with symptoms or disease.

Candida sp. is dimorphic. Carriage is associated with the yeast ('blastospore') form and only the invasive hyphal form causes disease. The reasons for the organism switching to a pathogenic form are unclear, but disease seems to follow some change to the oral environment. Thus, host factors are probably more important than fungal factors.

The most common pathogenic species is *Candida albicans*; *Candida glabrata, tropicalis* and *krusei* and other less frequent species account for some 25% of disease between them. Some of the less frequent isolates are reported to be more likely to develop resistance to antifungal drugs, but this remains a relatively rare problem clinically.

The concept that candidosis is a 'disease of the diseased' dates back to 1868, and many medical factors are recognised to predispose to infection (Box 15.4). These are likely to

---

Box 15.4 **Oral candidosis: important predisposing factors**

- Extremes of age
- Immunodeficiency (diabetes mellitus, HIV infection, chemotherapy)
- Immunosuppression (including steroid inhalers)
- Anaemia, of any type
- Suppression of the normal oral flora by antibacterial drugs
- Xerostomia
- Denture wearing
- Smoking
- High carbohydrate diet
- Epithelium with increased keratin, for instance in lichen planus
- Almost any severely debilitating illness

---

*Candid*osis* not 'candid*iasis*' because it is a my*cosis*. Named fungal infections usually end in –osis, for instance histoplasmosis and cryptococcosis. The '-iases' are in general parasitic infections such as trypanosomiasis.

influence adhesion of the yeast form to the epithelial cells, which seems to trigger development of invasive hyphae. When the yeasts adhere, they trigger host cell receptors to activate an innate host response and attract neutrophils into the epithelium. Hyphae are only able to invade a limited distance into the epithelium, only within keratin and the upper prickle cell layer. Oral candidosis is a very superficial infection, explaining its mild symptoms.

Microbiology candida biofilms PMID: 21134239

Controversies in candidosis PMID: 22998462

There are various classifications of candidosis, but in reality these diseases merge into one another and can coexist. Thus, infection causes a spectrum of presentations, rather than many diseases (Box 15.5). The commonest forms are thrush, chronic hyperplastic candidosis and denture stomatitis. Chronic mucocutaneous candidosis is discussed later in this chapter and in Chapter 36.

Thrush → Summary chart 15.1 and 19.1 pp. 252, 314

Thrush**, a disease recognised by Hippocrates, is also sometimes called the acute pseudomembranous type of candidosis because of the thick white layer of candidal hyphae, dead and dying epithelial and inflammatory cells and debris that covers the mucosa like a membrane.

Thrush is common in neonates, caused by lack of an immune response and infection acquired during passage through the birth canal. It is also common in the very elderly and the very debilitated and on the soft palate of asthmatic steroid inhaler users who spray their palate rather than inhale the drug. It may also follow antibiotic treatment.

Rarely, persistent thrush is an early sign of chronic mucocutaneous candidosis or candida-endocrinopathy syndrome (Ch. 36).

Clinical features

Although classified as acute, thrush may have a rapid onset or develop insidiously from a chronic infection and in the immunosuppressed it may become chronic. Thrush forms soft, friable and creamy coloured plaques on the mucosa (Fig. 15.17), and the pseudomembrane can be scraped or wiped off exposing the erythematous mucosa below. This differentiates thrush from chronic forms of candidosis in which the white surface layer is keratin. The extent of pseudomembrane varies from isolated small flecks to

---

Box 15.5 **Spectrum of oral candidosis**

Acute candidosis

- Thrush
- Acute antibiotic stomatitis

Chronic candidosis

- Denture-induced stomatitis
- Chronic hyperplastic candidosis
- Chronic mucocutaneous candidosis
- Erythematous candidosis

Angular stomatitis

**Thrush is not a mere nickname or household term but is a medical term of respectable antiquity though its origin is uncertain.

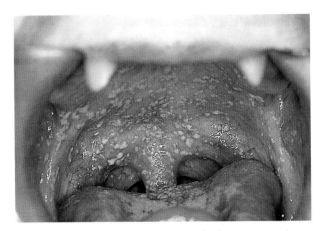

Fig. 15.17 **Thrush.** The lesions consist of soft, creamy patches or flecks lying superficially on an erythematous mucosa. This soft palate distribution is particularly frequent in those using steroid inhalers.

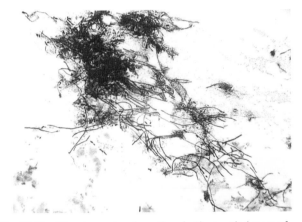

Fig. 15.18 **Direct scraping from thrush.** The tangled mass of gram-positive hyphae of *Candida albicans* is diagnostic. A few yeast cells may be present as well, but it is the large number of hyphae that is diagnostic.

widespread confluent plaques and the buccal mucosa, palate and dorsal tongue are the most commonly affected sites. Angular stomatitis is frequently associated, as it is with any form of intraoral candidosis.

The condition is not painful; rather it is uncomfortable, sometimes with a bad taste or burning sensation.

Pathology

A Gram- or periodic acid-Schiff (PAS)-stained scraping from the pseudomembrane shows large masses of tangled hyphae, detached epithelial cells and neutrophils (Fig. 15.18), and this test is diagnostic. Biopsy is not necessary but would show hyperplastic oedematous epithelium infiltrated by neutrophils. Staining with PAS shows many candidal hyphae growing down through the epithelial cells to the upper prickle cell layer (Fig. 15.19). More deeply, the epithelium is hyperplastic, with long slender rete processes extending down into the corium and a lymphoplasmacytic infiltrate below.

Key features are summarised in Box 15.6.

Management

The diagnosis is made on clinical features supported by microscopy of a scraping.

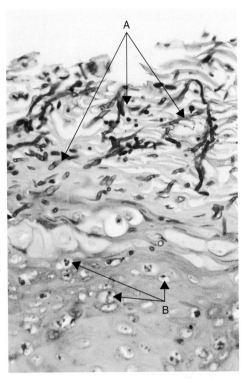

Fig. 15.19 **Thrush.** At high power the components of a plaque may be clearly seen. The surface layers of the epithelium are separated by inflammatory oedema and are colonised by fungal hyphae *(A)* and infiltrated by neutrophils *(B)*.

Box 15.6 Thrush: key features
- Acute candidosis
- Painful
- Secondary to various predisposing factors (Box 15.4)
- Common in HIV infection and indicates low immunity
- Creamy soft patches, readily wiped off the mucosa
- Smear shows many Gram-positive hyphae
- Histology shows hyphae invading superficial epithelium
- Responds to topical antifungals or itraconazole

The infection itself is managed by dealing with any identifiable predisposing factors, and this alone may allow thrush to resolve. However, usually a course of topical antifungal is first line treatment. The treatments for candida infection, and their indications are given in Appendix 15.1.

A search must also be made for the predisposing condition(s) in the medical history and oral examination, and they must be removed or ameliorated if possible. Denture wearers will benefit from the denture hygiene regime outlined below for denture-induced stomatitis.

Anaemia or some cause of immunosuppression, usually HIV infection, should be suspected when thrush is seen in an adult in whom there is no detectable predisposition. These are also suggested by failure to respond to treatment or recurrent disease. In immunosuppression specialised advice must be sought as recurrent thrush indicates marked suppression and extension to the oesophagus is a significant complication.

Web URL 15.3 NICE treatment guidance: http://cks.nice.org.uk/candida-oral

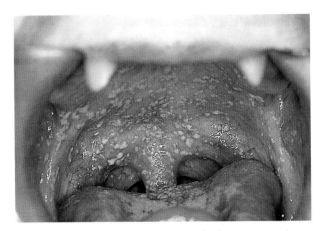

Angular cheilitis → Summary chart 15.1 p. 252

Angular cheilitis or angular stomatitis is an infection at the commissure of the lips, typically caused by leakage of candida-infected saliva at the angles of the mouth. It can be seen with thrush in infants, in denture wearers, in association with chronic hyperplastic candidosis or alone. It is a characteristic sign of candidal infection.

Clinically, there is mild inflammation at the angles of the mouth with painful fissuring or cracking and sometimes a soft crust.

The morphology of the lips, commissure and skin contribute to the condition. The commissure is normally dry and lightly keratinised, but in patients with angular cheilitis it is usually wet, either from saliva leakage or from deliberate licking or application of Vaseline or similar materials. This allows candida to infect the epithelium. In the elderly the commissure communicates with folds of skin caused by loss of elasticity and sagging of the facial tissues with age and angular cheilitis may then extend onto the skin (Fig. 15.20).

Management

Angular cheilitis is a mixed infection. Candida is found in as many as 90% of cases, but the proportion varies in different populations, being higher in denture wearers. Staphylococci, streptococci or other pathogens are frequently present and exactly which organisms are causative is unclear.

Treatment is targeted at treating the intraoral reservoir of candidal infection using local measures and antifungal drugs as appropriate. In mild cases this alone causes angular stomatitis to resolve. Miconazole gel is the ideal first-line treatment for the commissures as it has additional activity against several Gram-positive bacterial species including staphylococci and can be expected to successfully treat almost all cases. Failure is more likely due to incomplete treatment of the intraoral infection, but if this appears controlled, changing to 2% fusidic acid cream for the angles on assumption of staphylococcal or streptococcal infection is logical.

There is a particularly high proportion of patients with anaemia as a predisposing cause in angular cheilitis and iron, folate and B12 levels should be checked.

In the edentulous and those with loss of lip support with prominent skin folds, attempts to correct vertical dimension or thicken the labial flange cannot usually remove these susceptible areas. Dermal fillers haven been tried but so far remain without a good evidence base.

Erythematous candidosis

→ Summary charts 15.1 and 19.3 pp. 252, 316

This term is now applied to any candidal infection that produces red mucosa. Originally the name was used to describe the chronic red form of candidosis seen on the palate and gingiva of HIV-positive patients (see Fig. 29.5). However, the name was not very specific, and similar changes can arise in the immunocompetent.

The term is now taken to include a number of presentations with a primarily red mucosa, either localised or generalised. There may be occasional white flecks on the red background, but no 'pseudomembrane' (Fig. 15.21).

If a candidal infection produces a red area but does not fit the descriptions of the specific conditions listed in Box 15.7, it can simply be described as erythematous candidosis. Such lesions are usually on the hard palate, dorsum of the tongue and soft palate and are usually associated with immunosuppression or steroid inhalers as an underlying factor.

Web URL 15.3 NICE treatment guidance: http://cks.nice.org.uk/candida-oral

Acute antibiotic stomatitis

→ Summary chart 15.1 p. 252

This condition is also known as antibiotic sore mouth and acute atrophic candidosis. It follows overuse or topical oral use of antibiotics, especially broad-spectrum drugs such as tetracycline. These suppress the normal oral flora that competes with *Candida* in the mouth.

Clinically, the whole mucosa is red and sore, but the tongue is typically worst affected and appears smooth, having lost its filiform papillae. A few flecks of thrush may be present. Resolution may follow withdrawal of the antibiotic but is accelerated by topical antifungal treatment. A similar generalised candidal erythema can also be a consequence of xerostomia and is a typical complication of Sjögren's syndrome.

Box 15.7   Types of erythematous candidosis

- Acute antibiotic stomatitis
- Median rhomboid glossitis
- Denture stomatitis
- Erythematous candidosis

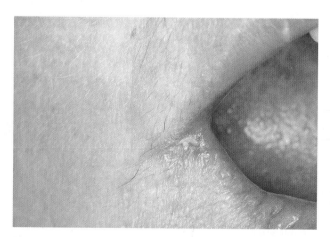

Fig. 15.20   Angular stomatitis. Cracking and erythema at the commissure is due to leakage of saliva containing *Candida albicans*, constantly reinfecting the saturated skin.

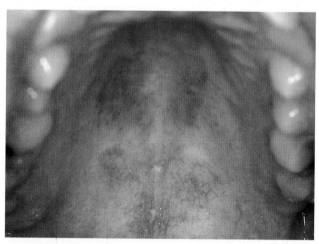

Fig. 15.21   Erythematous candidosis. Irregular patches of erythema on the palate of a patient using a steroid inhaler.

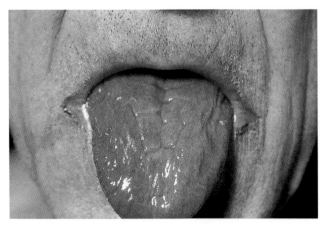

Fig. 15.22 Glossitis in antibiotic-induced candidosis. The tongue is red, smooth and sore as in anaemia, but the appearance results from inflammation and oedema. Similar changes affect other parts of the mouth, and there is angular cheilitis.

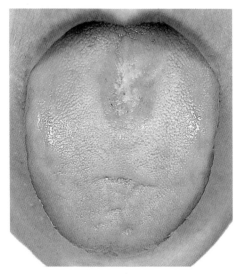

Fig. 15.24 Median rhomboid glossitis. There is a whitish patch of depapillation with sharply demarcated borders in the midline of the tongue.

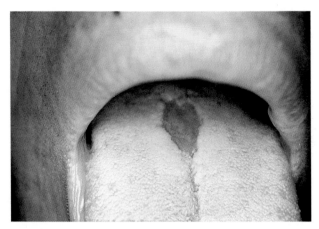

Fig. 15.23 Median rhomboid glossitis. The typical lozenge-shaped area of depapillation in the midline of the tongue.

Web URL 15.3 NICE treatment guidance: http://cks.nice.org.uk/candida-oral

Median rhomboid glossitis

→ Summary charts 15.3 and 19.3 pp. 252, 316

Median rhomboid glossitis produces a red patch in the midline of the dorsum of the tongue at the junction of the anterior two-thirds with the posterior third, classically in a diamond shape. It has previously been proposed to be developmental, but it is not seen in children and has nothing to do with persistence of the tuberculum impar or development of the thyroid. However, not all lesions can be shown to be infected with candida. It seems that this form is a very low level infection. Infection is probably intermittent and permanently damages the mucosa so that it loses its ability to form papillae and appears red even when infection is inactive.

Clinically, median rhomboid glossitis is seen in adults and is typically symptomless. Its colour ranges from pink to red, and the affected area loses its filiform papillae (Fig. 15.23). Usually the patch is flat or appears slightly depressed, but in longstanding lesions it may develop nodules. In the few cases with more intense infection, white flecks may be seen (Fig. 15.24). A florid lesion may appear worrying and be mistaken for a carcinoma, particularly when nodular, but squamous carcinoma virtually never develops at this site.

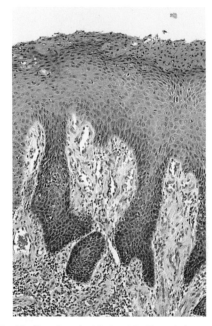

Fig. 15.25 Median rhomboid glossitis. There is hyperplasia with elongate rete processes, hyperparakeratosis and an inflammatory infiltrate of lymphocytes and plasma cells in the connective tissue. There are no signs of candidal infection.

One factor that may predispose to infection at this site is that, in many individuals, this part of the tongue rests against the soft palate, trapping saliva, and so is not as self-cleansing as the rest of the tongue. Sometimes a matching patch of candidosis is present on the soft palate.

Histologically, the appearances are variable. The primary change is epithelial atrophy with loss of filiform papillae and often broad parallel-sided rete process hyperplasia. Fungal hyphae should be sought but are often not found (Fig. 15.25). Below the epithelium in longstanding cases there is a broad band of dense scarred fibrous tissue (Fig. 15.26).

Case series and images PMID: 21912494

Case series PMID: 366496

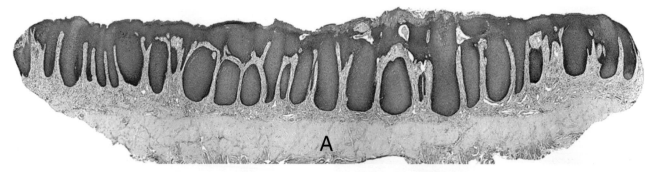

Fig. 15.26 Median rhomboid glossitis with epithelial hyperplasia, light inflammation below and a band of scar tissue *(A)*.

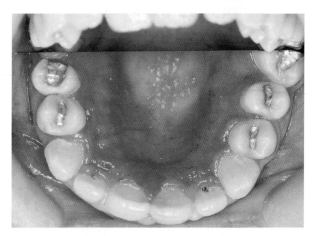

Fig. 15.27 Typical denture stomatitis. Clear demarcation between the erythema of the mucosa covered, in this instance, by an orthodontic appliance and the palate behind the posterior margin is clearly seen.

Management

Diagnosis is based on clinical appearance, and reassurance is usually the main requirement. Antifungal treatment does not usually resolve the lesion and should not be considered unless a scraping is positive for hyphae on microscopy. Nodular or lobulated lesions do not resolve on antifungal treatment. A biopsy should not be required.

Denture-induced stomatitis

→ Summary charts 15.1 and 19.3 pp. 252, 316

A well-fitting upper denture cuts off the underlying mucosa from the protective action of saliva and provides a space in which the oral flora, including candida, can proliferate freely. In susceptible patients, particularly smokers, this can promote candidosis, seen as a symptomless area of erythema. The erythema is sharply limited to the area of mucosa occluded by the upper denture or orthodontic appliance (Fig. 15.27). Similar inflammation is not seen under the more mobile lower denture, which allows a relatively free flow of saliva beneath it.

The exact relationship between the denture, candidal infection and denture-induced stomatitis remains somewhat contentious. In the past, the denture has been seen as the cause, either through poor fit, 'allergy' or irritation. *Candida* infection is definitely present, but hyphal forms are sparse and the inflamed mucosa may be reacting to either candida or bacteria in the biofilm adherent to the denture. Biopsy shows inflammation in the tissues and very sparse fungal hyphae at the surface. Evidence for the importance of candida comes from the fact that angular stomatitis is frequently associated.

> **Box 15.8 Denture-induced stomatitis: key features**
> - Candidal infection promoted by well-fitting upper denture
> - Enclosed mucosa is cut off from protective action of saliva
> - Mucosal erythema sharply restricted to area covered by the denture
> - Angular stomatitis frequently associated
> - Hyphae proliferate in denture–mucosa interface
> - Diagnosis by smear of mucosa or denture
> - Resolves after elimination of *Candida albicans* by antifungal treatment

Management

The clinical picture is distinctive, but the diagnosis can be confirmed by finding candidal hyphae in a smear from the inflamed mucosa or the fitting surface of the denture. Quantification of candida in saliva is of little value as candidal carriage is common and counts are higher in denture wearers.

The infection responds to antifungal drugs but recurs unless the denture factors are addressed. Topical agents such as nystatin can only gain access to the palate if the patient leaves out the denture while the medication is in the mouth. Systemic fluconazole is often used.

Porosity voids in methylmethacrylate denture bases also harbour *C. albicans* and dentures may therefore form a reservoir that can reinfect the mucosa. Elimination of *C. albicans* from the denture base is important and can be achieved by soaking the denture in dilute chlorhexidine mouthwash overnight. A key predisposing factor is night wear of dentures. Ceasing this alone may allow resolution.

A simpler alternative is to coat the fitting surface of the denture with miconazole gel while it is being worn. The denture should be removed and scrubbed clean at intervals and miconazole re-applied three times a day. This treatment should be continued until the inflammation has cleared and *C. albicans* has been eliminated. This is likely to take 1–2 weeks, but patients should be warned not to continue this treatment indefinitely. Resistance to miconazole is growing and the oral gel can be absorbed. This regime is contraindicated in patients taking warfarin or phenytoin because miconazole enhances their effects.

Lack of response may be due to poor patient compliance or to an underlying disorder, particularly iron deficiency. Systemic antifungal drugs without local measures are ineffective. Key features are summarised in Box 15.8.

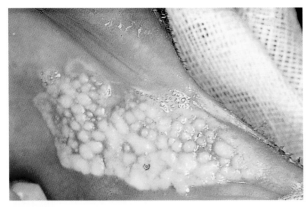

Fig. 15.28 Chronic hyperplastic candidosis. The typical site is the postcommissural buccal mucosa. This florid infection is white and nodular, clinically raising concern about potential malignancy. Most are flat and white only.

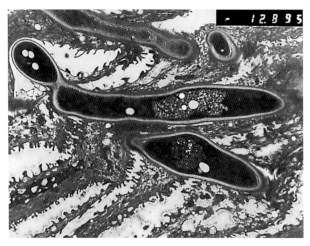

Fig. 15.30 Electron micrograph showing two candidal hyphae (very dark) growing through superficial keratinocytes of the oral mucosa. Note how they penetrate through the cells and do not grow around them.

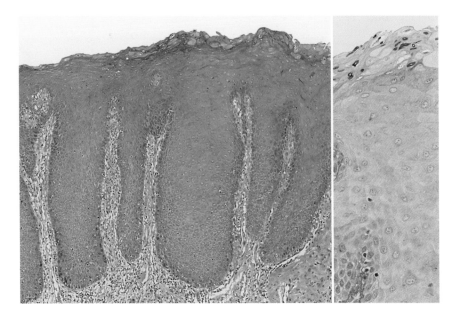

Fig. 15.29 Chronic hyperplastic candidosis. Thin parakeratin at the surface, long parallel-sided rete processes and a few inflammatory cells immediately below the epithelium (left). At higher power (right), a few candidal hyphae are in the keratin, appearing as magenta-coloured tubes in cross section in periodic acid Schiff (PAS) stain.

Web URL 15.3 NICE treatment guidance: http://cks.nice.org.uk/candida-oral

Treatment PMID: 24971864

Papillary hyperplasia of the palate

Extensive nodular fibroepithelial hyperplasia of the palate has often been considered a complication of candidosis, but candida alone is not the cause. This condition is discussed in Chapter 24.

Cause PMID: 6938680

Chronic hyperplastic candidosis

➔ Summary charts 15.1, 19.1 and 19.2 pp. 252, 314, 315

The alternative name of *candidal leukoplakia* reveals the controversial nature of this condition, in which chronic low level candidosis induces a localised zone of epithelial keratosis. Unfortunately, candida will also readily infect the keratotic lesions of true leukoplakia (Ch. 19) to produce the same clinical appearance. As many leukoplakias have no specific features, it may not be possible to tell these two situations apart. However, a white patch caused entirely by candidal infection carries a minimal risk of developing squamous carcinoma.

Clinical features

Adults, typically males of middle age or older, are affected, and most are smokers. The usual sites are the postcommissural buccal mucosa and the dorsum of the tongue. The plaque is variable in thickness, often rough or irregular in texture and tightly adherent. It will not rub off. Angular stomatitis may be confluent with plaques on the postcommissural mucosa.

When the candida infection is more florid, lesions develop an erythematous background or speckling and resemble speckled leukoplakia, a high-risk lesion for developing carcinoma (Fig. 15.28).

Pathology

The surface epithelium is parakeratotic and contains candidal hyphae. They are often sparse and elicit little or no inflammatory response, just a few neutrophils focally. PAS stain shows the hyphae growing (as in thrush) directly through the epithelial cells of the keratin layer (Figs 15.29 and 15.30) to the prickle cell layer, but no further. Candida induces mild hyperplasia, and often there is rete hyperplasia with long parallel-sided processes. Inflammation in the connective tissue is mild.

If dysplasia is present on biopsy, the lesion is a leukoplakia with superimposed candidal infection and not chronic hyperplastic candidosis.

Management

After confirmation of the diagnosis by histology or a scraping for hyphae, antifungal treatment is provided, but eradication of infection is difficult in this chronic infection. Usually miconazole gel is effective, but may need supplementing with a systemic antifungal drug such as fluconazole for two weeks. Accompanying angular cheilitis needs concurrent treatment, and denture hygiene and efforts to reduce the oral load of candida are required as described for denture stomatitis. Underlying anaemia may contribute and should be treated first, and ideally smoking should cease. These interventions not targeted to the lesion itself are often the key to success.

Long-term intermittent antifungal therapy may be required. Excision of the candidal plaque alone is of little value, as the infection can recur in the same site even after skin grafting.

If, after all these interventions, the plaque remains, consideration must be given to the fact that it may be a leukoplakia with superimposed candida infection and require follow up as a potentially malignant lesion. Although a potential for malignant change exists, the risk is low.

Review PMID: 12907694

Chronic mucocutaneous candidosis

syndromes → Summary chart 15.1 p. 351

These syndromes are all rare, but difficult to manage. Classification is complex now that many types can be classified by their causative genes.

The significance of these conditions is to recognise them when **chronic** *Candida* infection presents with very florid involvement, particularly of skin, nails and mucosa, proves resistant to treatment, or presents in childhood or adolescence.

All seem to be caused by immunodeficiency that is relatively selective for fungi or candida in particular, and one type is autoimmune. Family history is variable.

Review PMID: 20859203

Autoimmune polyendocrine syndrome I or endocrine candidosis syndrome is defined by hypoparathyroidism,

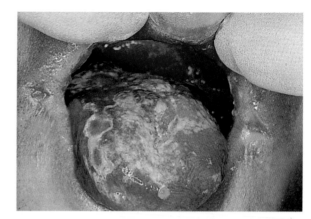

Fig. 15.31 Chronic mucocutaneous candidosis. Extensive red and white patches throughout the oral mucosa and angular cheilitis.

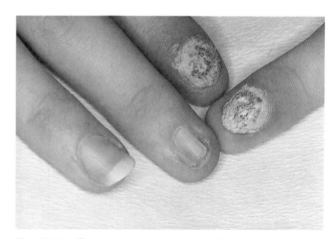

Fig. 15.32 Chronic mucocutaneous candidosis. Damage to fingernails through chronic infection in one of the more severe types.

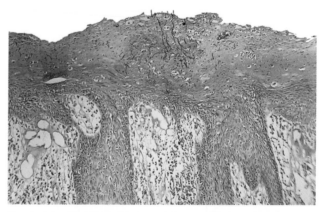

Fig. 15.33 Chronic mucocutaneous candidosis. At high power the thick parakeratin layer at the surface of this lesion is seen to be invaded by numerous fungal hyphae, as seen in simple chronic hyperplastic candidosis.

Box 15.9   Features of autoimmune polyendocrine syndrome I

- Genetic: usually autosomal recessive
- Hypoparathyroidism
- Adrenocortical insufficiency
- Chronic mucocutaneous candidosis
- Type 1 diabetes
- Autoimmune keratitis of the eye
- Malabsorption and diarrhoea
- Autoimmune hepatitis

adrenocortical insufficiency and chronic mucocutaneous candidosis, though many other features can present before the classical features are evident (Box 15.9). Inheritance can be autosomal recessive or dominant, and onset is in the first two decades of life. Failure of an immune regulator gene allows autoreactive T cells to escape deletion in the thymus during development. There are multiple autoantibodies to endocrine glands and against interferons, which are diagnostic. Candidosis is usually the presenting feature with thick plaques and red areas at any or all sites in the mouth, spreading to the pharynx and oesophagus.

This form of candidosis is potentially malignant, and 20% of patients may develop oral or oesophageal carcinoma.

Treatment of the candida infection must be aggressive and involves multiple agents. In children care must be taken to avoid finger sucking as infection will spread to wet skin and may be intractable. Hypoplastic dental defects are frequently also present.

General review PMID: 15141045

Other types of mucocutaneous candidosis are recognised, with variable inheritance, severity and specific gene defects. Some arise from autoimmune failure as a result of major histocompatibility complex gene mutations, and others are associated with autoantibodies to interleukin 17, STAT1 mutations reducing levels of interleukin (IL)-17 or other cytokines, or defects that compromise killing of candida by neutrophils. Mild forms are indistinguishable from sporadic cases of chronic hyperplastic candidosis (Figs 15.31–15.33). More severe forms may have susceptibility to bacterial infection or a range of other diseases. Thymoma and myasthenia gravis are associated with those types with autoantibodies against IL 17.

Summary chart 15.1   Summary of the types of oral candidal infection and their management.

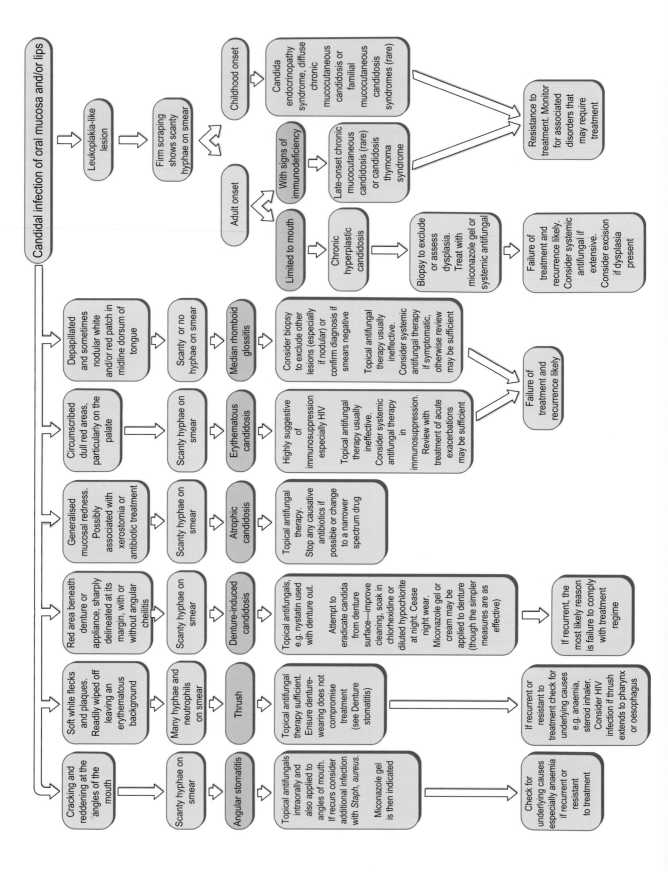

Summary chart 15.2   Differential diagnosis and management of the common and important causes of multiple oral ulcers with acute onset.

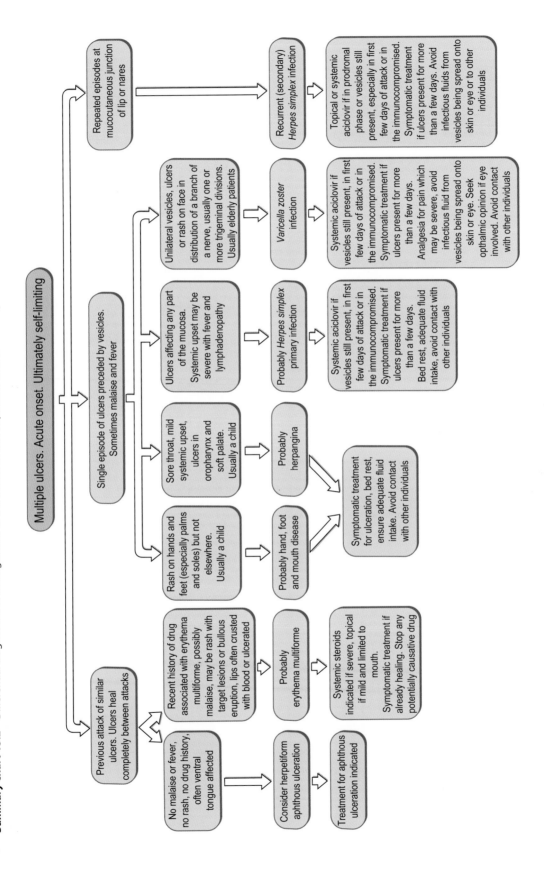

Appendix 15.1

Recommendations are aligned with NICE guidance http://cks.nice.org.uk/candida-oral

Confirm diagnosis with smear (most types) or biopsy (chronic hyperplastic candidosis) unless presentation is typical

Check history for predisposing causes which may require treatment

If candidosis is recurrent or not responsive to treatment, test for anaemia, folate and vitamin B_{12} deficiency and perform a urine test for diabetes

If a denture is worn:

* Stop night-time wear
* Check denture hygiene and advise
* Soak denture overnight in antifungal (dilute hypochlorite, chlorhexidine mouthwash) or, less effective, apply miconazole gel to denture fit surface while worn

If a steroid inhaler is used, check it is being used correctly, preferably with a spacer. Advise to rinse mouth out after use.

Drug treatments

Presentation	Generalised or severe	Localised or mild infection including chronic hyperplastic form	Angular stomatitis	Immunosuppression or otherwise resistant to treatment*
Drug of choice and regime	Fluconazole 50 mg/day for 7 days, repeated if necessary. *or* Nystatin suspension 100,000 units/mL (less effective)	Miconazole gel 20 mg/mL Apply QDS** if lesion localised	Apply miconazole gel 20 mg/mL QDS to the angles of the mouth 10 days or fusidic acid cream	Start with miconazole or nystatin, consider fluconazole 50 mg/day for 7–14 days
Notes	Amphotericin is no longer recommended as first-line treatment in primary care due to poor evidence base and is no longer available in the UK Fluconazole is reserved for severe infections because of the risk of resistance	Most effective if lesion accessible for application For recurrent infection in white patches fluconazole may be required simultaneously	Must treat intraoral infection simultaneously. This is always present even if not evident	Itraconazole has a higher risk of adverse effects and is not recommended for use in primary care
Cautions	Avoid in liver dysfunction and those taking drugs metabolised by the liver including warfarin, statins and some immunosuppressants. Avoid in pregnancy	Miconazole oral gel is absorbed, particularly if applied to denture fit surface. Avoid in liver dysfunction and those taking drugs metabolised by the liver including warfarin, statins and some immunosuppressants. Avoid in pregnancy	No adverse effects if only small amounts are applied as described above	Seek advice before prescribing for those on immunosuppressive drugs, especially ciclosporin

If there is conspicuous papillary hyperplasia of the palate, consider treatment (cryosurgery or excision) after treatment when inflammation has subsided. The irregular surface predisposes to recurrence of candidosis.

*Candidal resistance to azole drugs is possible, but failure of treatment is more likely to result from non-compliance with local measures such as denture wear and cleaning or an untreated underlying condition.

**Quater in die sumendus*, meaning take four times a day.

Diseases of the oral mucosa: non-infective stomatitis | 16

ULCERS

→ Summary charts 16.2 and 16.3 pp. 280, 281

Ulcers are breaks in the continuity of the epithelial covering of the body, and their general features are discussed at the start of Chapter 15.

Clinically, dividing ulcers into those that are persistent and those that are recurrent is a useful first step in differential diagnosis. Most oral ulcers heal after a few days to 2 weeks depending on their size, more rapidly on the floor of mouth or buccal mucosa than on the palate or gingiva. Recurrent oral ulcers are those that recur singly or in crops at the same or different sites. Recurrent ulcers have few common causes.

It is important to distinguish recurrent oral ulceration, which has a few causes, from recurrent aphthous ulceration (recurrent aphthous stomatitis), which is a specific condition.

General review diagnosis ulcers PMID: 26650694

TRAUMATIC ULCERS

→ Summary charts 16.2 and 16.3 pp. 280, 281

Traumatic ulcers are usually caused by biting, denture trauma or chemical trauma and arise at trauma-prone sites such as lip, buccal mucosa or adjacent to a denture flange. They are tender, have a yellowish-grey floor of fibrin slough and red margins (Fig. 16.1). Inflammation, swelling and erythema are variable, depending on the cause and time since trauma. There is no induration unless the site is scarred from repeated episodes of trauma. Occasionally, a large ulcer is caused by biting after a dental local anaesthetic (see Fig. 39.1). Biting trauma may produce two small adjacent ulcers matching cusps of upper and lower opposing teeth.

Chemical trauma is usually accidentally self-inflicted or iatrogenic. Etchant, hypochlorite and silver nitrate are just a few of the caustic agents used in dentistry that can cause mucosal ulcers after sometimes quite short contact time. Some patients continue to believe that aspirin is effective for toothache if held against the alveolus to dissolve. The result is local whitening caused by epithelial necrosis, followed by ulceration.

Traumatic ulcers heal in days after elimination of the cause. If they persist for more than 10 days without reduction in size and symptoms, or there is any other cause for suspicion as to the cause, biopsy should be carried out to exclude other diseases. Biopsy is not otherwise helpful because the histological features are of non-specific inflammation and repair only.

Eosinophilic ulcer (atypical or traumatic eosinophilic granuloma)

This condition may present as a deep ulcer or as a mass with an ulcerated surface. The cause is unknown, but an unusual response to trauma is suspected. A history of trauma is not always present.

Eosinophilic ulcers have a worrying presentation, often resembling carcinoma and exceeding 10 mm in diameter and enlarging rapidly before stabilising. The ulcers are usually on the tongue but also develop on the gingivae and, occasionally, other sites. Most are in adults of middle age or older, but a characteristic presentation is in infants in the first year of life where erupting lower incisors repeatedly traumatise the ventral tongue or lower lip on feeding (Riga-Fede disease). A concerning feature is failure to heal, and eosinophilic ulcers may persist for many months, during which the cellular inflammatory infiltrate below expands, raising the ulcer above the adjacent mucosa. Such nodular ulcerated lesions are sometimes called *traumatic ulcerative granulomas* (with stromal eosinophilia) and can mimic lymphoma histologically.

In practice, lesions usually heal spontaneously within 3–10 weeks, but biopsy will often trigger more rapid resolution.

Pathology

Biopsy is usually undertaken to exclude carcinoma or malignant disease because of size, induration and failure to heal. It is therefore unfortunate that the histological appearances can also be worrying and somewhat resemble some types of lymphoma. A mixed inflammatory infiltrate of eosinophils and pale macrophages and endothelial cells extends deeply, disrupting underlying tissues, and there may be suspicion of cytological atypia and mitotic activity.

Eosinophilic ulcer case series PMID: 8515985

Traumatic ulcerative granuloma PMID: 3884130 and 9415340

Factitious ulceration (self-inflicted oral ulcers)

Factitious ulcers in the mouth are rare and usually associated with psychosocial disorders in which the patient gains 'benefit' from producing their lesions in some way or

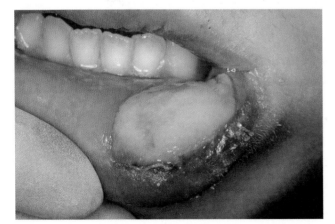

Fig. 16.1 A large traumatic ulcer on the lower lip. Note the colour of the fibrin slough, distinct from the keratin of a white patch, and the well-defined epithelial margin with minimal inflammation.

Table 16.1   Diseases in which the ulcers have the features of recurrent aphthous stomatitis (not including those associated through deficiency states)

Disease	Features
Behçet's disease	See text
MAGIC syndrome	Mouth And Genital ulcers with Inflamed Cartilage, a variant of Behçet's disease with relapsing polychondritis
PFAPA syndrome	Periodic Fever, Aphthous stomatitis, Pharyngitis, and cervical Adenitis, a disease of young children of unknown cause, usually treated with steroids, ultimately self-limiting. Probably a genetic auto-inflammatory disease. Monthly fever rising as high as 41°C for 3–5 days with mucosal inflammation and enlarged nodes
HIV infection	Often associated with ulcers of major aphthous type

another. Rarely, factitious oral ulceration has been a prelude to suicide.

The usual presentation is a non-healing ulcer in the anterior mouth, often easily visible, caused by repeated physical trauma, but presentation and methods of inducing the injury are diverse (Box 16.1). Even self-extraction of teeth has been reported.

Biopsy may be performed to exclude organic disease. Underlying emotional disturbance is typically well concealed, and definitive diagnosis is often difficult.

Self-harm is also a recognised manifestation of a variety of medical conditions: autism, familial dysautonomia, Lesch-Nyhan and Tourette syndromes and other causes of learning difficulties.

Unintended factitious injury can also follow repetitive habits such as picking at the gingival margin with a fingernail, but the degree of trauma is then minor and ulcers rarely develop.

RECURRENT APHTHOUS STOMATITIS

→ Summary charts 15.2 and 16.2 pp. 252, 280

Recurrent aphthae constitute the most common oral mucosal disease and affect as much as 25% of the population at some time in their life. Many cases are mild, and no treatment is sought.

There are three presentations of recurrent aphthous stomatitis (often called *recurrent aphthous ulceration* or just *recurrent aphthae*), each of which is defined by its clinical presentation.

Ulcers similar and sometimes identical to aphthous stomatitis can be a feature of other diseases or syndromes. Whether these are truly aphthous stomatitis is unclear (Table 16.1).

PFAPA case series PMID: 24237762 and 19889105

MAGIC case series PMID: 4014306

Clinical features

Ulcers frequently start in childhood. Recurrences increase in frequency until early adult life or a little later, then gradually wane. Recurrent aphthae are rare in the elderly, particularly the edentulous unless affected by a haematological deficiency. The great majority of patients are of high or middle socioeconomic status and are non-smokers.

Many patients have prodromal symptoms of pricking or sensitivity at the site for a few hours or a day before the ulcer forms. There is a brief period of erythema before the ulcer appears. The ulcers have a smooth sharply defined margin with an erythematous rim in the enlarging phase. The erythematous rim reduces once the ulcer reaches its full size, and while it heals, the margin becomes irregular or less well defined. Typical features common to all types of recurrent aphthae are summarised in Box 16.2.

Box 16.2   Typical features of recurrent aphthae

- Onset frequently in childhood but peak in adolescence or early adult life
- Attacks at variable but sometimes relatively regular intervals
- Most patients are otherwise healthy
- A few have haematological defects
- Most patients are non-smokers
- Usually self-limiting eventually
- Ulcers often preceded by a prodromal phase
- Ulcers almost never occur on keratinised mucosa

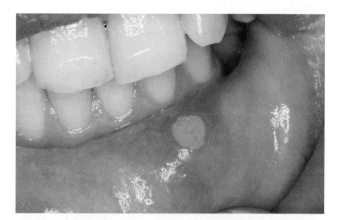

Fig. 16.2   Aphthous stomatitis, minor form. A single, relatively large shallow ulcer in a typical site. There is a narrow band of periulcer erythema. These features are non-specific, and the diagnosis must be made primarily on the basis of the history.

Minor aphthous stomatitis is the most common type, and the usual history is one or crops of several painful ulcers recurring at intervals of a few weeks. Aphthae typically affect only the non-keratinised mucosa, usually the labial and buccal mucosa, sulcuses, or lateral borders of the tongue (Fig. 16.2). Individual minor aphthae persist for 7–10 days, then heal without scarring. Often all ulcers in a crop develop and heal more or less synchronously. Unpredictable

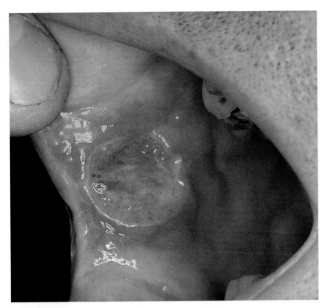

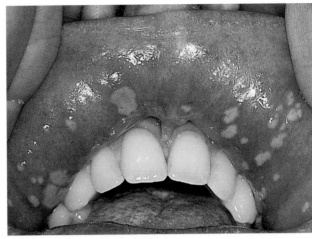

Fig. 16.5 Recurrent aphthous stomatitis, herpetiform type. There are numerous small, rounded and pinpoint ulcers, some of which are coalescing. The surrounding mucosa is lightly erythematous and the overall picture is highly suggestive of viral infection, but the attacks are recurrent and no virus can be isolated.

Fig. 16.3 Aphthous stomatitis, major type. This large, deep ulcer with considerable surrounding erythema has been present for several weeks.

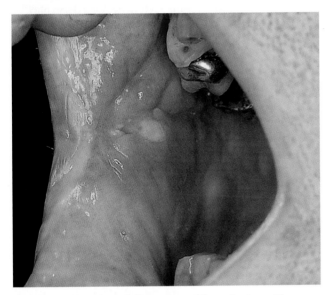

Fig. 16.4 Recurrent aphthous stomatitis, major type. The same ulcer shown in Fig. 16.3, but healing. The ulcer is much smaller, but there is scarring and puckering of the surrounding mucosa.

Box 16.3   Types of recurrent aphthae

Minor aphthae (Fig. 16.2)
- The most common type
- Non-keratinised mucosa affected
- Ulcers are shallow, rounded, 3–7 mm across, with an erythematous margin and yellowish floor
- One or several ulcers may be present

Major aphthae (Fig. 16.3)
- Uncommon
- Ulcers frequently several centimetres across
- Sometimes mimic a malignant ulcer
- Ulcers persist for several months
- Masticatory mucosa, such as the dorsum of the tongue or occasionally the gingivae, may be involved
- Scarring may follow healing (Fig. 16.4)

Herpetiform aphthae (Fig. 16.5)
- Uncommon
- Non-keratinised mucosa affected
- Ulcers are 1–2 mm across
- Dozens or hundreds may be present
- May coalesce to form irregular ulcers
- Widespread bright erythema round the ulcers

---

remissions of several months may be noted. In severe cases, ulcers are more numerous, and new crops may develop and heal continuously at different sites, without remission.

Major aphthous stomatitis is rare and causes single large ulcers or occasionally two or three at a time. These are much larger than in the minor form and persist for many weeks. They usually affect the soft palate, fauces, buccal mucosa and lateral tongue (Figs 16.3 and 16.4). This type may occasionally develop on keratinised mucosa. These ulcers heal with scarring. Ulcers can be designated as major form on the basis of either size or duration. A cut off of 10 mm is often taken as the upper limit of the minor form, but size should not be an absolute criterion. The pain of major aphthae can interfere with eating.

Herpetiform aphthous stomatitis is also rare and causes crops of many tiny ulcers, as many as 100 at a time, usually in the floor of mouth and ventral tongue (Fig. 16.5). The background mucosa is red, giving a resemblance to herpetic ulceration, but viral infection is not the cause.

The three types are summarised in Box 16.3.

Aetiology

The main factors thought to contribute are shown in Box 16.4. None completely explain the disease, but different factors may apply to different individuals or subgroups of patients

Genetic factors There is good evidence for a genetic predisposition. The family history is often positive, and the disease affects identical more frequently than non-identical twins. No genetic marker has been found. In the possibly related Behçet's disease (see later in this chapter), the evidence for a genetic predisposition is much stronger.

- Genetic predisposition
- Exaggerated response to trauma
- Infections
- Immunological abnormalities
- Gastrointestinal disorders
- Haematological deficiencies
- Hormonal disturbances
- Stress

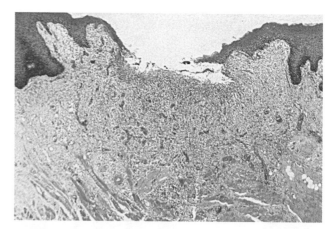

Fig. 16.6   Recurrent aphtha. Section of an early ulcer showing the break in the epithelium, the inflammatory cells in the floor and the inflammatory changes more deeply where numerous dilated vessels can be seen.

Trauma Patients often blame ulcers on trauma. There is some evidence that minor trauma is more likely to develop into an ulcer in a susceptible individual, and most ulcers are on the less trauma-resistant lining mucosa. The evidence for this is stronger in Behçet's disease.

Infections There is no evidence that aphthae are directly due to any microbes either causing infection or triggering immune reactions. An extensive range of oral commensals, pathogens, bacteria, viruses and unusual organisms such as mycoplasmas and L-forms have been investigated fruitlessly.

Immunological abnormalities The formation and healing of an ulcer involves inflammatory and immune mechanisms, but there is no evidence any are causal, and the disease is not autoimmune. There is no association with atopy or other known allergens despite many patients linking ulcers to dietary components. Aphthae lack virtually all features of typical autoimmune diseases. They also fail to respond reliably to immunosuppressive drugs and become more severe in the immune deficiency state induced by HIV infection.

Gastrointestinal disease Aphthae are only rarely associated with gastrointestinal disease such as coeliac disease, and then as a result of a deficiency secondary to malabsorption, particularly of vitamin B_{12} or folate.

Haematological deficiencies Deficiencies of vitamin B_{12}, folate or iron have been reported in as many as 20% of patients with aphthae. Such deficiencies are more frequent in patients whose aphthae start or worsen in middle age or later, have more than three ulcers at a time or very frequent or unremitting attacks. In many such patients, the deficiency is latent, the haemoglobin is within normal limits, and the main sign is micro- or macrocytosis of the red cells. In patients who thus prove to be vitamin B_{12} or folate deficient, remedying the deficiency may bring rapid resolution of the ulcers.

Hormonal factors In a few women, aphthae are associated with the luteal phase of the menstrual cycle, but there is no strong evidence that hormone treatment is reliably effective. Pregnancy is often associated with remission.

'Stress' Some patients relate exacerbations in times of stress, and some studies have reported a correlation. However, stress is notoriously difficult to quantify, and some studies have found no association.

HIV infection Aphthous stomatitis is a recognised feature of HIV infection. Its frequency and severity are related to the degree of immune deficiency, as discussed later.

Non-smoking It has long been established that recurrent aphthae are a disease, almost exclusively, of non-smokers, and this is one of the few consistent findings. Recurrent aphthae may also start when smoking is abandoned (but restarting does not induce remission), and quitting using nicotine supplements seems to prevent this. The reasons are unclear.

In brief, therefore, deficiencies of iron, folate or B_{12} are the most significant predisposing factors because these may be secondary to another more significant condition and because addressing them may cure or ameliorate the condition.

Pathology

Biopsy plays no role in the diagnosis except to exclude carcinoma in the case of clinically worrying major aphthae or to exclude viral infection in herpetiform aphthae.

If performed, biopsy in the prodromal phase reveals an initial lymphocytic infiltration of the epithelium, followed by destruction of the epithelium and non-specific acute and chronic inflammation (Fig. 16.6). Aphthae are not preceded by vesicles.

Diagnosis

Diagnosis is almost exclusively by history, primarily recurrences of self-healing intraoral ulcers at fairly regular intervals. Almost the only other condition with this history is Behçet's disease. Usually, increasing frequency of ulcers brings the patient to seek treatment. A detailed history of the ulcer number, shape, size, site, duration, frequency of attacks is required.

Most patients appear well, but haematological investigation is particularly important in older patients and those with recent exacerbations in frequency of crops, ulcer size or pain. Routine blood indices are informative, and usually the most important finding is an abnormal mean corpuscular volume (MCV). If macro- or microcytosis is present, further investigation is necessary to find and remedy the cause. Treatment of vitamin B_{12} deficiency or folate deficiency is sometimes sufficient to control or abolish aphthae. Applying the most sensitive tests of iron, folate and B_{12} deficiency identifies more patients who can benefit from treatment, and they will often respond to supplementation despite apparently having very mild or early deficiency.

Key features for diagnosis are shown in Table 16.2.

Medical conditions associated PMID: 9421219

Management

Apart from the minority with underlying systemic disease, treatment is empirical and palliative only. Despite

Table 16.2   Checklist for diagnosis of recurrent aphthae

	Check for	Comments
History	• Recurrences	The history is all-important
	• Pattern? Minor, major or herpetiform type?	
	• Onset as child or teenager	
	• Family history	
	• Distribution only on non-keratinised mucosa	
	• Signs or symptoms of Behçet's disease (ocular, genital, skin, joint lesions) (Box 13.4)	
Examination	• Discrete well-defined ulcers	Exclude other diseases with specific,
	• Scarring or soft palate involvement suggesting major aphthae	appearances, e.g. lichen planus or vesiculobullous disease
Investigations	• Anaemia, iron, red cell folate and vitamin B_{12} status	Used to exclude underlying conditions,
	• History of diarrhoea, constipation or blood in stools suggesting gastrointestinal disease, e.g. coeliac disease or malabsorption	especially in patients with onset in later life

numerous clinical trials, no medication gives completely reliable relief. Low-potency and topical agents should be tried first. Some patients report that changing toothpastes is helpful.

Reassurance and education Patients need to understand that the ulcers may not be curable but can be made bearable with symptomatic treatment. Reducing the number of attacks is more difficult to address, but some treatments are successful, particularly if attacks are frequent. The condition usually wanes eventually of its own accord, although after many years.

Corticosteroids Some patients get relief from hydrocortisone, 2.5 mg, oromucosal tablets allowed to dissolve next to the ulcer three times per day. These low-potency corticosteroids adhere to the mucosa to provide a high local concentration of drug and are suitable for use in dental practice. They probably reduce the painful inflammation but do not speed healing much or reduce frequency of attacks. They are best applied in the very early, asymptomatic stages.

Triamcinolone dental paste (Adcortyl in Orabase) is no longer available in the UK and is superseded by the previously mentioned mucosal adhesive tablets.

Tetracycline mouth rinses Trials in both Britain and the United States showed that tetracycline rinses significantly reduced both the frequency and severity of aphthae. Best reserved for herpetiform aphthae. The contents of a tetracycline capsule (250 mg) can be stirred in a little water and held in the mouth for 2–3 minutes, three times daily. However, there are few easily soluble tetracycline preparations, and use carries a risk of superinfection by *Candida albicans*.

Chlorhexidine A 0.2% solution has also been used as a mouth rinse for aphthae. Used three times daily after meals and held in the mouth for at least 1 minute, it has been claimed to reduce the duration and discomfort of aphthous stomatitis.

Topical salicylate preparations Salicylates have an anti-inflammatory action and also have local effects. Preparations of choline salicylate in a gel can be applied to aphthae. These preparations, which are available over the counter, appear to help some patients.

Local analgesics These provide only symptomatic relief, but benzydamine mouthwash or spray helps some patients. Topical lidocaine or benzocaine sprays and gels are more effective but can only be used in limited doses and for a short time. They do not require prescription in the UK.

Treatment of major aphthae Major aphthae, whether or not there is underlying disease such as HIV infection, may

sometimes be so painful, persistent and resistant to conventional treatment as to be disabling. Reportedly effective treatments include azathioprine, cyclosporin, colchicine and dapsone, but thalidomide is probably most reliably effective. Their use may be justified for major aphthae even in otherwise healthy persons if they are disabled by the pain and difficulty of eating. However, such drugs can only be given under specialist supervision.

Complementary and experimental treatments Common, relatively inconsequential diseases that are difficult to treat will always be used to promote treatments without a good evidence base. While the disease remits spontaneously and unpredictably, and measurement of symptoms is imprecise, it is difficult to prove whether treatments are either effective or ineffective.

Possible treatments for recurrent aphthae are summarised in Appendix 16.1.

RAS review PMID: 21812866 and 17850936

Disease associations PMID: 22233487

Cochrane review treatment PMID: 22972085

BEHÇET'S DISEASE

→ Summary chart 16.2 p. 280

Behçet's disease was originally defined as a triad of oral aphthous stomatitis, genital ulceration and uveitis. However, it is a systemic vasculitis of small blood vessels and affects many more organ systems than suggested by this limited definition.

The importance of making the diagnosis is indicated by the life-threatening risk of thrombosis, of blindness or brain damage.

Clinical

Behçet's disease is particularly common in Turkey (Behçet was a Turk), central Asia, the Middle East and Japan but is less common in emigrants from these areas and is rare in those from Europe, the Americas and Africa. This matches the geographic incidence of the human leukocyte antigen (HLA) B51 allele (see later in this chapter).

Patients are usually young adult males between 20 and 40 years old. Patients suffer one of four patterns of disease:

Mucocutaneous Oral aphthae are the most consistent feature, are not distinguishable from common aphthous stomatitis and may be of any of the three types. There is

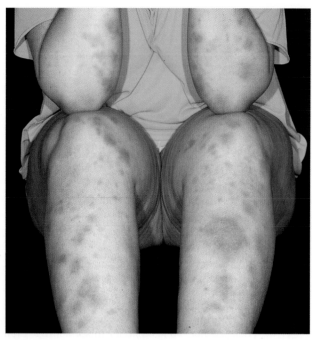

Fig. 16.7 Erythema nodosum. This is the commonest skin manifestation of Behçet's disease. *(From Habib, F., 2004. Clinical Dermatology: A colour guide to diagnosis and therapy, fourth ed. Mosby, Philadelphia.)*

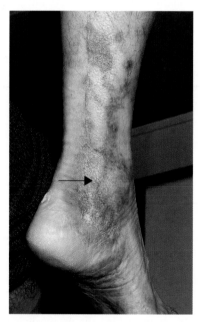

Fig. 16.8 Thrombophlebitis in Behçet's disease. Inflammation and pigmentation highlight the sites of veins *(arrow)* and their valves.

often genital ulceration and a variety of rashes including erythema nodosum (Fig. 16.7) and vasculitis (Fig. 16.8).

Arthritic Joint involvement with or without mucocutaneous involvement. The large weight-bearing joints are most affected. There is pain, but no destructive arthritis and only a few joints are involved. The pain may be relapsing or constant.

Neurological This type may occur with or without other features and is usually a late stage. Vasculitis within the brain causes a variety of neurological symptoms including sensory and motor disturbances, confusion and fits.

Table 16.3	The International Criteria for Behçet's Disease 2010 together with their overall incidence in all patients*		
Sign group	Criteria	Points	Incidence
Oral aphthous stomatitis	Three attacks or more in one year	2	80%†
Genital ulceration	Recurrent ulcers or scarring	2	80%
Ocular lesions	Uveitis or retinal vasculitis	2	50%
Skin lesions	Follicular pustular rash or erythema nodosum	1	75%
Central nervous system involvement	Any involvement	1	10%
Vascular manifestations	Superficial phlebitis, deep vein thrombosis, large vein thrombosis, arterial thrombosis, and aneurysm	1	30%
Positive pathergy test (optional to include)		1	5-60%‡

*A score of 4 or more points predicts Behçet's disease with 95% certainty, 98% if the pathergy test is performed. Incidence of features varies between populations.
†100% using older criteria, previously a requirement for diagnosis.
‡The higher figure is for patients from the middle East and central Asia.

Thrombosis of vessels causes raised intracranial pressure, blurred vision and headache.

Ocular This type may also be solitary or accompany other types. There may be uveal inflammation or vasculitis and thrombosis of the retinal arteries, either of which can lead rapidly to blindness if not treated.

Behçet's review PMID: 23597962 and 23007742

Aetiology

The aetiology is unknown, but the disease has features including circulating immune complexes, high levels of cytokine secretion and activation of lymphocytes and macrophages in the circulation. These suggest an immune-mediated reaction, and it is presumed that this may be a response to an unknown infectious agent, possibly through immune cross reaction between pathogen and host heat shock proteins.

The racial distribution suggests a strong genetic component and HLA tissue types are linked, most strongly to HLA-B51. This is a common allele and so is not of use in diagnosis but can predict ocular lesions.

Behçet's update PMID: 26487500

Diagnosis and management

Oral aphthae are frequently the first manifestation. Behçet's disease should therefore be considered in the differential diagnosis of aphthous stomatitis, particularly in patients in a racial group at risk, and the medical history should be checked for the features shown in Table 16.3. The frequency of other manifestations is highly variable.

Box 16.13   Pemphigus vulgaris: pathology

- Loss of intercellular adherence of suprabasal prickle cells (acantholysis)
- Formation of clefts immediately superficial to the basal cells
- Extension of clefts to form intraepithelial vesicles (Fig. 16.27)
- Rupture of vesicles and bullae to form ulcers
- High titre of circulating antibodies to desmogleins
- Binding of antibodies to desmosomes detectable by immunofluorescence staining

Box 16.14   Mucous membrane pemphigoid: typical features

- Females mainly affected and usually elderly
- Oral mucosa often the first site
- Involvement of the eyes, may cause scarring and blindness
- Skin involvement absent or minimal
- Indolent, non-fatal disease
- Oral bullae are subepithelial and sometimes seen intact

of circulating autoantibody. Oral lesions respond more slowly than skin lesions. Almost all immunosuppressive drugs can be effective. The anti-CD20 drug rituximab depletes B lymphocytes, reducing autoantibody titres, and is effective in treatment-resistant cases. Eventually severity wanes, and patients may be maintained on low doses of steroid or immunosuppressants.

Pemphigus vulgaris review PMID: 15888101

Controversies PMID: 22335787

Treatment PMID: 25934414 and skin 14632796

Pemphigus variants

These resemble pemphigus vulgaris clinically, but differ in their histological features, target antigens and response to treatment. Pemphigus vegetans is a benign localised form of pemphigus vulgaris. IgA pemphigus has autoantibodies of IgA class instead of the usual IgG_4, and mucosal involvement is rare. Pemphigus foliaceous has no mucosal involvement because the target antigen is only desmoglein 1.

Occasionally drugs trigger pemphigus; many can, but penicillamine is the usual cause.

Paraneoplastic pemphigus

Paraneoplastic pemphigus is a rare type of pemphigus seen in patients with malignant neoplasms, particularly lymphomas, leukaemias and Castleman's disease. There is severe mucosal but variable skin involvement, often with extension to nasal or oesophageal mucosa or the eye. The pathogenesis is the same except that, in addition to the desmoglein autoantibodies, there are antibodies against other desmosome components such as desmoplakins and also antibasement membrane antibodies, producing a confusing clinical picture with features of pemphigus, pemphigoid and erythema multiforme.

Histologically, the biopsy shows correspondingly mixed features with both suprabasal acantholysis and splitting along the basement membrane. Immunofluorescence is required for diagnosis. Indirect immunofluorescence using rat bladder as a substrate is the most specific test because it detects autoantibodies against the desmoplakin proteins.

The malignant neoplasm is usually known, but a third of cases present with pemphigus and a search for an underlying malignancy must be made. This type of pemphigus is very difficult to treat, may be intractable and often fatal. Aggressive immunosuppression is required.

Review PMID: 15063382 and 18940624

MUCOUS MEMBRANE PEMPHIGOID

→ Summary charts 16.2, 16.3 pp. 280, 281

Diseases of the pemphigoid group are uncommon chronic autoimmune diseases causing bullae and painful erosions as a result of separation of epithelium from the connective tissue (Box 16.14). An obsolete name for mucous membrane pemphigoid is *cicatricial pemphigoid*, meaning scarring pemphigoid, but scarring is not a prominent feature in the mouth, unlike in the eye.

Aetiology

In mucous membrane pemphigoid, the autoantibodies are directed against several basement membrane components, mostly against the BP180 antigen or less frequently integrins, laminin and type VII collagen. The antibodies are of IgG class and fix complement. Binding to the basement membrane causes complement activation, attracting and activating neutrophils to degrade the basement membrane. The result is that the epithelium falls off the connective tissue on the slightest trauma.

Clinical

Mucous membrane pemphigoid affects mostly women and has onset between the ages of 50 and 80 years. Blisters develop on the oral mucosa and in the eye, and less frequently in the vagina, pharynx, nose, pharynx and oesophagus.

Intraorally the common sites are gingivae, buccal mucosa, palate and tongue. Vesicles and blisters form and may be seen for a short while before they burst (Fig. 16.29) because the roof of the blister is formed by an intact resilient full thickness layer of epithelium, unlike the blisters in pemphigus. Bleeding into bullae can cause them to appear as blood blisters. However, the blisters soon break down to leave shallow ulcers with ragged margins (Fig. 16.30), sometimes with small flaps or tags of separated epithelium at their edges. Desquamative gingivitis (page 262) is a common manifestation (Fig. 16.31) and occasionally the only intraoral sign in mild disease.

The severity is very variable. Individual erosions are very painful and heal slowly over several weeks, but new blisters and erosions develop continuously.

The eye is involved less frequently that the mouth, producing conjunctivitis, erythema and erosions. Blisters inside the eyelids and over the sclera heal with scarring, distorting the lids and causing adhesions between the lids and the sclera. Approximately one-quarter of patients will develop eye lesions in the first 5 years of disease. Severity of eye involvement determines treatment because ultimately scarring can lead to blindness.

The skin is very rarely involved.

Clinical features are summarised in Box 16.14.

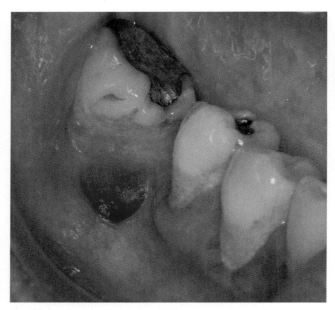

Fig. 16.29 Mucous membrane pemphigoid, an intact bulla at the junction of the attached gingiva and alveolar mucosa. The bulla fluid is lightly blood stained and visible through the intact pale yellow epithelial roof.

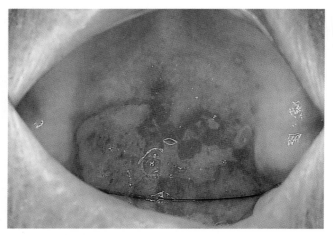

Fig. 16.30 Mucous membrane pemphigoid. Typical oral presentation with persistent erythema and ulceration of the palate. On close examination tags of epithelium are sometimes seen at the ulcer margins.

Diagnosis and management

In addition to the typical presentation, Nikolsky's sign (page 272) is typically positive.

The diagnosis is confirmed by biopsy and immunofluorescence microscopy and requires either an intact vesicle or a sample from the margin of a blister for best chance of positive immunofluorescence findings. Unfortunately, biopsy of such involved tissue is difficult because the epithelium may separate from the underlying tissue during biopsy, rendering it useless for diagnosis. Great care must be taken to obtain an intact specimen. A skin biopsy is preferable if skin lesions are present.

Histologically, there is loss of attachment and separation of the full thickness of the epithelium from the connective tissue at basement membrane level. The roof of a bulla is formed by intact full thickness epithelium (Fig. 16.32). The floor is formed by connective tissue alone, infiltrated by inflammatory cells.

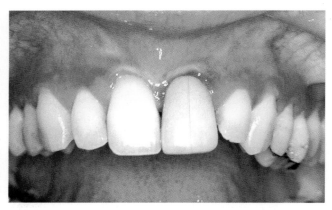

Fig. 16.31 Desquamative gingivitis as a result of mucous membrane pemphigoid. There is patchy reddening involving the attached gingivae around several teeth and in places the erythema extends to the alveolar mucosa. Unlike desquamative gingivitis caused by lichen planus, no white flecks or striae are present. Occasionally, tags of separating epithelium may be found.

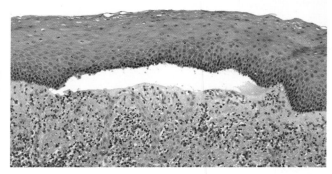

Fig. 16.32 Mucous membrane pemphigoid. Biopsy from clinically normal mucosa. The full thickness of the epithelium has separated cleanly from the underlying connective tissue to form a microscopic fluid-filled bulla. The weakened attachment of epithelium to connective tissue has separated with the slight trauma involved in biopsy.

Direct immunofluorescence reveals the site of autoantibody binding, its immunoglobulin class and any complement activation. In almost all cases immunoglobulin IgG and/or complement component 3 can be found along the basement membrane (Fig. 16.33). When both IgA and IgG antibodies are present, the clinical course is usually more severe and resistant to treatment.

Indirect immunofluorescence is less useful than in pemphigus as the autoantibodies circulate only at very low concentration. It is positive in just more than half of cases. Indirect immunofluorescence can be used to differentiate the target antigen by using a substrate of normal skin split along its basement membrane zone by incubation in concentrated salt solution. Whether the autoantibodies bind to the floor or roof of the split gives information on the localisation of the target antigen. Binding to the floor indicates the variant called *epidermolysis bullosa acquisita* (discussed later).

Mild disease or disease in remission can often be effectively controlled with topical corticosteroids. Doses are low and without systemic effects, and application in a vacuum-formed tray enhances effectiveness for gingival lesions. Moderate disease requires a high-potency steroid topically or dapsone if this is ineffective. If there is severe oral disease or involvement of other sites, systemic steroids with

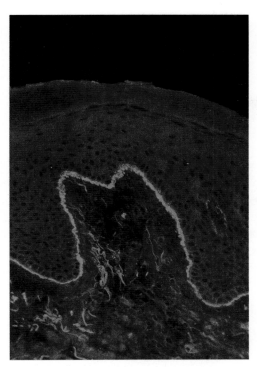

Fig. 16.33 Mucous membrane pemphigoid. Frozen tissue stained with fluorescent anti-C3 shows a line of fluorescence along the basement membrane indicating complement activation there. Intact mucosa is required for immunofluorescence, and biopsy is best performed in apparently normal mucosa, not in a lesion. (See Fig. 1.6.)

azathioprine as a steroid-sparing agent are used to induce remission before moving to less potent drugs. Non-responsive disease requires immunosuppressants such as mycophenolate.

Because of the possible risk to sight, ocular examination is necessary if early changes in the eyes are suspected. Minor eye involvement also responds to dapsone, but severe eye disease requires potent immunosuppression with steroids and azathioprine, cyclophosphamide, mycophenolate mofetil or infliximab to induce remission.

General review PMID: 15984952

Treatment PMID: 22727107

Bullous pemphigoid

Bullous pemphigoid is the commonest blistering disease of skin. It affects a similar population to mucous membrane pemphigoid, and the signs are similar. However, it affects the mouth in less than 10% of patients, producing the same superficial erosions as mucous membrane pemphigoid, and is treated in the same way. The eye is involved only very rarely.

Other pemphigoid variants

Linear IgA disease or linear IgA bullous dermatosis is a form of pemphigoid in which the autoantibodies binding to the basement membrane are of IgA class. Half of patients have intraoral blistering, and the eye may be involved. It can also arise in children.

Lichen planus pemphigoides is a hybrid condition resembling both lichen planus and pemphigoid, usually affecting the skin and very occasionally the mouth.

Epidermolysis bullosa acquisita is unrelated to the developmental condition epidermolysis bullosa and presents in

the same way as bullous pemphigoid. The autoantibodies are directed against the collagen type VII anchoring fibrils below the basement membrane. Both skin and mouth are often involved, and there is a mucosa-predominant form.

ERYTHEMA MULTIFORME

→ Summary charts 15.2 and 16.2 pp. 253, 280

This mucocutaneous hypersensitivity reaction affects the mouth in many cases and, in patients presenting to dentists, oral lesions may be the only sign. Erythema multiforme is one of the few causes of *recurrent* oral ulceration and also produces blisters.

Aetiology

Though the mechanism is unclear, erythema multiforme appears to be a cell-mediated hypersensitivity reaction. It is more likely in immunosuppression, HIV infection, systemic lupus erythematosus and during radiotherapy and chemotherapy.

Erythema multiforme may be triggered by many agents (Box 16.15), but 90% of attacks are precipitated by an infection, usually *herpes simplex* infection. Patients with herpes infections as the trigger have a genetic predisposition, the HLA DQw3 allele.

When patients have a triggering stimulus, it is usually 9–14 days before onset.

Clinical

Most patients are aged between 20 and 40 years, with a slight male predominance. Two forms are recognised. In the *minor form* only skin is involved and this is a relatively mild self-limiting condition. In the *major form* there are florid lesions on skin and oral, nasal and genital mucosae.

There is acute onset, sometimes preceded by vague arthralgia or slight fever for a day in the major form. Then the characteristic 'target' lesions appear, initially on arms and legs and spreading centrally. Each is a well-defined red macule a centimetre or more in diameter. During a period of a few hours to days, the centre becomes raised, with a bluish cyanotic centre. In severe cases, skin lesions blister and ulcerate centrally. New crops of lesions develop during a period of approximately 10 days. Oral and lip lesions appear a few days into the attack, most commonly anteriorly in the mouth on the buccal and labial mucosa and tongue. Target lesions are not seen intraorally; the oral lesions are inflamed patches with irregular blistering and broad, shallow irregular ulcers. On the lips, fibrin oozes continually and forms haemorrhagic crusts. There is severe pain.

Features are summarised in Box 16.16 and shown in Figs 16.34–16.36.

General review PMID: 22788803

Oral review PMID: 17767983 and 24034067

Difference from Stevens Johnson PMID: 7741539 and 15567361

Box 16.15 Triggers for erythema multiforme

- *Herpes simplex* infection, usually a cold sore
- Genital recurrent herpes
- Mycoplasmal pneumonia
- *Varicella zoster* infections
- Rarely drugs, penicillins

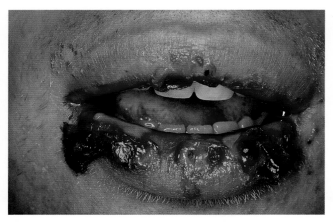

Fig. 16.34 Erythema multiforme. Ulceration of the vermilion of the lip with bleeding, swelling and crusting is characteristic.

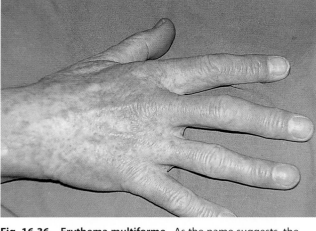

Fig. 16.36 Erythema multiforme. As the name suggests, the rash is variable and here shows only patchy erythema.

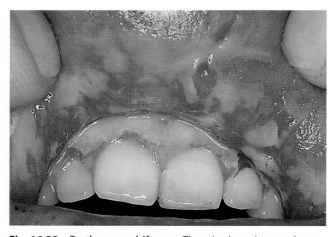

Fig. 16.35 Erythema multiforme. There is ulceration, erythema, sloughing of epithelium and a small vesicle centrally. The anterior part of the mouth and the lips are typically affected.

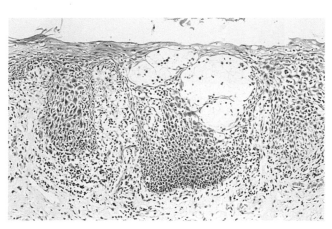

Fig. 16.37 Erythema multiforme. In this example there is necrosis of prickle cells, producing intraepithelial vesicles, much oedema but few inflammatory cells.

Box 16.16 Erythema multiforme: typical clinical features

- Adolescents or young adults, particularly males, mainly affected
- Lips frequently grossly swollen, split, crusted and bleeding (Fig. 16.34)
- Widespread irregular fibrin-covered erosions and erythema in the mouth (Fig. 16.35)
- Conjunctivitis may be associated
- Cutaneous target lesions or erythematous patches (Fig. 16.36)
- Attacks may recur at intervals of several months
- Recurrent but usually ultimately self-limiting

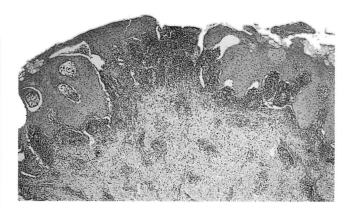

Fig. 16.38 Erythema multiforme. In this example there is a dense inflammatory infiltrate immediately below the epithelium and around blood vessels in the deeper corium. The epithelium is separating from the connective tissue, here along the basement membrane, and there is ulceration centrally.

Diagnosis and management

Diagnosis relies on the typical presentation, history of previous recurrent episodes and a trigger, if present. When only the mouth is involved, a biopsy may be required, but the appearances are very variable and this aids most by excluding alternative causes.

The histological appearances are variable. There are lymphocytes below the epithelium and basal cell degeneration with apoptosis similar to that in lichen planus, but with additional acute inflammation and accumulation of oedema fluid in and below the epithelium, producing intraepithelial vesicle or bulla formation (Figs 16.37 and 16.38).

The attack usually lasts for 3 or 4 weeks and is self-limiting without treatment in the minor form. However, oral lesions are painful, interfere with eating and fluid intake must be maintained. Unless already resolving, lesions seem to benefit from treatment with corticosteroids. A short reducing dose of prednisolone starting at around 60 mg/day for 3 days, tapering off over a week, is frequently given but has no good evidence base. Chlorhexidine will prevent secondary mucosal infection and maintain gingival health while tooth brushing is impossible. Eye lesions require specialist treatment.

Recurrences, usually at intervals of several months, for a year or two are characteristic and are sometimes increasingly severe. An attempt should be made to identify the trigger, though often none is identifiable. It is considered that recurrent *herpes simplex* infections trigger most cases, and whether or not this can be confirmed, treatment with continuous aciclovir for several months will suppress any triggering infection and confirm the link. In patients who have only oral lesions, mycoplasmal infection should be suspected and suppressed instead.

Web URL 16.1 Treatment: http://emedicine.medscape.com/article/1122915-treatment

Web URL 16.2 Guideline: http://www.pcds.org.uk/clinical-guidance/erythema-multiforme

STEVENS JOHNSON SYNDROME

→ Summary charts 15.2, 16.2 pp. 253, 280

This severe hypersensitivity reaction has many features in common with erythema multiforme but is now considered a separate entity on the basis of its severity, extent and causes. Toxic epidermal necrolysis is its most severe presentation. The mouth is always involved.

Unlike erythema multiforme, the trigger is usually a drug and sometimes mycoplasmal infection. Many drugs are implicated, but the most frequent causes are sulphonamides, allopurinol, and anticonvulsants. Some genetic predispositions are known for individual drugs.

Skin lesions are erythematous patches, target lesions or raised blisters that break down into ulcers with widespread detachment and loss of epithelium, sometimes in large sheets. Other organs may also be involved. Histopathology shows necrosis of the whole skin thickness by apoptosis with little inflammation.

Treatment is controversial, with immunosuppressants, cyclosporine and antibiotics to control skin infection and cessation of causative drugs. There is a high risk of death when the area of skin involved in toxic epidermal necrolysis is great.

Review PMID: 26769645

Web URL 16.3 Management guideline Stevens Johnson Syndrome: http://www.bad.org.uk/healthcare-professionals/clinical-standards/clinical-guidelines

TOOTHPASTE-INDUCED EPITHELIAL PEELING

Superficial epithelial desquamation can be mistaken for blistering by patients. It may be caused by detergents in toothpastes, particularly sodium lauryl sulphate, and is best managed by patient education and acceptance, or changing brand. However, the sloughing is often unnoticed or blamed on astringent or sharp foods. This condition appears to be of no significance, and it is not established whether it is an irritant or allergic phenomenon. The common sites are the lingual alveolar mucosa and buccal mucosa.

Experimental series PMID: 8811477

OTHER MUCOSAL ALLERGIC RESPONSES

Oral mucosa is rarely the site of allergic responses. Oral allergy syndrome is discussed in the next chapter.

Case series PMID: 1437060

ORAL SIGNS IN REACTIVE ARTHRITIS

The 'classical' presentation of reactive arthropathy, previously known as Reiter's disease, comprises arthritis, urethritis and conjunctivitis. Sexually transmitted *Chlamydia*

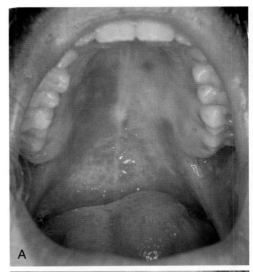

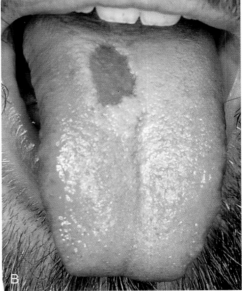

Fig. 16.39 Reactive arthritis oral signs. There is erythema and patches of depapillation on the tongue, which when multiple resemble erythema migrans. *(From Fehrnbach, M.J., Phelan, J.A., 2004. Immunity. In: Ibsen, O.A.C., Phelan, J.A. (Eds.), Oral Pathology for the dental hygienist, fourth ed. St Louis, Saunders.)*

infection or gut infections such as with *Salmonella sp.* or *Shigella sp.* usually precede arthritis by about 1–3 weeks. Patients are typically males between the ages of 20 and 40 years; 80% of them are HLA-B27 positive. Pain and swelling typically affect the knees, ankles and feet.

Antibiotics are given to eliminate the gut or other triggering infections; non-steroidal anti-inflammatory drugs are frequently effective for controlling joint pain. The disease may be self-limiting or recurrent and progressively debilitating.

Dental aspects

The temporomandibular joints can be involved with erosions but are not a major source of symptoms.

Oral manifestations develop in 15% of patients and are characteristic and consist of scalloped or circinate white lines somewhat resembling erythema migrans but involving all or any part of the mouth and the genital mucosa. In other cases there may be shallow erosions. Lesions are typically painless and frequently unnoticed.

General review: 18436339

MUCOCUTANEOUS LYMPH NODE SYNDROME (KAWASAKI'S DISEASE)

Kawasaki's disease is a self-limiting necrotising systemic vasculitis of children with a particular propensity to attack the coronary arteries. It presents with stomatitis and cervical lymphadenopathy.

Kawasaki's disease is endemic in Japan, Taiwan, Korea and adjacent countries and affects patients with these genetic backgrounds living elsewhere. It is increasingly recognised in European Caucasian populations and is the leading cause of childhood-acquired heart disease in Europe since the decline of rheumatic fever. It affects 8 in every 100,000 children in the UK.

The aetiology remains unknown. An infection is thought to trigger an immune reaction in those genetically predisposed, but many infections are implicated.

Small and medium-sized arteries are involved, infiltrated by neutrophils that destroy the elastic lamina and endothelial lining, weakening the artery, which dilates to produce aneurysms.

The features are summarised in Box 16.17.

In a dental setting, presentation mimics childhood viral illnesses but the involvement of lips and diffuse erythema of tongue without ulcers are characteristic. The tongue is bright red with prominent papillae, producing the strawberry appearance (Fig. 16.40). The cervical lymphadenopathy is

obvious, with nodes palpable and distinctively affecting only one side of the neck anterior to sternomastoid muscle. Almost every kind of rash except blisters can occur, but involvement of the soles and palms with peeling of skin from the tips of fingers and toes is a characteristic, but late, sign (Fig. 16.41).

Oral changes arise early in the disease. Suspected cases should be referred to hospital urgently without waiting to

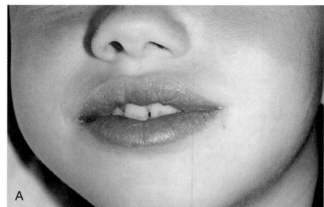

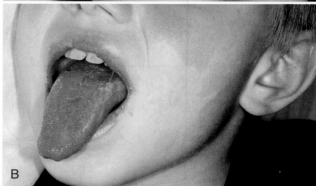

Fig. 16.40 Kawasaki's disease. Hyperaemia, crusting and cracking of the lips (A), bright red tongue with prominent papillae (strawberry tongue, B) and facial rash. *(From Paller, A.S., Mancini, A.J., 2016. Vasculitic disorders. In: Paller, A.S., Mancini, A.J. Hurwitz clinical pediatric dermatology. Elsevier, Amsterdam, pp. 495-508.e3.)*

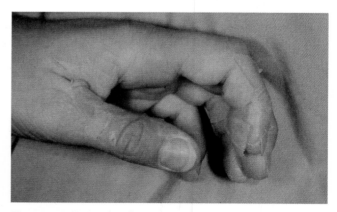

Fig. 16.41 Kawasaki's disease. The desquamative rash that characteristically affects the fingers and toes and perineum 7–10 days after onset of fever. The fingers are red and swollen before peeling starts. *(From Baselga, E., Hernandez-Martin, A., Torrelo, A., 2015. Immunologic, reactive, and purpuric disorders. In: Eichenfield, L.F., Frieden, I.J., Mathes, E.F., Zaenglein, A.L. (Eds.), Neonatal and infant dermatology. Saunders, Philadelphia, pp. 303-335.e10.)*

Box 16.17 Typical features of Kawasaki's disease

- Children under 5 years old affected
- Fever persisting for more than 5 days
- Marked irritability and malaise ('extreme misery')
- Generalised rash of variable type
- Red, swollen and peeling palms and soles
- Erythematous stomatitis with 'strawberry tongue'
- Swelling and cracking of the lips and pharynx
- Unilateral mass of swollen cervical lymph nodes
- Abdominal symptoms frequently
- Heart involvement in approximately 20%

see whether the fever persists more than 5 days, usually considered a required diagnostic criterion. Some patients have incomplete presentations with no fever, so a high index of suspicion is required.

There is no diagnostic test. Intravenous immunoglobulin and steroids are the main treatment. Aspirin is still used despite the risk of Reye's syndrome but without evidence of effect. Tumour necrosis factor blockade with infliximab is experimental but shows promise. Recovery takes many weeks or months, and the significant complications are coronary artery aneurysms and myocardial infarction. Treatment significantly reduces these complications, and early recognition and referral could be lifesaving. The overall mortality is around 1%.

Dental presentation PMID: 10230100 and 2717153

Treatment PMID: 26547265

MISCELLANEOUS MUCOSAL ULCERS

Wegener's granulomatosis

Mucosal ulceration is occasionally a feature of this disease but mainly in its established stage (Ch. 33). Clinically, ulceration may be widespread but is otherwise nonspecific.

Oral reactions to drugs

A great variety of drugs (see Box 16.9, Table 42.1 can cause mucosal reactions, either as local effects (Fig. 16.42) or

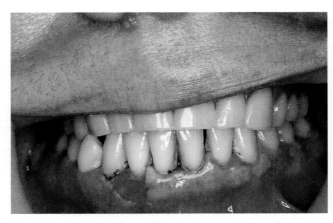

Fig. 16.42 Chemical burn. The gingivae are white and necrotic following injudicious use of a caustic agent. On the patient's right side full-thickness ulceration is present.

through systemic mechanisms that are often obscure. Systemically mediated reactions include ulceration, lichenoid reactions and erythema multiforme.

More uncommon mucocutaneous diseases

In many of these conditions, the oral lesions are rare or insignificant in comparison with the skin disease (Table 16.5).

Table 16.5 Some uncommon mucosal diseases

Disease	Cause	Oral features	Treatment
Epidermolysis bullosa PMID: 19945630	Autosomal recessive – gravis type due to type VII collagen defect (junctional type usually lethal at birth)	Subepithelial bullae leading to severe intraoral scarring after minimal trauma especially in recessive types	None wholly effective. Protect against any mucosal abrasion
Pyostomatitis vegetans (see page 456) PMID: 14723710	Complication of inflammatory bowel disease particularly ulcerative colitis	Yellowish miliary pustules in thickened erythematous mucosa release pus, leaving shallow ulcers. Suprabasal clefting and intraepithelial vesiculation or abscesses containing eosinophils. Peripheral eosinophilia up to 20% of white cells	Control of inflammatory bowel disease or systemic prednisolone
Gonorrhoea PMID: 806627	*N. gonorrhoeae* sexually transmitted	Oropharyngeal erythema or ulcers, rarely seen	Requires specialist referral
Leprosy PMID: 17223587 and 17119765	*Mycobacterium leprae*	Oral ulcers or nodules. Seen mainly in Asia	Dapsone
Keratosis follicularis (Darier's disease; warty dyskeratoma) PMID: 1931295	Genetic. Autosomal dominant	Intraepithelial bullae containing granulocytes and acantholytic cells. Pebbly lesions mainly of palate due to hyperkeratosis, acantholysis with 'corps ronds' and 'grains' (dyskeratosis) Can cause parotid duct stenosis	Oral lesions not troublesome but respond to retinoids

Summary chart 16.2   Differential diagnosis of the common causes of recurrent oral ulceration.

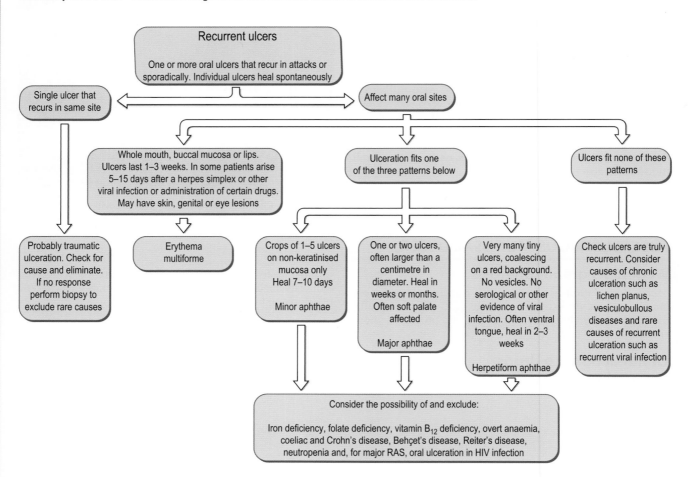

Tongue disorders

17

The tongue can be involved in generalised stomatitis, as discussed in the previous chapter, but is also the site of lesions or the source of symptoms peculiar to itself. Soreness limited to the tongue has few causes (Box 17.1).

Odd tongues, epidemiology PMID: 3466199

NORMAL STRUCTURES

The tongue is easily visible, and normal structures may concern patients and healthcare professionals.

Furred tongue

Some degree of furring is normal, caused by the filiform papillae and is more intense near the midline and posteriorly. Filiform papillae elongate continually from the base and are abraded by the diet. Bacteria adhere to the keratinised tips much more easily than to other parts of the mucosa, so that increased furring may be associated with a bad taste or halitosis.

Furring is increased in smokers, in many systemic upsets, especially of the gastrointestinal tract, and in infections in which the mouth becomes dry and little food is taken. A furred tongue is often seen in the childhood fevers. Many of these causes are reversible, but a tongue scraper is an effective intervention.

Filiform papillae also become long in black hairy tongue, discussed later.

Foliate papillae

These bilateral, pinkish soft nodules on the lateral borders of the tongue contain taste buds and minor oral tonsils forming part of Waldeyer's ring. They lie at the junction of the anterior two-thirds and the posterior third and sometimes become hyperplastic or inflamed and sore (see Figs 1.1 and 1.2).

Lingual varicosities

Dilated tortuous veins are normal along the ventral surface of the tongue and tend to become more prominent with age (see Fig. 17.1). They lie superficially and raise the covering thin mucosa into soft sessile nodules and generally cause no problems, being only extremely rarely the site of thrombus formation.

Case series PMID: 19540027

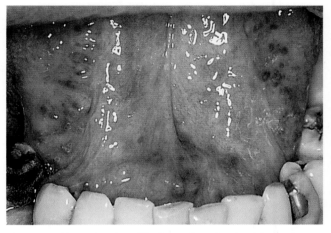

Fig. 17.1 Lingual varices. The formation of varicosities in the vessels of the undersurface of tongue and floor of mouth is a common finding with age.

ERYTHEMA MIGRANS

→ Summary charts 19.1 and 19.3 pp. 314, 316

This common benign condition usually affects only the tongue, producing an appearance likened to a map of the world on the dorsum, hence its alternative common name of *geographic tongue*.

The cause is unknown, and the condition is very common. Approximately 2% of the population are affected at any one time, but more than 20% will have an episode at some time in their life. It is seen at all ages but seems more frequent in young and middle age. There is a familial tendency.

The condition has been postulated to be a manifestation of twenty or more diseases, but no association withstands scrutiny. One that is widely accepted in medical circles is that erythema migrans may be a subclinical manifestation of psoriasis, partly based on histological similarities. This remains unsubstantiated, and several lines of evidence suggest this is incorrect.

Clinically, there are irregular, smooth, red areas on the dorsal tongue caused by loss of filiform papillae. Each patch starts as a small area on or near the lateral border and extends for a few days before healing, only to appear again in another area. The patches have a curved or semicircular shape centred on the lateral margin, a red rim and an enhanced white line around the edge. Several of these areas often coalesce to form a scalloped or geographic pattern (Figs 17.2 and 17.3). While lesions expand, they heal by regrowth of filiform papillae from the centre, and the moving pattern over a period of weeks confirms the diagnosis.

Histologically, the centre of the patch shows thinning of the epithelium with loss of filiform papillae. At the periphery the epithelium has a zone of hyperplasia with long rete ridges and dense infiltration by neutrophils forming microabscesses in the superficial layers (Fig. 17.4). This keratin

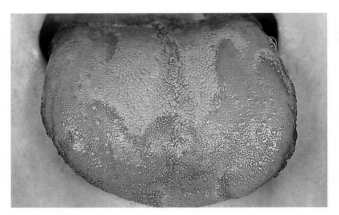

Fig. 17.2   Erythema migrans. Typical appearance with irregular depapillated patches centred on the lateral border of the tongue. Each patch has a narrow red and white rim.

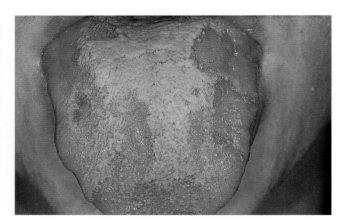

Fig. 17.3   Erythema migrans. The change of pattern can be seen, on a later occasion, in the same patient as in Fig. 17.2.

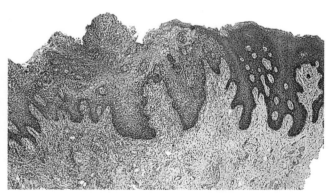

Fig. 17.4   Erythema migrans. The edge of a lesion showing normal mucosa to the right and, to the left, the epithelium densely infiltrated by neutrophils. This epithelium at the advancing edge will be shed, leaving the depapillated red patch.

is seen clinically as the white line around the margin. The superficial layers of epithelium die and desquamate, enlarging the central atrophic zone and enlarging the patch.

Most patients have no symptoms, but some complain of soreness, probably a result of epithelial thinning and inflammation. In such cases reassurance and precautionary exclusion of subclinical anaemia is prudent. Because there is no effective treatment, avoidance of spicy or astringent foods

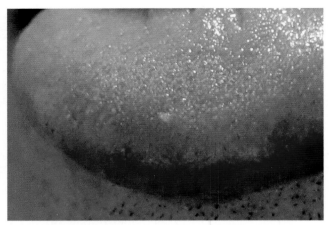

Fig. 17.5   Lingual papillitis. One fungiform papilla appears white and is intensely painful.

and toothpaste during the active phase is usually all that can be suggested. After a period the condition usually resolves, sometimes for long periods, but in most patients it is transient and recurrent for decades.

In a small minority of patients, other oral mucosae can be affected. The changes are not so obvious because there are no filiform papillae to lose, but the annular pattern of slowly moving white lines is the same.

Erythema migrans is unrelated to the rash of Lyme disease called *erythema chronicum migrans*.

Features PMID: 1804987

LINGUAL PAPILLITIS

This condition, also known as *transient lingual papillitis* or *fungiform papillitis*, is very common in the population, but patients rarely seek treatment. One or a cluster of fungiform papillae become slightly swollen, white and intensely painful to touch (Fig. 17.5). The condition resolves spontaneously after a few days, sometimes after only one, and without an ulcer developing. The cause is unknown, but trauma and certain foods are usually blamed. A few patients have more diffuse involvement.

Biopsy does not aid diagnosis and shows non-specific inflammatory changes.

Description PMID: 8899785 and 19774866

HAIRY TONGUE AND BLACK HAIRY TONGUE

The filiform papillae can become elongate and hair-like, forming a thick fur on the dorsum of the tongue. The filaments may be several millimetres long.

There is no clear distinction between a furred tongue and hairy tongue; this is a matter of degree. Hairy tongue is quite common, affecting as much as 1% of the population, and is commoner in heavy smokers and adults. No cause is known, but some patients report acute onset after radiotherapy, a stressful life event or debilitating illness.

The condition is more marked down the centre of the anterior tongue. The colour of the 'hairs' ranges from pale brown to black in colour (Fig. 17.6). When the papillae are dark brown or black, the cause is colonisation by adherent pigment-producing bacteria. Onset of dark colour can follow

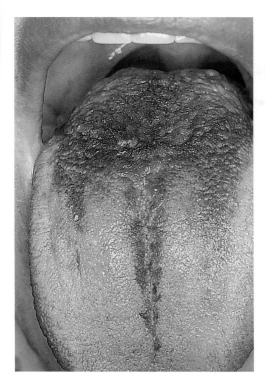

Fig. 17.6 Hairy tongue. In this patient there are numerous elongate papillae but a brown rather than black pigmentation.

antibiotic treatment that disturbs the normal ecology of the oral flora, allowing overgrowth of pigmented species. Like a furred tongue, trapping of food particles and adherent bacteria may produce halitosis and a bad taste. Otherwise the condition is asymptomatic, although papillae may be long enough to trigger gagging in susceptible patients.

Treatment is difficult. Pale hairy tongue may be mistaken for candidosis, but treatment with antifungals is inappropriate and ineffective. Tongue scraping is the best solution, with measures to reduce predisposing causes such as smoking or xerostomia.

Review PMID: 25152586

Black tongue

The dorsum of the tongue may sometimes become black without overgrowth of the papillae. This may be staining due to drugs, such as iron compounds used for the treatment of anaemia or bismuth from antacid preparations, but is then transient. Occasionally, the sucking of antiseptic lozenges causes the tongue to become black through overgrowth of pigment-producing organisms. Chlorhexidine mouthwash, coffee and other extrinsic agents also stain the dorsal tongue papillae preferentially.

Glossitis

Glossitis means no more than inflammation of the tongue, but the term is confusingly applied to many conditions, not all of which are inflammatory in origin or particularly inflamed.

Glossitis is used to describe erythematous changes, pain or burning, but these can also result from epithelial atrophy and several specific diseases.

Causes of glossitis are listed in Box 17.2, and anaemia is discussed in Chapter 27.

ANAEMIC GLOSSITIS

A red, smooth and sore tongue is particularly characteristic of anaemia, but anaemic patients may also have an asymptomatic red tongue or a normally appearing but sore tongue. A high index of suspicion for anaemia must therefore be maintained.

The cause is atrophy of the epithelium, which becomes thin and loses its filiform papillae, and therefore the keratinised parts of its surface. It then appears smooth and red.

The possibility that candidosis, predisposed to by anaemia, might cause some of the oral symptoms should also be considered. Patchy red zones suggest candidosis; the atrophy of anaemia is more widespread.

Iron deficiency

Three-quarters of patients with established iron deficiency have a painful tongue, and about a quarter have an atrophic tongue. Conversely, only 15% of patients with glossitis or soreness of the tongue are iron deficient when assessed by haemoglobin levels and reduced mean red cell volume. More sensitive measures of iron deficiency such as ferritin levels reveal deficiency before anaemia develops, and such subclinical deficiency is commonly found. It is also common in the normal population without symptoms, but those with a sore tongue are likely to benefit from supplementation.

The glossitis is mild, with minimal redness and loss of papillae around the outside of the dorsal surface (Fig. 17.7). There is often angular cheilitis associated.

Treatment is by supplementation. In severe cases there is rapid resolution of signs and symptoms with regrowth of papillae in a month, but mild cases require several months supplementation and respond slowly.

Though dietary deficiency is common, all patients with these signs or confirmed deficiency should be investigated for a cause of blood loss. The sore tongue may herald no more than menstrual loss or haemorrhoids, but occasionally signals loss from an intestinal carcinoma or other significant cause. Blood loss is a more likely cause in adult males.

Pain and iron deficiency PMID: 10555095

Paterson Kelly (Paterson Brown-Kelly) syndrome

This combination of iron deficiency, dysphagia and a post cricoid oesophageal stricture is known as Plummer-Vinson syndrome in the United States. It affects middle-aged

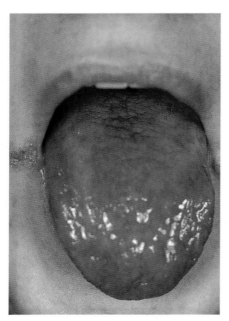

Fig. 17.7 **Glossitis in iron-deficiency anaemia.** The tongue is smooth, due to atrophy of the papillae, and is red and sore. Anaemia is the most common diagnosable cause of glossitis and must always be looked for by haematological examination.

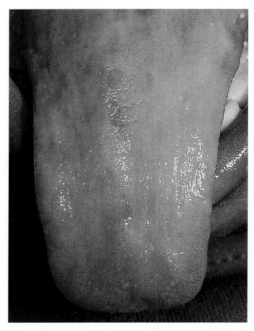

Fig. 17.8 **B$_{12}$ deficiency.** The tongue has generalised depapillation and toward the tip the typical 'beefy' appearance of severe deficiency. *(From Tersak, J.M., Malatack, J.J., Ritchey, A.K., 2002. Haematology and oncology. In: Zitelli, B.J., Davis, H.W. (Eds.), Atlas of Pediatric Physical Diagnosis, fourth ed. Mosby, St Louis.)*

women. Glossitis and angular cheilitis and obvious systemic signs of anaemia are usual.

Several decades ago the syndrome was found in 7% of patients with overt iron deficiency, but it has reduced dramatically in incidence and is now extremely rare. Its main significance is the association with subsequent carcinoma of the pharynx and oesophagus.

Review PMID: 16978405

B group vitamin deficiency

Glossitis of vitamin B$_{12}$ deficiency is particularly florid, and the tongue is described as 'beefy' (Fig. 17.8). However, as with iron, subclinical deficiency can cause burning and lingual discomfort and often there are no obvious signs (Fig. 17.9). More than half of patients with pernicious anaemia have glossitis on presentation, but less than 10% of patients with glossitis have B$_{12}$ deficiency. Patients may have macrocytosis without overt anaemia. If macrocytosis or deficiency are proven, symptoms usually resolve on supplementation by injection, pain rapidly and filiform papillae in a month or so.

The underlying cause is usually an absorption defect rather than dietary deficiency. B$_{12}$ deficiency is a particular risk after stomach bypass or other bariatric surgical procedures that reduce stomach mucosa, reducing intrinsic factor production. Other causes include proton pump inhibitors such as omeprazole, because they reduce stomach acidity, metformin, many antibiotics used long term, atrophic gastritis, small intestinal disease such as Crohn's disease, alcoholism and autoimmune diseases such as Grave's disease. The most common cause is lack of intrinsic factor in pernicious anaemia.

Folic acid ('folate', vitamin B$_9$) deficiency is the third most common deficiency to be associated with glossitis, affecting 2%–4% of patients. Again, subclinical deficiency can cause the signs and symptoms, and overt anaemia may not be present. Serum folate levels indicate the deficiency; red cell

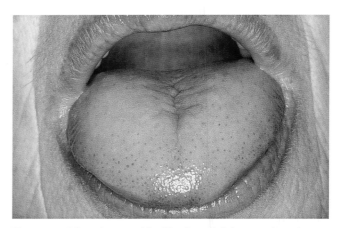

Fig. 17.9 A largely normal-looking but slightly smooth and persistently sore tongue in a patient who had repeated but inadequate haematological investigations that failed to detect early pernicious anaemia.

folate level reflects total body stores and is a second-line test. Treatment is by dietary adjustment, it being difficult to be folate deficient as many foods are supplemented. Deficiency tends to affect the very elderly or alcoholics. Folic acid supplementation may be useful in these cases of overt anaemia, provided B$_{12}$ deficiency is excluded first because supplementation in B$_{12}$ deficiency could precipitate neurological damage.

Riboflavin (vitamin B$_2$) deficiency classically causes glossitis with angular stomatitis and these may also be seen less frequently in **nicotinic acid** (Niacin, vitamin B$_3$) deficiency, but are rare.

Blind prescribing or self-medicating with B vitamins for oral symptoms in an otherwise healthy patient is virtually invariably ineffective, and investigation is required for all cases with these signs or symptoms.

General review nutritional deficiency PMID: 2693058 and 19735964

B₁₂ case report PMID: 17209796

Subclinical B₁₂ deficiency PMID: 8600284

GLOSSODYNIA AND THE SORE, PHYSICALLY NORMAL TONGUE

This presentation creates some of the most difficult problems in diagnosis and treatment. The symptoms are frequently part of the spectrum of burning mouth syndrome and atypical facial pain, but it is essential to exclude organic disease, particularly a haematological deficiency. These conditions are dealt with together in Chapter 38.

MACROGLOSSIA

Important causes of an enlarged tongue are summarised in Box 17.3. In many syndromes and in patients with poor neuromuscular control or muscle tone, the tongue may appear large, but be of normal size with a forward posture.

AMYLOIDOSIS

Amyloidosis is the deposition in the tissues of an abnormal protein with characteristic staining properties. Several different proteins have the ability to deposit as amyloid, which requires the molecules to align closely together and bind to form an insoluble and undegradable mass.

The amyloid protein may deposit at the site of production or circulate to deposit in remote sites, usually the kidneys,

around nerves, joints and in some organs. This interferes with function and can lead to organ failure.

In the head and neck, amyloid of AL type is commonly deposited in the tongue where it almost always signifies myeloma or a pre-myeloma plasma cell disorder (Ch. 12). Small deposits form asymptomatic nodules, usually along the lateral borders, but more extensive amyloidosis makes the tongue enlarged and stiff, affecting speech and eating (Figs 17.11 and 17.12). The tongue then feels firm and the

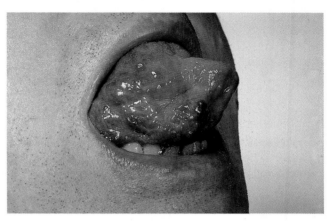

Fig. 17.10 Macroglossia due to a congenital haemangioma.

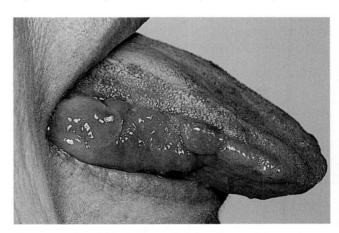

Fig. 17.11 **Amyloidosis.** These slightly yellow nodules on the lateral border of an enlarged tongue are characteristic of amyloidosis.

Box 17.3 Important causes of macroglossia

- Congenital haemangioma or lymphangioma (Fig. 17.10 and Ch. 25)
- Down's syndrome (Ch. 39)
- Cretinism (Ch. 36)
- Acromegaly (Ch. 36)
- Amyloidosis
- Lingual thyroid (Ch. 36)
- Mucopolysaccharidoses

Table 17.1 Selected types of amyloid*

Type	Protein	Source	Effect / significance
AL	Immunoglobulin light chains	The usual source is neoplastic plasma cells in myeloma.	Deposition mainly in kidneys, but common in the tongue, affecting about a third of patients
SAA	Serum 'amyloid A' protein, an acute phase serum protein	Produced in chronic infections and inflammatory conditions such as rheumatoid arthritis, Crohn's disease or tuberculosis	Rarely affects tongue, deposits mostly in liver and kidney
ATTR	Transthyretin, a serum protein	Usually a familial form associated with mutant protein	Deposits in muscle, kidney and heart, but rarely in tongue
AM	B2 microglobulin, a cell surface protein	Serum levels rise dramatically during renal haemodialysis	Deposits mostly in joints and occasionally in tongue. Lingual deposits affect about 2% of patients on long-term dialysis
ACal	Calcitonin	Secreted in excess by medullary thyroid carcinoma	Deposited only in the tumour, aids diagnosis
ODAM	Odontogenic ameloblast-associated protein	Odontogenic epithelium in the calcifying epithelial odontogenic tumour (Ch. 11)	Deposited in the tumour, aids diagnosis, mineralises focally to produce radiopacities

*Many more are known, but these are more common or more relevant.

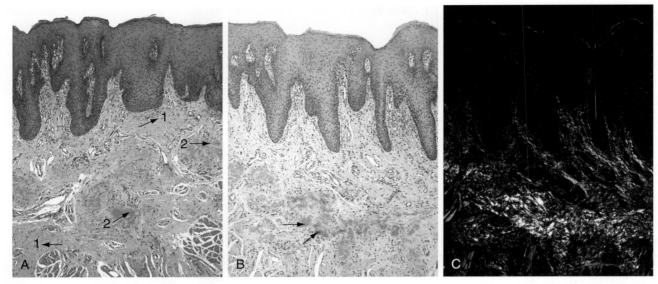

Fig. 17.12 **Amyloid deposited in tongue mucosa.** (A) The hematoxylin and eosin–stained section shows a broad band of amorphous tissue between the epithelium and underlying muscle *(1)*. This stains bright red with eosin where it is densest *(2)*. (B) Congo Red stain also stains the densest deposits red *(arrows)*. (C) When the Congo Red section is viewed under polarised light, the amyloid shows green birefringence.

mucosa appears pale and yellowish as surface blood flow is reduced by deposition around vessels. Vessels cannot constrict properly, and petechiae and ecchymoses are seen in involved mucosa.

Amyloid deposition in salivary glands produces xerostomia.

Management

Biopsy is diagnostic. Amyloid appears as weakly eosinophilic, hyaline homogeneous material replacing the collagen and muscle of the mucosa and tongue and surrounding vessels. Amyloid stains with Congo Red and has a characteristic, usually apple-green, birefringence under polarised light (see Fig. 17.12). Various specialised techniques are used to distinguish the various types of protein that form amyloid (Table 17.1).

Treatment is for the underlying condition, if that is possible. Surgical reduction has been required for massive macroglossia caused by amyloid.

Reviews PMID: 15124168 and 23715681

OTHER DISEASES AFFECTING THE TONGUE

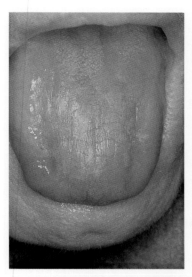

Fig. 17.13   Smooth atrophic tongue due to lichen planus. This is a late change due to longstanding disease. (See Ch. 16.)

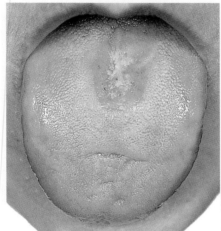

Fig. 17.14   Median rhomboid glossitis, Median rhomboid glossitis, an active candidal infection or evidence of past infection. (See Ch. 15.)

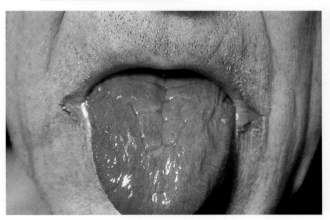

Fig. 17.15   Glossitis in antibiotic sore tongue, a candidal infection. (See Ch. 15.)

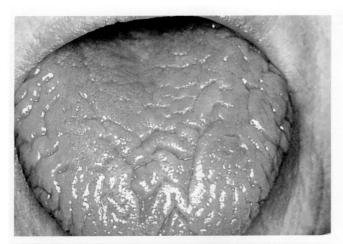

Fig. 17.16 Tongue in longstanding xerostomia. (See Ch. 22.)

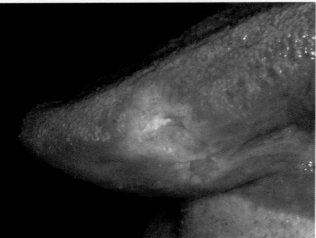

Fig. 17.17 **Traumatic ulcer.** The tongue is a common site, here due to biting.

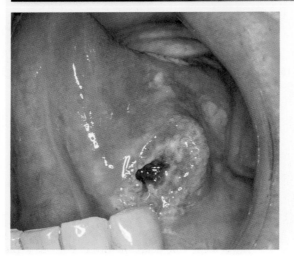

Fig. 17.18 **Squamous carcinoma.** The lateral tongue is a common site. (See Ch. 20.)

Benign chronic white mucosal lesions

18

There are many causes of white patches or diffuse whitening of the oral mucosa, and a small minority are potentially malignant. When confronted with a white lesion in the mouth, every clinician needs a list of oral white lesions in their mind for diagnosis so that the few with significant risk are identified quickly and accurately.

The appearance of most mucosal white lesions is due to hyperkeratosis. Keratin absorbs moisture from saliva and then appears white. Apart from the lingual filiform papillae, visible keratinisation of any significant degree is abnormal in the mouth.

Review oral white lesions PMID: 23600041

Leukoplakia

A leukoplakia is a clinical term for a white patch. Understanding how this term is used and avoiding misuse is important. A leukoplakia is a predominantly white patch of the oral mucosa that cannot be characterised clinically or pathologically as any other definable lesion. This states clearly that leukoplakia is idiopathic – no cause is known because the patch cannot be characterised as any other definable lesion.

Previous definitions included the fact that a leukoplakia cannot be wiped off, but the importance of this finding has been overemphasised. The intention is to exclude thrush (Ch. 15) in which the surface white pseudomembrane can be wiped off. However, not all types of *Candida* infection produce loosely adherent plaques, and this feature is of minimal diagnostic value.

Unfortunately, the term *leukoplakia* is widely misused. To many it means a white patch that has a risk of malignant transformation to squamous carcinoma. This is true of only a tiny small minority, but a patient searching the internet with the term could easily become very frightened. The term also appears in the names of many specific diseases, such as *oral hairy leukoplakia* or *candidal leukoplakia* where the cause is known. Some prefer not to use the term at all, and simply saying 'white patch' instead avoids much of the confusion.

Leukoplakia is only a clinical description, and it can be a useful label for a white patch on first presentation. However, once investigations and biopsy are complete, either a specific cause is known or a histological diagnosis can be given. The term is then redundant, unless used in the name of a specific entity.

The majority of white patches, without malignant potential, are discussed here (Table 18.1).

Current definition PMID: 17944749

New definition proposal PMID: 26449439

FORDYCE SPOTS → Summary chart 19.2 p. 315

Fordyce spots or granules are sebaceous glands in the oral mucosa. They are normal rather than ectopic, appearing in at least 80% of adults, but perform no function in mucosa.

Table 18.1	Important causes of benign mucosal white lesions	
Prevalence	Lesion	Cause
Common	Leukoedema	Normal variation
	Frictional keratosis	Friction
	Cheek biting	Cheek biting
	Fordyce's granules	Developmental
	Stomatitis nicotina	Pipe smoking
	Thrush	Candidal infection
	Lichen planus	Unknown
Uncommon	Chemical trauma	Caustic chemicals
	Hairy leukoplakia	Epstein–Barr virus
	White sponge naevus	Genetic
	Oral keratosis of renal failure	Uncertain
	Verruciform xanthoma	Uncertain
	Skin grafts	Iatrogenic

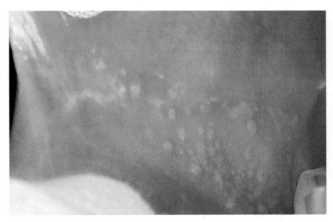

Fig. 18.1 Fordyce's spots. Clusters of creamy, slightly elevated papules on the buccal mucosa.

They are soft, symmetrically distributed, creamy white spots from 0.5–2 mm in diameter, grow in size with age and are more prominent in the elderly (Fig. 18.1). The buccal and labial mucosa are the main sites, but sometimes the lips and, rarely, even the tongue are involved. Fordyce spots are more or less evenly spaced, but in some patients they are very prominent and can form a creamy white slightly raised plaque that is mistaken for a leukoplakia. However, they do not show the bright white colour of keratin, and the lightly yellow colour of the fat in the gland can be seen to be below the surface.

Patients can be reassured that they are of no significance. If a biopsy is carried out, it shows normal sebaceous glands with two or three lobules but no hair follicle, as would be present in sebaceous glands on the skin (Fig. 18.2).

And other oral sebaceous lesions PMID: 8355222

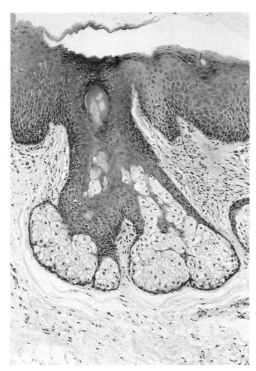

Fig. 18.2 Fordyce's spots. Each spot is a histologically normal superficial sebaceous gland without a hair follicle.

LEUKOEDEMA → Summary chart 19.2 p. 315

Leukoedema is a bilateral, diffuse, translucent white greyish thickening of the surface layers of the epithelium with an increase in thickness of parakeratin at the surface. The characteristic feature for diagnosis is that it disappears on stretching the mucosa. The buccal and labial mucosae are affected.

Leukoedema is possibly normal; it is present to some degree in 90% of those of African descent. It is also sometimes seen in other races but is rarely as intense. It has been claimed to be caused by some unknown environmental insult, such as smoking, but is seen in non-smokers and children.

Histologically, there is thickening of the surface layers of the epithelium with irregular parakeratinisation and the upper prickle cells show an enhanced 'basket weave' pattern caused by vacuolation of their cytoplasm. There is no oedema, intracellular or otherwise, and no inflammation.

Treatment is unnecessary. The main significance is not to overreact and perform a biopsy without good reason.

Review PMID: 1460680

Epidemiology and causes PMID: 3926975

FRICTIONAL KERATOSIS

→ Summary charts 19.1 and 19.2 pp. 314, 315

White patches can be caused by prolonged mild abrasion of the mucous membrane by such irritants as a sharp tooth or dentures.

At first, the patches are pale and translucent (Fig. 18.3), but with prolonged friction become dense and white, usually with a smooth surface. Common sites are buccal mucosa and edentulous alveolar ridge, particularly behind the last

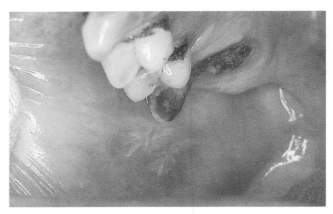

Fig. 18.3 Frictional keratosis. A poorly defined patch of keratosis on the buccal mucosa is due to friction from the sharp buccal cusp of a grossly carious upper molar.

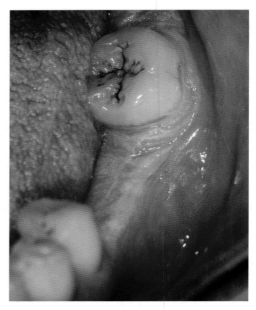

Fig. 18.4 Frictional keratosis. Some degree of frictional keratosis is almost universal on edentulous alveolar ridges when teeth are not replaced.

standing molar (Fig. 18.4). The buccal *linea alba* is a normal frictional keratosis.

Excessive trauma will cause an ulcer, and the margins of a traumatic ulcer are often surrounded by a zone of frictional keratosis where the degree of trauma is less.

Diagnosis and management

The diagnosis is usually obvious from the cause. The patch fades gradually into surrounding normal mucosa without sharply defined margins.

Removal of the irritant causes the patch to disappear. Frictional keratosis is completely benign. Biopsy is necessary only if the patch persists or there are other clinical indications, such as smoking. If performed, the epithelium shows hyperplasia, thickening of the prickle cell layer and para or orthokeratosis but no dysplasia (Fig. 18.5). More intense friction may be associated with mild inflammation, but often there is none.

Ridge keratosis PMID: 18158926

General review white lesions PMID: 23600041

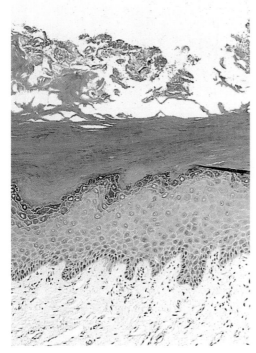

Fig. 18.5   Frictional keratosis. There is a slight hyperplasia of the basal cells and a thick layer of orthokeratin at the surface.

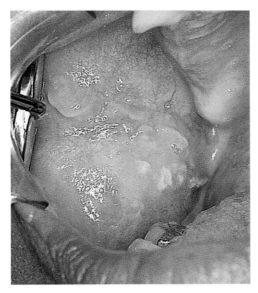

Fig. 18.6   Cheek biting. There is whitening of the buccal mucosa and a shredded surface.

CHEEK AND TONGUE BITING

→ Summary charts 19.1 and 19.2 pp. 314, 315

Habitual biting trauma is distinct from frictional keratosis and traumatic ulceration. Unlike the smooth surface of frictional keratosis, biting produces small indentations and shredded tags where the habitual chewer nips off small pieces of the superficial epithelium. The background epithelium undergoes even keratosis in response.

Biting causes an area of mucosa to appear patchily red and white with a rough surface (Fig. 18.6). The margin of the bitten zone is well demarcated as only a limited amount

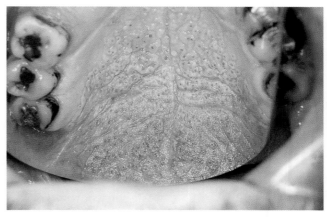

Fig. 18.7   Stomatitis nicotina (smoker's palate). There is a generalised whitening with sparing of the gingival margin. The inflamed openings of the minor salivary glands form red spots on the white background.

of the buccal, labial and lateral tongue mucosa can be interposed between the teeth. The damage is very superficial and usually along the occlusal line.

The diagnosis should be obvious from the clinical appearance and history of the habit, which is rarely unconscious.

Biopsy is not indicated. If performed on a tongue lesion, care must be taken not to mistake the histological features for those of oral hairy leukoplakia as both conditions induce enlarged pale epithelial cells in the prickle cell layer.

Review PMID: 19070760

STOMATITIS NICOTINA

→ Summary chart 19.1 p. 314

Previously known as *smokers' palate*, or *pipe smoker's keratosis*, this condition has become rare now that pipe and cigar smoking have declined. It appears to be a reaction to the heat of smoking, which in these habits is directed at the posterior palate. Changes take many years to develop. Only the heaviest of cigarette smokers can produce similar alterations.

Clinical features

The appearances are distinctive in that the palate is affected, but any part protected by a denture is spared. There is diffuse whitening of the palate caused by hyperkeratosis and inflammatory swelling of minor mucous glands. The openings of the minor gland ducts are seen as red spots against the white, and in marked cases they are umbilicated swellings with red centres and a distinct line of keratosis around them (Fig. 18.7). The white plaque is sometimes distinctly tessellated (crazy paving appearance).

Diagnosis and management

The clinical appearance and history are so distinctive that biopsy should not be necessary. If the patient can be persuaded to stop smoking, the lesion resolves within a few weeks or months.

Unlike other oral white lesions associated with smoking, stomatitis nicotina carries no risk of malignant transformation. Management can therefore be conservative, and no biopsy is usually taken unless there are other concerning features.

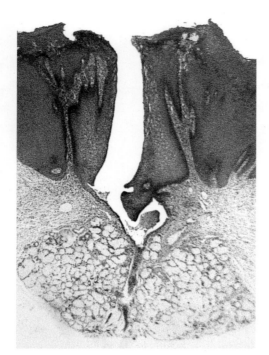

Fig. 18.8 Stomatitis nicotina (smoker's palate). The epithelium is hyperplastic and hyperkeratotic, especially around the orifice of the duct where there is inflammation.

Box 18.1 Stomatitis nicotina
- Affects palatal mucosa exposed to smoke and heat
- Areas protected by denture unaffected
- Palate is white from keratosis
- Umbilicated swellings with red centres are inflamed salivary ducts
- Responds rapidly to abstinence from pipe smoking
- Benign despite being tobacco-induced

If performed, biopsy shows hyperorthokeratosis and acanthosis of the epithelium with a variable inflammatory infiltrate in underlying glands and around ducts but no dysplasia (Fig. 18.8).

Although the condition is benign, its presence indicates prolonged heavy smoking and the possibility of carcinoma developing at another site in the mouth, pharynx, larynx or lung should be considered.

Key features are summarised in Box 19.1.

Reverse smoking PMID: 9081765

Caused by hot drinks PMID: 2234881

ORAL HAIRY LEUKOPLAKIA

→ Summary chart 19.2 p. 315

This Epstein–Barr virus infection of oral mucosa was originally considered to develop only in HIV infection. However, it is now recognised in other immunosuppressed patients and in a small number of apparently normal individuals. The name causes some confusion. The lesion is not hairy and, having a known cause, is not a leukoplakia.

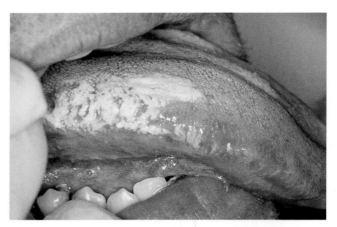

Fig. 18.9 Hairy leukoplakia in a patient with early symptomatic HIV infection. The surface of the lesion is corrugated, accentuating the normal anatomy of the lateral border of the tongue.

Clinical features

In HIV infection, hairy leukoplakia is usually a late sign and is 'strongly associated' (Ch. 29). Men who have sex with men are predominantly affected, and highly active antiretroviral treatment reduces the incidence. Hairy leukoplakia is occasionally the presenting sign in unsuspected HIV infection. Renal transplant patients are also predisposed.

Hairy leukoplakia produces an asymptomatic vertically corrugated or shaggy soft keratosis of the lateral borders of the tongue (Fig. 18.9). It may also rarely affect the buccal mucosa, soft palate and pharynx, but tongue lesions will then also be present. The vertical ridging is enhancement of the normal epithelial morphology on the posterolateral tongue, and not a useful feature for diagnosis.

Diagnosis

Biopsy is required for diagnosis unless other features and a cause of immunosuppression are known. Hairy leukoplakia shows hyperkeratosis or parakeratosis, or both, with a ridged or shaggy surface. Koilocyte-like cells are the site of the infection. They are vacuolated and ballooned prickle cells with shrunken, dark (pyknotic) nuclei, chromatin pushed to the nuclear rim, and surrounded by a clear halo in the cytoplasm (Fig. 18.10). The infected cells form bands parallel with the surface in alternating layers with parakeratin. The presence of Epstein–Barr virus is demonstrated by using either immunohistochemistry to detect virus particles or in situ hybridisation to demonstrate their DNA (see Fig. 18.10).

Secondary infection of the surface by candidal hyphae is common in examples from HIV-positive patients; fungal hyphae are then very numerous and not accompanied by an inflammatory response because of the immunosuppression.

Management

No treatment is required. Hairy leukoplakia has a remittent course and can regress when immunosuppression improves. Antiviral drugs are effective only while being taken, but these, and topical podophyllin, have been used in HIV infection when the lesions become very extensive.

Hairy leukoplakia in HIV infection indicates advanced immunodeficiency, a more rapid progression to AIDS and a

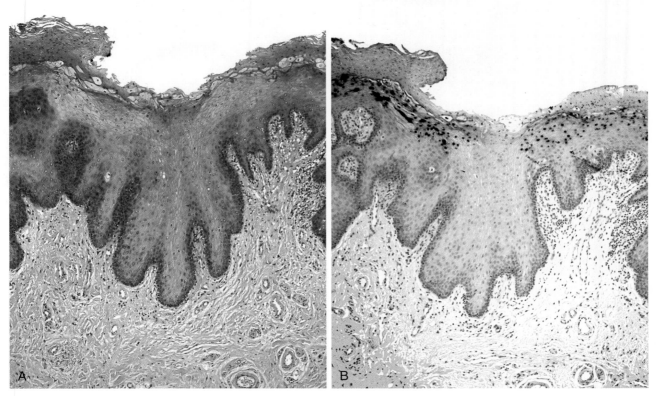

Fig. 18.10 Hairy leukoplakia. (A) There is thickening of the epithelium and a thick superficial layer of parakeratin, below which the pale-staining layer of 'koilocyte-like' cells lies. Because this patient is severely immunosuppressed, there is no inflammatory reaction to the numerous candidal hyphae which are present in the surface layers of the epithelium. (B) In situ hybridisation using probes complementary to the Epstein–Barr virus. The presence of viral DNA is shown by the dark brown staining in the upper prickle cells and koilocyte-like cells. Details of this technique are included in Chapter 1.

Box 18.2 Hairy leukoplakia: key features

- Usually in males and a sign of HIV infection, but occasionally in normal individuals
- Typically forms soft, corrugated, painless plaques on lateral borders of tongue
- Diagnosis by biopsy
- Histologically, koilocyte-like cells in prickle cell layer are typical
- Epstein–Barr virus antigens detectable in epithelial cell nuclei by in-situ hybridisation
- Indicates advanced immunodeficiency and poor prognosis but not premalignant
- May regress spontaneously or with HIV antiretroviral treatment (Ch. 29)

---

poor prognosis. Known HIV-positive patients who develop it should be referred back to their HIV clinic for reassessment of their anti-HIV medication.

In those few patients without known immunosuppression, it resolves spontaneously and often has a more localised distribution.

Key features are summarised in Box 18.2.

Description PMID: 1312689

Non-HIV cases PMID: 25600979

WHITE SPONGE NAEVUS

➜ Summary chart 19.2 p. 315

White sponge naevus is a developmental anomaly inherited as an autosomal dominant trait, caused by mutation in genes for keratins 4 and 13. These keratin molecules are only expressed in the upper layers of non-keratinised mucosal epithelium.

Clinical features

The lining mucosa becomes white, soft and irregularly thickened (Fig. 18.11). The abnormality is usually bilateral on the buccal mucosa, and changes become more prominent with age, often presenting in the second or third decade. There are no defined borders, and the edges fade imperceptibly into normal tissue. Any non-keratinised mucosa can be affected; involvement of multiple sites such as nose or vagina constitutes Cannon's syndrome.

Pathology

The epithelium is very thick, with uniform acanthosis and shaggy hyperparakeratosis. The upper prickle cells are vacuolated with prominent epithelial cell membranes producing an enhanced basket-weave appearance (Fig. 18.12). The abnormal keratin cytoskeleton can sometimes be seen collapsed around the nucleus. There is no dysplasia or inflammation.

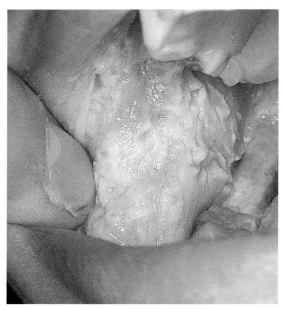

Fig. 18.11   White sponge naevus. The keratosis is irregular and folded and extends into areas which are not subject to friction.

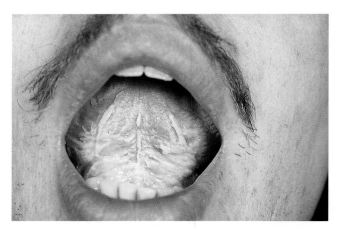

Fig. 18.13   Oral keratosis of renal failure. The white lesions are symmetrical, soft and wrinkled.

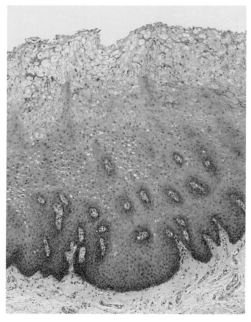

Fig. 18.12   White sponge naevus. The epithelium is acanthotic, and the prickle cell layer is composed of large vacuolated cells.

Management

The family history and appearance are virtually diagnostic, but biopsy can confirm the diagnosis if required. The condition requires no treatment.

Key features are summarised in Box 18.3.

And other keratin diseases review PMID: 12688839

Web URL 18.1 Genetics: http://omim.org/entry/193900

CANDIDOSIS

Three types of candidal infection cause white patches and are relatively common.

Box 18.3   White sponge naevus: key features

- Genetic – autosomal dominant trait
- Shaggy whitish thickening can involve all lining mucosa
- White areas lack sharp borders
- Histologically, epithelial thickening
- Defective parakeratinisation
- No dysplasia or inflammation
- No treatment other than reassurance

Thrush (acute candidosis) is readily distinguishable from other white lesions. The patches can easily be wiped off, and the condition is sore (Ch. 15).

Chronic hyperplastic candidosis and **chronic mucocutaneous candidosis** form discrete white plaques similar clinically to other types of leukoplakia (Ch. 15).

ORAL KERATOSIS OF RENAL FAILURE

Leukoplakia-like oral lesions are an unexplained complication of longstanding renal failure. However, this complication is rarely seen, and some similar presentations may be accounted for by diseases such as oral hairy leukoplakia.

Clinically, the plaques are soft and are typically symmetrically distributed (Fig. 18.13). Biopsy is useful to exclude adherent plaques of bacteria and desquamated epithelium and debris, which also form in late renal failure (Fig. 18.14).

Case renal keratosis PMID: 9084198

Review oral findings PMID: 15723858

SKIN GRAFTS

Split skin grafting is relatively rarely used in current surgical practice, and only to cover relatively small excision sites.

Skin grafts typically appear sharply demarcated, smooth and paler than the surrounding mucosa and occasionally grow hairs (Fig. 18.15). After many years grafts change in appearance and are less easy to differentiate from a leukoplakia (Fig. 18.16).

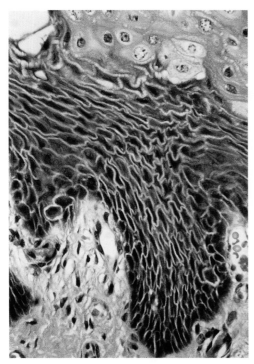

Fig. 18.14   Oral keratosis of renal failure. Microscopy shows acanthosis and a picture somewhat similar to hairy leukoplakia.

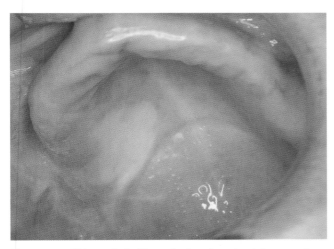

Fig. 18.15   Skin graft. A skin graft placed on the right posterior hard palate appears as a scar-like, pale patch. Hair follicles occasionally survive transplantation to the mouth.

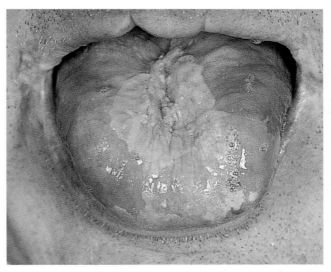

Fig. 18.16   Skin graft. This graft placed on the anterior dorsum of the tongue has contracted to produce an irregular margin and surface and might be mistaken for leukoplakia.

PSORIASIS

Psoriasis is a very common skin disease estimated to affect 2% of the population, but cases with convincing oral lesions are extremely rare and some doubt their existence. A relationship with erythema migrans is often stated but unproven.

The diagnosis should only be considered when there is cutaneous psoriasis and lesions wax and wane in severity with them. The appearance of the oral lesions is reported to vary from translucent plaques, mild stippled erythema to that of erythema migrans. Biopsy appearances are not specific.

OTHER WHITE LESIONS

A number of other conditions can cause localised white lesions. These include lichen planus (Ch. 16), chemical burns (see Fig. 16.42), verruciform xanthoma (Ch. 24) and papillomas (Ch. 24).

Potentially malignant disorders | 19

Various oral mucosal lesions indicate that a patient is at risk of developing an oral squamous cell carcinoma. Such lesions are usually red or white in appearance. Their risks of developing into cancer vary quite widely.

Terminology

The current preferred term for these conditions is *oral potentially malignant disorders*. This is meant to emphasise that the risk is only potential and may never materialise. 'Premalignancy' and 'precancer' imply that cancer will definitely develop, and these terms are best avoided, although they are widely used.

Current understanding also makes the difference between a premalignant lesion and a premalignant disease redundant. It used to be thought that some conditions indicated a risk of carcinoma at the site of the lesion itself ('premalignant lesion'), whereas others might indicate a risk elsewhere in the mouth ('premalignant disease'). We now understand that all potentially malignant disorders are indicators of genetic 'field change'. They indicate a risk not just at the site of the lesion itself but throughout the mouth and, in smokers, more widely in the upper aerodigestive tract.

Other useful definitions for this chapter are shown in Table 19.1.

The oral potentially malignant disorders

In general, the oral white lesions have the lowest risk of malignant transformation and red and speckled lesions the highest risk, but there are completely benign white and red lesions.

It is the role of the dentist to recognise these lesions, assess their risk and refer when that risk is significant. The process of identifying 'at risk' lesions is fundamental to diagnosis and treatment planning.

The oral potentially malignant disorders are listed in Table 19.2, with their risk and causes, as far as is known.

Nomenclature and classification PMID: 17944749

Review PMID: 18674954

Field change

Potentially malignant disorders are thought to result from field change or field cancerisation. This is a process whereby a wide area of tissue becomes genetically altered, making it prone to develop cancer anywhere within the field. In heavy smokers, mutations predisposing to cancer can be found throughout a large field including the mouth, pharynx, larynx and lung. Examples are loss of function of cell cycle control proteins or DNA repair enzymes.

Defects are not limited to individual genes. The cells in the field may also show chromosome abnormalities, usually amplifications or duplications of whole or part chromosomes. This results from chromosomal instability, a

Table 19.1 Key definitions for potentially malignant disorders

Erythroplakia	A predominantly red lesion of the oral mucosa that cannot be characterised clinically or pathologically as any other definable lesion
Leukoplakia	A white plaque of questionable risk having excluded other known diseases or disorders that carry no increased risk for cancer
Precursor lesion	Any identifiable lesion or altered mucosa with a risk of transformation. A relatively non-specific term

Table 19.2 Oral potentially malignant disorders

Disorder	Aetiology	Risk of malignant change*	Prevalence in UK
Leukoplakia	Idiopathic/smoking	Varies with dysplasia grade	Uncommon
Erythroplakia	Idiopathic/smoking	Very high	Rare
Speckled leukoplakia	Idiopathic/smoking	Very high	Rare
Oral submucous fibrosis	Betel quid chewing	High	Uncommon
Dyskeratosis congenita	Genetic	High	Very rare
Pipe smoker's keratosis	Pipe smoking	Low and not in the keratotic area	Now uncommon
Snuff-dippers' keratosis	Smokeless tobacco	Low	Uncommon
Chronic candidosis	*Candida albicans*	Low	Uncommon
Lichen planus	Idiopathic	Low	Common
Discoid lupus erythematosus	Autoimmune	Unclear (mainly lip)	Uncommon
Tertiary syphilis	*Treponema pallidum*	Very high	No longer seen

*Risks of malignant change are difficult to determine accurately and vary with many factors discussed later in this chapter. If more than 25% of patients with a specific disorder develop carcinoma in 10 years, this is considered an exceptionally high risk. Malignant change in 1% of lesions in 10 years is considered a relatively low risk. High-risk disorders are uncommon. Common disorders appear in between 1% and 5% of the population.

continuous process of worsening genetic damage. The genetic changes in the altered field are not in themselves sufficient to cause cancer, but they increase the likelihood of cancer developing.

Within an area of field change in the mouth, not all the epithelial cells have the same DNA defects. There are overlapping areas of slightly different changes making up the field. Each patch is a clone of cells that has a survival advantage over normal cells and grows too slowly replace surrounding tissue. Different parts of the field will therefore have different risks for developing into cancer.

Field change has several implications. The first is that the extent of the field may or may not be visible clinically or histologically depending on the particular combination of genetic changes present. The size of the field at risk, therefore, cannot be easily determined. Second, the size of the field affects the success of surgical treatment because excision could only be effective for a small field. Third, patients at risk of one carcinoma are at risk of multiple potentially malignant lesions and cancers in different sites in the field.

Dysplasia, features of abnormal growth seen histologically, is the best predictor of risk (page 308). It is not necessarily detectable throughout the area of field change, but it often is.

In tobacco users PMID: 12949809

'Mapping' fields PMID: 16757199

ERYTHROPLAKIA

→ Summary charts 19.1 and 19.3, p. 314, 316

An erythroplakia is a predominantly red lesion of the oral mucosa that cannot be characterised clinically or pathologically as any other definable lesion. The term *erythroplasia* is sometimes used to indicate that these lesions are often not raised plaques like leukoplakias, but flat or slightly depressed (Fig. 19.1).

Pure red lesions are rare and usually affect the floor of mouth, lateral and ventral tongue and soft palate of the elderly, often smokers. The surface is frequently velvety in texture and ranges from dull matte red to bright scarlet. The margin may or may not be sharply defined. Erythroplasia is uncommon in the mouth but carries the highest risk of malignant transformation.

Almost half of lesions turn out to be malignant on first biopsy, and the remainder show some degree of dysplasia, often severe. The epithelium is atrophic and non-keratinised, and these features, together with inflammation, account for the red colour seen clinically.

Review PMID: 15975518

SPECKLED LEUKOPLAKIA

→ Summary chart 19.1, p. 314

Also known as *erythroleukoplakia*, this term applies to lesions with both red and white areas, usually white flecks or nodules on an atrophic erythematous base (Fig. 19.2). They can be regarded as a combination of leukoplakia and erythroplakia.

The clinical features otherwise resemble erythroplakia, and there is a similar risk of finding carcinoma in a first biopsy. Speckled leukoplakia more frequently shows dysplasia than pure white lesions. The histological characteristics are intermediate between leukoplakia and erythroplasia.

Some cases of chronic candidosis have a similar appearance, but without the high risk of developing carcinoma.

LEUKOPLAKIA

→ Summary chart 19.2, p. 315

Leukoplakia is defined as a white plaque of questionable risk having excluded other known diseases or disorders that carry no increased risk for cancer. Like erythroplakia and speckled leukoplakia, the diagnosis is therefore by exclusion of other diseases. Many completely benign conditions form similar white patches (Ch. 18).

Leukoplakia is common, accounting for over three-quarters of all potentially malignant conditions and being present in 1%–5% of the population, more in India and other countries with many tobacco users.

In the UK, the risk of a leukoplakia undergoing transformation to carcinoma is approximately 0.3% each year if no dysplasia is present and 6% each year if severe dysplasia is

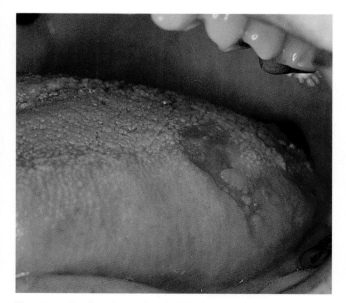

Fig. 19.1 Erythroplasia. This slightly depressed, well-defined red patch on the dorsolateral tongue showed squamous carcinoma on biopsy.

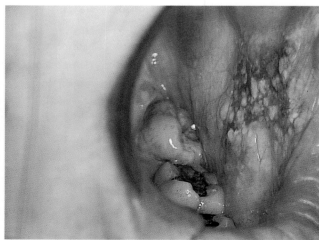

Fig. 19.2 Speckled leukoplakia. A poorly-defined speckled leukoplakia on the cheek of an elderly female. Carcinoma was present at the first biopsy. See also Fig. 19.11.

present. Homogeneous, flat leukoplakias have a lower risk than those with a nodular or verrucous surface clinically. Large patches, those on the lateral or ventral tongue and floor of mouth, and those in older patients have a higher risk. Nevertheless, the malignant transformation rate of leukoplakia is relatively low, and, even in smokers, the vast majority of leukoplakias show no dysplasia histologically and carry no risk of malignant transformation.

Current definition PMID: 17944749

New definition proposal PMID: 26449439

Clinical features

Idiopathic leukoplakias and dysplastic lesions do not have any specific clinical appearance but are tough and adherent white plaques whose surface is slightly raised above the surrounding mucosa. The surface is usually irregular. Small and innocent-looking white patches are as likely to show epithelial dysplasia as large and irregular ones (Figs 19.3 and

19.4). However, lesions with red, nodular or verrucous areas (Fig. 19.5) should be regarded with particular suspicion. The most common sites are the posterior buccal mucosa, retromolar region, floor of mouth and tongue.

Pathology

The histopathology is highly variable, but there is always keratinisation, which gives the lesion its white appearance (Figs 19.6 and 19.7). Features of dysplasia and its assessment are considered later in this chapter.

Most leukoplakias, 85%, show no dysplasia histologically, whereas 8% show mild dysplasia, 5% moderate and 2% show severe dysplasia.

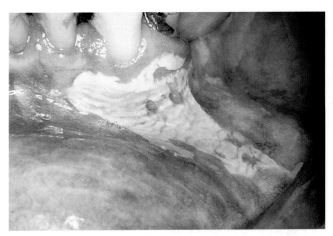

Fig. 19.3   Homogeneous leukoplakia. There is a bright, white, sharply-defined patch extending from the gingiva on to the labial mucosa. The surface has a slightly rippled appearance, and no red areas are associated.

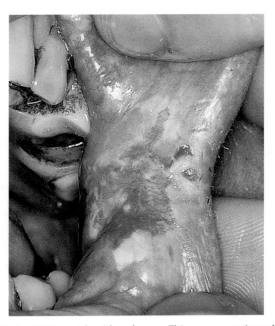

Fig. 19.5   White patch with red areas. This post-commissural lesion is poorly defined. Lesions at this site are frequently due to candidosis, but this example showed dysplasia on biopsy rather than simple candidosis.

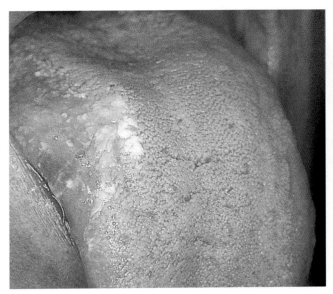

Fig. 19.4   An innocent-looking, poorly-defined inconspicuous white patch which showed dysplasia on biopsy. Despite excision, malignant transformation followed several months later.

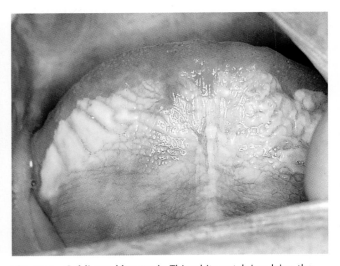

Fig. 19.6   Sublingual keratosis. This white patch involving the entire ventral tongue and floor of mouth has a uniformly wrinkled appearance. No red areas are associated, but the site alone may possibly indicate a high risk of malignant transformation.

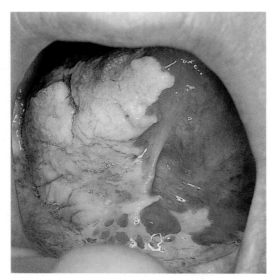

Fig. 19.7 Sublingual keratosis. This more irregular white patch is associated with some reddening in the floor of the mouth.

Sublingual keratosis

The term 'sublingual keratosis' is sometimes applied to leukoplakia on the floor of mouth and ventral tongue, a high-risk site for malignant change. Sublingual keratosis is not a specific entity, but white patches at this site do show some unusual features; they are often extensive, form a soft plaque with a finely wrinkled surface and often show a low grade of dysplasia despite having significant risk of developing carcinoma (see Figs 19.6 and 19.7). The histology and treatment are as for leukoplakia.

PROLIFERATIVE VERRUCOUS LEUKOPLAKIA

This is a distinctive presentation of multiple white lesions with a very high risk of transformation. Patients are older than 55 years of age, mostly female, and most are non-smokers.

They develop flat leukoplakias that, over a period of decades, develop a nodular or verrucous surface and progress inexorably to verrucous or squamous carcinoma. Common sites affected are buccal mucosa, gingiva and tongue (Fig. 19.8). Many patches may be present, each at a different stage in its evolution. Patients can suffer several separate carcinomas over many years. Lesions are difficult or impossible to eradicate surgically and recur or develop in new sites.

The histological features of the lesions are those of leukoplakia, with or without dysplasia, but it is striking that these lesions often display an apparently innocuous lack of dysplasia or only mild dysplasia that can lead to underestimation of the risk.

In order for the diagnosis to have any value, it is important that the criteria are strictly applied. Not all verrucous leukoplakias are proliferative verrucous leukoplakia, regardless of how verrucous they become or how much they enlarge. It is usually said that the ultimate diagnostic criterion is that all cases develop carcinoma. However, recognition must be much earlier to benefit the patient, and identifying the unusual clinical presentation allows close monitoring and targeted intervention.

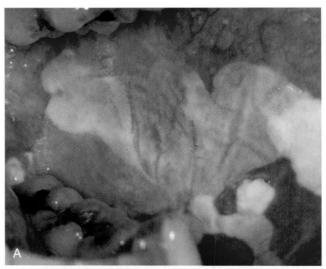

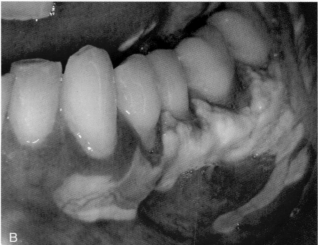

Fig. 19.8 Proliferative verrucous leukoplakia. There are large white patches affecting the typical sites, and on the lower gingiva the leukoplakia has a nodular surface.

Patients with proliferative verrucous leukoplakia often have a surprisingly good long-term prognosis, developing well-differentiated carcinomas, often on the gingiva or buccal mucosa.

Review PMID: 20233330 and 17448134

STOMATITIS NICOTINA

→ Summary chart 19.2, p. 315

Palatal keratosis due to pipe-smoking is itself benign (Ch. 18) but may be an indicator of risk elsewhere in the aerodigestive tract.

SMOKELESS TOBACCO-INDUCED KERATOSES

The majority of tobacco used worldwide is dried, cured and then smoked in cigarettes or cigars. However, many cultures have traditional tobacco habits that use snuff, crude tobacco or commercial preparations topically on the oral mucosa. These may be 'dipped', chewed or dissolved in the mouth and are termed *smokeless* tobacco habits. A dedicated smokeless tobacco user can consume several kilogrammes of tobacco each year in this way. Most smokeless tobacco habits have a limited geographic spread, but international travel and emigration have brought them to new populations and use is increasing dramatically in the United States, with 6% of males being users.

Betel quid is widely used in the UK by immigrant communities, and further details are given in the section on oral submucous fibrosis. Some smokeless tobacco habits are listed in Table 20.1 and are discussed further in the next chapter.

Web URL 19.1 Review habits and carcinogenicity: http://monographs.iarc.fr/ENG/recentpub/mono89.pdf

Clinical features

Application of pure tobacco to the mucosa induces hyperkeratosis and inflammation. Changes are limited to the site where the tobacco is held, usually in the buccal sulcus, and lesions do not have sharply defined margins. These changes seem to take prolonged periods to develop and, in the early stages, there is only erythema and mild, whitish thickening of the epithelium. Later there is extensive white thickening and wrinkling of the mucosa. Before developing carcinoma, the mucosa will usually show varying degrees of dysplasia on biopsy, but even a non-dysplastic lesion at a site of tobacco application signifies a risk of carcinoma.

Betel quid users show distinctive features from the various other components of the quid. In addition to the features mentioned previously, frequent users may develop erythematous areas or erythroplakia. There is often also some localised fibrosis that need not signify submucous fibrosis (discussed later), but makes the lesion firm on palpation. Areca nut in the quid produces a dark red stain on the teeth, and in heavy users, of the mucosa too.

Malignant change follows at the site of tobacco placement but only after many years of use. Most habits induce squamous cell carcinoma, but snuff dippers develop verrucous carcinomas (Ch. 20) much more frequently and after a longer exposure. If these remain untreated, invasive squamous carcinoma may develop.

Lesions associated with *snus*, Swedish moist snuff, are characteristic. Unlike other habits, the site is often the anterior buccal sulcus. The mucosa is greatly thickened, wrinkled and appears oedematous with a keratotic surface. This habit appears to carry a very low or minimal risk. Snus is sold as a loose powder and in a small paper pouch like a teabag, and is popular in Sweden and the United States.

Smokeless tobacco products have other adverse effects including gingival and alveolar bone recession at the site. The oesophagus and pharynx are also exposed to carcinogens, and carcinoma may also develop there. Betel quid use has also been linked to diabetes and exacerbation of asthma.

Pathology

The main changes are thickening of the epithelium with varying degrees of hyperorthokeratosis or parakeratosis. Regular and heavy users develop a thickened basement membrane and superficial fibrosis in the area where the tobacco is held and atrophy of underlying salivary glands. Later, there may be epithelial atrophy and the features of dysplasia may eventually be seen.

Management

Diagnosis is based on the history of smokeless tobacco use and the lesion in the area where the tobacco is held. It is important to ascertain exactly what type of tobacco is used and how it is prepared. Biopsy is required to exclude dysplasia or early malignant change.

The most effective and important intervention is to stop the tobacco habit by patient education.

Lesions that are dysplastic may resolve completely or may regress, although there is a risk of delayed progression and malignant transformation. Non-dysplastic lesions in snuff dippers will resolve on stopping the habit even after 25 years of use. If the habit continues, regular follow up and biopsies are required. Most smokeless tobacco users also smoke, and this also needs to be addressed with smoking cessation advice.

Harm reduction for smokers Scandinavian moist snuff sachets (snus) have a lower carcinogen content than other tobacco products. This is because the tobacco is cured in steam and is not fermented, unlike the kiln-dried tobacco for cigarettes. The risk of developing carcinoma from these products appears negligible, some claim non-existent.

This has led to the proposal that smokers could reduce their risk of smoking-induced disease by switching to this type of smokeless tobacco. Statistically this makes some sense. The risk of lung and laryngeal carcinoma, of cardiovascular disease and other risks of inhaled tobacco are abolished and replaced by a low risk that affects a more readily examined site. Smokers also find this type of tobacco more acceptable than nicotine patches (and even nicotine patches have adverse health effects).

Opponents of this view point out that no tobacco product is safe, no use should be encouraged and that this is not a safe alternative to smoking. They worry that children and adolescents will develop this habit and progress to become smokers, although the Swedish experience suggests the opposite. There is no doubt that these products are still addictive and should never be recommended outside a smoking cessation programme with regular oral examination.

The concept of promoting a harmful product as an alternative to an even more harmful one has generated intense argument, similar to that which still surrounds the use of methadone for heroin users. This is a difficult ethical area, and the interpretation of the evidence is still a matter of debate. Certainly there is a risk of sending conflicting messages to the public. Use of such products is rising dramatically in the United States, but they are banned, although readily available, in Europe outside Sweden.

Topical tobacco lesions review PMID: 17238967

Snuff dipping PMID: 6808102

Snus PMID: 24314326 and snus lesions PMID: 16470839

Electronic cigarettes and 'vaping' raise similar issues. Use has become very widespread in a few years. Nicotine vapour is safer than smoke but is addictive, carries cardiovascular risks and contains other toxins including formaldehyde and metals, though at lower levels than smoke. Evidence shows that vaping can be an effective smoking cessation aid, and it has been suggested that it should be available on prescription like nicotine patches. Oral effects are little studied, dry mouth and throat being reported. Nicotine is easily absorbed through oral mucosa, and further studies are needed. Most users smoke as well, and it is easy to assimilate high doses of nicotine using these devices. To date no distinctive oral lesion appears to be linked to vaping.

Vaping PMID: 27705269

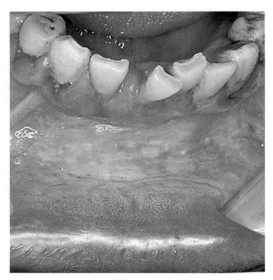

Fig. 19.9 **Tobacco pouch or snus lesion.** Keratosis with wrinkling of the sulcus mucosa where the pouch is held. Although this type of tobacco has a very low risk of cancer, note the inflammation and recession of the gingiva in contact with the pouch. *(From Pediatric Dentistry, 2005, 'Examination, Diagnosis, and Treatment Planning for General and Orthodontic Problems')*

CHRONIC HYPERPLASTIC CANDIDOSIS

A detailed description of this condition is in Chapter 15, and the difficulty of distinguishing a 'pure' chronic candidal infection from a leukoplakia with superimposed candidosis was noted. If a white plaque is suspected from its clinical presentation to be candidal but fails to respond to treatment, or if there is dysplasia on biopsy, the lesion must be treated as a leukoplakia.

The clinical appearance of chronic hyperplastic candidosis can be very worrying, with a florid speckled appearance.

Whether candida itself is a carcinogen is controversial, but it can produce known chemical carcinogens, induce hyperplasia and activate epithelial cells. Leukoplakia infected by candida has an increased risk of transformation, and it is usual to try to treat the infection. However, any risk of transformation is very low.

The chronic candidosis of autoimmune polyendocrine syndrome 1 and the forms of mucocutaneous candidosis are different and have significant risk (Chs 36 and 15).

Is candidal infection oncogenic PMCID: PMC3084579

ORAL SUBMUCOUS FIBROSIS

Oral submucous fibrosis is an important and readily recognised condition in which the oral mucosa becomes fibrotic, immobile and contracts progressively causing limitation of opening. More significantly, oral submucous fibrosis undergoes malignant transformation in 4%–8% of cases and makes a significant contribution to the high incidence of oral cancer in the Indian subcontinent and in Asian emigrant populations.

The cause of oral submucous fibrosis has long been known to be the chewing of betel quid (*paan* or *pan*), and its primary ingredient areca nut is the causative agent. The relative risk for users is almost 100 times, and betel quid is an extremely potent carcinogen. The simplest quid comprises chopped or grated areca nut mixed with slaked lime (CaOH) and wrapped in a leaf from the betel vine. There

are enormous regional variations in additional ingredients, which include tobacco, spices and flavourings. The quid is folded tightly or tied, held in the buccal sulcus and occasionally chewed.

Areca nut contains alkaloids and the habit is addictive. However, it also has cultural significance, is associated with tradition and religious rituals and is regarded by many users as a general tonic with beneficial medicinal effects. Similar mixtures of ingredients may be used as toothpastes. For these reasons, the habit is often acquired young, between the age of 5 and 12 years in India and 10–20 years in the UK. In the UK, between 13% and 30% of immigrant children chew betel quid, more in lower socioeconomic classes, and half use it daily though rarely with tobacco included. A heavy user may consume 20 or 30 quid each day, and some will sleep with a quid in the mouth. Betel quid use is prevalent throughout the Indian subcontinent, Southeast Asia, Malaysia, the Philippines, Taiwan and parts of China, as well as in their emigrants. Different combinations of ingredients are used in these different countries.

The two main adverse effects of betel quid use are oral cancer and submucous fibrosis. However, other risks include carcinoma of the pharynx and oesophagus and possibly diabetes. Quid containing tobacco carries the highest risk for carcinoma. Areca nut alone carries the highest risk for submucous fibrosis, but also causes carcinoma at a lower rate.

In the United Kingdom and United States, it appears that most users add tobacco to the quid, even though they develop the habit using tobacco-free quid. Particularly worrying is the emergence of cheap commercially prepared quid ingredients *paan masala* and *gutka*, the latter a flavoured and sweetened product aimed at children that can be imported legally into the UK.

Clinical features

Clinically, users of all types of quid show some common features. The teeth are typically stained dark brown by a dye extracted from the nut by the lime. At the site of quid placement there is usually erythema, keratosis and a flaking surface ('betel chewer's mucosa'), and sometimes erythroplakia or leukoplakia. Long-term users have periodontitis and recession of the adjacent gingiva.

Symmetrical fibrosis develops in the buccal mucosa, soft palate or inner aspects of the lips. In the earliest stages, there may be a burning sensation and scattered small vesicles. Later, fibrosis and loss of vascularity cause extreme pallor of the affected area, which then appears almost white and marble-like. The fibrosis starts immediately below the epithelium but extends to deeper tissues until they eventually become so hard that they cannot be indented with the finger (Fig. 19.10). Muscles of mastication are eventually involved. At this stage, the epithelium appears smooth, thin and atrophic. Ultimately, mouth opening may become so limited that eating and dental treatment become difficult, and tube feeding may become necessary.

Erythroplakia and leukoplakia may develop in oral submucous fibrosis (Fig. 19.11), and the epithelium may show dysplasia on biopsy. Later, there is a very high risk of carcinoma and, if these changes develop when opening is limited, they may easily be missed.

Pathology

The minority of areca users that develop submucous fibrosis are genetically predisposed. Occasionally, there is a familial incidence. Those that are most susceptible can develop the

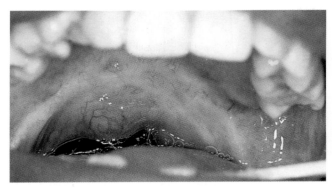

Fig. 19.10   Oral submucous fibrosis. Typical appearance in a relatively advanced case with pale fibrotic bands of scarring running across the soft palate and down the anterior pillar of the fauces. Similar fibrous bands were present in the buccal mucosa bilaterally.

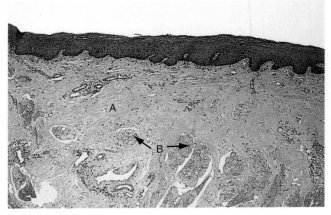

Fig. 19.12   Oral submucous fibrosis. There is fibrosis *(A)* extending from the epithelium down into the underlying muscle *(B)*, which is replaced by hyalinised fibrous tissue.

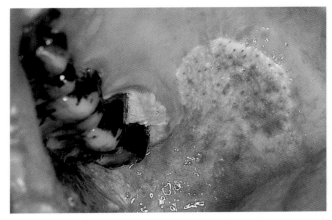

Fig. 19.11   High-risk potentially malignant lesion in a betel quid chewer. The classical appearance of a speckled leukoplakia such as this is almost always associated with either severe dysplasia or invasive carcinoma. Note also the brown betel quid staining on the teeth.

disease in childhood, but most cases follow years of exposure to areca.

An alkaloid component of areca nut, arecoline, can induce fibroblast proliferation and collagen synthesis and may penetrate the oral mucosa to cause progressive cross-linking of collagen fibres.

The cause of the carcinomas and dysplastic lesions is presumed to be the carcinogens from the tobacco and nitrosamines from the areca nut. Similar molecular changes have been identified in the DNA of epithelial cells in quid users and smokers. The epithelial atrophy, relative avascularity and inflammation may also play a role.

Histologically, the subepithelial connective tissue becomes thickened, hyaline and avascular and there may be infiltration by modest numbers of chronic inflammatory cells. The epithelium usually becomes thinned and may show dysplasia. Underlying muscle fibres undergo progressive atrophy and replacement by dense fibrous tissue (Fig. 19.12).

Management

Treatment is largely ineffective. Patients must stop the causative habit, but no regression usually follows; only stabilisation of the trismus can be expected. Intralesional injections of corticosteroids may be tried in association with muscle stretching exercises or a 'trismus screw' between the teeth

forcibly to stretch the bands of scar tissue, but these require dedication in use and the benefit is not usually great. Wide surgical excision of the affected tissues including the underlying buccinator muscle together with skin grafting or various flap procedures can be carried out, but are likely to be followed by relapse.

The most important measure is to slow progression and reduce the risk of malignant progression by stopping the betel quid habit. Regular follow-up and biopsy of red or white lesions is essential but, even so, the risk of malignant change is reported to be about 5%–8%. Carcinomas also arise in the posterior tongue and pharynx, and in severe cases these can only be examined under anaesthetic or using endoscopy.

Submucous fibrosis review PMID: 23107623

Oral lesions in betel users PMID: 9890449

Gutka hazards PMID: 20382045

Risks internationally PMID: 24302487

Betel quid use UK PMID: 11309868

Risk of transformation PMID: 3866655

LICHEN PLANUS

Lichen planus is accepted as a potentially malignant disorder, but the risk must be extremely low. Some of the problems in proving this controversial association are discussed in Chapter 16.

A number of patients develop carcinoma in a background of keratosis and atrophy that either is lichen planus or is indistinguishable from it, but the overall transformation rate in lichen planus seems unlikely to exceed 0.05% in 10 years.

Review of cases of carcinoma developing in lichen planus often reveals the presence of mild dysplasia or unusual clinical features from the outset, either of which should have favoured a diagnosis of leukoplakia or erythroplakia rather than lichen planus. A significant contribution to the difficulty is that mild dysplasia is recognised by the immune system, which mounts a cell-mediated host response against the abnormal epithelium. As much as a quarter of dysplastic lesions show this feature to some degree. Histologically, it is characterised by T cells migrating into the basal cells and

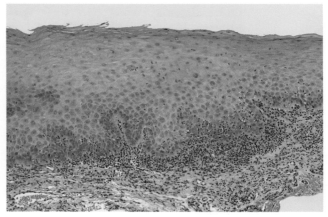

Fig. 19.13 Dysplastic lesion mimicking lichen planus. This sample comes from a lesion described as being a white patch with striae, suggesting lichen planus, and the histological appearances suggest lichen planus, with a well-defined infiltrate of lymphocytes below the epithelium and lymphocytes in the basal cell layer inducing apoptosis. However, note that the basal cell layer survives for the most part. The lichen planus-like features arise from a cell-mediated response against the abnormal epithelial cells. Such lesions are good mimics of lichen planus and easily misdiagnosed.

killing them by inducing apoptosis, exactly the same process as causes lichen planus (Fig. 19.13). Some have called this process *lichenoid dysplasia*, but it is not a specific condition, and any lesion that shows dysplasia is best diagnosed as such, and not as lichen planus, however convincing the clinical picture.

Apparent lichen planus with unusual features, such as lesions in the floor of mouth or soft palate, late onset or unusual red areas should be regarded with suspicion, submitted for biopsy and followed up closely. Many cases of proliferative verrucous leukoplakia are initially misdiagnosed as lichen planus.

LUPUS ERYTHEMATOSUS

Lupus erythematosus, discussed in Chapter 16, is associated with a small risk of malignant change, especially in lesions of the lower lip.

DYSKERATOSIS CONGENITA

Dyskeratosis congenita is a rare disease with several inheritance patterns caused by loss of chromosomal telomeres. The main oral feature is dysplastic white or red lesions of the buccal mucosa, tongue and soft palate (Fig. 19.14). Other features include cutaneous pigmentation, dystrophies of the nails and haematological abnormalities. Oral carcinoma develops in up to a third of cases.

Causes of death include cancers of the mouth or other sites, bleeding (gastrointestinal or cerebral), but in 50% from infections resulting from bone marrow failure.

General review PMID: 23782086

Oral features review PMID: 18938267

HPV-ASSOCIATED DYSPLASIA

During the early years of the AIDS epidemic, oral white patches caused by infection with human papillomavirus

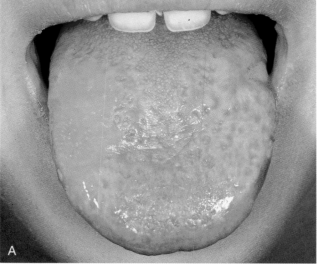

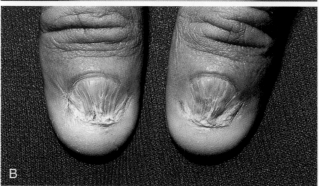

Fig. 19.14 Dyskeratosis congenita. A young patient with diffuse keratosis of the dorsum of the tongue (*A*) and another patient showing the typical nail dystrophy (*B*). *(From Paller, A.S., Mancini, A.J., 2011. Hurwitz clinical pediatric dermatology: a textbook of skin disorders of childhood and adolescence. Saunders, Philadelphia.)*

were recognised, but these became very rare following introduction of antiretroviral treatment. These were originally called *koilocytic dysplasia*.

More recently, similar white patches have been increasing in incidence in non-immunocompromised patients. They are indistinguishable clinically from other leukoplakias but histologically distinctive (Fig. 19.15). Almost all are infected by high-risk HPV subtypes, as found in oropharyngeal carcinomas (Ch. 21). The viral DNA may be in the cytoplasm or integrated into the host DNA, and there is also low-level viral replication. There have been insufficient cases reported to understand the natural history of this new disease, but it is clear that at least some cases develop carcinoma, and from first principles this is to be expected.

Although it might be expected that papillomavirus infection in dysplastic lesions would produce a papillomatous appearance, clinically this is not so, although some are slightly verrucous. HPV is not associated with proliferative verrucous leukoplakia or the majority of verrucous leukoplakias.

Description PMID: 8843454

SYPHILITIC LEUKOPLAKIA

Leukoplakia of the dorsum of the tongue is a characteristic complication of tertiary syphilis, but is so rare now as to be

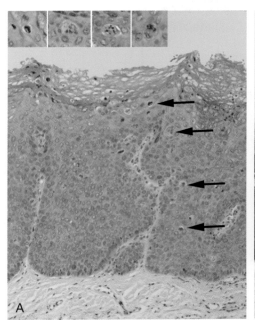
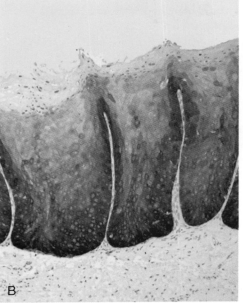
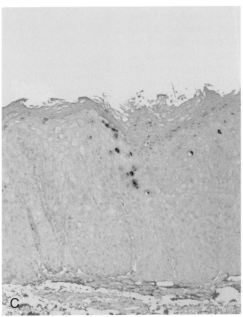

Fig. 19.15 Human papillomavirus–associated dysplasia. There are numerous mitoses and unusual degenerate and apoptotic cells at all levels including the upper prickle cell layers (*A*). These cells often have a chromatin pattern suggesting that they are degenerate mitoses (*inset*). Immunohistochemistry for p16 cell cycle regulatory protein is positive (*B*, brown stain), indicating that the virus is transcribing its oncogenic E6/E7 proteins (see Ch. 21). DNA in situ hybridisation reveals high-risk viral DNA in some of the cells (*C, blue stain is positive*).

of little more than historical interest in the UK. Few patients reach the tertiary stage in developed countries but may do so in some parts of the world. Syphilitic leukoplakia was a feared complication because of its very high malignant transformation rate of 50% or more.

Syphilitic leukoplakia has no distinctive features but typically affects the dorsum of the tongue and spares the margins. The lesion has an irregular outline and surface. Cracks, small erosions or nodules may prove on histology to be foci of invasive carcinoma.

On biopsy there is hyperkeratosis, dysplasia and the characteristic late syphilitic chronic inflammatory changes with plasma cells, granulomas and endarteritis of small arteries.

The diagnosis depends on serological findings. The presence of syphilitic endarteritis may be a contraindication to radiotherapy, making treatment difficult.

Treatment of syphilis does not cure the leukoplakia, which persists and can undergo malignant change many years later.

MANAGEMENT OF POTENTIALLY MALIGNANT DISORDERS

As will be noted in Chapter 20, the prognosis in oral carcinoma is good only when the diagnosis is made early and the tumour is small. The principles of management are

> **Box 19.1 Principles of management of dysplastic lesions**
>
> - Stop any associated habits, e.g. betel quid or smoking
> - Dietary intervention
> - Treat candidal infection and/or iron deficiency if present
> - Biopsy to assess dysplasia
> - Assess risk of transformation on clinical and histological findings
> - Consider ablation of individual lesions (see Box 19.3)
> - Maintain observation for signs of malignant change

> **Box 19.2 Clinical risk factors for malignant change in erythroplakia and leukoplakia**
>
> **History**
> - Betel quid usage
> - Tobacco smoking or topical tobacco habit*
> - High alcohol intake
> - Specific genetic disorders
>
> **Clinical aspects**
> - Advanced age
> - Female gender[†]
> - Areas of reddening in the lesion
> - Areas of speckling in the lesion
> - Nodular or verrucous areas or ulceration
> - High-risk site:
>   - posterolateral tongue
>   - floor of mouth
>   - retromolar region
>   - anterior pillar of fauces
> - Large lesions
> - Lesions present for long periods
> - Enlargement or change in character of pre-existing lesion
>
> *Nevertheless, surveys indicate that the risk of malignant change in white lesions is higher in non-smokers, because tobacco induces very many low-risk lesions. Thus, both non-smokers and heavy smokers with red and white patches are at risk.
> [†]Surveys indicate that malignant change in white lesions is more frequent in women. This is partly accounted for by the fact that women have many fewer lesions, smoke less, but develop proliferative verrucous leukoplakia in which carcinoma is highly likely. Male heavy smokers and female non-smokers with red and white patches thus both carry a relatively high risk.

therefore to prevent carcinoma developing, or if already present, to detect it when small. Ideally, cancer could be prevented by detecting potentially malignant lesions and treating them.

Red or white lesions in the mouth should never be ignored. Have a high index of suspicion that an oral lesion may be potentially malignant and investigate appropriately. It may turn out to be innocuous but must be assessed with the possibility of future carcinomatous change borne in mind.

The management of dysplastic oral lesions remains controversial because very large numbers must be treated to prevent malignant transformation in a small minority. For all practical purposes, dysplasia seen on biopsy has to be considered a possible early stage in the development of carcinoma. Detecting dysplasia provides an opportunity to treat carcinoma at an exceptionally early and potentially curative preinvasive stage. Unfortunately, the assumption that surgical removal will prevent carcinoma is not well supported by clinical evidence.

The principles of the management of dysplastic lesions are summarised in Box 19.1. The first step is to assess the risk of malignant transformation.

Review PMID: 17257863

Risk assessment

Clinical

The first stage in management is clinical assessment. The patient should be questioned, and the lesion should be examined for the features in Box 19.2. Risk habits, tobacco use, betel quid and alcohol should be recorded by type amount and frequency.

Potentially malignant disorders indicate field change (mentioned previously), so a full and detailed examination of the mouth is required, with an attempt made to visualise the pharynx. All cervical lymph nodes should be palpated in case carcinoma is already present and has metastasised. Any additional lesions found must be managed in the same way as the initial lesion.

The size of the lesion, colour, homogeneity, any areas of nodular or verrucous change, ulceration, redness or speckling and whether or not it lies in a high-risk site for developing carcinoma (see Fig. 19.8) must be recorded. A photographic or diagrammatic record is very useful for monitoring changes during follow up. Large and longstanding lesions are at higher risk, and those in the elderly. A change in nature of a lesion is a worrying sign.

Induration, a feeling of firmness on palpation caused by fibrosis of the underlying connective tissue, is an early sign of carcinoma, signifying invasion into underlying tissues. If induration is present a carcinoma is likely and the patient should be referred directly to a cancer centre for further investigation. Apart from induration and ulceration, the features of carcinoma in its earliest stages may be identical to those of red, white and speckled patches (see Fig. 19.6). Elicit all features likely to indicate increased risk (Box 19.2).

Size is important PMID: 23521625 and 12945594

A number of adjuncts to clinical diagnosis are available that are claimed to either identify lesions more effectively, identify higher risk lesions or aid diagnosis of carcinoma. Tolonium chloride rinsing and brush biopsy are considered in Chapter 20 with oral cancer screening. Some 'visualisation' techniques claim to make dysplastic lesions more readily identifiable on examination. Some illuminate the mucosa with a wavelength of light that is normally absorbed but reflected by abnormal epithelium. Others use autofluorescence patterns or more complex laser reflectance. These techniques are sometimes used in conjunction with dyes. All occasionally identify lesions missed in routine examination, but none has yet been proved cost effective in appropriately designed trials.

Biopsy

Biopsy is the key investigation. It excludes or confirms whether carcinoma is already present and, if not, allows dysplasia to be detected and graded. The term dysplasia

Table 19.3   Epithelial dysplasia: histological features

Architectural features	Cytological features
These are changes in the organisation of maturation and normal layering of the epithelium	These are changes in individual cells reflecting abnormal DNA content in the nucleus, failure to mature and keratinise correctly and increased proliferation
Irregular epithelial stratification	Abnormal variation in nuclear size
Loss of polarity of basal cells	Abnormal variation in nuclear shape
Drop-shaped rete ridges	Abnormal variation in cell size
Increased number of mitotic figures	Abnormal variation in cell shape
Abnormally superficial mitotic figures	Increased nuclear-cytoplasmic ratio
Premature keratinisation in single cells	Atypical mitotic figures
Keratin pearls within rete ridges	Increased number and size of nucleoli
Loss of epithelial cell cohesion	Nuclear hyperchromatism

(literally, abnormal growth) is the single best indicator of risk of transformation to carcinoma.

It is often said that every red or white patch in the mouth should be subject to biopsy, and this is certainly a logical precaution. In practice, some red and white lesions do not merit biopsy because their clinical features allow confident diagnosis as benign lesions. Examples would be median rhomboid glossitis or stomatitis nicotina. In further cases a response to treatment may avoid biopsy, for instance a suspected chronic hyperplastic candidosis may resolve on antifungal therapy. However, in most other cases, biopsy is considered best practice.

Selection of the correct site is critical to obtaining the most informative report. Biopsy must include the highest risk areas, those with erythema or speckling, verrucous or nodular change or induration. The centre of ulcers should be avoided. A biopsy from the margin rather than the centre avoids ulcer slough and non-specific inflammation. When several areas in the lesion appear at risk, or when several lesions are present, more than one biopsy may be necessary.

Techniques for biopsy are discussed in Chapter 1.

Dysplasia grading

Epithelial dysplasia is the combination of architectural and cytological abnormalities seen in tissues that indicate a risk of developing carcinoma (Table 19.3). All the features of dysplasia may also be seen in a carcinoma, the only difference between the two is the way the tissues are arranged. In epithelium with dysplasia the structure of the epithelium is retained, but deranged. In a carcinoma, epithelial cells no longer form a covering layer but invade the underlying connective tissue.

Note that dysplasia means only growth disturbance, and is used in the names of other completely benign conditions such as fibrous dysplasia or cemento-osseous dysplasia. It is only epithelial dysplasia that indicates potential malignancy.

The more abnormal the epithelium, the higher is the risk of carcinoma developing. The features seen in individual specimens vary, but there are common themes.

Mild dysplasia is diagnosed when the basal cells show slight disorganisation. There is increased proliferation with several layers of basaloid cells with large nuclei, and among them are scattered cells with very abnormal shape or size (Fig. 19.16).

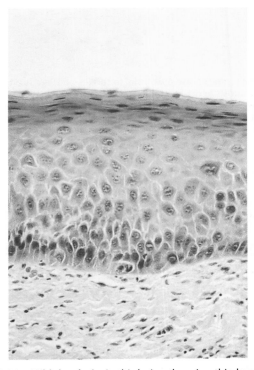

Fig. 19.16   Mild dysplasia. In this lesion there is a thin layer of parakeratin and the structure, maturation and orderly differentiation of the epithelial cells is largely unaffected. However, there is a degree of irregularity of basal cells with variation in size and hyperchromatism.

Moderate dysplasia has more layers of basaloid cells and usually increased intercellular spaces as a result of loss of cohesion. There is a disorganised higgledy-piggledy appearance in the basal layers. Mitotic figures and very abnormal cells may be seen not only in the basal cells but in the middle of the epithelium where basal cells proliferate upward at the expense of prickle cells (Fig. 19.17).

Severe dysplasia contains cells with the most marked abnormalities and loss of the normal layered structure of the epithelium. Most of the thickness is occupied by basal-type cells. There are few or no prickle cells or organised keratin layer, but individual cells may keratinise at any level (dyskeratosis). Loss of cohesion is usually marked. The

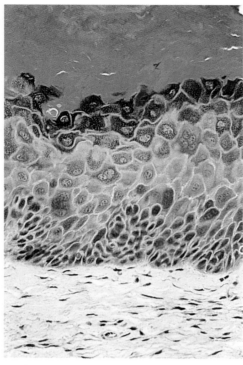

Fig. 19.17   Moderate dysplasia. In this lesion there is prominent orthokeratosis and a keratohyalin layer immediately below it. Dysplasia is more prominent than in the previous figure, with enlarged hyperchromatic and bizarre cells in the basal and lower prickle cell layers.

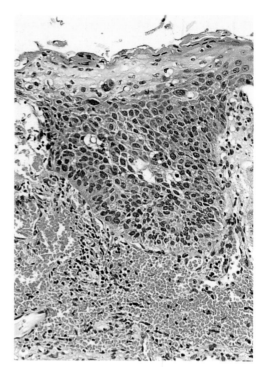

Fig. 19.19   Severe dysplasia. This rete process is composed almost entirely of cells with dark and irregularly shaped nuclei. Only the most superficial layers of cells show maturation to squamous cells, and the orderly maturation and differentiation of epithelial cells has been lost.

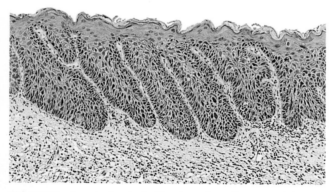

Fig. 19.18   Severe dysplasia. The dermal papillae extend close to the surface, and there are elongate rete processes, some of which are broader deeply. Enlarged and hyperchromatic cells are visible at this low power in rete processes and in most of the prickle cell layer.

Table 19.4	Proportion of the grades of dysplasia in oral red and white lesions in 1401 patients and the number developing carcinoma during 15 years follow up		
Grade	Number with each grade	Number developing carcinoma	Predictive value of the grade %
No dysplasia	1182	14	1
Mild dysplasia	105	6	6
Moderate dysplasia	76	14	18
Severe dysplasia	38	15	39

features are almost those of carcinoma; only invasion is missing. The term *carcinoma in situ* is sometimes used for this most severe dysplasia ('top-to-bottom change'; Figs 19.18 and 19.19).

Any degree of dysplasia may be accompanied by an immune host response. Potentially, this could kill the dysplastic cells, but in practice seems to have no protective effect.

Despite the fact that dysplasia is the best indicator of transformation, the exact relationship between grade and transformation is ill defined. Any grade signifies some risk. Whether different grades provide further useful information is a matter of considerable debate. The histological assessment of oral epithelial dysplasia is notoriously unreliable because it is subjective, there are no well-defined grading criteria and it is therefore not very reproducible. It also depends on the correct high-risk area being biopsied. Several large studies from different countries have shown no difference in malignant transformation rates between the grades, but this may be because they are performed on hospital patients who all tend to have relatively high risk.

In a recent UK study of 1401 patients with red or white lesions referred to hospital, 49 developed an oral carcinoma in 15 years. The value of dysplasia in predicting this is shown in Table 19.4.

Dysplasia grading works PMID: 23761273

Dysplasia grade not useful PMID: 9813722 and 16316774

Biopsy not representative PMID: 17448135

Grading is subjective PMID: 16931119

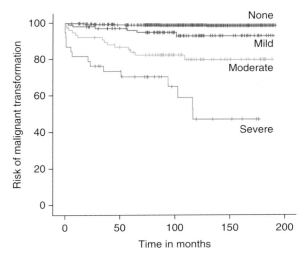

Fig. 19.20 Risk and time course of developing carcinoma in patients with mild, moderate, severe or no dysplasia in white lesions referred to hospital.

It can be seen that the majority of patients referred to hospital have benign conditions with no dysplasia, such as lichen planus. In this study, the risk of developing carcinoma rose with worsening grade. Patients with severe dysplasia are also at risk of carcinoma developing more quickly, and many patients with severe dysplasia develop a carcinoma in months (Fig. 19.20). This may well be because the carcinoma was present at the time of biopsy, but the invasive areas were not sampled. However, the diagnosis of severe dysplasia successfully identified that risk. Note that even some patients with no dysplasia develop oral carcinoma, so clinical risk assessment is still important. Note also that it can take years to develop carcinoma.

What happens to the dysplastic lesions that do not transform to cancer? Some resolve, some stay unchanged and others may remain and constitute a risk over an even longer period.

Transformation risk UK PMID: 12945594

Transformation risk Europe PMID: 9813722 and 16316774

Transformation risk United States PMID: 10815888 and 6537892

Transformation risk Taiwan PMID: 17181738

Transformation risk India PMID: 1056293

Other investigations

As dysplasia grading is an imperfect risk assessment, there is interest in molecular investigations that might be better predictors. Detecting abnormalities in chromosome numbers and loss or gain of function of genes is relatively easy, but no marker has yet proved a good predictor. Loss of heterozygosity (reflecting loss of a gene copy, probably due to a deletion) at various chromosomal loci is often found in oral carcinoma and potentially malignant epithelium. A panel of molecular markers identifying loss at 12 sites on chromosomes 3, 4, 8, 9, 11, 13 and 17 can be used to divide samples into low, medium and high risk groups from which 2, 15 and 64% of lesions transformed to carcinoma. These results are slightly better than for dysplasia grading, but the test is not yet available outside a research environment.

DNA ploidy analysis, a measure of total nuclear DNA content, is also a good predictor of malignant transformation. Nuclei from the biopsy are stained with a DNA binding dye that allows the total DNA content of each cell to be measured (Fig. 16.21). It is well known that dysplastic and malignant cells show chromosomal instability; their chromosomes have numerous deletions and duplications, sometimes of whole chromosomes. These changes can even be detected in epithelium that does not show dysplasia on routine light microscopic examination. Tissue with abnormal DNA content (aneuploidy) has a risk of transformation of 34% in 15 years, about the same risk as a diagnosis of severe dysplasia.

The value of such tests is that they can often detect risk when dysplasia is not present, so a combination of both assessments produces the most useful result.

Review diagnostic aids PMID: 17825602

Predictive biomarkers PMID: 19442563 and 21249481

Cochrane review diagnostic tests PMID: 26021841

DNA ploidy analysis PMID: 23761273

Treatment

The management of potential malignancy is controversial. It must be appreciated both that transformation has serious consequences for the patient, often culminating in death, but that the vast majority of such lesions will never transform.

After biopsy, the clinical features, dysplasia grade and any other information are compiled into a risk assessment.

Low-risk lesions can be managed conservatively. Patients' risk factors must be addressed, usually by smoking cessation advice or other habit intervention. Candidal infection should be eliminated and follow up instituted, ensuring a detailed and complete oral examination at every visit. Change in lesions is suspicious, and comparison with photographs or diagrams aids detection of changes.

Many patients, particularly those with heavy tobacco and alcohol intakes, have diets deficient in fruit and vegetables, a known risk factor for oral carcinoma. Dietary intervention to establish a balanced diet is known to reduce cancer development. It has been estimated that each portion of fruit or vegetables consumed each day reduces the risk of oral cancer by around 50%, and diet supplements induce regression of as much as 30% of oral white lesions. Dietary intervention is potentially extremely valuable.

High-risk lesions, on the basis of clinical features or dysplasia grade, should receive all the aforementioned interventions, but in addition may be ablated, by one of several methods (Box 19.3).

If lesions are of manageable size, it is tempting to excise them. However, evidence of disease eradication on prevention of carcinoma is very limited, and surgical removal of

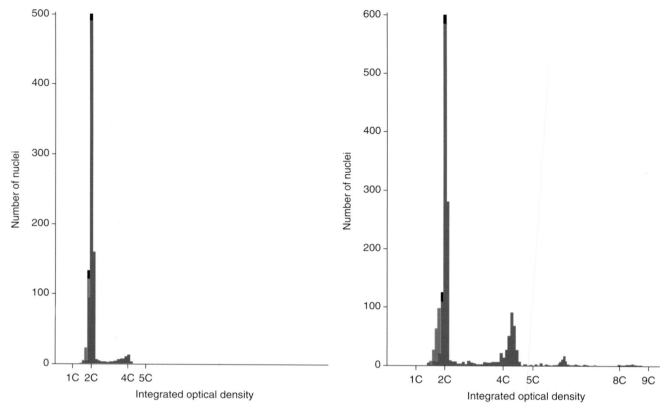

Fig. 19.21 **Ploidy analysis of normal and dysplastic epithelium.** Each graph shows the number of cells on the Y axis and the DNA content of each cell on the X axis. In normal mucosa (*left graph*) epithelial cells (*blue*) almost all have a normal diploid DNA content (called 2c, equivalent to 2 sets of chromosomes or diploid) with a few cells having doubled their DNA content because they are about to divide (small peak at 4c). Lymphocytes (*red*) and fibroblasts (*black*) act as a normal control. Dysplastic epithelium (*right graph, blue*) has peaks at abnormal DNA content (main peak between 4c and 5c) and many cells with grossly abnormal DNA content, up to 9c. Such a lesion may carry a high risk of malignant transformation.

large lesions carries morbidity. Visible mucosal changes are seen in only parts of the genetically altered field, making excision of the entire potentially malignant area impossible. Only areas of highest risk can be removed. Lesions in the highest risk areas in the posterior floor of mouth are technically difficult to excise.

Nevertheless, an attempt is usually made to excise all small lesions with moderate dysplasia and any lesions with severe dysplasia. Removal by laser surgery is well tolerated and heals well with limited scarring. Surgical excision provides a specimen that can be examined for the extent of dysplasia and for possible carcinoma. Early microscopic carcinoma may be found in 5%–10% of severe dysplasia when the whole lesion is excised.

Laser vaporisation, photodynamic therapy and medical treatments such as topical chemotherapeutic agents or systemic retinoids have proved unsuccessful and provide no specimen to detect unsuspected carcinoma, worsening the outcome.

After excision and reassessment of the risk following pathological examination, long-term follow up is required because carcinoma may not develop for 10 years or more (see Fig. 19.20). Three monthly appointments for 2 years are usual, gradually extending appointment intervals if lesions remain unchanged, habits and diet are addressed and the patient is educated about the risk.

An alternative approach for high-risk lesions is to observe closely for signs of deterioration, in the hope of detecting carcinoma as early as possible. Once carcinoma develops, the treatment options are much more clear cut. Such watchful waiting appears neglectful but avoids morbidity of treatment of little value and is supported by the natural history of the disease. However, the evidence that excision does have some benefit makes this difficult to justify, and patients need to be well informed if this path is to be chosen. Though surgical trials are small, meta-analysis shows that patients who have surgical treatment reduce their risk of malignant transformation from 15% to 5% independent of dysplasia grade.

In the absence of alternative treatments, surgical excision remains the treatment of choice for high-risk lesions, but recurrence of as many as 30% is reported.

Treatment effect PMID: 16316774

Treatment review PMID: 23159193

Treatment has some effect PMID: 19455705

Laser excision PMID: 12102411

Cochrane review PMID: 17054142

SMOKING CESSATION

Approximately 1 in 5 adults in the UK smoke, half the number that smoked in the 1970s. However, this reduction is mostly among older smokers; the number of young new smokers has remained stable, and two-thirds start the habit

Box 19.4 Oral adverse effects of smoking

- Lip, oral and oropharyngeal squamous carcinoma
- Oral potentially malignant lesions
- Predisposition to periodontitis
- Increased risk of implant failure
- Predisposition to candidal infection
- Predisposition to osteomyelitis
- Staining of teeth
- Taste impairment
- Halitosis

Recurrent aphthous stomatitis may worsen on smoking cessation, but not when nicotine replacement is used.

as teenagers. As half of cigarette smokers will eventually be killed by their habit, it is not surprising that almost three-quarters would like to stop.

Nicotine is powerfully addictive, having dopaminergic effects similar to cocaine. Even those who have had a laryngectomy or are dying of lung cancer will continue to smoke. Only 3% of smokers can quit smoking by willpower alone, and smokers are encouraged to seek professional support to help them quit.

Dentists are well placed to help. They screen a large proportion of the UK population, and oral adverse effects of smoking enable them to raise the issue with patients (Box 19.4). Smoking cessation in dental practice is as effective as in medical primary care. Three minutes' advice will help an additional 2% to quit and 10 minutes' advice a further 6%. These may seem small proportions, but they represent a significant health benefit for individuals.

Smoking cessation advice must be provided as part of a structured programme to be effective. A simple approach is to *Ask* about smoking at every consultation, *Advise* on oral and health effects, *Assist* with health promotion material and offer support and *Arrange* follow up or referral for specialist advice. A team approach is most effective at reinforcing the message. Smoking cessation literature should be available in the waiting room, but referral to a specialised cessation service has the highest success rate.

Some patients find nicotine replacement helpful in weaning themselves off tobacco. Chewing gum, skin patches, nasal spray, inhaler, tablets, lozenges and electronic cigarettes are available. When used as part of an individualised cessation plan, nicotine replacement increases the success rate to 1 in 6. Such products are available over the counter and may be provided in dental surgeries. Bupropion (Zyban) may also help some patients.

See also the section on oral cancer aetiological factors in Chapter 20.

Cochrane review role in dentistry PMID: 22696348

Dental patients' views PMID: 26609892

Web URL 19.2 UK NHS guidance dentistry: https://www.gov.uk/government/publications/smokefree-and-smiling

or, search NHS smokefree smiling

Water pipes (shisha) PMID: 27932840

Summary chart 19.1   Differential diagnosis and management of the common causes of red and white patches of the oral mucosa.

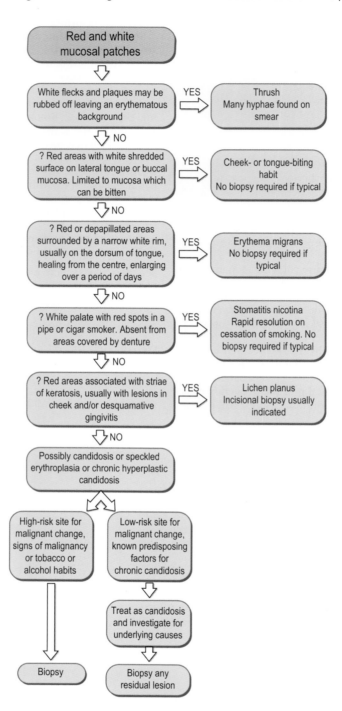

Summary chart 19.2 Summary of the key features of the common and important oral white patches.

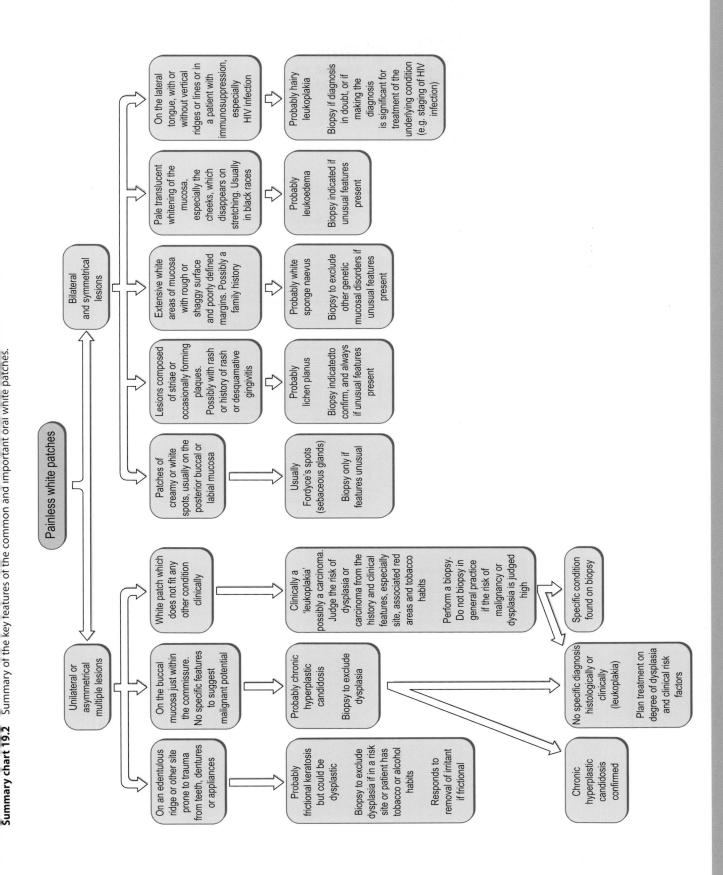

Summary chart 19.3 Differential diagnosis of common and important red patches affecting the oral mucosa.

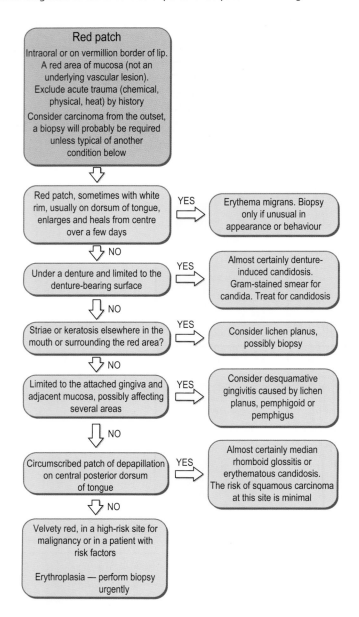

Oral cancer

20

More than 90% of malignant neoplasms in the mouth are squamous cell carcinomas arising from mucosal epithelium. Most of the remainder arise in minor salivary glands (Ch. 23), and a few are metastases. The term *oral cancer* is therefore used loosely to mean oral squamous carcinoma. Carcinomas of tonsil, pharynx and lip are considered in the next chapter.

EPIDEMIOLOGY

Oral carcinoma accounts for only approximately 2% of all malignant tumours in such countries as the United Kingdom and the United States. In most countries where reliable data are available, the incidence of cancer of the mouth, although variable, is low. India, Pakistan, Bangladesh and Sri Lanka are, however, exceptional, and cancer of the mouth accounts for approximately 40% or more of all cancer there, although the incidence varies widely in different parts of this subcontinent. Relatively high rates are found in parts of China, Southeast Asia, France, Brazil and Eastern Europe. This variation is largely due to tobacco and other habits, and incidence is rising in these areas. Those who neither drink nor smoke, such as Mormons and Seventh Day Adventists, have very low rates of oral carcinoma.

Approximately 4500 cases of intraoral carcinoma are registered each year in the UK. For the last 50 years, the incidence of oral cancer has been falling in many developed countries such as the United States and in Europe. In the United Kingdom, unusually, oral carcinoma incidence is slowly rising (Fig. 20.1). Claims that oral carcinoma is increasing dramatically are accounted for by inclusion of oropharyngeal and tonsil carcinomas in the total. These cancers are not oral, present and behave differently and are discussed in the next chapter. Cancer registry data often compile lip, oral and oropharynx together, and together these account for more than 7300 cases each year in the UK.

Web URL 20.1 International epidemiology: http://globocan .iarc.fr/

Web URL 20.2 UK National audit reports: http://www.hscic.gov.uk/ and use search facility for 'head and neck cancer audit'

Web URL 20.3 US epidemiology: http://www.oralcancer foundation.org/cdc/

India epidemiology PMID: 23410017

Web URL 20.4 UK incidence, mortality: Web search for: ncras head and neck cancer hub

Age and gender incidence

Oral cancer is an age-related disease, and 95% of patients are older than 40 years, with median age at diagnosis of just older than 60 years. There is a sharp and virtually linear rise in mouth cancer with age, as with carcinoma in many other sites, and oral cancer will become more common with an ageing population.

Cancer of the mouth is considerably more common in men than women in most countries, but this is tobacco and alcohol related. In the UK the male:female ratio has sunk to 1.5:1, and figures for southeast England show little difference in incidence between the genders. The change is the result of the progressive decline in oral cancer in men, but a low rate in women. However, there is a worrying but relatively small increase in rates in the young, particularly women.

Key epidemiological features of cancer of the mouth are summarised in Box 20.1.

Health inequality and oral cancer PMID: 21490236

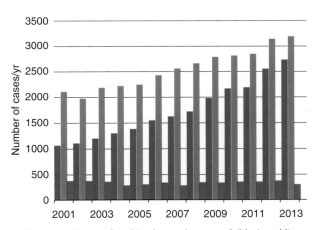

Fig. 20.1 Incidence of oral (*red*), oropharyngeal (*blue*) and lip carcinoma (*green*) for the UK until 2013, it taking several years to finalise incidence data at cancer registries. Current incidence reflects these rising trends. *(Data from National Cancer Intelligence Network (England), Information Services Division (Scotland), Welsh Cancer Intelligence Surveillance Unit and Northern Ireland Cancer Registry.)*

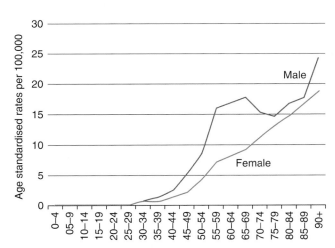

Fig. 20.2 Age-specific incidence graph showing incidence in different age groups. *(Data from the UK National Cancer Registration Service Cancer Analysis System.)*

Box 20.1   Cancer of the mouth: key features

- Accounts for approximately 2% of all cancers in the UK
- One of the most common cancers in the Indian subcontinent
- Males more frequently affected
- Most patients are older than 40 years and incidence rises with age
- Tongue, posterolaterally, is the most common site within the mouth
- Some arise in pre-existing white or red lesions
- Tobacco and alcohol are the main causes
- In the Indian subcontinent and Southeast Asia, betel quid is the main cause

Box 20.2   Possible aetiological factors for oral cancer

- Major factors
  - Tobacco smoking
  - Smokeless tobacco
  - Betel quid habit
  - Alcohol
  - Sunlight (lip only)
- Low risk factors
  - Diet
  - Candidosis
  - Human papillomavirus*
  - Lichen planus
- Rare in the UK, but significant
  - Oral submucous fibrosis
  - Dyskeratosis congenita
  - Fanconi's anaemia
  - Syphilis
- Speculative factors
  - Radiation
  - Immunodeficiency

*Human papillomavirus infection seems to carry a low risk in the oral cavity but is a high-risk infection in the oropharynx and nose.

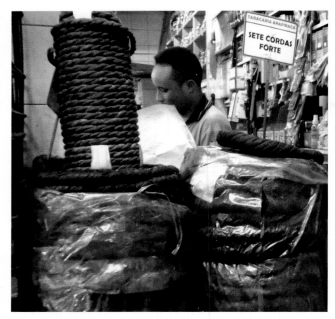

Fig. 20.3   Tobacco for sale in Brazil. Thick ropes of tobacco leaves for smoking and chewing. Such tobacco has been hardly processed, and carcinogenicity varies with the origin of the tobacco and the way the leaf is cured and processed. *(Kindly provided by Dr C Gomes.)*

carcinogenicity (Fig. 20.3). Nearly 6 trillion cigarettes are smoked each year worldwide, and consumption continues to rise, with the highest intakes in Russia, China, Central Asia, Southern and Eastern Europe. In much of the world, smokeless tobacco predominates.

Tobacco use should always be included in a medical history, and the best way to express cumulative tobacco exposure is in pack years (units of 1 pack (of 20 cigarettes or equivalent) smoked every day for 1 year; multiply packs per day by years smoked).

Web URL 20.5 Pack year calculator: http://smokingpackyears .com/

AETIOLOGY

Defining the contributions of different causative factors is difficult; the disease is complex and multifactorial, and patients must be exposed to causative factors for a prolonged period to develop cancer. Risk factors for oral squamous cell carcinoma are summarised in Box 20.2. Worldwide, tobacco is the main cause.

Tobacco use

The earliest recorded tobacco-related death, although unsuspected at the time, was in 1621 when Thomas Herriot, who introduced clay pipe smoking to England, died of lip cancer. It has taken many years to finally establish beyond doubt that tobacco is the major aetiological factor for oral carcinoma.

Tobacco may be smoked or used in various smokeless tobacco habits and effects of each are different. Methods of processing tobacco before use also vary widely and affect its

Cigarette smoking

Smoking is the major aetiological factor, particularly in association with alcohol, and its importance is that it is preventable. Large epidemiological studies of over 1 million individuals in the United States reveal that smokers' risk of cancer is proportional to the amount smoked and years spent smoking. Smokers overall have 30 times the risk of oral cancer versus those who never smoked. It is estimated that 80%–90% of all oral cancers can be attributed to smoking.

Smoking continues to be more common in men, and one in five adults in the UK smoke, and this level has remained unchanged for several years after a long slow decline. The average smoker smokes 31 cigarettes a week. The higher risk habit of hand-rolled cigarettes has doubled in incidence and carries a higher risk of lip carcinoma. Over 2 million smokers have switched to electronic cigarettes in just a few years (Ch. 19) with potential risk reduction.

Smoking is also in decline in the United States, Australia and northern Europe. Improvement in cancer incidence lags behind changes in smoking habits, and it will take decades for these changes to take effect. In the meantime, consumption is increasing in the developing world.

Table 20.1 Some common smokeless (topical) tobacco habits, many more exist but are geographically restricted

Name	Habit	Where used	Carcinogenicity in oral mucosa
Chewing tobacco ('spit' tobacco)	Chewing a damp plug of cured leaf tobacco or loose strips of leaf. Often flavoured or sweetened	Historically widely used in Europe and United States, now mainly in the United States	Moderate to low for oral cancer
Snuff dipping with dry snuff	Placing a pinch of dry snuff in the buccal sulcus	Southeastern United States and Scandinavia	Relatively low. Associated with verrucous rather than squamous carcinomas
Betel quid (and pan masala; supari, paan) with tobacco	Areca nut, slaked lime, betel vine leaf with or without tobacco, sweeteners, flavourings and spices, rolled freshly or produced commercially as premixed dry powder sachets	Indian subcontinent, Southeast Asia, Philippines, New Guinea and China	Very high when tobacco is included. Areca nut is associated with submucous fibrosis in addition
Nass	Tobacco, ash, cotton oil quid held in sulcus	Central Asia and Pakistan	High
Khaini	Tobacco and lime quid placed in sulcus	India and Pakistan	High
Dry (nasal) snuff	Dry snuff inhaled through nose	Historically widespread in Europe but now used mainly in Africa	Low, associated with nasal and sinus carcinoma
Gutka	Commercially prepared powder of areca nut, tobacco, lime and other flavourings and sweeteners	Indian subcontinent, Southeast Asia	Probably high, also risk of submucous fibrosis
Toombak	Rolled ball of tobacco and sodium bicarbonate placed in sulcus or floor of mouth	Sudan	High
Snus (moist snuff sachets; Scandinavian snuff)	Teabag-like pouch of moist unfermented snuff, sometimes with flavouring. Also some rolled leaf products	Originally Scandinavia but now prevalent in the United States	Thought to be low or very low. See section on harm reduction (Ch. 19)
Dissolvable tobacco	Tablets, strips or sticks of completely dissolvable tobacco for oral use, usually sucked, contains flavourings	A novel product	Unknown, carcinogen content variable

Unlike pipe smoking or smokeless tobacco use, there are no specific oral lesions related to cigarette smoking, although cigarette smokers develop patchy mucosal pigmentation and light keratosis if they smoke heavily.

Marijuana smoking is widespread, and the smoke contains many of the carcinogens and co-carcinogens as tobacco smoke. It is suspected that it may be a more potent carcinogen than tobacco alone, but this has proved difficult to separate from the effects of alcohol and tobacco smoking.

Tobacco-induced cancers and deaths are preventable. Smoking cessation is discussed in Chapter 19 with management of potentially malignant disorders, but is equally important in managing patients who already have a carcinoma.

It is unclear how much the risk reduces after quitting smoking. There are substantial reductions in risk of 50% after stopping smoking for 5 years, but data on lung cancer suggest that the risk will never drop back to that of someone who has never smoked. Nevertheless, stopping smoking significantly reduces risk, reduces comorbidity that can impact on treatment outcome, and reduces the risk of a second primary cancer.

Smoking and alcohol PMID: 17647085

Smoking and smokeless tobacco review PMID: 20361572

Pipe smoking

Pipe smoking has steadily declined in most Westernised countries and has never become popular with women. The risk is statistically equal to cigarette smoking, and the lip is considered at high risk. Heavy pipe smokers may also develop stomatitis nicotina of the palate (Ch. 18), a white patch with no malignant potential. Recently water pipe (shisha or narghile) has become popular with adolescents and young adults but is more damaging than cigarette smoking.

Water pipe smoking: PMID: 27932840

Smokeless tobacco

Much of the world's tobacco consumption is in smokeless form. Tobacco habits and their risks are shown in Table 20.1, and Chapter 19 describes the habit's effects on mucosa in relation to potentially malignant lesions.

The risk varies with the habit but can be extremely high. In the southern United States, the habit of 'snuff dipping' causes extensive hyperkeratotic plaques and, after decades of continuous use, may lead to verrucous carcinoma (discussed later), as well as squamous carcinoma. This is a very slow process, and the relative risk of developing carcinoma arises to about ×12 after 15 years and ×50 after 50 years use. Conversely, Scandinavian moist snuff (snus) appears to carry a very low risk.

For all smokeless tobacco habits, carcinomas tend to arise at the site in the mouth where the tobacco is habitually held and carcinomas are often preceded by red or white lesions or dysplasia. However, carcinogens are also swallowed, and the pharynx and oesophagus are also at risk.

Most smokeless tobacco users also smoke.

Smokeless tobacco review PMID: 15470264

Smoking and smokeless tobacco review PMID: 20361572

Snus PMID: 17498797

Betel quid

Betel quid habit is practised widely in the Middle East, Indian subcontinent, Southeast Asia and parts of China. The composition of the quid (Table 20.1) varies geographically and between users, changing the risk, but overall, this habit is one of the most carcinogenic known. Addition of tobacco carries the highest risk, but areca nut without tobacco is also carcinogenic. In Thailand, where use has recently declined, the rates of oral carcinoma have fallen. Use also causes oral submucous fibrosis (Ch. 19).

Web URL 20.6 Betel quid general information: https://monographs.iarc.fr/ENG/Monographs/vol85/mono85.pdf

Betel use in Asia PMID: 22995631

Association premalignancy PMID: 22390524

Alcohol

Many oral cancer patients smoke and drink heavily. The relative risks for alcohol and tobacco consumption are shown in Fig. 20.4.

The increasing rates of oral cancer in the UK despite reduction in smoking have increased interest in alcohol as a cause. In Denmark there is good epidemiological evidence to link alcohol intake with oral carcinoma, and in the Bas

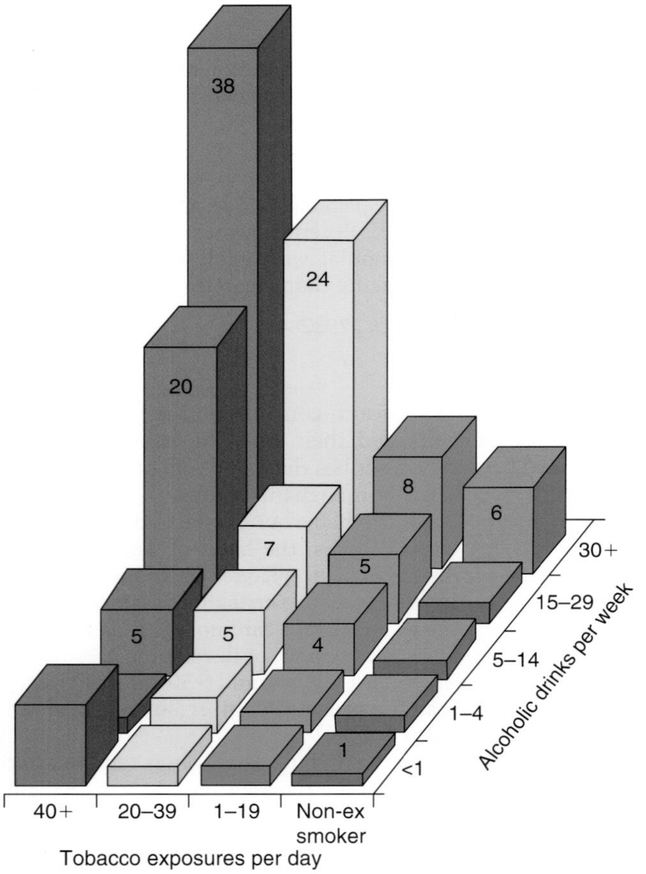

Fig. 20.4 **Relative risks of developing oral cancer in consumers (males in a Western population) of tobacco and alcohol.** The relative risk for a non-smoker and non-alcohol consumer is taken as one. A smoker consuming 30 cigarettes a day and 20 alcoholic drinks a week is seven times more likely to develop carcinoma.

Rhin area of France, alcohol is responsible for the highest oral and pharyngeal cancer incidence in Europe.

Drinks with the highest content of congeners, such as raw home-brewed spirits, have the closest association with carcinoma in some countries, whereas in others beer-drinking is implicated. As with smoking, total consumption is probably a critical factor. Recommended maximum intakes relate primarily to liver disease, and no safe limit for oral cancer is recognised.

In the UK, alcohol consumption had doubled in 50 years to an average intake of 8 litres pure ethanol each year in 2005, but has shown recent decline. The highest intakes are in the elderly and in low socioeconomic groups. One in five of those older than 65 years drink alcohol five times or more each week, more frequently if male. Those aged 16–25 years drink most, and there is no sex difference in the younger drinkers, but even in the binge drinking population there is a definite decline in intake since 2005.

Alcoholic drinks do not reside in the mouth for long, and there is no specific alcohol-related oral lesion. The mechanisms by which alcoholic drinks might cause carcinoma are unclear but include direct damage and increasing permeability to other carcinogens.

Some mouthwashes contain more than 25% alcohol, but any link to oral cancer remains speculative, with a possible weak association only in heavy users.

Alcohol effect review PMID: 20679896

Alcohol and potential malignancy PMID: 16614123

Smoking and alcohol PMID: 17647085

Infections and immunosuppression

Human papillomavirus (HPV) types 16 and 18 are now well-established causes of tonsil and oropharyngeal carcinomas (see next chapter), but their role in oral carcinomas is poorly understood and the subject of considerable research. Approximately 5% of oral carcinomas contain DNA from high-risk HPV subtypes and show p16 expression to suggest this is biologically active and potentially oncogenic.

Currently it seems that HPV is a minor factor in oral carcinoma, but there is some evidence that those carcinomas associated with the virus may have a slightly improved prognosis. HPV does not account for the recent increase in oral carcinoma in younger individuals.

Syphilitic leukoplakia is no longer a significant risk factor (Ch. 19).

Chronic candidosis causes hyperkeratotic plaques or speckled leukoplakias (Ch. 15), but outside the mucocutaneous candidosis syndromes carries a very low risk.

Immunosuppression is not a significant factor for intraoral carcinoma; incidence is not increased in HIV infection. However, lip carcinoma is more frequent in the immunosuppressed (Ch. 21).

Diet and malnutrition

Oral carcinoma is more frequent in those with low intake of fruit and vegetables. Vitamin A, C and carotenoids and other antioxidants are key protective factors, together with zinc and selenium. Though these are epidemiologically linked, evidence that dietary intervention could prevent carcinoma is limited, though it can induce regression of red and white potentially malignant lesions.

In India, malnutrition is widespread and may contribute, together with betel quid chewing, to the high incidence of carcinoma.

Diet and oral cancer PMID: 24937666

Folate and oral cancer PMID: 24974959

Diet in Sri Lanka and oral cancer PMID: 23601045

Other habits

Mate, or chimarrão, is an herbal tea made from the *Yerba mate* plant, a species of holly. It is drunk mostly in South and Central America, traditionally through a metal straw at a very high temperature. Use is weakly associated with carcinoma of the oesophagus, pharynx and palate, probably largely as a result of the high temperature, though it also contains known carcinogens.

Mate PMID: 20036605

Poor oral health

Oral sepsis, trauma from teeth, tooth loss and poor oral health have traditionally been regarded as contributing factors but are interrelated in complex ways with habits and socioeconomic factors. Chronic trauma has an effect in animal studies, probably by promoting constant proliferative activity, but in humans, such links remain speculative.

Genetic predisposition

Dyskeratosis congenita (Ch. 19) is rare, has oral precursor lesions and a distinctive presentation, so diagnosis is usually straightforward and established before any oral carcinoma develops.

Fanconi anaemia is an important but rare cause of oral carcinoma in the young, and oral carcinoma may be the presenting feature. Defects in several causative genes that are required for DNA repair are known, and inheritance is recessive. Patients develop aplastic anaemia and leukaemia and have a reduced lifespan. They are also at risk of many types of cancer, and one in three patients surviving till 50 years of age will develop one, even more among those treated by bone marrow transplantation. Squamous carcinomas of mouth, pharynx and oesophagus are relatively frequent, and any young patient with oral carcinoma should be screened for this condition. Clues for diagnosis include pigmented skin patches, short stature and a range of other developmental anomalies, but these features are very variable and genetic screening is required for diagnosis.

Case series PMID: 18831513

Potentially malignant disorders

These were discussed in the previous chapter and can be considered to fall into three groups:

- High-risk lesions associated with the same aetiological factors as oral carcinoma, such as speckled leukoplakia, erythroplasia and lesions with dysplasia.
- Specific high-risk conditions independent of risk factors such as proliferative verrucous leukoplakia and dyskeratosis congenita
- Chronic candidosis or lichen planus that are not associated with risk habits and are of very low risk

The proportion of carcinomas that arise in clinically recognisable potentially malignant diseases is unknown.

Patients without risk factors

A small proportion of patients appear to have no risk factors. Most are elderly and female, and they tend to have carcinomas of the buccal mucosa, alveolus and tongue. Many have the clinical presentation of proliferative verrucous leukoplakia (Ch. 19).

For the remainder, random mutation, background radiation, atmospheric pollution and passive smoking remain speculative aetiological factors. There is an increased risk for those with a first-degree relative who had oral carcinoma, but the relative risk is very low.

In young patients, those under 35 years of age, one in five have no identifiable risk factor.

Oral cancer in young PMID: 24103389

'EARLY' AND 'LATE' ORAL CARCINOMA

→ Summary charts 19.1, 19.2 and 19.3

pp. 314, 315, 316

It is important to recognise oral carcinomas at their earliest stages because this is the most important factor determining success of treatment.

It is often assumed that small carcinomas are early in their development, but carcinomas vary widely in their aggressiveness. Some very small carcinomas are detected small because they are slow growing and stay small and localised for a prolonged period. Conversely, some large carcinomas may have grown in a few weeks. Early carcinoma is usually taken to mean a carcinoma at a low Tumor Node Metastasis (TNM) stage.

The smallest carcinomas appear as painless red, speckled or white patches and only a minority are ulcerated (Figs 20.5 and 20.6). They are indistinguishable clinically from potentially malignant diseases, and approximately half of erythroplasias and speckled leukoplakias are already carcinomas on first biopsy.

After enlarging, a carcinoma may develop into a raised nodule, become ulcerated or both. Induration results from inflammation and fibrosis and infiltration of the tissues. By the time a carcinoma has formed an indurated ulcer with the typical rolled border, it will have been present for some months (Fig. 20.7).

Pain is generally considered of little value in the diagnosis of carcinoma. Certainly early carcinoma is often painless, but some patients are seen with a burning or sharp stinging

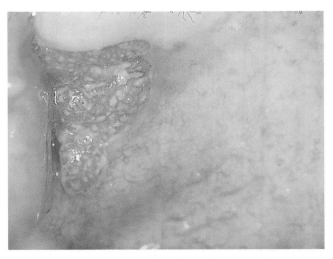

Fig. 20.5 Squamous carcinoma of the soft palate and mucosa posterior to the tuberosity appearing as a speckled leukoplakia.

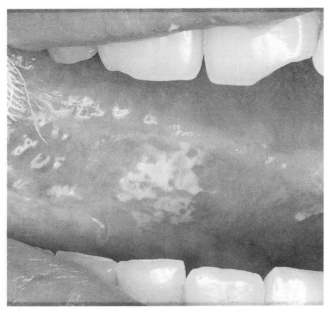

Fig. 20.6 Early squamous carcinoma. Despite its inconspicuous appearance, this small white patch on the lateral border of the tongue was found to be a squamous carcinoma on biopsy.

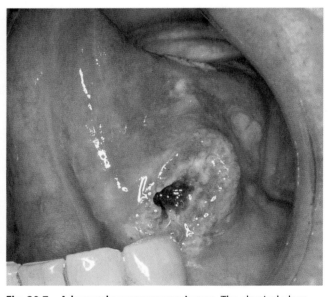

Fig. 20.7 Advanced squamous carcinoma. The classical ulcer with a rolled border and central necrosis is a late presentation. Note the surrounding areas of keratosis and erythema which had been present for many years before the carcinoma developed.

pain localised to the carcinoma, so unexplained pain should not be discounted. Ulceration may be associated with soreness or stinging pain when sharply flavoured food is eaten. Involvement of nerves by a carcinoma produces neuropathic pain, paraesthesia or anaesthesia in that nerve's distribution. Larger carcinomas may present with referred pain to the ear, through complex cranial nerve pathways. Pain increases with carcinoma size and is typically severe only in the late stages.

Presenting symptoms are diverse. Maintaining a high index of suspicion is critical to early diagnosis, and any unexplained lesion that fails to respond to treatment or does not heal spontaneously should raise suspicion of carcinoma.

Table 20.2 Clinical features of oral squamous carcinoma	
Superficially invasive	Established carcinoma
Low stage or 'Early'	High stage or 'Late'
Red patch	Indurated
Speckled patch	Ulcerated
White patch	Rolled ulcer margins
Soft or minimally firm	Nerve pain
Flat or slightly depressed	Paraesthesia or anaesthesia
Superficial non-healing ulcer	Loose teeth
	Bone loss
	Pain
	Reduced mobility of tissue/ tongue
	Spontaneous bleeding
	Palpable lymph node in neck
	Non-healing tooth socket

The features of early and late carcinoma are shown in Table 20.2.

Clinical features early carcinomas PMID: 20860767

Erythroplakia as early sign PMID: 273632

ORAL CANCER DISTRIBUTION

Overall, the tongue is the most frequently affected site in the mouth and the majority of cancers are concentrated in the lower part of the mouth, particularly the lateral borders and ventral tongue, the adjacent floor of the mouth and lingual aspect of the alveolus and retromolar region, forming a U-shaped area extending back toward the oropharynx (Fig. 20.8).

This accounts for only approximately 20% of the whole area of the interior of the oral cavity, but 70% of oral cancers are concentrated there. This distribution may be due to pooling of carcinogens in saliva and concentration in the lower mouth before swallowing. Possibly for the opposite reason, the hard palate and central dorsum of tongue are very rarely affected.

PATHOLOGY

The essential features of carcinoma are invasion and spread to lymph nodes and distant sites.

Oral carcinoma histopathology

The key feature is invasion (Figs 20.9 and 20.10). The epithelial cells lose their organisation into a surface layer and grow into the underlying tissues. Invasion is a complex cellular process in which the cells lose their polygonal shape and rigid cytoskeleton and become spindle shaped and motile. They induce surrounding fibroblasts and endothelial cells to aid their invasion by producing a fibrous tissue that is rich in proteoglycan ground substance and is easy to migrate through (tumour stroma). Growth of new vessels is induced to supply the increased nutrient requirements of the malignant cells. These actively invading cells are short lived and rarely, if ever, seen microscopically, but in late stage poorly differentiated carcinomas almost all cells can show this aggressive nature.

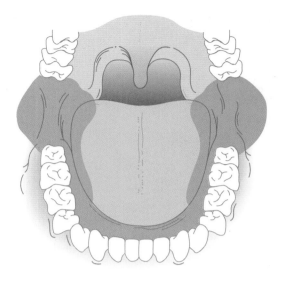

Fig. 20.8 High-risk sites for development of oral carcinoma. The shaded U-shaped area accounts for only approximately 20% of the whole area of the interior of the mouth, but is the site of more than 70% of oral cancers.

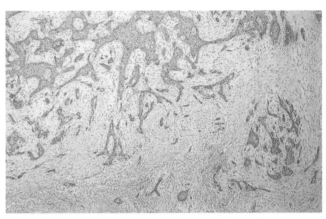

Fig. 20.10 Squamous carcinoma. Higher power shows strands of malignant epithelium invading the connective tissue.

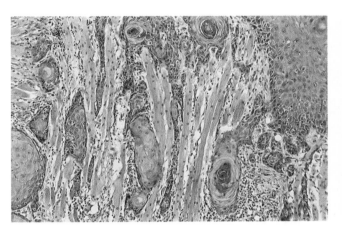

Fig. 20.11 Squamous carcinoma. At high power, a group of tumour cells shows typical cytological irregularity. Surrounding and beneath the tumour, muscle fibres are being destroyed.

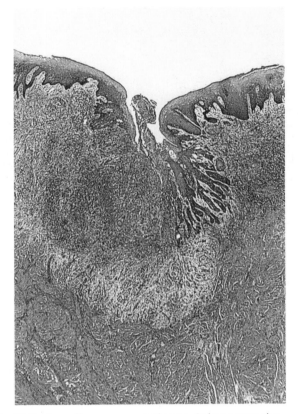

Fig. 20.9 A small squamous carcinoma. At low power, the epithelium is seen to invade deeply into the connective tissue and underlying muscle. At this early stage, there is no ulceration.

Each carcinoma comprises many genetically different clones of cells coexisting in an ecosystem in which each clone can only survive with nutrients or signals from its neighbouring cells, whether part of the carcinoma or normal cells in the tumour stroma. With time and continuous proliferation of the genetically damaged cells, there is increasing chromosomal instability and development of a more genetically diverse population of clones of cells with slightly different properties and survival abilities. Eventually a clone with metastatic ability emerges. Only a small proportion of cells may eventually do this.

Histologically, the individual cells show the features of malignancy: large and irregularly shaped nuclei, darkly stained nuclei (hyperchromatism), frequent and sometimes abnormal mitoses (Fig. 20.11). These are essentially the same cytological changes as are seen in dysplastic epithelium (Table 19.3); only invasion differentiates the two processes.

Squamous carcinoma is graded according to its degree of differentiation, the degree to which the malignant cells differentiate to form prickle cells and keratin. In well-differentiated tumours, the cells have cytoplasm that stains palely with eosin or may form concentric layers of keratin (cell nests or keratin pearls; Fig. 20.12). In poorly differentiated tumours, the cells tend to be more irregular and darkly staining and show little evidence of prickle cell differentiation or keratinisation. In the most poorly differentiated carcinomas, the cells have little cytoplasm and may not be recognisable as epithelial cells by routine microscopy (Fig. 20.13). Poorly differentiated carcinomas tend to infiltrate more widely at an early stage, are more likely to metastasise and carry a poorer prognosis. The majority of oral carcinomas are moderately differentiated.

Local spread

The invading cells grow into the tissues by direct extension. Irregular branching processes penetrate the tissue, the tips of which are often cut off in a histological section to give

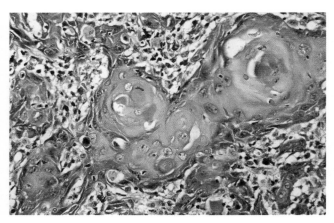

Fig. 20.12 Squamous carcinoma. In this moderately well-differentiated tumour, many of the neoplastic epithelial cells are forming keratin pearls.

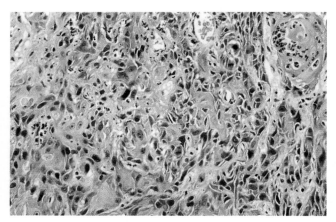

Fig. 20.13 Squamous carcinoma. In this poorly differentiated carcinoma, there is little or no keratin formation, and the malignant cells show great pleomorphism with variably sized nuclei, many of which are hyperchromatic, and frequent mitotic figures.

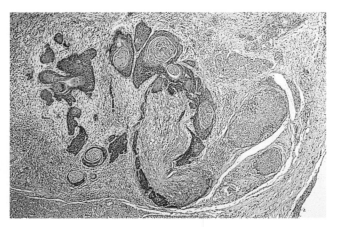

Fig. 20.14 Squamous carcinoma. In this carcinoma, malignant epithelium is invading around nerve sheaths. Although this is infrequent, occasionally carcinoma may spread some distance from the main tumour mass along nerve trunks.

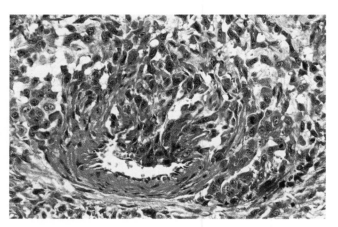

Fig. 20.15 Squamous carcinoma. Less frequent than perineural invasion is vascular invasion. Here a cluster of poorly-differentiated malignant epithelial cells have eroded the wall of the vessel and entered the circulation.

the appearance of separate islands of tumour (see Fig. 20.11). In the more infiltrative, poorly differentiated carcinomas, single cells and small clusters of cells detach along the invasive front of the lesion forming a discohesive invasive front. This carries a higher risk of metastasis than a cohesive invasive front of large islands of epithelium.

Aggressive carcinomas may show perineural infiltration, selective spread along nerves, or vascular invasion (Figs 20.14 and 20.15) both of which are adverse prognostic features. Carcinomas that spread along nerves are less likely to be excised and more likely to recur because of their unpredictable outline. Those with vascular invasion are more likely to metastasise.

Tumour cells invade all tissues (Fig. 20.10). Muscle, fat, nerves and eventually bone are infiltrated and destroyed. Carcinoma induces resorption of the bone by normal osteoclasts across a broad front, 'saucerising' the cortex until it can invade the medullary cavity.

Invading cancer cells excite an inflammatory and immune reaction and become surrounded by lymphocytes and plasma cells. Tumour-infiltrating lymphocytes kill the carcinoma cells, but unfortunately, the immune response provides no significant protection.

Perineural infiltration PMID: 25457832

Pattern of invasion PMID: 23250819 and 8039106

Metastasis

Lymphatic metastasis to the regional lymph nodes is the most likely form of distant spread. Clones of cells in the tumour eventually acquire the range of abilities required to migrate, penetrate lymphatics, survive as single cells during transit, lodge in a lymph node and proliferate to form a metastasis.

The specific sites of metastasis depend on the drainage of the tumour site but, because most carcinomas arise posteriorly in the lower mouth, the submandibular and jugulodigastric nodes are those most frequently involved. Lymphatic drainage from the tongue is shown in Fig. 20.16. Floor-of-mouth carcinomas and others involving or crossing the midline may spread bilaterally.

Metastases develop progressively down the jugular lymphatic chain (Fig. 20.17), reaching level IV supraclavicular lymph nodes at a late stage. Although these patterns of spread are relatively predictable overall, there is great difficulty in identifying and predicting metastatic spread to the neck when planning treatment for an individual case. Spread of cancer may be by an abnormal route, and all the lymph nodes of both sides of the neck must be examined and imaged.

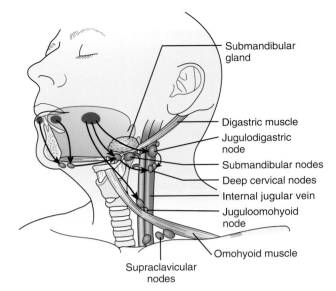

Submandibular
gland

Digastric muscle

Jugulodigastric
node

Submandibular nodes

Deep cervical nodes

Internal jugular vein

Juguloomohyoid
node

Omohyoid muscle

Supraclavicular
nodes

Fig. 20.16 Typical routes of lymphatic spread from lip and intraoral squamous carcinomas.

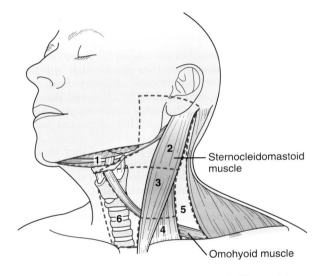

Sternocleidomastoid
muscle

Omohyoid muscle

Fig. 20.17   Neck levels for assessing metastasis. The neck is conventionally divided into level 1, the submandibular and submental region nodes, three levels 2, 3 and 4 down the jugular chain, 5 in the posterior triangle and 6 in the anterior neck. Metastasis patterns follow lymphatic drainage, and lower neck levels carry a poorer prognosis. In contrast, thyroid carcinomas metastasise to levels 6 first, then 3 and 4, while metastases in level 5 are usually from the skin or pharynx.

Metastatic carcinoma is initially limited to the affected node but, in time, grows through the capsule into the tissues of the neck. Excision is then difficult, and the chances of survival are diminished. This extranodal spread is evident clinically as fixation of the node.

Metastatic carcinoma forms a hard mass when small, but in larger masses the central area becomes necrotic. The centre may then break down, so that the metastasis becomes cystic and fluctuant clinically.

Bloodstream metastasis is an uncommon, late feature of the disease and often after several episodes of treatment.

Box 20.3   Oral cancer: clinicopathological features and behaviour

- Early cancers appear as white or red patches or shallow ulcers and are painless or only slightly sore
- Later carcinomas appear as ulcers with prominent rolled edges and induration and become painful
- More than 70% of oral cancers form on the lateral borders of the tongue and adjacent alveolar ridge and floor of mouth
- Over 95% are well- or moderately well-differentiated squamous cell carcinomas
- Spread is by direct invasion of surrounding tissues and by lymphatic metastasis
- The submandibular and jugulodigastric nodes are most frequently involved
- The prognosis deteriorates sharply with local spread and nodal involvement

Metastases then develop most frequently in lung, followed by liver and bone, heralding a terminal phase.

Key features are summarised in Box 20.3.

Tumour thickness and metastasis PMID: 16240329

Metastasis poor prognosis PMID: 20406474

Site variation

Tongue

The lateral border of the anterior two-thirds of the tongue and the adjacent ventral tongue are common sites. Conversely, a carcinoma arising centrally on the dorsum is extremely rare.

Carcinomas of the tongue only have to invade a millimetre or so before they enter muscle, a vascular tissue that seems to promote carcinoma growth. Carcinoma in the tongue is renowned for its unpredictable spread, in part because growth is directed along muscle bundles, which in the tongue radiate all directions. Carcinomas sometimes show selective sarcolemmal spread along muscle fibres and grow out long thin extensions of tumour, often reaching the midline at a relatively early stage. The tongue becomes progressively stiffer and more painful. Eating, swallowing and talking become difficult.

Carcinoma of the tongue is also known for its unpredictable metastasis. In addition to drainage to lymph nodes around the submandibular gland in level 2, carcinoma of the lateral border will metastasise directly the juguloomohyoid or other nodes in level 3. One in five carcinomas generate such 'fast track' metastases, directly to level 3 without involving level 2 first.

Once the midline is reached, metastases may develop bilaterally. Tongue carcinoma develops metastases at an early stage.

Floor of mouth

Unlike tongue carcinomas, floor of mouth carcinomas tend to spread laterally producing broad relatively superficial tumours. If they extend to the alveolar mucosa, they may erode bone, and if they extend up onto the ventral tongue, they may then extend into underlying muscle. Most arise anteriorly.

Treatment is difficult, and this site carries a poor prognosis. More carcinomas here are poorly differentiated, and there are

Table 20.4 Tumour Node Metastasis (TNM) staging for oral carcinoma.

T Tumour size	N Lymph node metastasis	M Distant metastasis
Tis Carcinoma in situ, not invasive, dysplasia only	N0 No regional lymph node metastasis	M0 No distant metastasis
T1: Tumour 2 cm or less greatest dimension and 5 mm or less depth of invasion	N1 Metastasis in a single ipsilateral lymph node, 3 cm maximum diameter without extranodal extension	M1 Distant metastasis present
T2: Tumour 2 cm or less in greatest dimension and with 5-10 mm depth of invasion or 2–4 cm in greatest dimension with depth of invasion up to 10 mm	N2a as N1 but with extranodal extension or, 3–6 cm maximum diameter without extranodal extension pN2b Metastasis in multiple ipsilateral lymph nodes, none more than 6 cm maximum diameter, without extranodal extension pN2c Metastasis in bilateral or contralateral lymph nodes, none more than 6 cm in maximum diameter, without extranodal extension	
T3: Tumour more than 4 cm in greatest dimension or more than 10 mm depth of invasion	N3a Metastasis in a lymph node more than 6 cm maximum diameter without extranodal extension N3b Metastasis in a lymph node more than 3 cm maximum diameter with extranodal extension or, multiple ipsilateral, contralateral or bilateral, with extranodal extension	
T4a: Tumour invades through the cortical bone of the mandible or maxillary sinus, or invades the skin of the face T4b: Tumour invades masticator space, pterygoid plates, or skull base, or encases internal carotid artery		

Stage 1	T1 N0 M0	
Stage 2	T2 N0 M0	
Stage 3	T3 N0 M0 T1-3 N1 M0	
Stage 4A	T4a N0 or 1 M0 T1-4a N2 M0	
Stage 4B	Any T N3 M0 T4b Any N M0	
Stage 4C	Any T Any N M1	

Note the importance of lymph node metastasis in determining the stage.
Adapted from UICC TNM version 8 (2017).

Box 20.5   Unwanted effects of radiotherapy to the oral region

During treatment

- Severe xerostomia
- Mucositis and ulceration
- Acute candidosis
- Skin erythema

Long term

- Xerostomia
- Mucosal and skin atrophy
- Risk of osteomyelitis (osteoradionecrosis)
- Scarring and fibrosis of tissues
- Cataract if eye irradiated (e.g. antral carcinoma)
- Risk of late radiation-induced malignancy

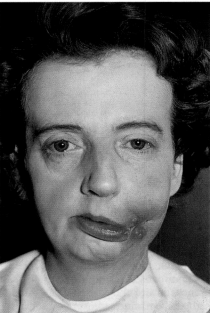

Fig. 20.18.   Late-stage presentation of oral carcinoma, about to ulcerate through the cheek.

Box 20.6 Potential adverse effects of cancer surgery to the oral region

Immediate

- Wound breakdown
- Reconstructive flap failure

Late complications at the primary site

- Disfigurement
- Loss of function
- Pain
- Dysphagia
- Difficulty with mastication
- Poor nutrition and weight loss
- Difficulty with speech
- Trismus
- Scarring and fibrosis of tissues
- Oronasal, oroantral and skin fistulae
- Numbness in mouth
- Traumatic neuroma formation
- Frey's syndrome

Complications of neck dissection

- Shoulder weakness if accessory nerve sacrificed in radical neck dissection
- Inability to abduct the arm if cervical plexus damaged in neck dissection
- Sensory loss over neck and chest
- Lymphoedema
- Lymphocoele

grafting or bypassing of many structures in the oral regions. However, a margin of more than a few millimetres is rarely achieved in practice because carcinomas have unpredictable irregular outlines or extend close to important anatomical structures. Also, wider excision may make reconstruction difficult.

Reconstructive surgery is normally performed at the same operation as excision, to provide a better cosmetic and functional result, and utilises a range of donor tissue sites. Excision by a few millimetres is insufficient to guarantee removal of the carcinoma, which may recur at the original site, and post-operative radiotherapy is, therefore, usually recommended.

Surgery also has adverse effects (Box 20.6).

All oral cancer radiotherapy in the UK is now delivered as intensity-modulated radiotherapy, a technologically complex system of linear accelerators allowing precisely controlled doses accurately conforming to the 3D shape of the tumour determined from imaging. This allows higher doses to be delivered to the carcinoma while reducing dose and adverse effects to surrounding normal tissue, particularly the eye, bone and salivary glands. Damage to surrounding tissues is further limited by fractionating the dose over many visits. A dose in the region of 60 Gy is usual for oral lesions, delivered in 30 daily fractions. A mask is made to fit the patient's head and immobilise it during treatment to allow reproducible beam angulation at each visit. Radiotherapy planning and mask construction are complex and involve a short delay before treatment can start.

Chemotherapy is less widely used in the UK than in Europe. Alone it gives good initial control, but relapse will always occur without surgery or radiotherapy. For best effect, it is carried out *concomitantly* with radiotherapy and gives approximately a 10% improvement in survival at best. The usual agent is cisplatin. All regimens have significant adverse effects, particularly with mucositis and immunosuppression, and these are compounded by radiotherapy. Only the fittest patients are able to tolerate concomitant chemotherapy.

The targeted therapy cetuximab has received much attention. It blocks activation of epidermal growth factor receptor (EGFR), which controls cell cycle and apoptosis and has indirect effects in invasion and metastasis. It is used for advanced disease with radiotherapy and provides a 10% improved survival.

Management of the neck

When surgery is to be recommended and lymph node metastases have been detected, neck dissection will be performed. Neck dissection removes all the cervical lymph nodes along the jugular chain from the base of skull to the clavicle, together with those in the submandibular and submental triangles and posterior triangle of the neck. Depending on the type of resection, the sternomastoid muscle, internal jugular vein and accessory nerve may also be sacrificed. Neck dissection may also be required to allow reconstructive flap surgery.

However, when no cervical lymph nodes appear involved, small deposits of carcinoma may already have spread to lymph nodes. If left in place, they will grow during a period of months or years to form a recurrence. A decision must be made whether or not to perform a neck dissection as an elective procedure to ensure any potential microscopic metastases are removed. However, the value is a matter of statistical chance, and many patients suffer an elective neck dissection and its consequences for no benefit.

Alternatively, a sentinel node biopsy may be performed. In this technique, a radioisotope is injected around the tumour the night before surgery, followed by a blue dye at the time of surgery. These drain via lymphatics to the sentinel lymph nodes, those that are first in the drainage pathway and are most likely to be involved by metastasis. These nodes are identified at surgery by using a radiosensitive probe and by their blue colour (Fig. 20.19), removed and examined histologically. If no metastasis is present, the rest of the neck is almost certainly uninvolved and a neck dissection and its adverse effects can be avoided. If metastasis is present, a neck dissection is performed separately. As metastasis is confirmed in only approximately 80% of therapeutic neck dissections and 33% of elective (apparently metastasis-free) neck dissections, this technique saves many patients from unnecessary neck dissections and the resultant morbidity.

Sentinel node biopsy trial PMID: 26597442

Outcome

The highest mortality from oral cancer is in the first 2 years after diagnosis. The disease then continues to claim victims but at a slower rate, and those few that survive for 10 years are likely to have been cured. As a guide to survival rates, more than 90% of patients with stage 1 and 2 disease survive the first year and approximately 75% survive for as long as 5 years. Stage 3 and 4 carcinomas will kill almost half of the patients by 2 years and as many as 60% at 5 years (Fig. 20.20).

As to the site of the cancer, the best results are seen in cancer of the lip, where the 5-year survival rate is 85%. For

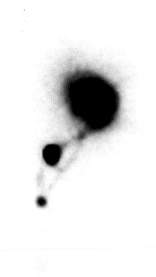

A

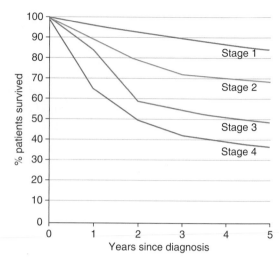

Fig. 20.20   Survival from oral carcinoma. The markedly different survival of stages 1–4 can be seen (see Table 20.4) and therefore the benefit of early diagnosis. These figures are for all oral sites; those in posterior sites have a worse prognosis than shown. *(Data from England until 2013, National Cancer Registration Service Cancer Analysis System.)*

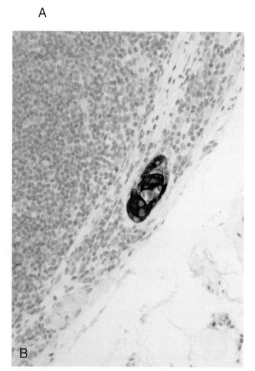

B

Fig. 20.19   Sentinel node biopsy. (A) lymphoscintigraphy, an image captured by a gamma camera (or scintillation camera) to localise the injected radioisotope. The tongue tumour at the top is the largest signal, where isotope remains at the injection site. Drainage to sentinel nodes can be traced to two nodes in the jugular chain. (B) Biopsy of the sentinel node reveals a microscopic metastasis comprising only a few cells, detected using immunohistochemistry for keratin. The dense brown positive stain aids discovery of single cells and small clusters that could be missed on routine hematoxylin and eosin stains. *(A courtesy of Dr G Tartaglione).*

Box 20.7   Some factors adversely affecting survival from oral cancer
• Delay in treatment
• Advanced age
• Male gender
• Poor general health, usually smoking-related diseases
• Tumour size
• Posterior location
• Lack of histological differentiation (high histological grade)
• Lymph node spread
• Blood-borne metastasis

prognosis. The quality of life in the terminal stages is also poor.

The poorer survival of older people is probably because they are less able to withstand radiotherapy or surgery. The reason for the poorer survival rates for males is uncertain, although later presentation is a possibility.

Development of radiation-induced sarcoma is a risk that has been estimated to be 1.6% after 10 years but carries a very poor prognosis.

Web URL 20.8 UK incidence, mortality: Web search for: ncras head and neck cancer hub

Second primary carcinomas

About 5% of patients develop a second primary carcinoma each year somewhere in the upper aerodigestive tract or lung. With better treatment and longer survival, this is an increasing problem. Young patients and smokers and those treated by radiotherapy alone are at highest risk. Patients with proliferative verrucous leukoplakia (Ch. 19) may develop several primary carcinomas, but the main cause in most oral cancer patients is field change from tobacco smoking. Treatment of a second primary may be made more complex by previous surgery or radiotherapy for the first carcinoma.

cancer of the tongue it is 60%, but for late-stage carcinomas in adverse sites, only 20%. In general the more posterior the tumour is, the poorer the survival.

Duration of survival after treatment depends on many factors (Box 20.7). In comparison with malignant neoplasms at other body sites, oral carcinoma has a poor

Treatment failure

Approximately 40% of patients suffer treatment failure and recurrence, either at the primary site, in lymph nodes or in distant sites such as lung, liver or bone.

Primary site recurrence usually signifies a poor prognosis because either a full course of radiotherapy or as large an excision as practical will already have been performed. Recurrence in lymph nodes usually appears within 2 years after treatment. The metastases probably arise from microscopic deposits of carcinoma already in the lymph nodes at the time of initial therapy (occult metastases). Neck recurrences may be treated surgically by neck dissection or by radiotherapy and do not necessarily indicate failure of treatment as further treatment is often curative.

Recurrent carcinoma is often less well differentiated and more aggressive. It invades more widely and unpredictably in the tissues, particularly if previously irradiated, and is difficult to localise. Re-excision is often impossible.

Primary and recurrent disease have been treated more aggressively and more successfully in recent years so that more patients than previously now survive, but succumb to distant blood-borne metastases later. Distant metastases are usually multiple, and there is no effective treatment.

Metastasis and death PMID: 20406474

Undetected metastasis and treatment failure PMID: 25074731

Distant metastasis PMID: 25883102

Palliative care

Palliative treatment is given to patients who have advanced tumours or for treatment failures. It is an active multidisciplinary treatment, not only pain control, that aims to reduce symptoms of all types and provide psychological, social and other holistic needs. Radiotherapy is the most frequent method for active palliative treatment, but surgery is occasionally used when a large tumour compromises the airway or becomes grossly necrotic.

Causes of death

The combination of pain, infection and difficulty in eating cause loss of weight, anaemia and deterioration of general health. This state (malignant cachexia) is ultimately fatal. In other patients, aspiration of septic material from the mouth causes bronchopneumonia.

In the terminal stages, oral carcinoma recurrent at the primary site can form a large fungating mass that erodes major vessels or the cranial cavity. Extranodal spread from affected lymph nodes may ulcerate through the skin and erode the jugular or carotid vessels.

A small, but possibly growing, proportion of patients survive treatment of the primary carcinoma but die later from distant metastases.

Novel treatments

A wide range of new treatments is under trial to determine the role for new agents such as small molecule tyrosine kinase inhibitors, new anti-EGFR antibodies or antiangiogenic agents. Talimogene laherparepvec (T-Vec) is an engineered virus targeting cancer that showed promise in an early trial and awaits full evaluation. A number of molecular targeted immunotherapy approaches are in trial including engineering patients' own lymphocytes to react to their carcinoma and boosting natural immune responses. Robotic surgery holds promise to excise carcinomas more accurately with smaller but disease-free margins, avoid large facial and neck incisions and provide a better functional outcome. However, its use is limited to small carcinomas.

Survivorship

Improved survival has produced many patients who live long term with the adverse effects of treatment and with a risk of second primary carcinoma. Psychological effects, usually depression, disfigurement and other long-term medical effects cause poor quality of life. Support for survivors is becoming increasingly important, and their complex medical needs are ideally managed outside cancer centres. Some of these patients are vocal advocates for research, reducing morbidity of treatment and awareness of cancer, but the survivorship agenda is in its infancy.

ROLE OF THE DENTIST

Early diagnosis is critical. Small carcinomas are more easily excised, less likely to have metastasised and have the best prognosis. Unfortunately, healthcare workers, including dentists, frequently either fail to make the diagnosis or actively delay referral.

Dentists must be alert to the possibility of carcinoma, despite its rarity, perform a risk assessment on any chronic ulcer, white or red lesion, or swelling of the mucous membrane and perform, or refer for, a biopsy. Indecision or trying the effect of local measures or antibiotics can prove fatal. It is better if the biopsy is performed by the cancer management team. Never perform an *excisional* biopsy of a possible small carcinoma. Once the biopsy site has healed, there may be no clue to its site or size, making further treatment difficult. Survival is reduced in such circumstances.

In the UK every practice is within a cancer network that has an urgent referral system for suspected cancer for UK National Health Service (NHS) patients. Referral criteria are published by the NHS of the devolved nations and in England and Wales by the National Centre for Clinical Excellence. In each country, every dentist is expected to be familiar with the relevant criteria. Patients meeting the criteria in Table 20.5 can be referred direct to rapid access clinics and, at least in England, be guaranteed an appointment within 2 weeks. Note that the dentist provides a key 'gatekeeper' role in this referral pathway and is expected to be able to risk assess oral lesions so that patients with trivial or benign lesions are not needlessly referred to hospital. This role is specifically included in the criteria for England, Wales and Northern Ireland. This places great responsibility on all dentists to be able to do this accurately.

The 2-week wait system is for *suspected* cancers, and it is expected that only a small proportion of referred patients will have cancer. Referral criteria are based on having more than a 3% chance of indicating cancer. If you were highly suspicious or confident that a lesion was either a high-risk potentially malignant disorder or already a carcinoma, a direct referral on the same day would be appropriate. For some cancers, even a 2-week wait is too long.

The dental practitioner is likely to see many more patients with white or red mucosal patches than carcinomas. As noted in Chapter 15, the vast majority of such lesions are benign and may be biopsied in a practice setting. However, it is inadvisable to perform a biopsy of a high-risk lesion (for instance, an erythroplasia or speckled leukoplakia) because the practitioner may be forced into the unenviable

Table 20.5 General practice referral criteria in the UK for head and neck cancer (excluding thyroid)

England and Wales 2015	Scotland 2014*	Northern Ireland 2012
Consider a suspected cancer pathway referral (for an appointment within 2 weeks) for oral cancer in people with either: • unexplained ulceration in the oral cavity lasting for more than 3 weeks or • a persistent and unexplained lump in the neck. Consider an urgent referral (for an appointment within 2 weeks) for assessment for possible oral cancer by a dentist in people who have either: • a lump on the lip or in the oral cavity or • a red or red and white patch in the oral cavity consistent with erythroplakia or erythroleukoplakia. Consider a suspected cancer pathway referral by the dentist (for an appointment within 2 weeks) for oral cancer in people when assessed by a dentist as having either: • a lump on the lip or in the oral cavity consistent with oral cancer or • a red or red and white patch in the oral cavity consistent with erythroplakia or erythroleukoplakia.	• Persistent unexplained head and neck lumps for >3 weeks. • Ulceration or unexplained swelling of the oral mucosa persisting for >3 weeks. • All red or mixed red and white patches of the oral mucosa persisting for >3 weeks. • Persistent hoarseness lasting for >3 weeks (request a chest X-ray at the same time). • Dysphagia or odynophagia (pain on swallowing) lasting for >3 weeks. • Persistent pain in the throat lasting for >3 weeks.	Red Flag referral, patients with: • an unexplained lump in the neck, of recent onset, or a previously undiagnosed lump that has changed over a period of 3 to 6 weeks • an unexplained persistent swelling in the parotid or submandibular gland • an unexplained persistent sore or painful throat • unilateral unexplained pain in the head and neck area for more than 4 weeks, associated with otalgia (ear ache) but a normal otoscopy • unexplained ulceration of the oral mucosa or mass persisting for more than 3 weeks • unexplained red and white patches (including suspected lichen planus) of the oral mucosa that are painful or swollen or bleeding. For patients with persistent symptoms or signs related to the oral cavity in whom a definitive diagnosis of a benign lesion cannot be made, refer to follow up until the symptoms and signs disappear. If the symptoms and signs have not disappeared after 6 weeks, make an urgent referral. **Red Flag referral to a dentist:** • patients with unexplained tooth mobility persisting for more than 3 weeks – monitor for oral cancer patients with confirmed oral lichen planus, as part of routine dental examination. Advise all patients, including those with dentures, to have regular dental checkups. **Non-urgent referral:** • a patient with unexplained red and white patches of the oral mucosa that are not painful, swollen or bleeding (including suspected lichen planus).

*Comment in accompanying text: With the changing pattern of disease, age, non-smoking or non-drinking status should not be a barrier to referral.

position of having to tell the patient that they have cancer, a task for which most dentists are not trained.

Although much of a patient's treatment has to be performed in hospital, patients often continue to see their practitioner after treatment.

The dental practitioner is also ideally placed for the prevention of oral cancer and can contribute in other ways (Box 20.8).

Role of dentist in United States PMID: 24192734

Dentist in diagnosis PMID: 26682494

Dental team diagnosis PMID: 12973333

Web URL 20.9 UK NICE referral criteria: https://www.nice.org.uk/guidance/csg6

ORAL CANCER SCREENING

Screening is the process of applying a rapid test or examining a population to identify a group at risk from a disease. This group can then be referred for accurate and earlier diagnosis. Oral carcinoma screening should be possible because the mouth is accessible and because those at most risk (elderly persons, smokers) are readily identified. A simple effective screening test is an examination of the mouth for red and white lesions.

Screening is not intended to provide an accurate diagnosis and may be performed by trained healthcare workers in the community. Such oral cancer screening schemes have

Box 20.8 Role of the dental practitioner in cancer prevention and diagnosis

Prevention
• Actively discourage smoking and betel quid use
• Encourage moderation of alcohol intake
• Health promotion and education on oral carcinoma
• Provide check-ups for the edentulous and/or institutionalised elderly and other high-risk non-attenders

Early diagnosis
• Be vigilant and suspicious
• Always examine all of the mucosa and the teeth
• Monitor low-risk premalignant lesions
• Refer all high-risk lesions on discovery
• Perform biopsy appropriately

After treatment
• Manage simple denture problems after surgery
• Alleviate the effects of post-irradiation dry mouth, e.g. preventing caries
• Monitor for recurrence, new premalignant lesions and second primary tumours
• Monitor for cervical metastasis
• Maintain morale of and provide additional support to patients and their relatives

proved successful in several countries with a high incidence. In the UK, such a scheme might reach the highest risk individuals who tend to be irregular dental attenders and would provide an opportunity for preventive advice.

The benefits of a national screening scheme for the UK have been evaluated. Such a scheme would be effective in identifying cancers but would not to be cost effective. No study has shown that screening improves life expectancy. Oral cancer screening thus remains within the remit of general dental and medical practitioners.

Cochrane review screening PMID: 24254989 and methods: 24258195

Status screening in United States PMID: 24276469

Patient view screening in dental practice PMID: 23249393

Screening effective in dental practice PMID: 16707071

Web URL 20.10 UK screening recommendation: http://legacy .screening.nhs.uk/oralcancer

Screening and detection aids

Several tests are marketed, some without a clear distinction as to whether they are for screening or diagnosis (the latter would demand a much higher predictive value). All require evaluation in properly controlled trials before any could be recommended. In the meantime all produce significant false-positive and negative results. Incisional biopsy is still the correct approach when there is any doubt about a lesion.

Tolonium chloride (toluidine blue) rinsing

Tolonium chloride is a dye that binds to nucleic acids and can be used as an oral rinse in the hope of staining carcinoma and dysplastic lesions blue.

The technique is not an accurate test for either carcinoma or premalignancy and is no more than an adjunct to clinical diagnosis. If used indiscriminately on white lesions, lichen planus and ulcers, the technique has a high false-positive rate. It may be of value when deciding which part of an extensive lesion should be biopsied or when the clinician does not feel confident about a clinical diagnosis. Any suspicious lesion must be subjected to biopsy as soon as possible, regardless of the pattern of staining with toluidine blue.

Brush biopsy

This technique is relatively non-invasive and therefore attractive for screening or long-term follow-up. It uses a round stiff-bristle brush to collect cells from the surface and subsurface layers of a lesion by vigorous abrasion. The brush is rotated in the fingers in one spot until bleeding starts, to ensure a sufficiently deep sample. There is little or no pain, minimal bleeding and no need for sutures. The cells collected are transferred to a microscope slide and the smear is scanned to identify abnormal cells.

Once collected, the cells can be subjected to several different test systems. A high degree of sensitivity and specificity for carcinoma is claimed, but studies have shown widely varying accuracy. It may have a role in follow-up for patients with potentially malignant lesions after definitive diagnosis.

Saliva tests

It is an attractive possibility that oral cancer or potential malignancy might be diagnosed by a simple saliva test. More than 100 different salivary biomarkers have been investigated. Despite claims for high sensitivity, none has yet been proven in a well-designed trial including patients with the many inflammatory and benign conditions with which cancers can be confused.

Review screening 'aids' PMID: 17825602

VERRUCOUS CARCINOMA

This variant of squamous cell carcinoma is a low-grade carcinoma. In the UK it is more frequent in the elderly, particularly males, and has a characteristic white, warty appearance, forming a well-circumscribed mass raised above the level of the surrounding mucosa (Fig. 20.21). If small, it may easily be mistaken for a papilloma. Verrucous carcinoma in other countries is particularly associated with the habit of snuff dipping (mentioned previously).

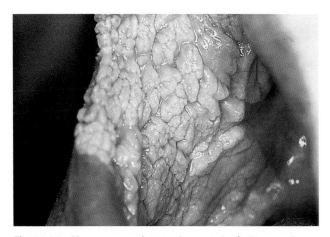

Fig. 20.21 Verrucous carcinoma. An extensive lesion covering most of the buccal mucosa and starting to involve the skin at the commissure. Such longstanding lesions are likely to develop invasive squamous carcinoma and may then metastasise. *(By kind permission of Professor SJ Challacombe.)*

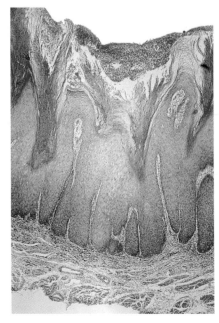

Fig. 20.22 Verrucous carcinoma. The epithelium is thickened and thrown into a series of folds with a spiky parakeratotic surface. Deeply, the carcinoma retains a broad pushing front.

Pathology

Verrucous carcinoma consists of close-packed papillary masses of well-differentiated squamous epithelium that are heavily keratinised. The lower border of the lesion is well defined and formed by blunt rete processes that indent the underlying tissues (Fig. 20.22), a process called *pushing* invasion.

Verrucous carcinoma is slow-growing and spreads laterally rather than deeply, so it can be excised relatively easily unless it is extensive. If left untreated for a period of years, a focus within verrucous carcinoma may progress to invasive squamous carcinoma and must then be treated as a conventional squamous carcinoma.

Review PMID: 18088849

Review and treatment outcome PMID: 11443616

Treatment PMID: 18620896

DIAGNOSTIC CATCHES

A number of conditions resemble oral squamous carcinoma clinically and histologically, and may be misdiagnosed as carcinoma. These lesions are discussed at the end of the next chapter.

Other mucosal and lip carcinomas

21

LIP CARCINOMA

Lip carcinoma is relatively common, with approximately 400 cases each year in the UK, but rarely presents directly to a dentist unless it is a chance finding. However, dentists should be able to recognise a sun-damaged lip and the early signs of potentially malignant change.

Aetiology

Exposure to ultraviolet light is the primary cause (Fig 21.1), usually sunlight, because the lip vermilion does not produce protective melanin. Lip cancer is predominantly a disease of outdoor workers, and fair-skinned persons are at most risk. The relationship between exposure to sunlight and lip cancer has been clearly shown in Australia and the United States with large immigrant, fair-skinned populations of European origin. In the United States, for example, the risk of lip cancer approximately doubles for every 250 miles nearer the equator of the site of residence.

Sunbed use is also a risk because high doses of ultraviolet light can be achieved. Legal limits on ultraviolet light output are equivalent to tropical sun. Sunbed use is thought to account for 8% of skin cancer in the United States and is more damaging in the young.

Changes due to ultraviolet light are preventable, and dentists should encourage the use of a high-factor sunblock when exposed to strong sunlight and avoidance of sunbeds.

Smoking, particularly of roll-your-own cigarettes without a filter, cigars or pipes, are the next most important factors, supplying heat and carcinogens to the lip.

The immunosuppressed, particularly organ transplant recipients, have an increased risk of lip carcinoma.

Pathology

More than 90% of lip carcinomas arise on the lower lip, to one side of the midline. Men are affected twice as frequently as women, and the elderly are predominantly affected.

An area of thickening, induration, crusting or shallow ulceration of the lip, less than a centimetre in diameter, is a typical early presentation (Fig. 21.2).

All are squamous carcinomas, and most are well differentiated. Spread to lymph nodes tends to be late and is seen in only 10% of patients, usually to the submental nodes. These factors, combined with relatively easy excision, give lip carcinoma a good prognosis, and 90% of patients survive 5 years and are cured. Carcinomas over 2 cm diameter; those that recur, metastasise or occur in the young or in the upper lip are more likely to be fatal.

Approximately half of cases are preceded by a zone of keratosis with dysplasia seen histologically, equivalent to an intraoral leukoplakia. All keratosis on the lip should be subject to biopsy. A sun-damaged lip may be identified clinically by its loss of elasticity, atrophic epithelium and telangiectasia (Fig. 21.3).

Lip carcinoma is treated by excision if small; larger tumours may receive multimodality treatment.

Skin cancer for dentists PMID: 24852988

Solar damage for dentists PMID: 8150192

HUMAN PAPILLOMAVIRUS–ASSOCIATED OROPHARYNGEAL CARCINOMAS

Since 1990, an epidemic of carcinoma of the oropharynx has been identified in many countries, particularly Canada, Eastern Europe, North America and the UK (Figs 21.4 and 20.1). Oropharyngeal carcinoma is the fastest increasing cancer in parts of the UK.

In the UK, 80% or more of these cancers are caused by viral infection. This section describes the virus-induced

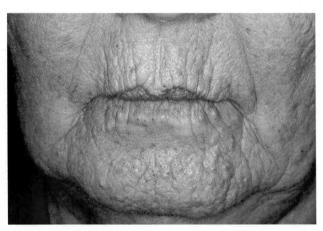

Fig. 21.1   Photoaged skin. Severe sun damage causing leathered wrinkling. Smoking exacerbates solar skin damage independently of any carcinogenic effect on the lip.

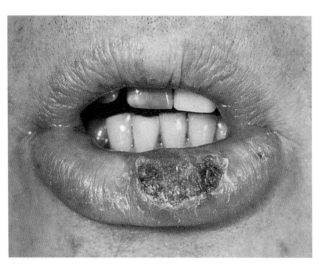

Fig. 21.2   Squamous carcinoma of lip. There is an indurated, crusted ulcer with keratosis at one margin in the centre of the lower lip.

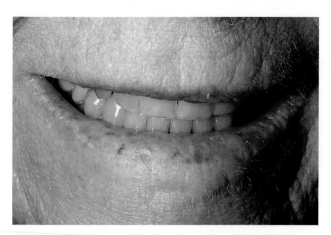

Fig. 21.3   Sun-damaged lip. There is atrophy of the epithelium, producing increased redness, loss of wrinkles and definition of the skin-vermilion boundary and telangiectasia. White flecks or patches of keratosis may also develop. Any nodule or ulcer developing in this background should be regarded with suspicion.

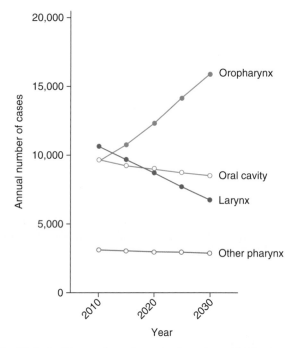

Fig. 21.4   Incidence of oropharyngeal carcinoma in the United States. Observed (until 2007) and projected (till 2030) number of new patients with oropharyngeal, oral cavity, larynx and other pharynx cancers per year. Larynx and oral carcinoma are in slow decline, pharynx cancer rates are stable but oropharyngeal carcinoma is predicted to rise dramatically. See also data from the UK in Fig. 20.1. *(Data from Chaturvedi, A.K., Engels, E.A., Pfeiffer, R.M., et al,. 2011. Human papillomavirus and rising oropharyngeal cancer incidence in the United States. J. Clin. Oncol. 29 (32), 4294–4301.)*

carcinomas because these differ in many respects from oral carcinoma. The remainder are usually caused by smoking and alcohol and present in a similar fashion to oral carcinoma.

Aetiology

The cause of the dramatic increase in incidence is human papillomavirus (HPV) infection. There are more than 150 subtypes of human papillomavirus, some of which cause warts and benign disease, and others of which can infect

and cause carcinoma in the uterine cervix. The most common carcinogenic types by far are types 16 and 18. These viruses are relatively widespread in the population and are the most common sexually transmitted infection with more than 6 million new infections each year in the United States and 20 million people infected at any one time. However, most patients' immune systems clear the infection in under a year, and the overall risk of developing carcinoma is very low.

Genital papillomavirus types can be transmitted to the mouth, primarily through oral sex though transmission across the placenta, during birth or shortly after is also possible. Clearance of oral infection takes several years and, as in the cervix, infection is common, but the risk of carcinoma is very low. It appears that persistent or repeated infection carries the highest risk, and it is possible that the few patients who develop carcinoma have a genetic or immunological predisposition to infection. The current increase in incidence started in about 1990 and appears to be a delayed effect of changes in sexual practices since the 1960s. In the United States, human papillomavirus now causes carcinoma more frequently in the oropharynx than in the cervix.

Incidence PMID: 24248688

Transmission PMID: 25873485 and 26908748

Pathogenesis

Human papillomavirus–associated carcinomas almost always arise in the oropharynx, specifically in the tonsil and minor tonsils of Waldeyer's ring, around the base of tongue, soft palate and pharynx. Tonsil crypts are lined by non-keratinised and permeable epithelium designed to allow antigens to penetrate into the lymphoid tissue below. HPV infects the epithelium, and the viral DNA either integrates into the DNA of the crypt lining epithelial cells or remains in their cytoplasm. Viral proteins E6 and E7 bind to and inactivate the tumour suppressor proteins p53 and retinoblastoma protein respectively, inhibiting apoptosis, increasing cell proliferation and generating genomic instability. After a prolonged latent period of 20–30 years, carcinoma may result. The mechanisms are slightly different from the way HPV causes cancer of the uterine cervix, but the differences are not yet understood.

General review HPV carcinogenesis PMID: 15479788

Clinical

It is often said that papillomavirus–associated carcinomas arise in young patients. However, the age of onset is only approximately 5–7 years younger than for oral cancer, at a mean of 55 years. HPV does not account for cancers in young patients.

The presenting signs of HPV–associated oropharyngeal carcinomas are very different from those of other oral and upper aerodigestive tract carcinomas. Half of patients are seen with a cervical lymph node metastasis producing a mass in the neck (Figs 21.5 and 21.6) and a third with a sore throat. Only 15% will have a visible lesion because the carcinoma arises inside the tonsil crypts without producing a surface mass (Figs 21.7 and 21.8). This type of carcinoma typically metastasises very early, and the primary tumour may only be a few millimetres across when metastasis becomes evident. Clinical examination is therefore unlikely to detect the primary carcinoma.

The cervical node metastases are unusual. Virus-associated carcinomas produce metastases that are soft,

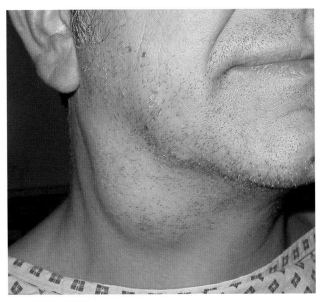

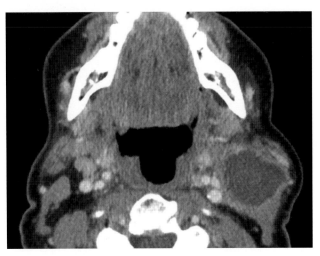

Fig. 21.6 Metastatic tonsil carcinoma in a computed tomography (CT) scan. On the patient's left is a large cystic lymph node metastasis several centimetres in diameter, but there is no mass at the site of the adjacent tonsil. CT with contrast.

Fig. 21.5 Metastatic tonsil carcinoma in a cervical lymph node. This is often the presenting symptom.

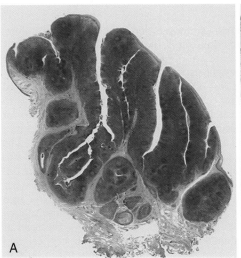

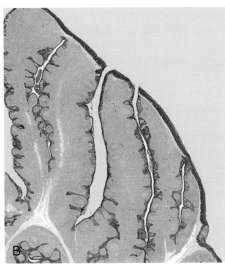

Fig. 21.7 Normal tonsil. (A) Stained in haematoxylin and eosin, the crypts can be seen as deep clefts surrounded by lymphoid tissue. (B) At slightly higher magnification and stained immunohistochemically for keratin (brown stain positive), the epithelial covering and crypt lining epithelium is highlighted.
(Kindly provided by Dr S Thavaraj.)

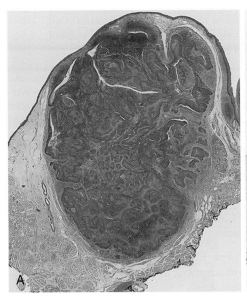

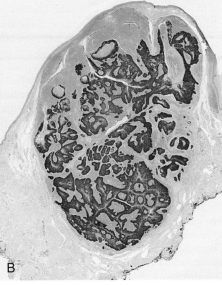

Fig. 21.8 Carcinoma of the tonsil. (A) Stained with haematoxylin and eosin, the carcinoma that has arisen in the crypt; epithelium is difficult to see. (B) Stained immunohistochemically for p16 as a marker of human papillomavirus, the carcinoma is highlighted. Note that the surface epithelium is not involved, not ulcerated and would appear normal clinically.
(Kindly provided by Dr S Thavaraj.)

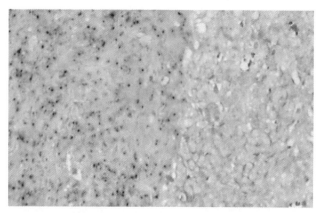

Fig. 21.9   HPV in a carcinoma of the tonsil. DNA in situ hybridisation reveals the presence of viral DNA as blue dots (see Fig. 1.10). HPV DNA is present in the nuclei of the carcinoma cells in an island of carcinoma on the left, but not in the connective tissue on the right. Red counterstain is for orientation, but the process partly degrades the tissue so that cells are not clearly seen.

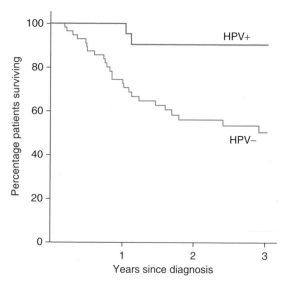

Fig. 21.10   Survival of patients with oropharyngeal carcinoma. Patients with human papillomavirus (HPV)-positive carcinomas survive much better than those with HPV-negative carcinomas. *(Data from Schache, A.G. Liloglou, T., Risk, J.M., et al., 2011. Evaluation of human papillomavirus diagnostic testing in oropharyngeal squamous cell carcinoma: sensitivity, specificity, and prognostic discrimination. Clin. Cancer Res. 17 (19), 6262–6271.)*

usually single, and often cystic and only become fixed at a late stage, unlike the hard, fixed, multiple lymph nodes of other carcinomas. Metastases are frequently mistaken for branchial or other cysts. They are also often the first sign of the disease.

Review for clinical practice PMCID: PMC4299160

Histopathology

The primary carcinoma is often undetected before it metastasises. Fine needle aspiration of the presenting neck mass will show squamous carcinoma and trigger a search for the primary site. If the appearances suggest an oropharyngeal primary, or if papillomavirus is detected in the sample, imaging, bilateral tonsillectomy, adenoidectomy and biopsies of the posterior tongue are performed to search for the primary if it is not evident.

The carcinoma comprises sheets, ribbons and islands of pale squamous epithelium with only microscopic foci of keratinisation (see Figs 21.7 and 21.8). There is often central necrosis in the islands ('comedo' necrosis) and infiltration by numerous lymphocytes ('lymphoepithelial carcinoma').

Viral infection is demonstrated by in situ hybridisation for viral DNA and overexpression of p16 protein, a cell cycle regulatory protein. Inactivation of retinoblastoma protein by the E7 viral protein triggers overexpression of p16 protein by the cancer cells. Demonstration of excess p16 protein indicates that the virus is driving carcinoma growth. Alternatively, in situ hybridisation against the E6 or E7 mRNA indicates both viral presence and activity (Fig. 21.9).

Testing cancers for HPV PMCID: PMC3394162

Treatment

Human papillomavirus–associated carcinomas have a much better prognosis than carcinomas induced by tobacco and alcohol. However, this link between virus and good prognosis appears limited to oropharynx carcinomas. More than 95% of patients with virus-positive carcinomas survive 3 years compared with only 60% of patients with conventional carcinomas (Fig. 21.10). Chemoradiotherapy is the usual treatment, but surgery, if the carcinoma is accessible, is also highly effective. If patients smoke and drink, they

have an additional carcinogenic effect that generates a more aggressive carcinoma, and the response to treatment is slightly worse.

The better prognosis is probably explained by the carcinomas having less DNA damage than smoking-induced carcinomas. The cells retain intact signalling pathways to trigger apoptosis when exposed to chemotherapy or radiation-induced DNA damage.

This type of carcinoma should eventually be prevented by vaccination against human papillomavirus. There are two vaccines, which are very safe and licensed in more than 100 countries. In the UK, the quadrivalent vaccine against types 6, 11, 16 and 18 is currently recommended for girls aged 12–13. Vaccine uptake is high, with 91% of those offered the vaccine having at least one course, above the level at which there should be an impact on both cervical and oropharyngeal carcinoma. Vaccination is offered to boys in some countries such as Australia, but the additional benefit is small if vaccine uptake by girls is high. The main benefit in males is to prevent anal carcinomas. Vaccine uptake in the United States is much lower. The vaccine is only effective if given before first sexual contact, and it has minimal protective effect in adults.

The concern that this cancer is caused by a sexually transmitted disease has led to considerable confusion and misinformation about the risks, transmission and prevention. Testing patients' saliva for papillomavirus has no value in predicting the risk of carcinoma. The virus does not replicate in the cancer, which is not infectious. By the time a cancer develops, 20–30 years may have passed since the original infection, and it will take this long for vaccination to have an impact on the incidence.

Good outcome PMID: 23606404 and 21969383

Description PMID: 20530316

Web URL 21.1 NICE referral criteria all head neck cancers: https://www.nice.org.uk/guidance/csg6

Web URL 21.2 UK incidence, mortality: Web search for: ncras head and neck cancer hub

HPV in oral carcinoma

Human papillomavirus can be found in approximately 5% of intraoral carcinomas. However, because infection in the population is so common, the significance is unclear. There is no evidence yet that papillomavirus plays a role in inducing oral carcinomas, and only very early evidence that it may be associated with a better response to treatment.

Key features of human papillomavirus–associated oropharyngeal carcinomas are shown in Table 21.1.

NASOPHARYNGEAL CARCINOMA

Nasopharyngeal carcinoma arises high in the nasopharynx, specifically in the minor tonsil tissue in the fossa of Rosenmuller at the pharyngeal opening of the Eustachian tube. The significance to dentists is that it often presents as an enlarged lymph node in the neck following metastasis, when the primary carcinoma is still unsuspected.

Aetiology

The cause is infection with Epstein–Barr virus in a genetically predisposed individual, often a patient with family origin in China, Southeast Asia or North Africa. Dietary factors may contribute. Patients are usually middle-aged males, except in Africa where they are usually children. A small number of cases are caused by human papillomavirus types 16 or 18.

Pathology

Presenting symptoms are often vague and include deafness or tinnitus from blockage of the Eustachian tube. Eighty-five per cent of cases present with a cervical lymph node metastasis, almost always to level 2 (see Fig. 20.17). Diagnosis is by fine needle aspiration, aided by identifying Epstein–Barr virus DNA in the carcinoma.

Treatment is usually by radiotherapy, with or without chemotherapy, but only 50% of patients survive 5 years because diagnosis is often late.

Web URL 21.1 NICE referral criteria all head neck cancers: https://www.nice.org.uk/guidance/csg6

Web URL 21.2 UK incidence, mortality: Web search for: ncras head and neck cancer hub

Table 21.1 Features of human papillomavirus–associated and other carcinomas of the oropharynx compared

Tobacco and alcohol-induced carcinomas, oral carcinoma and human papillomavirus–negative oropharyngeal carcinomas	Human papillomavirus–associated oropharyngeal carcinomas
Often have precursor dysplastic lesions	No precursor dysplastic lesion known
Present as visible ulcer or mass	Primary carcinoma often invisible
Usually symptomatic	Usually asymptomatic
Late metastasis	Early metastasis
Hard, fixed, multiple lymph node metastases	Soft cystic solitary lymph node metastases
Metastasise to any level in the neck	Usually metastasise to level 2 in the neck
Primary is large	Primary is small
Poor response to treatment	Good response to treatment

PSEUDOCARCINOMAS AND DIAGNOSTIC CATCHES

Various conditions can mimic oral malignant neoplasms either clinically or histologically. Those that are both clinical and histological mimics are particularly prone to be misdiagnosed as a cancer, to the detriment of the patient. This is best avoided by being aware of the conditions and always providing full clinical information to the pathologist who reports the biopsy. The fact that many of these conditions are relatively rare only increases the risk of misdiagnosis.

Many oral lesions are heavily inflamed, and others are prone to trauma. These processes may confuse the histological interpretation of a biopsy, and clinicians must always follow up a mismatch between clinical findings and biopsy results in case an error has been made.

The features of these lesions are summarised in Table 21.2.

In addition to these pseudomalignant lesions, the dental follicle can also be mistaken for the benign odontogenic myxoma (see Ch. 11).

Table 21.2   Oral conditions that may resemble malignant neoplasms

Condition	Clinical features	Histological features	Further information
Median rhomboid glossitis	Red and white, sometimes nodular appearance midline dorsum tongue	Usually readily distinguished from carcinoma	See Chapter 15
Traumatic and eosinophilic ulcer (and traumatic ulcerative granuloma with stromal eosinophilia and CD30 positive lymphoproliferative disease of mucosa)	Repeated trauma may prevent ulcers from healing and induce fibrosis mimicking carcinoma.	Simple traumatic ulcers are usually readily distinguished from carcinoma. Eosinophilic ulcers and traumatic ulcerative granuloma with stromal eosinophilia resemble lymphoma	See Chapter 16
Granular cell tumour	Smooth surfaced nodule, not usually suggestive of carcinoma clinically	Induces pseudocarcinomatous hyperplasia of overlying epithelium in a minority of cases. A biopsy that is superficial risks misdiagnosis.	See Chapter 25
Oral keratoacanthoma	Nodular lesion, usually on gingiva or palate, grows rapidly and ulcerates to form a keratin-filled crater appearing exactly as carcinoma, but usually in child or young adult. May resorb underlying bone	Almost identical to well-differentiated squamous carcinoma	Very rare. Probably not analogous to keratoacanthoma of skin or lip, but a similar self-healing epithelial proliferation. Untreated lesions resolve but are often excised through uncertainty of diagnosis. PMID: 6961343
Epstein–Barr ulcers in immunosuppression and acute EBV ulcers in glandular fever	Not usually concerning clinically, except EBV ulcers in immunosuppression, which can be very chronic	Resemble lymphoma	PMID: 26254983
Papillomas	Normally readily identifiable but large lesions resemble verrucous carcinoma	Superficial biopsy may be indistinguishable from verrucous carcinoma	The main risk is misdiagnosis of verrucous carcinoma as papilloma because of inadequate biopsy or clinical information
Necrotising sialometaplasia	Nodular inflamed lesion on palate, becoming ulcerated	Biopsy may resemble squamous or mucoepidermoid carcinoma, although usually readily identifiable.	Eventually heals without intervention. Small or superficial biopsies risk misdiagnosis. See Chapter 22
Lupus erythematosus of vermilion border	Ulcers, erythema and keratosis	Resembles dysplasia	Diagnosis aided by skin lesions elsewhere

Non-neoplastic diseases of salivary glands

22

DUCT OBSTRUCTION

→ Summary charts 12.1 and 22.1 pp. 202, 353

Salivary calculi

A stone can form in a salivary gland or duct. At least 80% of salivary calculi form in the submandibular gland, approximately 8% in the parotid and approximately 2% in the sublingual and minor salivary glands.

Clinical features

Adults are mainly affected, males twice as often as females. Calculi are usually unilateral. Symptoms are absent until the stone causes obstruction. Intermittent obstruction causes the classical symptom of 'meal time syndrome', pain and swelling of the gland when the smell or taste of food stimulates salivary secretion. Persistent obstruction leads to infection, pain and chronic swelling of the gland.

Otherwise there are no symptoms unless the stone passes forward and can be palpated or seen at the duct orifice (Fig. 22.1). Alternatively, the stone may be seen in a radiograph. However, approximately 40% of parotid and 20% of submandibular stones are not densely radiopaque, and sialography or ultrasound may be needed to locate them.

Pathology

Saliva is supersaturated, and calcium and magnesium phosphates deposit around a nidus, probably cell debris. Degenerate cells within the gland can also mineralise and may enter the duct system to act as a nidus. Mineralisation proceeds incrementally producing a layered structure (Fig. 22.2). An adherent layer of microbial flora often grows on stones and this, their rough surface and obstruction trigger inflammation and fibrosis around the duct.

Calculi are not a cause of dry mouth, but factors increasing the saturation of saliva including dry mouth, dehydration, obstruction and sialadenitis all predispose to stones, producing a vicious cycle in which the effects of a calculus contribute to its further growth. Established stones probably never redissolve. Stones are frequently multiple.

Parotid saliva is less saturated and so produces fewer stones. These have a higher organic content, making them less radiopaque and sometimes completely lucent.

Minor gland stones are unusual and present as a hard mass in the mucosa or with infection.

Management

The stone should be identified by plain radiography or ultrasound and the degree of damage to the gland from ascending infection and sialadenitis assessed by sialography.

Occasionally, small stones may sometimes be manipulated out of the duct orifice. Larger or distally placed stones must be treated starting with the least invasive method likely to succeed. Lithotripsy uses an ultrasonic shock wave applied extraorally and focused on the stone. A series of treatments may fracture the stone into small pieces that will pass out of the duct orifice. If this fails, stones in the duct but outside the gland can be removed using a 'basket' of fine wire manipulated down the duct and around the stone under radiological control. Alternatively, microendoscopy can be combined with laser disruption of the stone. These conservative techniques are often successful and, perhaps surprisingly, the gland will often recover normal function despite a history of repeated attacks of chronic sialadenitis.

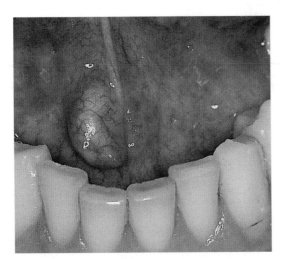

Fig. 22.1 Salivary calculus. This stone has impacted just behind the orifice of the submandibular duct forming a hard nodule. The yellow colour of the stone is visible through the thin mucosa.

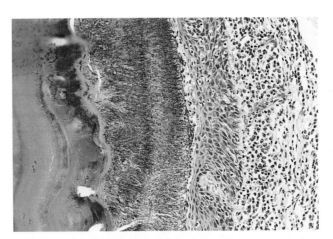

Fig. 22.2 Salivary calculus in a duct. To the left is the salivary calculus which has a lamellar structure and an irregular surface. On the surface is a thick layer of microbial flora filling the space between the stone and the epithelial lining. In the surrounding wall, there is an infiltrate of lymphocytes and plasma cells and neutrophils are migrating through the duct epithelium into the lumen.

If conservative measures fail and the stone is within the duct, the duct has to be opened, usually under local anaesthesia. A temporary suture should be put around the duct behind the calculus to prevent it from slipping backward and the stone released through an incision along the line of the duct. The opening should be left unsutured or sutured to the mucosa to prevent scarring and a fibrous stricture forming.

When stones are within the gland or a sialogram reveals that the gland is severely damaged by recurrent infection and fibrosis, the gland will probably have to be excised.

Key features of salivary calculi are summarised in Box 22.1.

Management review PMCID: PMC2640028

Salivary duct strictures

→ Summary chart 22.1 p. 353

The usual cause of strictures at the parotid papilla is chronic trauma (from such causes as projecting denture clasps, faulty restorations or sharp edges of broken teeth) leading to fibrosis.

Strictures of the duct itself are almost always caused by fibrosis resulting from inflammation round a calculus or scarring following surgery.

Obstruction from strictures presents with meal time syndrome in the same way as when caused by calculi.

Sialography should show the zone of narrowing with dilatation behind. Once any causative calculus has been removed, no further treatment may be required, but persistent obstruction may require dilatation of the duct with bougies, excision of the narrow segment or the whole gland.

Management review: PMCID: PMC2640028

MUCOCELES AND SALIVARY CYSTS

A mucocele is a cavity filled with mucus. Salivary mucoceles can be of two types, but these cannot be distinguished clinically and the difference is of little practical importance.

Review PMID: 20708324

Mucous extravasation

The most common type is the extravasation mucocele of minor glands, often called a *mucous extravasation cyst* even though it has no epithelial lining. The cause is trauma causing duct rupture so that saliva can escape into the tissues. Mucous extravasations most often form in the lower lip because it is more prone to trauma. They are commonest in children and young adults.

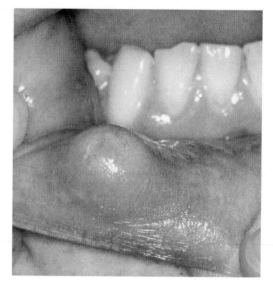

Fig. 22.3   Mucous extravasation cyst. The typical presentation at the commonest site: a rounded bluish, translucent cyst in the lower lip.

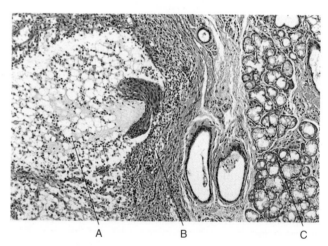

Fig. 22.4   Extravasation mucocele. To the left is a cavity of spilt mucin with the remnants of the ruptured duct lining epithelium at its edge. To the right is the associated minor mucous salivary gland. (A) Saliva and macrophages. (B) Compressed connective tissue wall. (C) Minor salivary gland.

The collection of secretion is superficial and rarely larger than 1 cm in diameter. In the early stages, they appear as rounded fleshy swellings. Later, they are obviously cystic, hemispherical, fluctuant and bluish due to the thin wall (Fig. 22.3).

The saliva leaking into the surrounding tissues excites an inflammatory reaction (Figs 22.4 and 22.5), and the pools of saliva gradually coalesce to form a rounded collection of fluid, surrounded by compressed connective tissue. Gradually macrophages infiltrate and degrade the mucin, the duct heals and a scar remains. However, extravasation mucoceles often recur at the same site, probably because of recurrent trauma.

In a superficial mucocele, the saliva pools just below the epithelium, mimicking a vesicle and potentially presenting similarly to pemphigoid. The translucent blisters are a few millimetres in diameter and usually affect the soft palate.

Superficial mucoceles PMID: 3174068

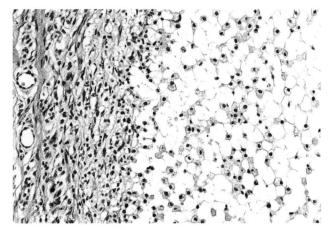

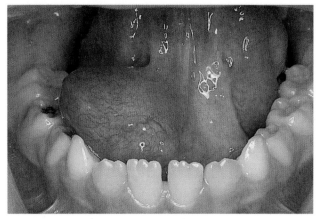

Fig. 22.5 **Extravasation mucocele.** Higher power showing the lining of the mucin-filled space. Macrophages are migrating into the mucin, and in phagocytosing it develop a foamy or vacuolated cytoplasm.

Fig. 22.7 **Ranula.** A large bluish, translucent swelling in the floor of the mouth caused by a mucous extravasation cyst.

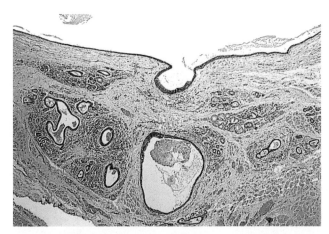

Fig. 22.6 **Mucous retention cyst.** Remnants of the minor mucous salivary gland are visible, together with its dilated duct, the epithelium of which is continuous with the epithelial lining of the cyst (*above*).

Mucous retention cysts

These cysts are less common and have an epithelial lining because they are salivary ducts that become very dilated following obstruction (Fig. 22.6). Retention cysts arise both within major glands, usually the parotid, and minor glands. There is less inflammation because the saliva does not escape into the tissues, and the pool of mucin is surrounded by duct epithelium. The epithelium often shows hyperplasia or oncocytic metaplasia.

Key features are summarised in Box 22.2.

Ranula

A ranula* is an uncommon and distinctive type of mucous extravasation arising in the floor of mouth from the sublingual gland. The structure is the same as other salivary extravasation cysts. The cause is damage to, or obstruction of, one of the several ducts of Rivinius that drain into the submandibular duct or floor of mouth.

Ranulae are usually unilateral and 2 or 3 cm in diameter (Fig. 22.7). Occasionally, they extend across the whole of the floor of the mouth. They are soft, fluctuant and bluish, typically painless but may interfere with speech or mastication.

Sublingual glands secrete continuously, unlike the larger glands, and ranulae can therefore reach a very large size in the loose tissue. A *plunging ranula* arises when the mucus passes through the mylohyoid muscle, which is a discontinuous sheet in many individuals, or around its posterior margin. Large volumes of mucus can then collect in the submandibular space and extend down into the neck, sometimes with minimal intraoral swelling.

Review ranula PMID: 20054853

Treatment

Untreated mucoceles rupture, often repeatedly, and some eventually heal spontaneously. Otherwise they should be excised with the underlying gland. The latter is usually found to have been removed with the cyst, but if not, recurrence is likely.

Ranulae do not require excision. If the cavity is drained and decompressed by marsupialisation, it will heal spontaneously provided the causative gland, always the sublingual, is removed. The sublingual gland comprises as many as 20 small glands, each with a separate duct, and only the involved segment needs to be removed if it can be identified.

An important diagnostic point is that what appears to be a mucocele in the upper lip is much more likely to be a salivary neoplasm and has a significant chance of being malignant (Ch. 23, Fig. 23.1). Some salivary neoplasms

---

*The name ranula means frog and comes from the clinical resemblance of the thin dilated wall to the air sac of a frog, together with the croaking speech ranulae can cause by displacing the tongue.

contain mucous-filled cysts, producing a similar appearance. Upper lip nodules should not be excised without this possibility having been investigated.

SIALADENITIS

Mumps → Summary chart 22.2 p. 354

Mumps† is due to a paramyxovirus (the mumps virus) and causes painful swelling of the parotids and other exocrine glands. It is highly infectious and is the most common cause of acute parotid swelling.

In the UK, mumps vaccination (in the MMR (measles-mumps-rubella) combination) was introduced in 1988. Before this there were epidemics every 3 years. MMR vaccination is given at around 1 and 4 years of age and is also available to adults. Concerns over side effects have proved unfounded, and uptake in the UK is now approximately 95%, but small clusters of cases still occur and in 2005 there was an epidemic of more than 70,000 cases. Several hundred cases occur each year. Almost all are 15–30-year-olds, and a quarter will have had at least one dose of vaccine, suggesting it is not as effective as natural mumps immunity (which is lifelong after infection). The mumps component of MMR is known to be less effective than the measles and rubella components.

Vaccination is with a live virus, and a small minority of recipients develop a mild presentation of mumps with salivary gland swelling 3 weeks after the first dose.

Clinical features

Classically, children were affected in epidemics. The disease is highly infectious and spread by saliva. Headache, malaise, fever and tense, painful and tender swelling of the parotids follow an incubation period of about 21 days.

Currently cases are adolescents or young adults, who unlike children may have severe and prolonged malaise and are prone to complications including orchitis, oophoritis pancreatitis, arthritis, mastitis, nephritis, pericarditis or meningitis.

Classical presentations are easily recognised, but adults may have only one or two glands swollen, raising possible misdiagnosis as dental infection, sialadenitis or lymphadenitis. A history of mumps, but not of vaccination, excludes the diagnosis. Immunised adults have reduced disease severity and often atypical presentations (Fig. 22.8). Many are subclinical, with mild non-specific malaise and tender glands without swelling.

If necessary, the diagnosis can be confirmed by a rise in titre of immunoglobulin (IgM) antibodies in the unvaccinated. Unfortunately, vaccination prevents development of the IgM antibodies in 90% of cases, and laboratory diagnosis is difficult.

Mumps review PMID: 18342688

Mumps post vaccination PMID: 20517181

Bacterial parotitis

Acute suppurative parotitis historically affected debilitated patients, particularly post-operatively, as a result of dehydration. This is now effectively prevented. Currently, suppurative parotitis is more commonly seen in patients with severe

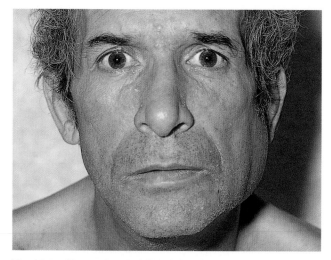

Fig. 22.8   Mumps in an adult. Adults often have atypical presentations such as this patient with unilateral parotitis. *(From General Medical Conditions in the Athlete, Mosby, 2012, Fig. 15-6.Source: Jarvis C: Physical examination and health assessment, ed 5, Philadelphia, 2008, Saunders.)*

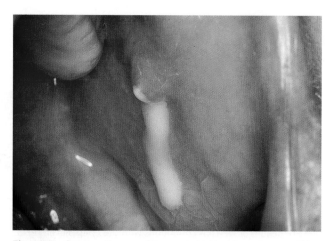

Fig. 22.9   Suppurative parotitis: pus is leaking from the parotid papilla.

xerostomia, particularly Sjögren's syndrome or as an uncommon complication of tricyclic antidepressant treatment.

Important bacterial causes include *Staphylococcus aureus*, streptococci and oral anaerobes. Typical clinical features are pain in one or both parotids with swelling, redness and tenderness, malaise and fever. The regional lymph nodes are enlarged and tender, and pus exudes or can be expressed from the parotid duct (Fig. 22.9). The progress of the infection depends largely on the patient's underlying physical state. Biopsy plays no role in diagnosis, but shows abscess formation, pus in ducts and acute inflammation.

In view of the potentially virulent pathogenic organisms involved, aggressive antibiotic treatment is required, usually with flucloxacillin, but only after pus has been obtained for culture and sensitivity testing because of the wide range of possible causative organisms. The antibiotic can be changed if necessary. Drainage is rarely necessary.

Acute parotitis case series PMID: 3468465

Salivary gland infection review PMID: 19608046

Tuberculous sialadenitis is very rare and seen mostly in the parotid gland in HIV infection and immunosuppression.

---

†Mumps comes from an old English word meaning to look miserable, describing well the marked malaise felt by sufferers.

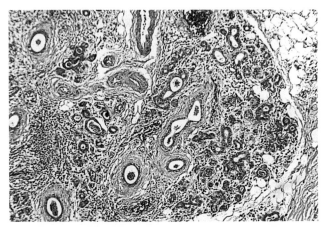

Fig. 22.10 **Chronic sialadenitis resulting from obstruction.** The ducts contain casts of mucin and neutrophils and are surrounded by a layer of fibrosis. There is severe acinar atrophy, and the space previously occupied by acinar cells now contains infiltrates of lymphocytes and plasma cells.

It presents clinically as a mass resembling a tumour or as a slowly and diffusely enlarging gland over many years. Fine needle aspiration will usually be diagnostic. Involvement of the gland probably follows spread from an intraparotid lymph node.

Chronic sialadenitis

→ Summary chart 22.1 p. 353

Chronic sialadenitis is usually a complication of duct obstruction, and the commonest cause by far is calculi. It is usually unilateral and asymptomatic or with intermittent painful swelling of one gland. Sialography may show dilatation of ducts behind the obstruction, with tortuous distorted ducts compressed by fibrosis.

Pathology

There are varying degrees of destruction of acini, duct dilatation and a scattered chronic inflammatory cellular infiltrate, predominantly lymphoplasmacytic (Fig. 22.10). Extensive interstitial fibrosis and, sometimes, squamous metaplasia in the duct epithelium follow.

Untreated sialadenitis progresses over many years until the gland is almost completely fibrotic. This terminal fibrosis produces a hard gland, easily mistaken for a lymph node metastasis or neoplasm‡.

Once any obstruction is removed, mild sialadenitis may resolve and the gland recover. If extensively damaged, the gland has to be excised.

Salivary gland infection review PMID: 19608046

XEROSTOMIA

Xerostomia is dry mouth. There are many causes, as summarised in Box 22.3. Dry mouth is not associated with ageing itself but is common in the elderly because of their disease burden and medications.

Though the mouth is dry and saliva sparse, stringy or frothy, many patients with mild xerostomia make

‡This end stage of chronic sialadenitis with sclerosis is sometimes called a *Küttner tumour*, although it is not neoplastic. However, this term has also been incorrectly and confusingly applied to other causes of fibrosis in the gland, such as IgG4 disease.

Box 22.3   Causes of xerostomia

Organic causes

- Sjögren's syndrome
- Irradiation
- Mumps (transient)
- HIV infection
- Hepatitis C infection
- Sarcoidosis
- Amyloidosis
- Iron deposition (haemochromatosis, thalassaemia)

Functional causes

- Dehydration
  - Fluid deprivation or loss
  - Haemorrhage
  - Persistent diarrhoea and/or vomiting
- Psychogenic
  - Anxiety states
  - Depression
- Drugs

Drugs

- Diuretic overdosage
- Drugs with antimuscarinic effects
  - Atropine, ipratropium, hyoscine and other analogues
  - Tricyclic and some other antidepressants
  - Antihistamines
  - Antiemetics (including antihistamines and phenothiazines)
  - Neuroleptics, particularly phenothiazines
- Some older antihypertensives (ganglion blockers and clonidine)
- Drugs with sympathomimetic actions
  - 'Cold cures' containing ephedrine, etc.
  - Decongestants
  - Bronchodilators
  - Appetite suppressants, particularly amphetamines

---

no complaint of dry mouth, but rather of difficulty eating or speaking. Some complain of an unpleasant taste in the mouth. Most find severe dryness almost unbearable.

Conversely, some with a subjective sensation of dry mouth have normal salivary flow rates on objective testing and the problem may be psychogenic. Mucosal diseases that cause roughening, particularly lichen planus, are often interpreted as dryness. Such patients are said to have *false xerostomia*. Before detailed investigation for xerostomia, a measurement of salivary flow is required to differentiate true from false xerostomia (see Sjögren's syndrome in the following section). Alternatively, a clinical assessment is reasonably accurate (Table 22.1).

Xerostomia, calculi and ascending infection are related in some patients, as shown in Fig. 22.11.

Significant sequelae of xerostomia are caries, often root caries, and candidosis. Treatment is discussed under Sjögren's syndrome.

Review PMID: 14716254

Table 22.1   The Challacombe scale for assessing dry mouth clinically*

Feature	Total score
• Mirror sticks to buccal mucosa • Mirror sticks to tongue • Saliva frothy	Total score of 1–3 indicates mild dryness. May not need treatment or management. Sugar-free chewing gum for 15 mins, twice daily and attention to hydration is needed. Many drugs will cause mild dryness. Routine checkup monitoring required.
• No saliva pooling in floor of mouth • Tongue shows generalised mild depapillation • Gingival architecture is smooth	Total score of 4–6 indicates moderate dryness. Sugar-free chewing gum or simple sialogogues may be required. Needs to be investigated further if reasons for dryness are not clear. Saliva substitutes and topical fluoride may be helpful. Monitor at regular intervals especially for caries and symptom change.
• Glassy appearance of oral mucosa, especially palate • Tongue lobulated / fissured • Cervical caries in more than two teeth • Debris on palate or sticking to teeth	Total score of 7–10 indicates severe dryness. Saliva substitutes and topical fluoride usually needed. Cause of hyposalivation needs to be ascertained and Sjögren's syndrome excluded. Refer for investigation and diagnosis. Patients then need to be monitored for changing symptoms and signs, with possible further specialist input if worsening.

*Features often appear in sequence as the mouth becomes dryer, but the sequence is not important. Each feature scores 1 and the significance of the total score is shown on the right.

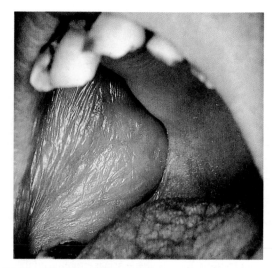

Fig. 22.12   Sjögren's syndrome. The mucosa is dry, red, atrophic and wrinkled and sticks to the fingers or mirror during examination. These changes are common to all causes of xerostomia.

Box 22.4   Oral effects of Sjögren's syndrome
- Discomfort
- Difficulties with eating or swallowing
- Disturbed taste sensation
- Disturbed quality of speech
- Predisposition to infection

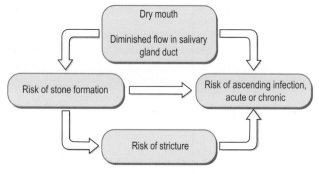

Fig. 22.11   Interrelationships between dry mouth, calculi and their complications. Note: dry mouth may promote stone formation, but stones do not cause dry mouth.

SJÖGREN'S SYNDROME

→ Summary chart 22.2 p. 354

In 1933, Sjögren noticed the association of dryness of the mouth and dryness of the eyes. Later, he found that there was a significant association with rheumatoid arthritis. These combinations of complaints are caused by two closely related but distinct diseases.

Primary Sjögren's syndrome comprises dry mouth and dry eyes not associated with any connective tissue disease. 'Sicca syndrome' is a poorly defined term that is best avoided because it can be used for any cause of dry eyes and mouth, as well as primary Sjögren's syndrome.

Secondary Sjögren's syndrome comprises dry mouth and dry eyes associated with rheumatoid arthritis or other connective tissue disease.

Primary Sjögren's syndrome causes more severe oral and ocular changes and has a higher risk of complications than secondary.

Clinical features

Females are affected nearly 10 times as frequently as males. Sjögren's syndrome affects 10%–15% of patients with rheumatoid arthritis, possibly 30% of patients with lupus erythematosus and a variable proportion of patients with or without other connective tissue diseases. Sjögren's syndrome is therefore relatively common.

Major oral effects of Sjögren's syndrome are summarised in Box 22.4.

Onset is in middle age. In the early stages, the mucosa may appear moist, but salivary flow measurement shows diminished secretion. In established cases, the oral mucosa is obviously dry, often red, shiny and parchment-like (Fig. 22.12). The tongue is typically red, the papillae characteristically atrophy and the dorsum becomes lobulated with a cobblestone appearance (Fig. 22.13). With diminished salivary secretion, the oral flora changes, and candidal infections are common. The latter are the main cause of soreness of the mouth in Sjögren's syndrome and cause generalised erythema of the mucosa, often with angular stomatitis. Plaque accumulates, and there may be rapidly progressive dental caries (see Fig. 22.14). The most severe infective complication is suppurative parotitis.

Parotid swelling is found at some stage in about 30% of patients but is not a common finding because it is often intermittent. Swollen glands are not inflamed clinically and are rarely painful (Fig. 22.15). A hot, tender parotid swelling with red, shiny overlying skin would indicate suppurative

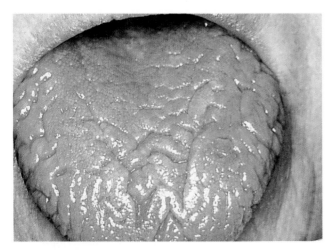

Fig. 22.13   Tongue in Sjögren's syndrome. Longstanding dry mouth and repeated candidal infection produce this depapillated but lobulated tongue.

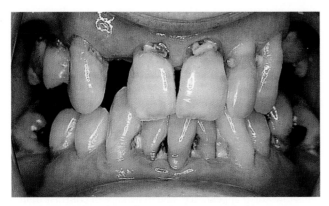

Fig. 22.14   Sjögren's syndrome. Extensive cervical caries is a frequent complication of dry mouth. In addition to the lack of saliva, patients may attempt to stimulate salivary flow with sweets or chewing gums.

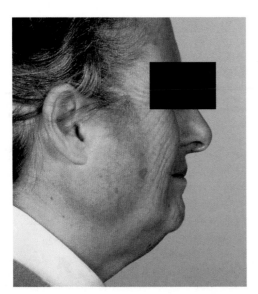

Fig. 22.15   Salivary gland swelling in primary Sjögren's syndrome. The outline of the parotid gland is clearly demarcated.

Box 22.5   Ocular effects of Sjögren's syndrome

- Failure of tear secretion
- Dried secretions stick to conjunctiva and cornea
- Failure of clearance of foreign particles from the cornea and conjunctiva
- Gritty sensation in the eyes
- Keratinisation and loss of goblet cells in conjunctiva
- Abrasions, ulcers and inflammation
- Risk of impairment or loss of sight

Box 22.6   Histological changes in salivary glands in Sjögren's syndrome

- Polyclonal infiltration mainly by CD4 lymphocytes
- Infiltrate initially periductal
- Progressive spread of infiltrate through the glandular tissue
- Progressive destruction of secretory acini
- Proliferation of ducts to form epimyoepithelial islands

---

parotitis. Bilateral parotid swelling strongly suggests lymphoma (discussed later).

Patients have increased incidence of allergy to antibiotics, particularly allergy to trimethoprim which causes fever, headache, backache and meningeal irritation.

Sjögren's syndrome can have serious ocular effects (Box 22.5). Dryness leads to keratinisation, splitting and inflammation of the conjunctiva and cornea. Ulceration, corneal scarring and induction of blood vessel ingrowth can lead to visual impairment.

Primary Sjögren's syndrome is not just a localised form of the disease. Although patients lack a connective tissue disorder, they have other systemic manifestations including involvement of all exocrine glands and features such as Raynaud's phenomenon.

General review PMID: 16039337

Review causes and prognosis PMID: 23993190

Extraglandular features primary disease PMID: 26231345

Aetiology and pathology

The cause is unknown, but genetic predisposition exists and environmental triggers, possibly viral, are suspected. The process is an autoimmune attack on all exocrine glands, including those of the skin, vagina, lung and pancreas, though these other sites rarely cause significant problems clinically.

Histological changes are shown in Box 22.6. Lymphocytes infiltrate the glands and cluster around small ducts, proliferate and gradually replace acinar cells (Fig. 22.16). The mechanisms of acinar cell destruction are unclear but may be apoptotic and induced by cytokine secretion. Over many years, the lymphocytic infiltrates enlarge and replace more of the gland, and the types of lymphocyte change with disease progression. The ductal cells proliferate, possibly in response to cytokines released by the lymphocytes, to form islands and sheets of cells around the ducts. Although myoepithelial cells are not a feature, the islands are called *epimyoepithelial islands* (Fig. 22.17), and the overall appearance is sometimes called *myoepithelial sialadenitis*.

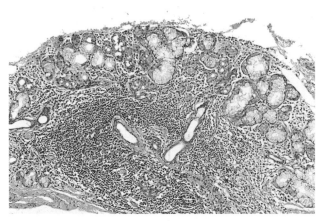

Fig. 22.16 Sjögren's syndrome. The histological appearance is typical. Dense, well-defined foci of lymphocytes surround the larger ducts in the centre of the lobules. In the area occupied by the lymphocytes, there is complete acinar atrophy and a rim of residual salivary parenchyma remains around the periphery of the lobule.

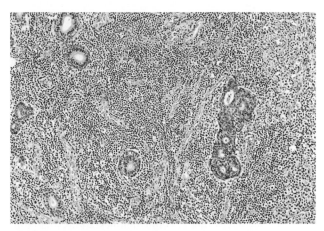

Fig. 22.17 Sjögren's syndrome. In late disease no salivary acini remain and the gland is replaced by a confluent infiltrate of lymphocytes. A few ducts remain and proliferate to form the epimyoepithelial islands. Such extensive changes sometimes suggest that there has been progression to a low-grade lymphoma.

The final result is destruction of acini and replacement of the whole gland by a dense lymphocytic infiltrate (Fig. 22.17). However, the infiltrate remains confined within the gland capsule and does not cross the intraglandular septa.

There is systemic polyclonal B cell activation, producing a variety of autoantibodies (Table 22.2) that aid diagnosis.

Diagnosis

No test is definitive; many may be required in early disease (Box 22.7). The least invasive tests are used first.

Salivary secretion should be assessed by testing unstimulated whole saliva flow by the patient drooling into a graduated container over 10 minutes. Normal salivary flow is between 1 and 2 mL/min but may be reduced to 0.2 mL/min or less. Reduction confirms a true xerostomia. Alternatively, dryness can be scored relatively accurately from clinical features (Table 22.1). If present, other causes of xerostomia must be excluded next (Box 22.3).

Table 22.2 Typical patterns of autoantibodies in primary and secondary Sjögren's syndromes

Autoantibodies	Primary SS	Secondary SS
Salivary duct antibody	10%–36%	67%–70%
Rheumatoid factor	50%	90%
SS-A (Ro) antibodies	5%–10%	50%–80%
SS-B (La) antibodies	50%–75%	2%–5%
Rheumatoid arthritis precipitin	5%	75%

Box 22.7 Diagnostic tests in Sjögren's syndrome

- Diminished total salivary flow rate
- Diminished tear secretion and ocular effects
- Raised immunoglobulin levels and erythrocyte sedimentation rate
- Antibody screen, especially rheumatoid factor and SS-A and SS-B
- Circulating CD4+/CD8+ lymphocyte ratio
- Sialectasis on sialography or ultrasound
- Labial salivary gland biopsy showing periductal lymphocytic infiltrate

Specialist ophthalmic examination is very sensitive to detect corneal drying and its effects. The Schirmer test, in which a filter paper strip tucked under the lower eyelid is used to measure tear production, is considerably less informative, extremely variable, uncomfortable for the patient and best avoided.

Serological support for the diagnosis should be sought next, using the tests in Table 22.2 while noting that none are specific to the disorder. A sialogram will usually show the snowstorm appearance, due to leakage of contrast material through the terminal duct walls (Fig. 22.18). Ultrasound examination may reveal similar features and is less invasive and more tolerable for the patient.

If no definitive diagnosis is yet possible, a labial gland biopsy may be performed. Pathological changes in labial salivary glands correlate closely with those in the parotid glands, and lip biopsy avoids the risks of damage to the facial nerve inherent in parotid gland biopsy. However, this test is considerably overrated. A harvest of 6–8 glands is required. The usual method for assessment is to count the number of foci of lymphocytes per 4 mm^2 of tissue. Although a score of 1 or more is highly suggestive, it is easy to misinterpret non-specific inflammation. The predictive value is probably no higher than 80% when correctly interpreted.

Several sets of international diagnostic criteria exist but are not completely accurate, do not identify the same cases and fail to identify early and subclinical cases.

Because there is no specific treatment for the underlying disease process, the effort, expense and morbidity of investigations have to be weighed against the certainty of diagnosis required.

Labial gland biopsy PMID: 21480190

Diagnostic criteria PMID: 22563590 and 23968620

Management

Many aspects need to be taken into account (Box 22.8).

Ophthalmological review is important to exclude or treat keratoconjunctivitis sicca, which is symptomless

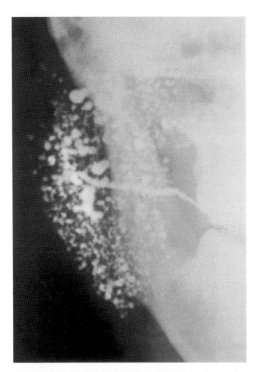

Fig. 22.18 Sjögren's syndrome. The sialogram shows the typical snowstorm appearance of blobs of contrast medium that have leaked from the duct system. Emptying and clearance of the contrast medium are also much delayed because of the reduced salivary flow.

Box 22.8 Principles of management of Sjögren's syndrome

- Salivary gland damage is irreversible
- Give reassurance and help with dry mouth
- Ophthalmological investigation for keratoconjunctivitis sicca
- Refer to specialist if connective tissue disease is untreated
- Check for any associated drug treatment contributing to dry mouth
- Alleviate dry mouth
  - Frequent small sips of water
  - Prescribe saliva substitutes
- Control caries in dentate patients
  - Avoid sweets (e.g. lemon drops)
  - Suggest sugar-free gum
  - Check diet for excess sugary foods
  - Maintain good oral hygiene
  - Fluoride applications
  - Chlorhexidine (0.2%) rinses
- Monitor for mucosal candidosis
  - Give antifungal mixtures (not tablets) as necessary
- Treat difficulties with dentures symptomatically
- Observe regularly for possible development of ascending parotitis or lymphoma

in its early stages. Dryness of the eyes is treated with artificial tears, such as methyl cellulose solution. Anaemia should be excluded, particularly when there is rheumatoid arthritis, because it contributes to candidosis.

Box 22.9 Types of artificial saliva currently available in UK and some European countries

- Bioextra moistening gel, Lactoperoxidase, Lactoferrin, Lysozymes and immunoglobulins
- Glandosane spray. Carmellose (carboxymethyl cellulose) solution with sorbitol and electrolytes
- Luborant spray. Carmellose solution with electrolytes and preservatives
- OralBalance gel. Lactoperoxidase, glucose oxidase and xylitol
- Saliva Orthana spray. Gastric mucin, xylitol, sodium fluoride with preservatives and flavouring
- Saliva Orthana lozenges. Mucin with xylitol in sorbitol base
- Salivace spray. Carmellose with xylitol, electrolytes and preservative
- Salivix pastilles. Sugar-free. Contain gum acacia and malic acid

Similar preparations are available in the United States and other countries as Oasis and Aquaoral spray, Caphosol solution, Salivasure lozenges and Xylimelt dissolvable disks.

Dryness of the mouth can be relieved to some degree by providing artificial saliva (Box 22.9), although these preparations are not very pleasant to use. Patients must conserve what little mucin they have in the mouth by sipping liquid, not rinsing and swallowing. Cholinesterase inhibitors, such as pilocarpine, are sometimes recommended to stimulate salivary secretion, but have unpleasant side effects such as nausea, diarrhoea and bradycardia.

In dentate patients, an aggressive preventive regime is required with topical fluorides and chlorhexidine mouth rinses to reduce plaque formation. Soreness of the mouth due to infection by *Candida albicans* can be treated with fluconazole or nystatin. Ascending parotitis should be treated as described earlier.

A dry and sore mouth and eyes, perhaps with pain from rheumatoid arthritis persisting over many years, is deeply distressing. Depression is a common consequence, and patients need support and reassurance.

Treatment PMID: 20664046

Ophthalmic assessment PMID: 20035924

Increasing salivary flow PMID: 15153695

Cochrane dry mouth topical treatment PMID: 22161442

Review xerostomia and treatment PMID: 25463902

Complications → Summary chart 22.2 p. 354

The risk to the eyes has been noted previously (Box 22.5).

Primary Sjögren's syndrome carries a relative risk of developing lymphoma of times 16, equivalent to 5% of patients, and higher in severely affected cases. The lymphomas are of B cell type, usually of the low-grade MALT (**M**ucosa-**A**ssociated **L**ymphoid **T**issue) type (Ch. 27), which are relatively indolent and carry a good prognosis. They arise in the affected glands and respond well to treatment while still localised there. Persistent swelling, particularly in long-standing disease, is suggestive, as is sudden enlargement of previously swollen glands, especially with cervical lymph

Review IgG4 head and neck PMID: 23068303

Rare cause salivary fibrosis PMID: 23692045

node enlargement. A low CD4$^+$ lymphocyte count or CD4$^+$/CD8$^+$ ratio is a strong risk factor for lymphoma. High-grade B cell lymphomas also arise and may develop from the low-grade lymphomas.

Key features are summarised in Box 22.10.

Lymphoma in Sjögren's PMID: 25316606

HIV-ASSOCIATED SALIVARY GLAND DISEASE → Summary chart 22.2 p. 354

This disease affects primarily children and young adults with HIV infection, causing chronic soft parotid enlargement of one or both glands, sometimes painful. It is discussed in detail in Chapter 29. Immunosuppression also leads to enlargement of intraparotid lymph nodes, which may be mistaken for parotid neoplasms.

IGG$_4$ SCLEROSING DISEASE

This recently recognised disease§ produces chronic focal inflammation and dense fibrosis. In the head and neck it is seen in salivary and lacrimal glands and the soft tissues but may affect almost any body site, particularly pancreas and lung. Either a single or multiple sites may be involved. Onset is after middle age. The disease is usually asymptomatic, and recurrent periods of activity are characterised by raised levels of serum IgG$_4$ in about half of cases. This subclass of immunoglobulin normally has a low serum concentration.

Fibrosis produces a firm enlarging mass, often mimicking a neoplasm, and the gland is progressively destroyed. Diagnosis is by biopsy showing fibrosis with obliteration of small veins, fibrosis and a dense lymphoplasmacytic infiltrate with numerous IgG$_4$ secreting plasma cells (Fig. 22.19).

When one salivary gland is affected, a search must be made for other sites, both other salivary glands and remote sites. The condition responds to steroids and other immunosuppressants, but if untreated, fibrosis will extend beyond the gland to adjacent tissues.

NECROTISING SIALOMETAPLASIA
→ Summary charts 23.1 and 23.2 pp. 365, 366

This tumour-like lesion mainly affects the minor glands of the palate and probably results from infarction or ischaemia triggered by thrombosis or trauma. The condition is commoner in males and in cigarette smokers and in the middle aged or elderly. Occasionally is it bilateral.

Typically, a relatively painless swelling 15–20 mm in diameter forms on the hard palate at the site of the minor glands (Fig. 22.20), growing rapidly. The surface becomes ulcerated, and the ulcer margins are irregular and heaped up or everted. Clinically, it resembles a salivary gland carcinoma.

There is necrosis of the gland acini, inflammation and, after a short period, a hyperplastic healing response of the duct epithelium. The duct epithelium forms squamous islands so that the condition can mimic a carcinoma histologically as well as clinically (Fig. 22.21).

Biopsy is often performed for diagnosis, although the clinical presentation is distinctive. Untreated, it heals in 6–8 weeks.

Review and case series PMID: 1923419 and 22921832

SARCOIDOSIS

This disease causes bilateral parotid enlargement with destruction of the gland and replacement by granulomatous inflammation (Fig. 22.22). It is discussed in detail in Chapter 30.

SIALADENOSIS → Summary chart 22.2 p. 354

Sialadenosis is a non-neoplastic, non-inflammatory enlargement of salivary glands, most noticeably of the parotids. There are many causes (Box 22.11). Enlargement is slow, and the process is usually bilateral (Fig. 22.23).

Histologically, there is hypertrophy of serous acini and the enlarged cells contain excess large secretory granules. The myoepithelial cells are atrophic. Both these effects are probably mediated by autonomic neuropathy caused by the underlying disease.

Cases and review PMID: 7551515

Minor gland involvement PMID: 15250838

Histological features PMID: 20580282

§Footnote: This disease is now recognised to be the common cause of several previously different diseases including lung pseudotumours, autoimmune pancreatitis and retroperitoneal fibrosis. However, it is not equivalent to Küttner tumour, the terminal fibrotic stage of chronic sialadenitis. Nor does it explain so-called *Mikulicz's disease*, which was probably MALT lymphoma. These confusing historical eponyms are best avoided. See PMID: 21707715.

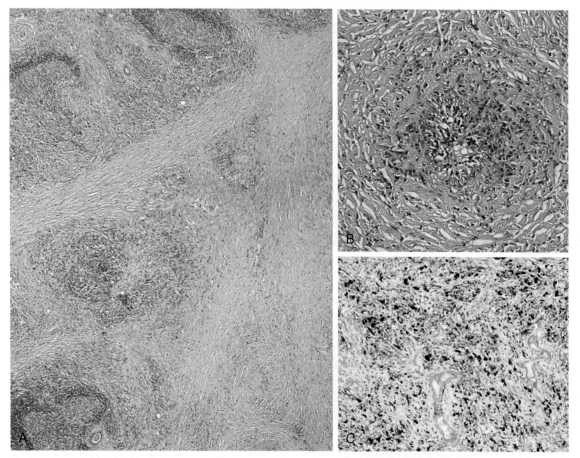

Fig. 22.19   IgG₄ sclerosing disease affecting a submandibular gland. The gland is destroyed by intersecting bands of 'storiform' fibrosis and inflammatory infiltrate including lymphoid follicles (*A*). Small veins are obliterated by inflammation (*B*). Immunohistochemistry against IgG₄ class immunoglobulin produces a brown positive reaction on numerous cells secreting IgG₄ (*C*). In a typical non-specific sialadenitis, such cells are rarely present in any numbers.

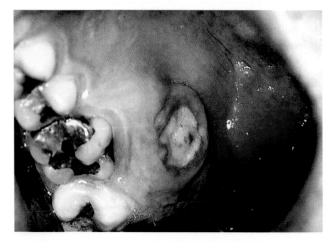

Fig. 22.20   Necrotising sialometaplasia. The clinical appearances are similar to those of a malignant salivary neoplasm.

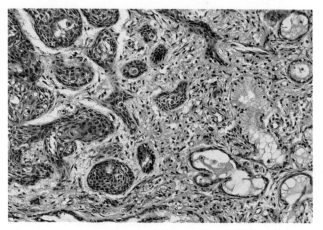

Fig. 22.21   Necrotising sialometaplasia. The histological features may also be mistaken for malignancy. There is necrosis of all the acinar cells and the islands of epithelium on the left are hyperplastic ducts showing squamous metaplasia.

OTHER SALIVARY GLAND DISORDERS

Irradiation Salivary tissue is highly sensitive to ionising radiation, which causes irreversible destruction of acini and fibrous replacement of glands in the irradiated field. Xerostomia is immediate in onset, severe, and recovers poorly. Management is as for Sjögren's syndrome. Radioiodine, used to treat thyroid carcinomas, is concentrated in salivary glands but causes minimal problems with dry mouth unless repeated doses have been used.

Salivary fistula, a communication between the duct system or gland with the skin or mucous membrane, is uncommon. Internal fistulae drain into the oral cavity and cause no symptoms. By contrast, parotid fistula on the skin is troublesome and often persistent. It may be the result of

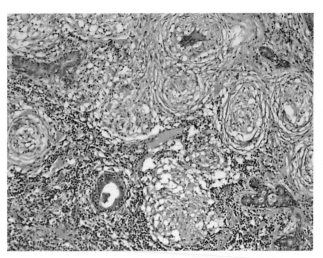

Fig. 22.22 Sarcoidosis of salivary gland. The acinar cells are completely effaced and only a few ducts remain, surrounded by fibrosis and pale staining rounded granulomas of loosely cohesive macrophages. The granuloma near the top centre contains a small multinucleate cell.

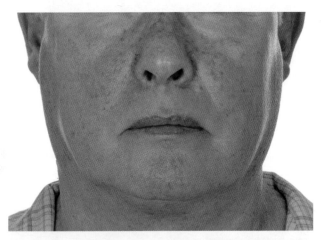

Fig. 22.23 Sialadenosis. Typical appearance of bilateral swelling of parotid glands.

an injury to the cheek or a complication of surgery. Infection often becomes superimposed, and persistent leakage of saliva prevents healing. The treatment is primarily by surgical repair but is difficult.

Sjögren's-like syndrome in graft-versus-host disease develops in approximately one-third of all cases of graft-versus-host disease (GVHD), particularly when severe, and mimics primary Sjögren's.

Juvenile recurrent parotitis is rare and poorly understood, possibly a low-grade recurrent infection. It starts

---

Box 22.12 Causes of ptyalism

Local reflexes

- Oral infections (e.g. acute necrotising ulcerative gingivitis)
- Oral wounds
- Dental procedures
- New dentures

Systemic reflexes

- Nausea
- Oesophageal disease (reflux oesophagitis)
- Rare effect of pregnancy

Toxic

- Iodine
- Heavy metals: mercury, copper arsenic

'False ptyalism' (drooling)

- Psychogenic
- Bell's palsy
- Parkinson's disease
- Stroke

---

before the age of 6 years and causes recurrent episodes of acute swelling lasting a few days with fever and malaise, usually unilaterally. It resolves around the time of puberty.

Cystic fibrosis is discussed in Chapter 33.

HYPERSALIVATION (SIALORRHOEA OR PTYALISM)

True ptyalism is rarely a significant complaint because excess saliva is swallowed. However, it is a symptom increasingly considered to merit medical investigation given its many causes (Box 22.12). Idiopathic paroxysmal sialorrhea, known to patients as 'waterbrash', is reflex secretion caused by oesophagitis, peptic ulcers, infections and other gastrointestinal irritation. There is a sudden rush of saliva, sometimes waking the patient because their mouth is suddenly full of saliva.

'False ptyalism', a sensation of excess saliva, is more common than true ptyalism and is either delusional or results from failure to swallow. Drooling in neurological disorders, or in those with syndromic presentations such as Down's syndrome, is due to faulty neuromuscular control, often with a forward head and tongue posture and weak swallowing.

Drooling PMID: 19236564

Botulinum toxin treatment PMID: 23112272

Summary chart 22.1   Differential diagnosis and management of a patient with 'mealtime syndrome'.

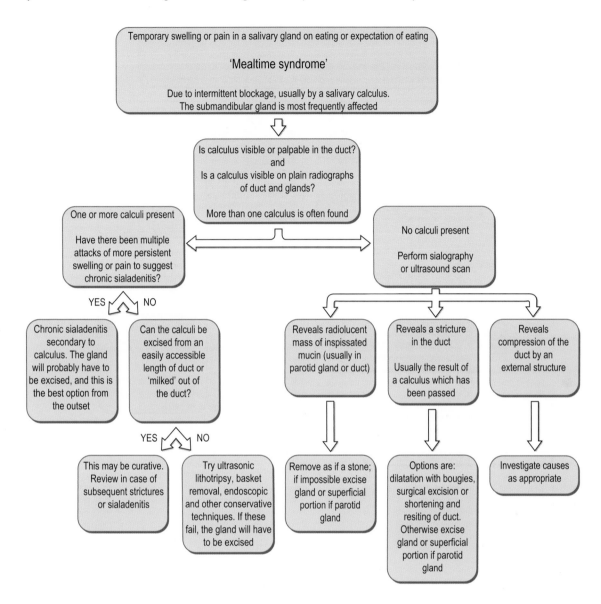

Summary chart 22.2   Summary of the diagnosis of persistent bilateral swelling of the parotid glands.

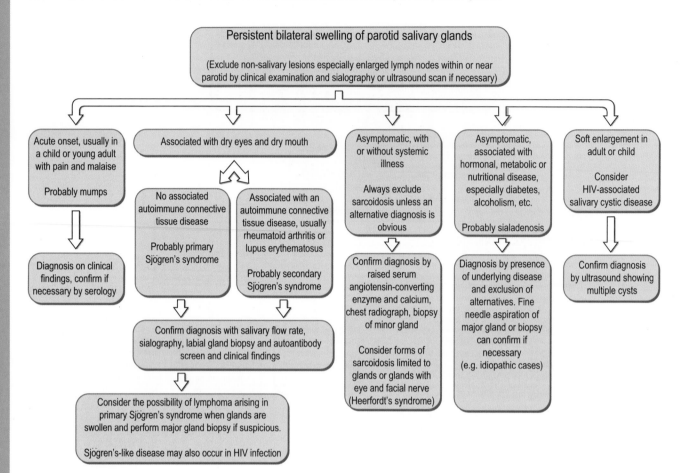

Salivary gland neoplasms

23

SALIVARY GLAND NEOPLASMS

Most salivary gland neoplasms arise in the parotid glands, but they are also frequent in intraoral minor glands, making them the second most common neoplasms of the mouth after squamous cell carcinoma. Neoplasms of salivary glands arise from the stem cell population that resides in the ducts and gives rise normally to duct lining epithelium, secretory acinar cells and myoepithelial cells. The histology of the tumours is therefore complex because all these lines of differentiation may appear in different proportions.

Occasionally lymphomas arise in the intraparotid lymph nodes and other soft tissue neoplasms arise from the supporting connective tissue of the gland. Although within the gland, these are not considered salivary gland neoplasms.

Mucous-secreting glands in the nose and nasal sinuses, pharynx and larynx can also give rise to the same types of neoplasm as those that develop in salivary glands.

Epidemiology and aetiology

The total incidence of salivary gland tumours is difficult to determine because benign tumours are not recorded by cancer registries. Taken together, benign and malignant tumours arise in at least 10 per 100,000 of the population so that several thousand cases arise in the UK each year. *Malignant* salivary neoplasms have a relatively stable prevalence of approximately 0.8 per 10,000 in the UK, and approximately 600 new salivary gland cancers are registered in England each year. Women are slightly more frequently affected, and the peak incidence for all types is in the fifth decade, although both benign and malignant neoplasms have a very broad age distribution. Although the numbers are small, the incidence of *malignant* salivary gland tumours in the UK is increasing.

The aetiology of most salivary gland tumours remains obscure. They can result from irradiation to the head and prevalence increased in survivors of the atomic blasts at Hiroshima and Nagasaki. Salivary tumours can also follow therapeutic irradiation for other head and neck cancers and, it is suggested, multiple dental diagnostic radiographs. Studies on association with mobile phone use suggest no risk of malignant tumours, but there are no good data to analyse for benign tumours.

Several salivary tumours are known to be caused by specific fusion genes. These arise through chromosomal breakage during mitosis, the fragments rejoining incorrectly as chromosomal translocations, deletions or inversions. Where the fragments rejoin, a new fusion gene is formed, a hybrid that links together parts of two previously unrelated genes. Such fusion genes are often oncogenic. Fusion genes can be detected by fluorescence in situ hybridisation to aid diagnosis of difficult cases (Ch. 1, Fig. 1.11).

There are large differences in the incidence of individual tumour types worldwide. In the United Kingdom, mucoepidermoid and acinic cell carcinomas are rarer than in the United States, and undifferentiated carcinomas are much more common in the Eastern countries.

Web URL 23.1 UK incidence: Web search for: ncras head and neck cancer hub

US incidence PMID: 19861510

Presentation of salivary gland tumours

Salivary neoplasms almost always present as a mass, sometimes with added symptoms of obstruction if the excretory duct is compressed. Often the lump may be longstanding, but that does not necessarily indicate that it is likely to be benign. Key symptoms to elicit in the history are those of nerve involvement. Facial nerve signs almost certainly indicate that a parotid mass is a malignant neoplasm. Adenoid cystic carcinoma has a particular propensity to spread along nerves and give rise to symptoms of facial palsy, pain or paraesthesia.

It is critically important to recognise the relationship between the gland of origin and risk of a neoplasm being malignant (Fig. 23.1) before planning a biopsy or excision. About 75% of salivary gland tumours develop in the parotid gland, most in the superficial lobe, and about 10% in the submandibular glands. These produce a visible or palpable mass. Tumours in the deep lobe of parotid present as a mass in the lateral wall of the pharynx, close to the tonsil. Tumours in the sublingual glands are rare but usually malignant. The usual intraoral site is the palatal glands at or near the junction of the hard and soft palate (Fig. 23.2), followed by the buccal mucosa or labial minor glands.

Typical clinical features of benign and malignant salivary gland tumours are shown in Table 23.1. However, in their early stages, benign and malignant salivary gland tumours usually cannot be distinguished clinically (Summary chart 23.2).

Types and classification

The classification of salivary gland tumours is complex. The current World Health Organization scheme lists 21 malignant, 11 benign tumours and 5 tumour-like conditions, but

Table 23.1	Typical clinical features of salivary gland tumours	
Benign salivary gland tumours	**Malignant salivary gland tumours**
Slow-growing	Some are fast-growing and painful, but many are slow growing and asymptomatic
Soft or rubbery consistency	Sometimes hard consistency
Comprise 85% of parotid tumours	Comprise 45% of minor gland tumours
Do not ulcerate	May ulcerate and invade bone
No associated nerve signs	May cause cranial nerve palsies, usually lingual, facial or hypoglossal depending on the site

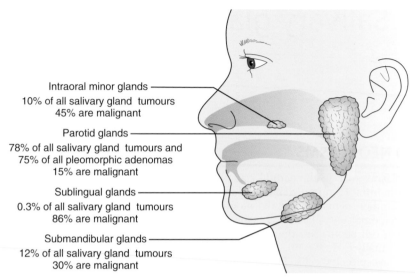

Fig. 23.1 The distribution of salivary gland neoplasms showing the approximate overall frequency of tumours in different sites and the relevant frequency of benign and malignant tumours by site.

Intraoral minor glands
10% of all salivary gland tumours
45% are malignant

Parotid glands
78% of all salivary gland tumours and
75% of all pleomorphic adenomas
15% are malignant

Sublingual glands
0.3% of all salivary gland tumours
86% are malignant

Submandibular glands
12% of all salivary gland tumours
30% are malignant

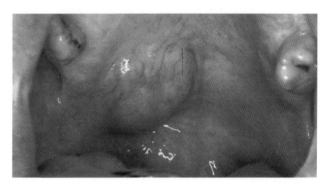

Fig. 23.2 Typical presentation of a salivary neoplasm. A mass lies at the junction of hard and soft palates, a common intraoral site. This particular example is a pleomorphic adenoma, which usually feels rubbery and firm on palpation.

still more have been described. However, many are rarities, and a simplified classification of the commoner and more important entities is shown in Box 23.1. The full classification, with a brief note on the rarer entities, is shown in Appendix 23.1 and is available online with detailed descriptions of each tumour type.

Investigations

Treatment depends on tumour type and extent, and either a definitive diagnosis or categorisation into benign or malignant is needed to plan surgery. The key investigation is fine needle aspiration. For pleomorphic adenoma, Warthin's tumour, adenoid cystic carcinoma and many common neoplasms, fine needle aspiration almost always gives the correct diagnosis. For other tumours, it can often determine whether neoplasms are benign or malignant, low or high grade, or can be used to narrow down a differential diagnosis. Most neoplasms in the superficial parotid gland are amenable to fine needle aspiration, and ultrasound guidance can be used to target more deeply seated tumours.

Imaging for suspected salivary neoplasms is best performed by magnetic resonance imaging (MRI), which is capable of detecting perineural spread and base of skull invasion by

---

Box 23.1   Salivary gland neoplasms (simplified World Health Organization classification, see also Appendix 23.1)

Epithelial tumours

Primary benign (adenomas)

- Pleomorphic adenoma and myoepithelioma
- Warthin's tumour
- Basal cell and canalicular adenoma
- Oncocytoma

Primary malignant (carcinomas)

- Acinic cell carcinoma
- Secretory carcinoma
- Mucoepidermoid carcinoma
- Adenoid cystic carcinoma
- Polymorphous adenocarcinoma
- Salivary duct carcinoma
- Epithelial-myoepithelial carcinoma
- Undifferentiated carcinoma
- Carcinoma ex pleomorphic adenoma
- Adenocarcinoma not otherwise specified

Secondary malignant (metastatic)

- Lymphatic spread: usually from head and neck
- Blood-borne: from other body sites

Non-epithelial tumours

- Hamartomas: haemangioma
- Lymphoma: in parotid lymph nodes

---

palatal and parotid cancers. Cone beam computed tomography (CT) or conventional thin slice CT is useful to detect palatal bone perforation below palatal tumours. Sialography no longer has any role in investigation of salivary neoplasms, and ultrasound scanning is the best way to differentiate salivary neoplasms from enlarged intraparotid lymph nodes. The thought processes underlying investigation and diagnosis are shown in Summary charts 23.1 and 23.2.

BENIGN TUMOURS

→ Summary charts 23.1 and 23.2 pp. 365, 366

Pleomorphic adenoma

Pleomorphic adenomas, or pleomorphic salivary adenomas, are benign salivary tumours characterised microscopically by an unusually broad range of types of tissue. The neoplastic cells are epithelial but differentiate to a connective tissue cell type and secrete connective tissue ground substance, collagen, form cartilage and sometimes bone. This mixture of epithelial and connective tissue types accounts for the old name of 'mixed tumour'.

These benign tumours are the commonest salivary tumours and account for about 75% of parotid tumours, and a further 20% are distributed equally between the submandibular gland and intraoral minor glands, usually on the palate (see Fig. 23.2). They can arise at any age but are most common in middle age.

Pleomorphic adenomas grow slowly and take several years to reach 2 cm in diameter. They are rubbery, firm swellings (see Figs. 23.2 and 23.3), smooth when small but often very lobulated when large (Fig. 23.4). The overlying skin or mucosa is mobile over the lump, although in the palate the more inflexible mucoperiosteum may appear fixed.

The cause of most pleomorphic adenomas is a chromosomal translocation that activates one of two genes, PLAG1 or HMGA2. These encode transcription factors important in normal development. Their constitutive activation results in cell proliferation and abnormal differentiation, explaining the varied tissues formed. In addition to these causative translocations, pleomorphic adenomas can have many other chromosomal abnormalities involving oncogenes and tumour suppressor genes. These additional changes increase with time and probably account for the risk of malignant transformation in longstanding tumours.

Each adenoma is circumscribed, and there is usually a capsule around most of the periphery. While it grows, the tumour pushes out large finger-like extensions or bulges out

to form a lobulated outline. Inside, there is a disorganised arrangement of tissues (Figs 23.5–23.8). The epithelial cells form ducts and small cysts and sheets. Around the ducts and detaching and migrating into the surrounding tissue are cells that show partial differentiation into myoepithelial

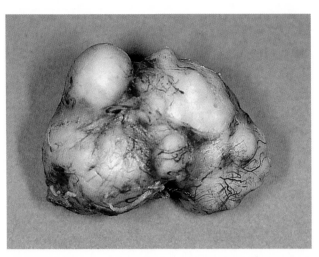

Fig. 23.4 This excised pleomorphic adenoma is 3 cm across, and the lobular shape is clearly seen.

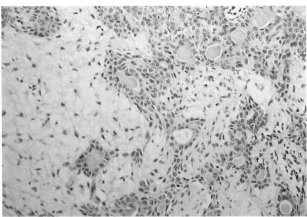

Fig. 23.5 **Pleomorphic adenoma.** The histological appearances are very varied. In this typical area, there are clusters of ducts containing eosinophilic material surrounded by stellate cells lying in a mucinous stroma.

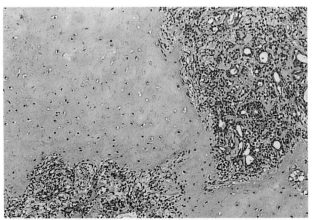

Fig. 23.6 **Pleomorphic adenoma.** In this area, there has been maturation of the mucinous stroma to form a cartilage-like material within which there are more cellular islands with ducts.

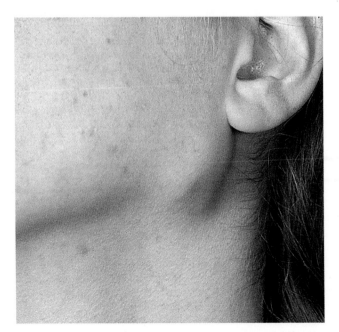

Fig. 23.3 **Pleomorphic adenoma.** This slowly enlarging lump in the lower pole of the parotid gland is caused by a pleomorphic adenoma, but the appearance is not specific and any benign and some low-grade malignant neoplasms could appear the same.

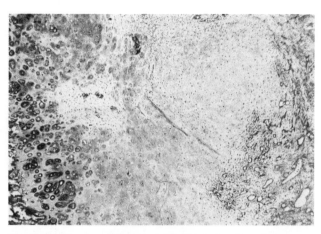

Fig. 23.7 Pleomorphic adenoma. In this lesion, there is formation of true cartilage which is undergoing calcification.

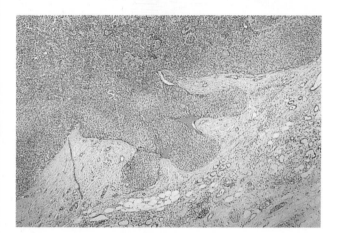

Fig. 23.8 Pleomorphic adenoma. At the margins of pleomorphic adenomas there are often extensions of the tumour into and beyond the capsule, rendering enucleation a risky treatment that is likely to be followed by recurrence.

cells. These cells can be identified immunohistochemically by their expression of cytokeratins and contractile proteins such as actin, but unlike normal myoepithelial cells around acini, they have no useful contractile function. Rather they take on the shapes and functions of connective tissue cells. Most are spindle or stellate in shape, secrete excess proteoglycan ground substance and become dispersed in it to form a myxoid (gelatinous) tissue. Some are rounded and look like plasma cells microscopically, and others form collagen, cartilage or bone (Box 23.2). The proportion of these tissues varies widely between tumours producing a confusing range of histological appearances. When no ducts are present and myoepithelial cells predominate or are the only cells present, the tumour is termed *myoepithelioma,* but the presentation, histological appearances and treatment are otherwise the same.

Pleomorphic adenomas are treated by excision with a margin of normal tissue; without this, recurrence is likely. The reputation of the pleomorphic adenoma for recurrence is due a combination of its structure and anatomical location. In the parotid gland, the facial nerve in particular makes dissection hazardous. Tumours in the deep lobe require complete parotidectomy, and it is not unusual for tumours to have to be peeled off nerves to preserve them.

The risk of recurrence also depends on the tumour. Those comprising almost exclusively the gelatinous myxoid tissue

can burst at operation, if not gently handled, and even a small disruption of the capsule can allow the semisolid contents to seed widespread recurrence in the tissues. Recurrence is most problematic for parotid tumours, where spillage of gelatinous tumour into the fascial planes of the neck can seed multiple nodules of tumour in tissues from the base of skull down to the clavicle. Unfortunately, almost all pleomorphic adenomas contain at least some of this myxoid component.

The strategy to avoid recurrence is to remove tumours intact with a margin of normal tissue. In the superficial parotid gland, this is normally considered to require removal of the whole superficial lobe. The whole gland is removed for those in the submandibular gland. Tumours in minor glands are excised with a few millimetres of normal tissue margin and rarely recur. There has recently been a suggestion that pleomorphic adenomas can be effectively treated by more conservative surgery, 'extracapsular dissection', removing a minimal amount of tissue beyond the capsule. This is controversial and risks both puncture of the capsule or failure to gain clearance in areas without a capsule, but seems to have a low recurrence rate when performed by those skilled in the procedure.

When recurrence develops, it is often multifocal and difficult or impossible to eradicate by surgery. Although the recurrent nodules are benign, radiotherapy is sometimes used as a last resort to control surgically unresectable tumour seedlings in the infratemporal fossa or more widespread in the neck.

If neglected, pleomorphic adenomas can grow to a great size, over 10 cm diameter is not unusual. Longstanding examples, regardless of size, occasionally undergo malignant change as described later in the section on carcinoma ex pleomorphic adenoma.

Review treatment PMID: 18376235

Warthin's tumour

This is the second commonest type of salivary tumour. Almost all arise in the parotid glands, usually the lower pole, and account for approximately 10% of parotid tumours. Although often said to be more common in males, this is not supported by current evidence. Almost all patients are aged older than 40 years, and there appears to be a close association with heavy smoking, particularly in multifocal tumours.

Warthin's tumours develop not only in salivary glands but also in the lymph nodes around the lower pole of the gland and in the upper third of the deep cervical lymphatic chain.

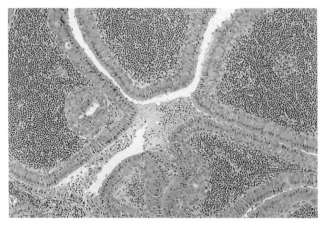

Fig. 23.9 Warthin's tumour. Tall columnar cells surround lymphoid tissue and line a convoluted cystic space.

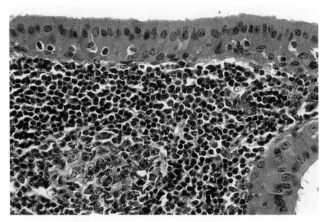

Fig. 23.10 Warthin's tumour. At higher power, the tall columnar epithelial cells are readily identified and beneath them the lymphoid tissue.

The lymph node tumours are not metastatic but arise from developmental rests of salivary gland ducts that are commonly found in lymph nodes at these sites. Approximately 15% of patients will have a second Warthin's tumour, and histologically there are often multifocal microscopic foci of developing Warthin's tumours in surrounding gland or lymph nodes.

The nature of this unusual multifocal tumour is unclear. Molecular analysis shows that the tumours are not clonal, suggesting that they are not true neoplasms despite findings of chromosomal translocations in some. The cause may be defects of mitochondrial genes.

The tumour is a cyst or part solid part cystic mass with a thin capsule and a highly characteristic histological appearance with a lymphoid and an epithelial component. The lymphoid tissue resembles lymph node, with many lymphoid follicles and germinal centres. The epithelial cells are tall, eosinophilic columnar cells that form a much-folded epithelium lining cysts and papillary projections into the cystic spaces (Figs 23.9 and 23.10). The bright pink appearance of the epithelial cells' cytoplasm is caused by abnormal large distorted mitochondria that almost completely fill the cell. Cells showing this change are referred to as *oncocytes* (see also oncocytoma later in this chapter).

Warthin's tumour is benign and cured by simple excision but may appear to recur because new tumours develop elsewhere in the gland. Preoperative diagnosis by fine needle aspiration (FNA) is accurate, and it has been suggested that,

after FNA diagnosis, surgery can be avoided and the lesion managed by repeated imaging. This may be an attractive option in a very elderly patient. However, Warthin's tumours can reach several centimetres diameter, and FNA results can be incorrect because similar oncocytic cells can be found in many types of salivary tumour. In practice, most are excised.

The older name of adenolymphoma should not be used as it risks confusion with lymphoma and other types of tumour.

Review PMID: 3458128

Infarcted Warthin's: PMID: 2743609

Canalicular adenoma

Canalicular adenomas affect particularly the upper lip and buccal mucosa, and some are multifocal in origin. They have a uniform cellular structure, comprising strands and trabeculae or duct-like rings of basaloid epithelial cells. They lack myoepithelial cells and do not form the myxoid or cartilaginous tissues of pleomorphic adenoma and do not recur on simple excision.

Basal cell adenoma

These adenomas arise mostly in the parotid glands of elderly patients. They are encapsulated and comprise basaloid cells arranged in strands, trabeculae and solid sheets. Like canalicular adenomas, they do not form myxoid tissue or cartilage. Basal cell adenomas do not recur on excision, but because they can be difficult to confidently differentiate from pleomorphic adenomas on FNA, they are often diagnosed only after a superficial parotidectomy undertaken for an assumed pleomorphic adenoma.

Oncocytoma

Oncocytoma is a rare benign tumour that almost always affects the parotid gland, particularly in the elderly. It consists of large eosinophilic cells with small compact nuclei ('oncocytes'), arranged in solid cords, nests or sheets. Oncocytes stain a granular bright pink in haematoxylin and eosin stains because their cytoplasm is packed with enlarged mitochondria. As in the oncocytic cells of Warthin's tumour, this may be caused by mutation of genes encoded by mitochondrial DNA controlling mitochondrial synthesis. Oncocytomas do not recur after complete excision.

Oncocytosis is the term given to the process of accumulating excessive mitochondria in cells of salivary glands, probably as a result of the same mitochondrial DNA mutations described above. Acinar and ductal cells may undergo oncocytosis as an age change forming small nodules like microscopic oncocytomas throughout several glands. When the change is extensive, the gland becomes swollen and soft, and individual nodules may enlarge significantly to develop into oncocytomas. Oncocytosis is otherwise asymptomatic and is often a chance finding histologically in the gland excised for an oncocytoma. Similar changes can develop in the kidney, thyroid gland and mucous glands in the mucosa of the upper aerodigestive tract.

MALIGNANT SALIVARY GLAND TUMOURS

→ Summary charts 23.1 and 23.2 pp. 365, 366

Malignant salivary gland neoplasms are rarer than benign neoplasms. More than 25 different types are recognised, and no one type stands out as particularly frequent. The average

age of patients with malignant neoplasms is almost the same as those with benign neoplasms; malignant salivary neoplasms can be found in the very young and the elderly.

Many are low-grade carcinomas, with slow growth and a clinical presentation that can be identical to that of benign neoplasms. Appreciating that these tumours are malignant preoperatively is critical to providing the correct treatment and achieving a good outcome. A key clue to malignancy is recognising how the risk of a salivary neoplasm being malignant varies between sites, as shown in Fig. 23.1. Most types present as an unremarkable firm mass. Conversely, some are aggressive and present with classical signs of malignancy: fixation to adjacent tissues, nerve signs, ulceration, bleeding, bone erosion or metastasis to regional lymph nodes. Trismus may result from infiltration of muscles of mastication when carcinomas arise in the parotid, soft palate and retromolar area.

The risk of metastasis varies widely between different types, but those that do metastasise usually spread to cervical lymph nodes and less frequently via the blood to lungs and other distant sites.

Diagnosis depends on histological examination. High-grade neoplasms are readily recognised on FNA, which can often provide an accurate diagnosis. However, many of the lower grade types are not amenable to diagnosis in this way and are only diagnosed after excision. For this reason, excision of any salivary mass without a diagnosis after FNA and imaging must be undertaken on the assumption that it may turn out to be malignant.

Malignant salivary gland tumours are treated by surgical excision, followed by radiotherapy if excision is incomplete or margins close. Recurrence is often difficult to manage; minor gland re-excision may require resection of facial skin, and parotid gland recurrences may involve the base of skull and infratemporal fossa. The prognosis depends on the size and extent of the carcinoma, its histological type and, for some types, its histological grade. Some types have specific causative genetic changes, and these are being explored as potential targets for new types of treatment. Others may express hormone receptors, making them suitable targets for the types of hormone therapy used for breast or prostate carcinomas.

Web URL 23.1 UK incidence, mortality: Web search for: ncras head and neck cancer hub

Mucoepidermoid carcinoma

Mucoepidermoid carcinoma is the most common single type of malignant salivary neoplasm, yet it accounts for less than 10% of salivary gland neoplasms. About half arise in a parotid gland, but all glands including minor glands can be affected. The carcinomas usually contain mucin-filled cysts and so are easily mistaken clinically for mucous extravasation or retention cysts when they develop in minor glands.

The cause is a t(11;19) translocation that brings the MECT1 gene together with the MAML2 gene, producing a novel fusion gene that activates the notch signalling pathway, an important developmental pathway that is deranged in several types of cancer.

The diagnosis requires histological examination and can be aided by identifying the translocation if required. Most contain numerous cysts lined by epithelium that resembles skin epithelium and is therefore called *epidermoid*. It has basal and prickle cells but does not keratinise. Scattered in the epidermoid sheets and cyst linings are variable numbers of mucus-secreting goblet cells, the two cell types explaining

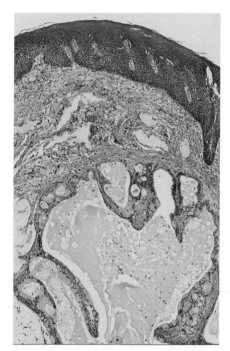

Fig. 23.11 Mucoepidermoid carcinoma. Palatal mucosa overlying a multicystic poorly defined lesion.

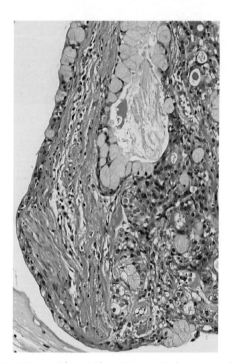

Fig. 23.12 Mucoepidermoid carcinoma. Higher power showing cysts lined by pale mucous cells and lower right a solid area of epidermoid and mucous cells.

the name mucoepidermoid (Figs 23.11 and 23.12). Either mucous or epidermoid cells may predominate.

The tumour usually grows slowly and infiltrates into surrounding tissues and so treatment is by wide excision. Mucoepidermoid carcinomas occasionally metastasise, and the risk is predicted, although not accurately, by histological grading, dividing the carcinomas into high, intermediate and low grade types. Approximately 40% of high-grade carcinomas metastasise and approximately 30% of patients with high-grade carcinomas die of the disease. Conversely, low-grade and intermediate- grade carcinomas metastasise in only a few per cent of patients and are almost never fatal.

Review PMID: 21371076

Genetics PMID: 23459841

Adenoid cystic carcinoma

The adenoid cystic carcinoma is distinctive among salivary carcinomas and must be appreciated for its unusual behaviour and poor outcome.

This carcinoma is almost as frequent as mucoepidermoid carcinoma and can affect any gland. Most arise in major glands, usually the parotid, but it accounts for almost a third of minor gland carcinomas (Fig. 23.13). They also arise in mucous glands in the nose and antrum and throughout the mucosa of the aerodigestive tract.

The cause of most cases is a t(6;9) translocation that fuses the proto-oncogene myb with a transcription factor gene NFIB, producing a novel fusion protein. The carcinomas overexpress myb protein, which can be detected immunohistochemically to aid diagnosis, and the translocation can be identified by fluorescence in situ hybridisation.

Adenoid cystic carcinomas grow slowly and have a peculiar propensity to invade along nerves - 'perineural spread'. In some cases the carcinoma can extend several centimetres along nerves beyond the clinically apparent mass (Fig. 23.14). Carcinomas in palatal glands or parotid are sometimes found to have reached the brain at presentation.

Perineural spread can produce unusual sensory symptoms, pain or facial weakness, and occasional patients present with these symptoms rather than a mass. Suspicion of adenoid cystic carcinoma may arise when nerves are seen to be thickened on magnetic resonance imaging.

The diagnosis can be made accurately by FNA, biopsy or after excision. There is a highly characteristic histological pattern consisting of rounded groups of small darkly staining cells of almost uniform size, surrounding multiple small clear spaces (cribriform or 'swiss cheese' pattern) (Fig. 23.15). Small ducts lie in the sheets of epithelium, and the carcinoma islands are widely infiltrative.

The prognosis in adenoid cystic carcinoma is poor. Although some small or well-circumscribed tumours are effectively excised, larger tumours and those with perineural spread and diffuse infiltration through bone and soft tissues are difficult or impossible to excise despite extensive surgery. Post-operative radiotherapy is usually given but cannot be relied on to kill this radio-resistant tumour. The slow growth means that a third of patients survive 5 years, but the outcome is ultimately fatal in most cases, although patients may live 15 years after diagnosis. Lymph node metastasis is unusual, but about a third of patients eventually develop blood-borne metastases in lung, liver or bone.

Review PMID: 25943783

Molecular genetics review PMID: 23821214

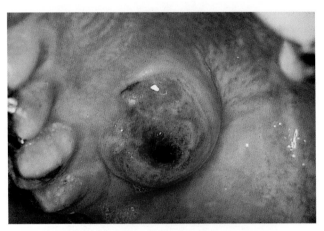

Fig. 23.13 Adenoid cystic carcinoma. There is an ulcerated mass arising from a minor gland in the palate. The clinical appearance would be the same as other malignant salivary neoplasms.

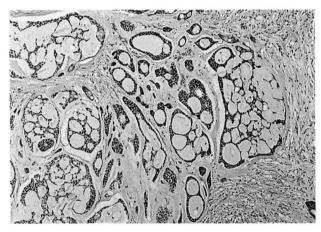

Fig. 23.15 Adenoid cystic carcinoma. The small darkly staining cells of the adenoid cystic carcinoma form cribriform islands with large holes which have been likened, rather inappropriately, to Swiss cheese.

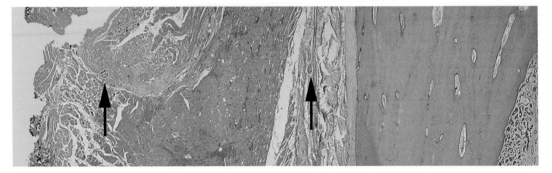

Fig. 23.14 Adenoid cystic carcinoma. In this panoramic photomicrograph taken from a resection, an adenoid cystic carcinoma in the floor of the mouth has infiltrated into the medullary cavity of the mandible and can be seen in the lower right corner. The extremely infiltrative nature of this carcinoma is demonstrated by the two small islands of dispersed carcinoma that have penetrated the intact cortical bone and now infiltrate the buccal muscle over 10 mm from the main tumour.

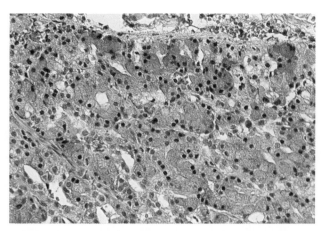

Fig. 23.16 **Acinic cell carcinoma.** The tumour is composed of granular acinar-type cells, sometimes arranged in acinus-like clusters and sometimes forming irregular sheets. Cytological atypia is uncommon.

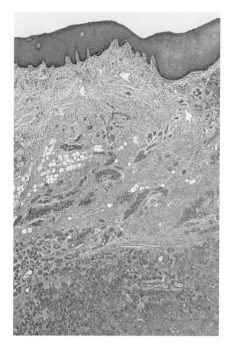

Fig. 23.17 **Polymorphous adenocarcinoma.** Low power showing a poorly circumscribed tumour with small islands invading upward into the overlying mucosa.

Acinic cell carcinoma

Acinic cell carcinomas are less common in Europe than in the United States. They arise almost always in the parotid gland and have an unpredictable behaviour despite their slow growth.

Histologically, they show an almost uniform pattern of large cells similar to serous cells, with granular basophilic cytoplasm. These are often arranged in acini (Fig. 23.16), though a variety of different histological patterns are recognised.

Despite apparently benign histological appearances, even sometimes including encapsulation, acinic cell carcinomas can be invasive and occasionally metastasise. Most are low grade.

Secretory carcinoma

This recently described low-grade carcinoma arises in all glands but usually in the parotid. It is caused by a translocation between the *ETV6* and *NTRK3* genes. The carcinoma is solid and cystic, with papillary areas, and contains many ducts and spaces filled with secretory material. Approximately 1 in 5 cases metastasise, but this is a relatively indolent carcinoma that responds to excision. A similar carcinoma in the breast is caused by the same translocation, so that this was previously called *mammary analogue secretory carcinoma*.

Polymorphous adenocarcinoma

Polymorphous adenocarcinoma arises almost exclusively in minor glands, particularly of the palate. It is the commonest or second commonest carcinoma in minor glands and, though most cases arise in those older than 50 years, it can develop over a broad age range.

The name derives from the presence of its many histological patterns, with sheets of cells, ducts, narrow strands and cysts, the last sometimes containing papillary projections (Figs 23.17 and 23.18). The cells themselves are small and bland with very infrequent mitoses, and only infiltration of surrounding tissues may indicate that these are malignant neoplasms. Polymorphous adenocarcinomas are mostly low grade, but they do metastasise in about 10% of cases, although the outcome is almost never fatal. Treatment is by complete local excision.

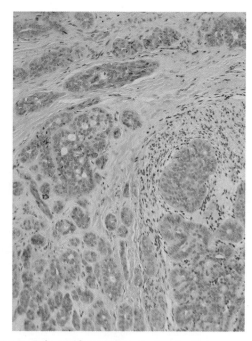

Fig. 23.18 **Polymorphous adenocarcinoma.** High power showing the cytologically bland cells organised as sheets, ducts and strands.

The many patterns can cause histological misdiagnosis, particularly confusing it with adenoid cystic carcinoma because both may contain cribriform islands and show perineural spread. Despite the histological similarity, the behaviour of the two carcinomas is very different. Perineural spread in polymorphous adenocarcinoma is very limited in extent, unlike in adenoid cystic carcinoma. To prevent histological misdiagnosis, it is important to obtain a good-sized incisional biopsy that includes part of the periphery for all minor gland neoplasms. Punch and needle core biopsies are often used on palatal tumours but are often inadequate to make a confident diagnosis.

Review PMID: 20403856

Salivary duct carcinoma

This aggressive high-grade carcinoma is so called because it resembles ductal carcinoma of the breast microscopically. It develops mainly in those older than 50 years of age, is significantly commoner in males and carries a poor prognosis. Lesions arise mainly in the parotid gland but can develop in other major and, occasionally, minor glands. This carcinoma usually presents as an obviously malignant tumour with rapid growth.

Perineural spread and lymphatic invasion are common, the latter accounting for the fact that many patients have lymph node metastases on presentation. The cells of the carcinoma are large and have very pink oncocytic cytoplasm and form ducts and cysts with the cribriform pattern known as 'Roman bridging'. Androgen receptor is strongly expressed by the carcinoma raising the possibility of targeted therapy, though this is not yet known to be effective. Currently more than half of patients die in less than 5 years from diagnosis as a result of metastasis to lungs, liver and bone. Perineural and dispersed infiltration also makes local recurrence frequent. Many carcinomas ex pleomorphic adenoma (discussed below) have this histological pattern.

Review PMID: 26939990

Epithelial-myoepithelial carcinoma

Epithelial-myoepithelial carcinoma is a low-grade carcinoma affecting mostly the major glands and the elderly. It has a striking microscopic pattern of ducts or small islands of epithelium, each with an outer layer of clear myoepithelial cells and a small duct centrally. This type often presents as a benign tumour clinically and, although most are effectively treated by local excision, local recurrence is frequent and approximately 10% develop distant metastasis.

Undifferentiated carcinomas

These have no definite histological features and resemble undifferentiated carcinomas arising in the nasopharynx and tonsil. Rapid spread and metastasis is typical. As with nasopharyngeal carcinoma, many cases are caused by Epstein–Barr virus infection.

Carcinoma ex pleomorphic adenoma

Pleomorphic adenoma is one of the few benign tumours that can undergo malignant change. It is estimated that as many as 5% of pleomorphic adenomas show some progression to carcinoma, but the process seems to take many years, so the diagnosis is usually made in the elderly. However, because pleomorphic adenomas may arise at any age, occasional carcinomas can present in young adults and the middle aged. As noted above, pleomorphic adenomas harbour a surprising range of genetic abnormalities for benign neoplasms. It seems that these lead to chromosomal instability, and the cells progressively become genetically more and more damaged until carcinoma develops.

The history is usually of a slow-growing mass that enlarges suddenly and rapidly and may develop the classical signs of malignancy, usually facial nerve palsy because most arise in the parotid gland. However, the initial adenoma may be small or deeply situated and unsuspected until carcinoma develops.

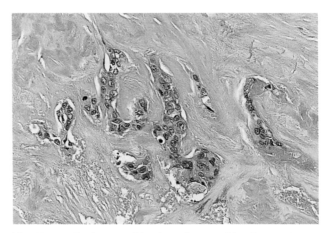

Fig. 23.19 Carcinoma arising in a pleomorphic adenoma. In longstanding pleomorphic adenomas, the stroma may become hyalinised, dense and acellular. In such tumours, there is a risk of transformation to carcinoma, as shown here by clusters of cells showing cytological atypia.

Histologically, the original pleomorphic adenoma may be detectable as a circumscribed benign tumour, but more often it is destroyed by the carcinoma and only a nodule of hyaline stroma or cartilage may remain. The carcinoma cells have obviously malignant features, infiltration is usually extensive and there is often necrosis (Fig. 23.19). The carcinoma that develops may be of a recognisable type, such as a salivary duct, mucoepidermoid, epithelial-myoepithelial type or be an unclassifiable carcinoma.

Carcinoma ex pleomorphic adenoma is an aggressive carcinoma, and over half of cases suffer distant metastases to lung, bone or brain. The further the carcinoma has invaded beyond the capsule of the original pleomorphic adenoma (not always easy to define histologically), the worse the prognosis. There is disagreement about exactly how far is critical, but those that invade more than a few millimetres require aggressive surgery and radiotherapy.

A minority of cases are termed *non-invasive carcinoma ex pleomorphic adenoma* (in a confusing oxymoron) meaning that the carcinomatous changes are detected histologically but remain confined within the capsule of the old pleomorphic adenoma. This is analogous to the concept of an in situ carcinoma or a pleomorphic adenoma with dysplasia. Such cases can be removed in the same way as a benign pleomorphic adenoma and carry no risk of recurrence or metastasis. Accurate histological assessment of any carcinoma ex pleomorphic adenoma is therefore essential to plan whether post-operative radiotherapy may be required.

Review PMID: 21744105

Adenocarcinoma not otherwise specified

Sometimes a salivary carcinoma cannot be classified into a specific type histologically. Under these circumstances it is classified as adenocarcinoma NOS (not otherwise specified) and graded as low, intermediate or high grade to plan treatment.

OTHER EPITHELIAL LESIONS

Sclerosing polycystic adenosis is a condition of uncertain nature, possibly a benign neoplasm, resembling sclerosing adenosis in the breast. It affects those of middle age and usually develops as a slow growing firm mass in the parotid gland. There is a fibrotic mass containing proliferating ducts that can recur if incompletely excised.

Intercalated duct hyperplasia or adenomatoid ductal hyperplasia is a nodular proliferation of ductal cells, usually in the parotid and probably of no significance.

METASTATIC NEOPLASMS

Metastatic neoplasms account for approximately 1 in 20 lumps in salivary glands and almost all occur in the elderly, matching the age distribution of the common malignant neoplasms at other body sites. Almost all metastases develop in the parotid gland by lymphatic spread to the intraparotid lymph nodes, and only involve the gland itself if they invade beyond the lymph node capsule. The primary carcinoma is usually in the sites drained by these nodes so that squamous carcinomas or melanoma of the scalp are likely primary tumours.

Very occasionally the parotid or submandibular gland is the site of a blood-borne metastasis from a more distant primary. The commonest example is renal cell carcinoma, which has a particular tendency to spread through central veins to the head and neck. Usually these tumours are readily recognised as metastases microscopically, though renal cell carcinoma can resemble some types of salivary carcinoma histologically. Diagnosis is usually suspected on the basis of the known cancer elsewhere.

Metastases to salivary glands are indistinguishable from primary salivary neoplasms in their clinical presentation.

NON-EPITHELIAL TUMOURS

Haemangioma of the parotids

Haemangiomas are easily recognised hamartomas that may present at birth or in childhood. Almost all salivary examples arise in the parotid gland, and they are relatively common causes of a salivary gland enlargement in children but rare in adults. Girls are more frequently affected.

Haemangiomas are soft, sometimes bluish, swellings. The salivary gland may be involved by localised lesions or as part of a more extensive vascular malformation of the head and neck.

Histologically, the parotid parenchyma is largely replaced by sheets of endothelial cells and small blood vessels of capillary type with a few clusters of residual acini and ducts scattered through (Fig. 23.20). Sometimes there are larger vessels, a higher blood throughput making the lesion feel warm or even an arteriovenous fistula producing a bruit.

Despite their dramatic appearance, especially if the skin is involved, these tumours are hamartomas not neoplasms. They grow initially but gradually regress in the first 5 years of life and may almost vanish by 10 years of age. Corticosteroids may delay their growth and facilitate later surgery but propanolol is currently the preferred treatment and is highly effective. Unless the eye or other important structures are threatened, most are treated conservatively depending on site and appearance.

Review PMID: 19910858

Lymphoma

The most common non-epithelial tumours of salivary glands are lymphomas. They can arise in the lymph nodes that lie within the gland and are identical to lymphomas arising in the cervical or other lymph nodes. The type is usually a high-grade non-Hodgkin lymphoma of B-cell origin or Hodgkin's disease. Salivary gland involvement is sometimes the first sign of these systemic diseases.

Conversely, the MALT (mucosa-associated lymphoid tissue) lymphomas arise in the gland parenchyma rather than the nodes. These are described in more detail in

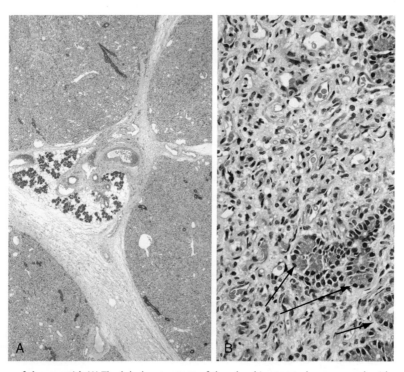

Fig. 23.20   Haemangioma of the parotid. (A) The lobular structure of the gland is seen to be preserved, with a small lobule of normal parotid centrally. (B) The tissue that replaces the lobules, closely packed small capillary vessels with a few scattered residual serous acini (*arrowed*).

Chapter 27. The majority arise as a complication of Sjögren's syndrome, and development of lymphoma is indicated by a persistent painless swelling of the gland, particularly in patients with longstanding disease. MALT lymphomas are usually low grade and indolent with an excellent prognosis, but more aggressive high-grade variants can also arise in salivary glands.

INTRAOSSEOUS SALIVARY GLAND TUMOURS

Salivary gland tumours can develop within the medullary cavity of the mandible or maxilla, so-called *central* or *intraosseous salivary tumours*. This is extremely rare and also difficult to explain. It is suggested that there are developmental rests of salivary tissue within the bone, although origin in odontogenic epithelium would appear a more likely explanation. Odontogenic epithelium lining dentigerous and other cysts often undergoes mucous metaplasia to form goblet cells, and so it is surmised that odontogenic epithelium might be able to undergo salivary differentiation if it

became neoplastic. This is supported by the fact that most of these tumours are mucoepidermoid carcinomas, a type that includes many mucous cells.

Radiographically, intraosseous salivary tumours produce cyst-like or poorly circumscribed areas of radiolucency. The diagnosis can only be made histologically, and a metastasis from a carcinoma elsewhere must be excluded before the rarer central tumour diagnosis is accepted. Wide excision is required.

Intraosseous salivary neoplasms do not arise in Stafne bone cavity (salivary inclusion 'cyst') at the angle of the mandible because this is merely submandibular gland in a depression or indentation of the cortex; the salivary tissue does not extend into the medullary cavity.

TUMOUR-LIKE SALIVARY GLAND SWELLINGS

Necrotising sialometaplasia and **IgG4 sclerosing disease can** mimic salivary gland tumours, both clinically and histologically. They are described in Chapter 22.

Summary chart 23.1 Management decisions and treatment for a lump in the parotid gland.

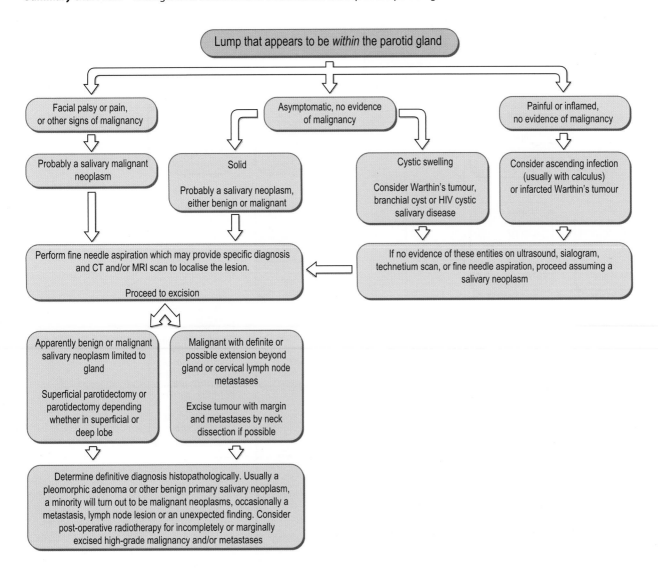

Summary chart 23.2   Considerations in differentiating salivary neoplasms. A mind map.

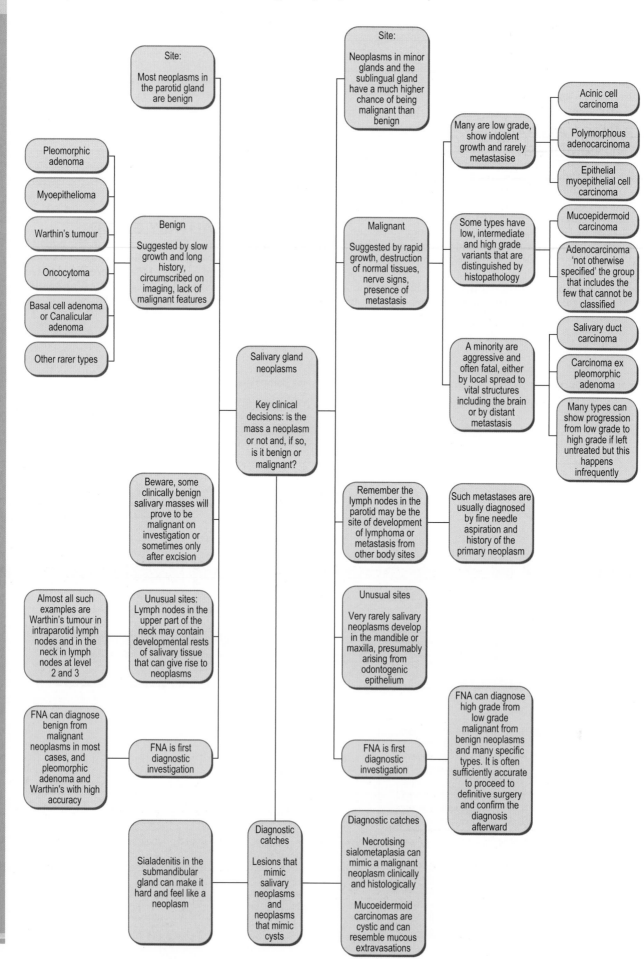

Site:

Most neoplasms in the parotid gland are benign

Site:

Neoplasms in minor glands and the sublingual gland have a much higher chance of being malignant than benign

Pleomorphic adenoma

Myoepithelioma

Warthin's tumour

Oncocytoma

Basal cell adenoma or Canalicular adenoma

Other rarer types

Benign

Suggested by slow growth and long history, circumscribed on imaging, lack of malignant features

Many are low grade, show indolent growth and rarely metastasise

Acinic cell carcinoma

Polymorphous adenocarcinoma

Epithelial myoepithelial cell carcinoma

Malignant

Suggested by rapid growth, destruction of normal tissues, nerve signs, presence of metastasis

Some types have low, intermediate and high grade variants that are distinguished by histopathology

Mucoepidermoid carcinoma

Adenocarcinoma 'not otherwise specified' the group that includes the few that cannot be classified

Salivary gland neoplasms

Key clinical decisions: is the mass a neoplasm or not and, if so, is it benign or malignant?

A minority are aggressive and often fatal, either by local spread to vital structures including the brain or by distant metastasis

Salivary duct carcinoma

Carcinoma ex pleomorphic adenoma

Many types can show progression from low grade to high grade if left untreated but this happens infrequently

Beware, some clinically benign salivary masses will prove to be malignant on investigation or sometimes only after excision

Remember the lymph nodes in the parotid may be the site of development of lymphoma or metastasis from other body sites

Such metastases are usually diagnosed by fine needle aspiration and history of the primary neoplasm

Almost all such examples are Warthin's tumour in intraparotid lymph nodes and in the neck in lymph nodes at level 2 and 3

Unusual sites: Lymph nodes in the upper part of the neck may contain developmental rests of salivary tissue that can give rise to neoplasms

Unusual sites

Very rarely salivary neoplasms develop in the mandible or maxilla, presumably arising from odontogenic epithelium

FNA can diagnose benign from malignant neoplasms in most cases, and pleomorphic adenoma and Warthin's with high accuracy

FNA is first diagnostic investigation

FNA is first diagnostic investigation

FNA can diagnose high grade from low grade malignant from benign neoplasms and many specific types. It is often sufficiently accurate to proceed to definitive surgery and confirm the diagnosis afterward

Sialadenitis in the submandibular gland can make it hard and feel like a neoplasm

Diagnostic catches

Lesions that mimic salivary neoplasms and neoplasms that mimic cysts

Diagnostic catches

Necrotising sialometaplasia can mimic a malignant neoplasm clinically and histologically

Mucoeidermoid carcinomas are cystic and can resemble mucous extravasations

Appendix 23.1

Salivary gland neoplasms

Malignant epithelial tumours

Acinic cell carcinoma	See text of Chapter 23
Secretory carcinoma	See text of Chapter 23
Mucoepidermoid carcinoma	See text of Chapter 23
Adenoid cystic carcinoma	See text of Chapter 23
Polymorphous adenocarcinoma	See text of Chapter 23
Epithelial-myoepithelial carcinoma	See text of Chapter 23
Clear cell carcinoma NOS*	Composed of clear cells and with no features of other tumours. Usually intraoral minor glands, especially the palate. Low-grade malignancy, prognosis good. Has a consistent translocation involving the EWSR1 and ATF-1 genes
Basal cell adenocarcinoma	Appear like basal cell adenomas but infiltrative. Recur locally but rarely metastasise
Sebaceous carcinoma	Very rare, usually in parotid and the elderly. High grade
Cystadenocarcinoma	Low-grade malignancy of parotid gland and intraoral glands. Contains many cysts, a few have recurred locally or metastasised
Intraductal carcinoma	Also known as low-grade salivary duct or cribriform cystadenocarcinoma, a mostly cystic carcinoma that is almost always in the parotid gland and responds well to excision
Adenocarcinoma NOS	See text of Chapter 23
Salivary duct carcinoma	See text of Chapter 23
Myoepithelial carcinoma	The malignant variant of myoepithelioma, high grade with recurrence and frequent metastases
Carcinoma ex pleomorphic adenoma	See text of Chapter 23
Carcinosarcoma	A highly malignant neoplasm containing both carcinoma, of any pattern, with a sarcoma, usually chondrosarcoma or osteosarcoma. Survival is very poor
Poorly differentiated neuroendocrine carcinoma	Very rare neuroendocrine carcinomas. Metastasis to a parotid node could be mistaken for a salivary primary. Poor prognosis.
Lymphoepithelial carcinoma	Common in Japan, Southeast China and in Inuit races, but otherwise very rare. Caused by Epstein–Barr virus infection. Usually parotid or submandibular glands, wide age range. Responds well to radiotherapy
Squamous cell carcinoma	Rare, resemble mucosal squamous carcinomas. Parotid and submandibular glands, wide age range
Oncocytic carcinoma	Very rare high-grade carcinoma, usually in parotid, fewer in submandibular gland metastasis, arise in all glands but particularly the parotid

Borderline tumours

Sialoblastoma	Very rare, often congenital or in first 2 years of life. Respond well to excision but can recur, mostly in parotid

Benign epithelial tumours

Pleomorphic adenoma	See text of Chapter 23
Metastasising pleomorphic adenoma	Very rare. An apparently benign pleomorphic adenoma that metastasises, to bone, lung or lymph node. Arise in the parotid, submandibular and palatal glands and seem to spread into vessels by surgical manipulation or to the lungs by aspiration of disrupted tumour rather than true metastasis. PMID: 25958295
Myoepithelioma	Similar to pleomorphic adenoma but without the varied histological appearances, formed of sheets of epithelial cells of various shapes.
Basal cell adenoma	See text of Chapter 23
Warthin's tumour	See text of Chapter 23
Oncocytoma	See text of Chapter 23
Lymphadenoma, sebaceous and non-sebaceous	Very rare lesions of the parotid and the elderly
Cystadenoma	Rare lesion of numerous duct-like cysts, arise in any gland and in middle aged and the elderly
Sialadenoma papilliferum	Papillary neoplasm of the excretory duct, usually on the palate in the elderly. Rarely recurs
Ductal papillomas, inverted, intraductal	Develop in or at the opening of minor gland ducts, wide age range, usually near the distal end of minor gland ducts and are readily excised.
Sebaceous adenoma	Circumscribed tumour of nests of sebaceous cells, do not recur on excision
Canalicular and other ductal adenomas	Minor gland tumour, often in upper lip, develop multicentrically, excision is curative

Other epithelial lesions

Sclerosing polycystic adenosis	See text of Chapter 23
Nodular oncocytic hyperplasia	See text of Chapter 23, oncocytoma
Lymphoepithelial lesions	See text of Chapter 22
Intercalated duct hyperplasia	See text of Chapter 23

Soft tissue lesions

Haemangioma	See text of Chapter 23
Lipoma / sialolipoma	Lipomas of salivary glands usually develop in the parotid glands
Nodular fasciitis	Rapidly growing lesion, probably reactive or borderline neoplasm of fibroblasts

Lymphoma

Extranodal marginal B-cell lymphoma	See text of Chapter 27 ('MALT lymphoma')

Secondary tumours

*NOS indicates 'not otherwise specified'.

Benign mucosal swellings

24

FIBROEPITHELIAL POLYP, EPULIS AND DENTURE-INDUCED GRANULOMA

→ Summary chart 24.2 p. 273

These hyperplastic swellings are the commonest oral swellings and develop in sites of chronic minor injury or low-grade infection. Although sometimes called *fibromas*, they are not benign neoplasms. The term *epulis* means only 'on the gingiva'.

Most epulides are fibrous epulides. Irritation of the gingival margin by the edge of a carious cavity, calculus or a plaque trap may lead to the formation of a fibrous epulis; irritation of alveolar or palatal mucosa by an overextended or rough area on a denture may provoke development of a denture granuloma. Although different names are given to these lesions, they are similar in origin and nature.

Key points are shown in (Box 24.1).

Clinical features

A fibrous epulis is most common near the front of the mouth on the gingiva between two teeth (Fig. 24.1).

Box 24.1   Fibrous nodules: practical points

- The most common oral tumour-like swellings
- Most frequently form at gingival margins (fibrous epulis) or on the buccal mucosa
- They are hyperplastic responses to chronic irritation
- Should be excised complete
- Histological examination confirms diagnosis and excludes unsuspected causes

---

Fibroepithelial polyps (fibrous polyps) usually form on the buccal mucosa along the occlusal line or on the lip at sites of biting (Fig. 24.2). Denture-induced hyperplasias ('denture-induced granulomas') often form in mucosa at the edge of dentures (Fig. 24.3). These swellings are pale and firm but may be abraded and ulcerated, and then inflamed.

'*Leaf fibroma*' is fibrous overgrowth which forms under a denture but has become flattened against the palate (Fig. 24.4). It may be difficult to see until lifted away from its bed.

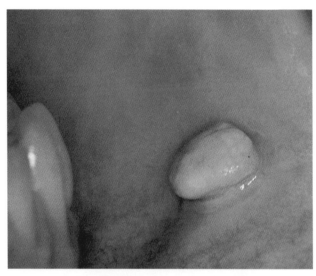

Fig. 24.2   Fibrous polyp. This lesion on the buccal mucosa has arisen as a result of cheek biting and is a firm, painless polyp covered by mucosa of normal appearance.

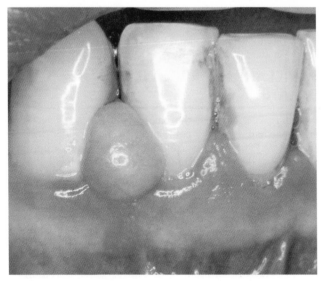

Fig. 24.1   Fibrous epulis. This lesion, arising from the gingival margin between the lower central incisors, is firm, pink and not ulcerated.

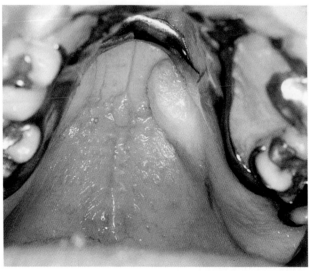

Fig. 24.3   Denture-induced granuloma. Fibrous hyperplasia at the posterior border of this upper partial denture has resulted in a firm mucosal swelling moulded to fit the denture.

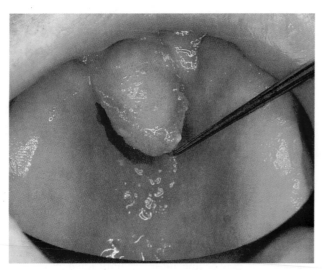

Fig. 24.4 'Leaf fibroma'. Flat lesions formed between the denture and mucosa are often termed *leaf fibromas* because of their shape. Raising this example with a probe reveals its pedunculated shape.

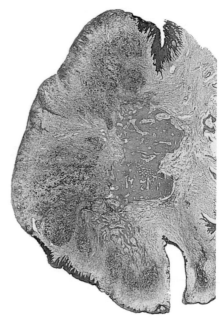

Fig. 24.6 **Fibrous epulis with ossification.** Much of the surface of this pedunculated nodule is ulcerated, and hyperplastic epithelium covers the margins. Centrally, the lesion is very cellular, partly as a result of inflammatory infiltrate, and trabeculae of woven bone are being formed and maturing into lamellar bone.

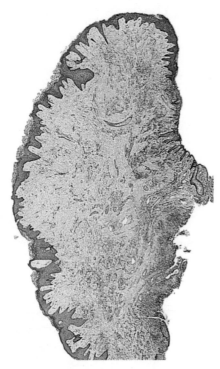

Fig. 24.5 **Fibrous polyp.** The lesion is composed of mature fibrous tissue covered by hyperplastic epithelium with spiky rete processes. A few inflammatory cells are present near the base.

Pathology

In their early stages, these nodules consist of hyperplastic, lightly inflamed, slightly myxoid fibrous tissue, but they mature to a dense collagenous mass. The surface is covered by epithelium, which is usually also hyperplastic (Fig. 24.5).

Bone formation is sometimes seen in a fibrous epulis (Fig. 24.6). In American usage, this combination is termed a *peripheral ossifying fibroma*, but this lesion has no relation to the ossifying fibroma of bone and is not a fibroma. Some consider that those containing bone are more likely to recur after excision, but there is little evidence for this. Mineralising fibrous epulis is a better name.

Fibrous nodules should be excised together with the small base of normal tissue from which they arise. In the case of a fibrous epulis, the underlying bone should be curetted. There should be no recurrence if this is done thoroughly and the source of irritation is removed.

Histological examination is needed to confirm that an epulis is fibrous and not a giant cell epulis, pyogenic granuloma or an unsuspected diagnosis. Several types of lesion occasionally form on the gingival margin and simulate a fibrous epulis.

The giant cell fibroma is a variant distinguished microscopically by scattered large, stellate, darkly staining multinucleate fibroblasts. Clinically, giant cell fibromas are typically pedunculated and usually arise from the gingivae or tip of tongue.

Review gingival lesions PMID: 6936553 and 2120653

All fibroepithelial hyperplasias PMID: 26355878

PAPILLARY HYPERPLASIA OF THE PALATE

Nodular overgrowth of the palatal mucosa is occasionally seen, particularly under complete dentures in older persons (Fig. 24.7). The exact cause is unclear, but a poor denture fit and poor denture hygiene are usual. Although candidosis is sometimes superimposed, it is not the cause. Mild palatal papillary hyperplasia is also occasionally seen in non-denture wearers.

Histologically, palatal papillary hyperplasia shows close-set nodules of vascular fibrous tissue with a variable chronic inflammatory infiltrate and a covering of hyperplastic epithelium (Figs 24.8 and 24.9).

Conservative treatment of denture hygiene, cessation of night wear, and treatment of any superimposed candidal infection is usually sufficient. In the most florid cases, with deep clefts between nodules or when new dentures are to be

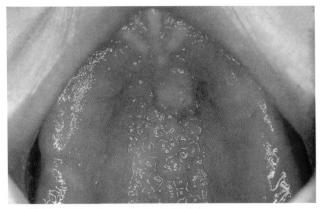

Fig. 24.7   Papillary hyperplasia of the palate. A small leaf fibroma is also present in the anterior palate.

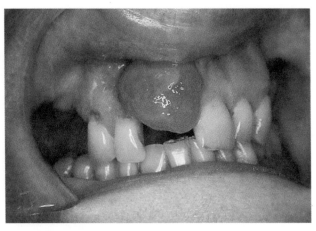

Fig. 24.10   Pyogenic granuloma. A bright-red polypoid swelling. The gingiva is a common site.

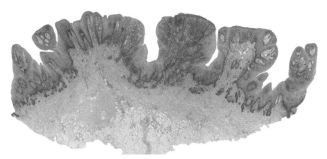

Fig. 24.8   Papillary hyperplasia. There are nodules, each similar to a fibrous polyp, and the subepithelial inflammatory infiltrate indicates probable candidal infection.

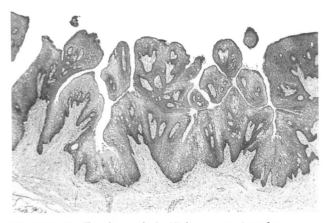

Fig. 24.9   Papillary hyperplasia. Higher-power view after antifungal treatment. The mucosa is now uninflamed, but the papillary structure remains.

constructed, surgical removal may be considered. After surgery, a temporary soft lining must be placed to prevent the healing tissue proliferating back into the space below the denture.

Case series PMID: 4917113

PYOGENIC GRANULOMA AND PREGNANCY EPULIS

→ Summary chart 24.2 p. 373

These are hyperplastic lesions of granulation tissue, proliferating masses of endothelial cells and fibroblasts.

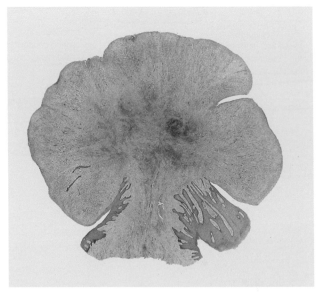

Fig. 24.11   Pyogenic granuloma. Lobular nodule of granulation tissue. Differences from a fibrous polyp (Fig. 24.5) include the ulcerated surface.

Clinically, they are usually painless, pedunculated, red and relatively soft (Fig. 24.10) and usually on the gingiva. Microscopically, they consist of many dilated blood vessels in a loose oedematous connective tissue stroma (Fig. 24.11) that matures with time to become more fibrous and less vascular. No true granulomas are present. Inflammation is variable, often scanty or absent. A pregnancy epulis can only be distinguished by patient's pregnancy and, usually, associated pregnancy gingivitis (see also Fig. 36.8). Treatment is as for fibrous epulis. Excision of pregnancy epulis may be delayed as they tend to regrow if removed during pregnancy. Improved oral hygiene may halt or slow growth until parturition.

Pyogenic granuloma pregnancy PMID: 1923399

GIANT-CELL EPULIS

→ Summary chart 24.2 p. 273

The giant-cell epulis, like the fibrous epulis, is a hyperplastic lesion. It arises only on the gingival margin, usually interdentally and anterior to the permanent molars. There

Summary chart 24.1 Differential diagnosis and management of the common localised gingival swellings.

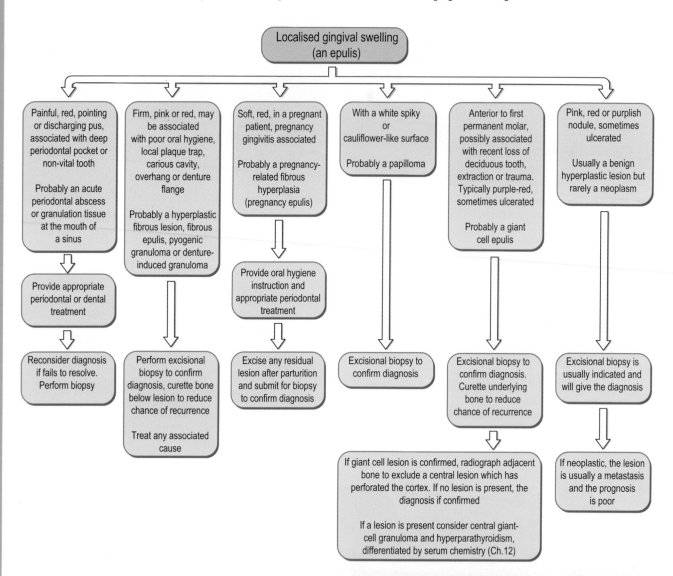

Localised gingival swelling (an epulis)

Painful, red, pointing or discharging pus, associated with deep periodontal pocket or non-vital tooth

Probably an acute periodontal abscess or granulation tissue at the mouth of a sinus

↓

Provide appropriate periodontal or dental treatment

↓

Reconsider diagnosis if fails to resolve. Perform biopsy

Firm, pink or red, may be associated with poor oral hygiene, local plaque trap, carious cavity, overhang or denture flange

Probably a hyperplastic fibrous lesion, fibrous epulis, pyogenic granuloma or denture-induced granuloma

↓

Perform excisional biopsy to confirm diagnosis, curette bone below lesion to reduce chance of recurrence

Treat any associated cause

Soft, red, in a pregnant patient, pregnancy gingivitis associated

Probably a pregnancy-related fibrous hyperplasia (pregnancy epulis)

↓

Provide oral hygiene instruction and appropriate periodontal treatment

↓

Excise any residual lesion after parturition and submit for biopsy to confirm diagnosis

---

With a white spiky or cauliflower-like surface

Probably a papilloma

↓

Excisional biopsy to confirm diagnosis

Anterior to first permanent molar, possibly associated with recent loss of deciduous tooth, extraction or trauma. Typically purple-red, sometimes ulcerated

Probably a giant cell epulis

↓

Excisional biopsy to confirm diagnosis. Curette underlying bone to reduce chance of recurrence

↓

If giant cell lesion is confirmed, radiograph adjacent bone to exclude a central lesion which has perforated the cortex. If no lesion is present, the diagnosis if confirmed

If a lesion is present consider central giant-cell granuloma and hyperparathyroidism, differentiated by serum chemistry (Ch.12)

Pink, red or purplish nodule, sometimes ulcerated

Usually a benign hyperplastic lesion but rarely a neoplasm

↓

Excisional biopsy is usually indicated and will give the diagnosis

↓

If neoplastic, the lesion is usually a metastasis and the prognosis is poor

---

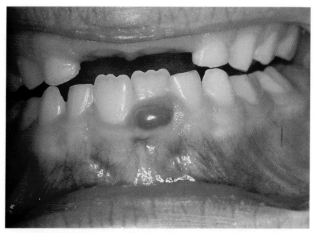

Fig. 24.12 Giant-cell epulis. Small lesion with a maroon colour in a child. *(Courtesy of Mrs H Pitt-Ford.)*

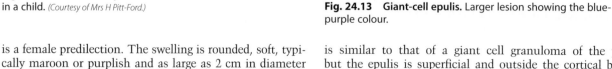

Fig. 24.13 Giant-cell epulis. Larger lesion showing the blue-purple colour.

is a female predilection. The swelling is rounded, soft, typically maroon or purplish and as large as 2 cm in diameter (Figs 24.12 and 24.13).

Histologically, numerous multinucleate cells lie in a vascular stroma of plump spindle-shaped cells. The appearance

is similar to that of a giant cell granuloma of the jaw, but the epulis is superficial and outside the cortical bone (Fig. 24.14).

A giant-cell epulis should be excised, together with its gingival base, and the underlying bone curetted. Adjacent

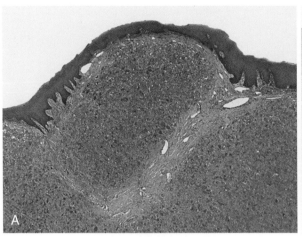
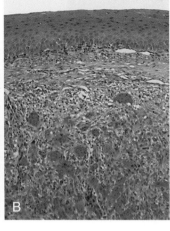

Fig. 24.14 Giant-cell epulis.
(A) The lobular structure can be seen. (B) A high-power view shows giant cells in vascular fibrous lying immediately below the covering epithelium.

Summary chart 24.2   Differential diagnosis of common and important causes of gingival enlargement.

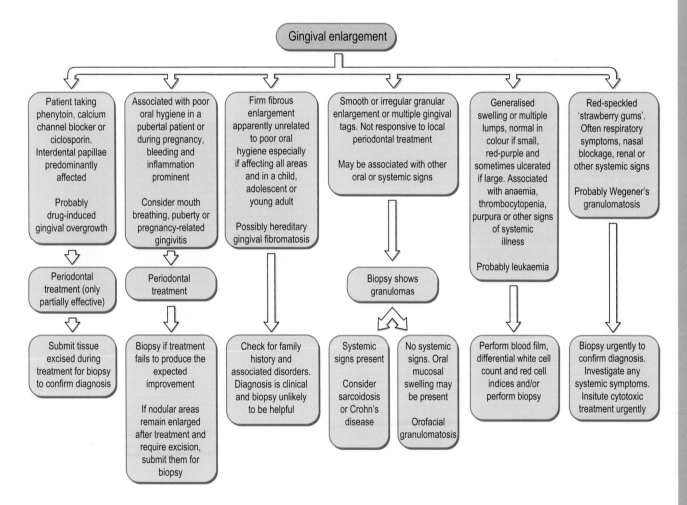

teeth need not be extracted if they are healthy and, if treatment is thorough, there should be no recurrence. A radiograph should be taken to exclude the possibility that the lesion is the superficial part of a central giant cell granuloma (see Ch. 12) that has perforated through the gingiva. Very rarely, similar lesions are a sign of hyperparathyroidism (see Ch. 13).

Case series review PMID: 3133432

PAPILLOMAS → Summary chart 24.1 p. 372

These benign lesions have spiky exophytic or rounded cauliflower-like shapes as large as a centimetre or so in diameter. Probably all are caused by human papillomavirus (HPV) even though it cannot be detected in some lesions.

Human papillomaviruses are ubiquitous, and almost all individuals harbour some of the more than 150 types as commensals. HPV types tend to infect particular

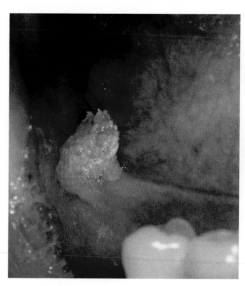

Fig. 24.15 Squamous papilloma arising on the alveolar ridge. Note the spiky white surface.

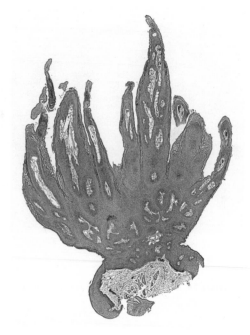

Fig. 24.16 Papilloma. The lesion consists of thickened fingers of epithelium. Slender vascular cores of connective tissue support each frond. The fronds are keratinised and so appear white clinically.

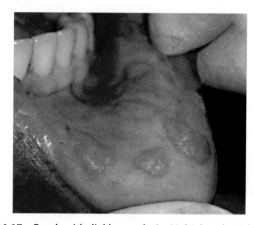

Fig. 24.17 Focal epithelial hyperplasia. Multiple pale pink slightly raised rounded nodules on the labial mucosa. *(Courtesy of Dr Braz Campos Durso.)*

anatomical sites. However, this is not absolute, and oral lesions containing genital types 6 and 11, and less commonly 16 and 18, are found. Papillomas with a rounded non-keratinised shape (condylomas) are not necessarily infections transmitted from genital warts, though they often are. These types of HPV can be transmitted at birth, in utero and vertically and horizontally in families without direct sexual contact.

Oral papillomas are not premalignant. Dysplastic lesions containing low-risk or high-risk HPV are increasingly recognised, but they present as white patches and are not papillomatous.

All oral papillomas are painless and of extremely low infectivity. All types respond to simple excision, including a small amount of normal mucosa at the base.

Oral papillomas of all types are occasionally multiple but, if numerous or confluent, HIV infection or other cause of immunodeficiency should be suspected. Extensive lesions in the immunosuppressed are difficult or impossible to eradicate.

Review PMID: 6154913

Squamous cell papilloma

Squamous papillomas mainly affect adults and have a distinctive, clinically recognisable, cauliflower-like or branched structure of finger-like processes (Fig. 24.15).

Histologically, the papillae consist of stratified squamous epithelium supported by a vascular connective tissue core (Fig. 24.16). Most are keratinised and so appear white.

Human papillomavirus (HPV) of various subtypes are associated, but koilocytes (infected keratinocytes producing virus and with crumpled nuclei, perinuclear space and condensed cytoplasm) are seen in only a minority. Probably either HPV is present at very low level or has disappeared from the lesion in its later stages. When present, it is usually of types 6 and 11.

Infective warts (verruca vulgaris)

Lesions caused by autoinoculation from warts on the hands are uncommon but seen particularly in children. The lesions may appear identical to squamous papillomas, be more rounded or even only slightly raised.

Histologically, the structure is generally similar to that of papillomas, but there are typically obvious koilocytes indicating active viral infection, which can be confirmed with immunohistochemistry. The causative HPV type is usually type 2 or 4.

Multifocal epithelial hyperplasia

Multifocal epithelial hyperplasia or Heck's disease causes numerous rounded mucosal papillomas as large as a centimetre across, usually clustered on the labial, buccal mucosa and tongue mucosa (Fig. 24.17). These may be confluent, producing raised plaques or a cobblestone appearance.

Children, adolescents and young adults are affected, often in familial clusters. The condition is an infection by human papillomavirus types 13 or 32, which spreads easily between family members under close living conditions. The condition is endemic in some parts of the world.

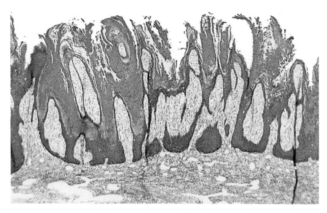

Fig. 24.18 Verruciform xanthoma. The epithelium is thin and parakeratotic and forms a series of spiky folds.

Unlike most other papillomas, the surface is smooth or slightly nodular without keratin so that the lesions appear pink rather than white. Histologically, the papillomas have a characteristic feature that the infected cells resemble mitotic figures (mitosoid bodies). No treatment is required and there is usually resolution, although only after many years. If appearance dictates, individual lesions are readily excised or removed by laser.

Description and series PMID: 8065729

Review PMID: 23061874

VERRUCIFORM XANTHOMA

Verruciform xanthoma is a rare hyperplastic lesion that can have a white, hyperkeratotic surface resembling a papilloma.

Verruciform xanthoma is most common in the fifth to seventh decades. It is usually found on the gingiva but can form in almost any site in the mouth. It can be white or red in colour, sessile, have a warty surface and range in size from one to several centimetres across. It may be mistaken for a papilloma, leukoplakia or carcinoma clinically, but is readily recognisable histologically. Verruciform xanthoma is benign and has no known associations with diseases such as hyperlipidaemia or diabetes mellitus that are associated with cutaneous xanthomas.

Pathology

The warty surface is due to the much-infolded epithelium which, in white variants, is hyperkeratinised or parakeratinised. In haematoxylin and eosin stained sections, the parakeratin layer stains a distinctive orange colour. The elongate rete ridges are of equal length and extend to a straight, well-defined lower border (Fig. 24.18).

The diagnostic feature is the large, foamy, xanthoma cells that fill the connective tissue papillae but extend only to the lower border of the lesion (Fig. 24.19). These cells are macrophages containing lipid and periodic acid–Schiff (PAS) positive granules.

Simple surgical excision is curative.

Review PMID: 12676251

CALIBRE-PERSISTENT ARTERY

Calibre-persistent artery is a loop or tortuosity of the labial artery that pushes superficially from its normal site deep in

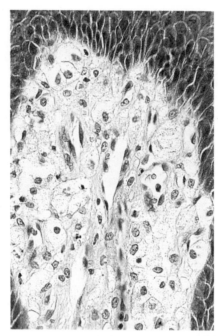

Fig. 24.19 Verruciform xanthoma. At higher power, dermal papillae within the folded epithelium can be seen to contain many large rounded cells with foamy or vacuolated cytoplasm.

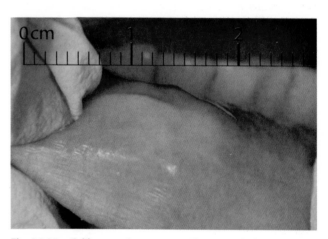

Fig. 24.20 Calibre-persistent artery. This example forms a raised linear firm and pulsatile swelling. *(From Awni, S., Conn, B., 2016. Caliber-persistent artery. J. Oral MaxFac. Surg. 74, 1391–1395.)*

the lip to lie just below the vermilion border or labial mucosa. It appears to be an age change seen in the elderly. It may be palpable, or if superficial, visible and forms a nodule or linear curved firm mass, sometimes pulsatile (Fig. 24.20). Some appear bluish, and they are frequently mistaken for mucoceles despite the site on the vermilion border (where mucoceles never form). Those on the lower lip are usually to one side of the midline, whereas those in the upper lip are usually near the midline.

Histology shows normal labial artery (Fig. 24.21), but ideally the condition should be recognised clinically as biopsy will cause considerable haemorrhage and produces no benefit.

The name comes from the fact that the lumen of the artery does not narrow while it passes up into the superficial tissues, as a normal artery would at the site. A similar vascular anomaly occurs in the stomach where it is a cause of gastric bleeding, but lip lesions do not cause this problem.

Cases and review PMID: 20646912 and 26868184

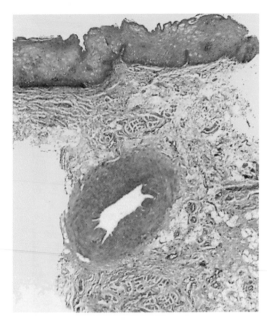

Fig. 24.21 Calibre-persistent artery. A loop of the labial artery ascends high into the mucosa, almost to the overlying epithelium.

COSMETIC IMPLANTS

Increasing demand for cosmetic procedures and lack of regulation in some countries have generated a small but steady stream of patients with adverse outcomes. Probably all implanted materials can induce an inflammatory reaction, a foreign body reaction or fibrosis in some patients, whether allergic or irritant (Fig 24.22).

The main irreversible outcome is fibrosis, producing skin puckering, hard nodules and tethering. The lips are a common site for injections, and fibrosis here can mimic orofacial granulomatosis or Crohn's disease and be very disfiguring. Surgical treatment is difficult or impossible.

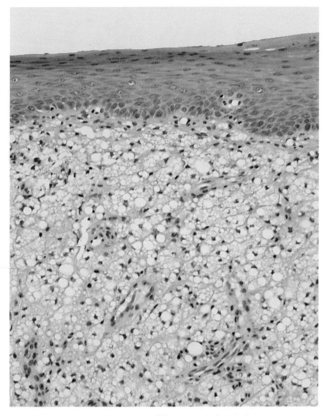

Fig. 24.22 Injected cosmetic filler material. All of the connective tissue is infiltrated by macrophages containing multiple small vacuoles of silicone. More deeply, the macrophage infiltrate had produced extensive fibrosis and the lower lip was hard and distorted by scarring.

Injected materials include collagen, hyaluronic acid, hydroxyapatites and synthetic materials including acrylates.

Web URL 24.1 Histological appearances materials: http://www .aaomp.org/atlas/

Soft tissue tumours

25

BENIGN TUMOURS

Benign nerve sheath tumours

Several types of benign neoplasm arise from peripheral nerve. All present as firm, mobile soft tissue lumps, are treated by excision and are differentiated histologically.

Traumatic neuromas are hyperplastic healing responses at the site of damage to a nerve and comprise a tangled mass of regrowing normal nerve bundles.

Neurilemmomas are benign neoplasms of Schwann cells. Histologically, they comprise an encapsulated mass of elongate spindle cells with palisaded nuclei (Antoni A tissue – Fig. 25.1) and a variable amount of myxoid loose connective tissue (Antoni B tissue).

Solitary circumscribed neuromas may be neoplasms or reactive lesions and comprise Schwann cells and neurites.

Neurofibromas are rare, and when seen in the mouth, neurofibromatosis should be suspected. Histologically, neurofibromas are cellular with plump nuclei separated by fine, sinuous collagen fibres among which mast cells can usually be found.

Mucosal neuromas are hamartomatous malformations often associated with syndromes, particularly multiple endocrine neoplasia. They are convoluted large nerves.

Lingual nerve traumatic neuromas PMID: 15772589

Schwannomas PMID: 10748827

Solitary circumscribed neuroma PMID: 20237984

Neurofibromatosis PMID: 21301902 and 1545973

Mucosal neuromas PMID: 21552134

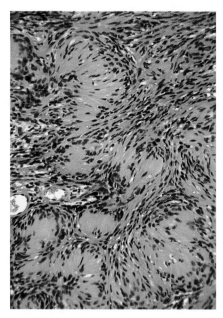

Fig. 25.1   Neurilemmoma. Antoni A tissue showing striking palisading of nuclei.

Lipoma and fibrolipoma

Lipomas, benign neoplasms of fat, are rare in the mouth and occur in the middle aged and elderly. They are smooth, soft, sometimes yellowish, asymptomatic, slow growing swellings, which may be pedunculated (Fig. 25.2). Tongue, lips and buccal fat pad are common sites.

Histologically, lipomas consist of apparently normal fat (Fig. 25.3) with a variable amount of supporting fibrous tissue and a partial fibrous capsule (Fig. 25.4). When fibrous tissue is prominent, the lesion is called a *fibrolipoma*. Lipomas should be excised.

Oral lipoma review PMID: 21447447

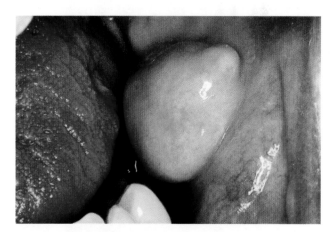

Fig. 25.2   Lipoma of the cheek. The tumour forms a pale, very soft yellowish swelling.

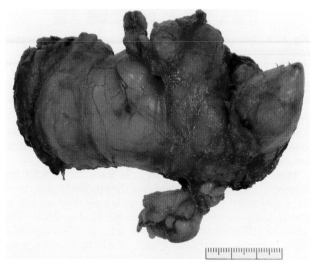

Fig. 25.3   Lipoma. The lobular structure of the fat is visible.

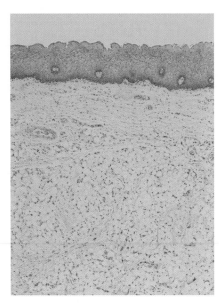

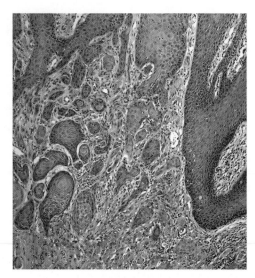

Fig. 25.4   Lipoma. A lipoma immediately below the oral mucosa; the fat appears normal and is often only partially encapsulated at the margin.

Fig. 25.6   Granular cell tumour. High power of a superficial area in Fig. 25.7 showing the small irregular islands of epithelium that appear to invade the fibrous tissue and superficial muscle. Some show keratin formation similar to keratin pearls in squamous carcinoma. Granular cells are only present along the lower edge of the figure.

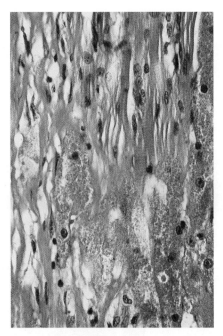

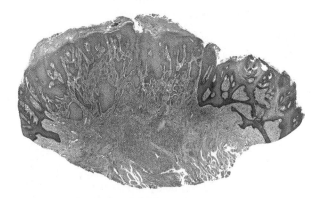

Fig. 25.7   Granular cell tumour. The irregular proliferation of the overlying epithelium (pseudocarcinomatous hyperplasia), which is very florid in this example, may mimic a squamous carcinoma in superficial biopsy specimens.

Fig. 25.5   Granular cell tumour. At high power, the granular cells apparently merging with muscle fibres are characteristic and indicate the diagnosis.

The granular cell tumour can induce striking pseudocarcinomatous ('pseudoepitheliomatous') hyperplasia of the overlying epithelium (Figs 25.6 and 25.7). Although only present in a minority, this has resulted in misdiagnosis as carcinoma, with resulting overtreatment. Such misdiagnosis is likely in an insufficiently deep biopsy that shows only the epithelium.

Simple excision is curative, often even when incomplete.

Description and case series PMID: 19192059

Granular cell tumour

Clinically, granular cell tumours typically form painless domed smooth swellings. The dorsum of tongue and buccal mucosa are the commonest sites.

Histologically, large granular cells form the bulk of the lesion. Their origin is unclear, but they probably arise from Schwann cells of small nerves, although they appear to merge with muscle around the periphery (Fig. 25.5). The granular cells are large, with clearly defined cell membranes, and the granular cytoplasm is explained by large eosinophilic lysosomes containing cell debris, mitochondria and degenerate cell membrane.

Congenital (granular cell) epulis

The rare congenital epulis is typically present at birth as a smooth soft nodule a few millimetres in diameter, usually on the upper alveolar ridge (Fig. 25.8) and very occasionally the tongue. A very large majority are in females.

Histologically, the mass comprises large pale granular cells that resemble those of granular cell tumour. Pseudocarcinomatous hyperplasia is not seen. If small, spontaneous resolution is likely. If large, interfering with feeding or respiration, conservative excision is curative even if incomplete.

Case series and review PMID: 21393037

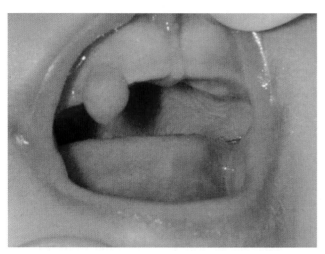

Fig. 25.8   Congenital epulis. A firm pink non-ulcerated nodule on the alveolar ridge of a neonate is the typical presentation. *(From Oda, D. 2005. Soft-tissue lesions in children. Oral Maxillofac Surg Clin North Am, 17:383, pp. 402.)*

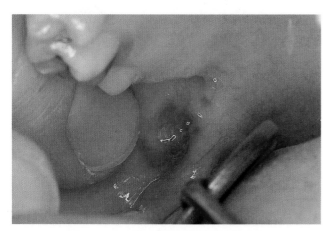

Fig. 25.9   Cavernous haemangioma of the cheek. The colour is deep purple, and the structure, a mass of thin-walled blood sinuses, is visible through the thin epithelium. A mass engorged with blood and as prominent as this is liable to trauma and to bleed profusely.

Haemangiomas → Summary chart 26.1 p. 390

Haemangiomas are difficult to classify. Some are developmental anomalies, some are hamartomas and others are benign neoplasms. A further group are vascular ectasias, developmental conditions in which the number of vessels is normal but they are constantly dilated. Few types are common, and the only frequent genuine vascular neoplasm is Kaposi's sarcoma (mentioned later in this chapter).

Capillary and cavernous haemangiomas form purple, flat or nodular superficial lesions that blanch on pressure (Fig. 25.9). The capillary type consists of innumerable minute blood vessels and vasoformative tissue – mere rosettes of endothelial cells (Fig. 25.10). The cavernous type consists of large blood-filled sinusoids. Some show both histological patterns. In infancy these will usually resolve without treatment. In adults they can usually be excised easily if required as they have low blood flow. Cryosurgery can be used to destroy a haemangioma without excessive bleeding.

Arteriovenous and venous malformations have higher blood flow, are hamartomas that are present from birth and

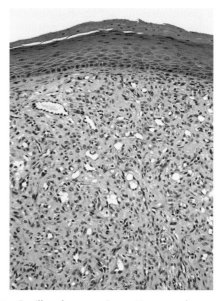

Fig. 25.10   Capillary haemangioma. Numerous large and small closely packed capillary vessels extend from the epithelium into the deeper tissues.

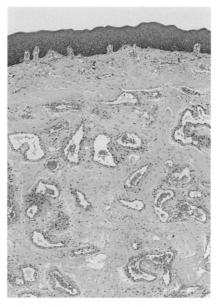

Fig. 25.11   Sturge-Weber syndrome. Biopsy from the gingiva affected by an intraoral port wine stain. The number of vessels and their distribution is normal, but all are markedly dilated, producing the appearance of many extra vessels.

grow with the patient. Thrombosis is common, causing pain. They affect deep and superficial tissues, and excision carries significant risks depending on blood flow. Embolisation is the first line of treatment.

Haemangiomas of bone are discussed in Chapter 12.

Port wine stains are non-inherited congenital vascular ectasias caused by mutation in a G-signalling protein gene. Vessels in the lesions are normal in number, but their defective walls cannot contract, so they are constantly dilated (Fig. 25.11). This causes prolonged bleeding on surgery. Port wine stains in the distribution of the trigeminal nerve, including intraoral haemangiomas, together with meningeal angiomas, epilepsy and sometimes learning difficulty constitute the Sturge-Weber syndrome. In this syndrome, the intracranial lesions often cause epilepsy in later life.

Pyogenic granulomas are not haemangiomas but hyperplastic nodules of endothelial cells and granulation tissue. However, they are often confusingly called lobular capillary haemangiomas.

Hereditary haemorrhagic telangiectasia is discussed in Chapter 28.

Head and neck vascular lesions review PMID: 25439548

Infantile haemangiomas PMID: 23338947

Arteriovenous malformations PMID: 20115972

Oral port wine stains PMID: 22226814

Lymphangiomas

These are uncommon vascular malformations arising before birth or in infancy. They form pale, translucent, smooth or nodular elevations of the mucosa in which the superficial dilated lymphatics can often be seen clinically. The commonest site is the tongue and, if large and diffuse, lymphangiomas cause generalised macroglossia. They are normally asymptomatic but may present due to bleeding into the lymphatic spaces.

Histologically, lymphangiomas consist of thin-walled lymphatics containing lymph, seen as a pinkish amorphous material in sections (Fig. 25.12).

Localised lymphangiomas can be excised if necessary, but larger and diffuse types are difficult to remove. Injection of sclerosing agents is then the first line of treatment.

Cystic hygroma is a large diffuse lymphangioma of very dilated lymphatics, each several millimetres in diameter, usually in the neck in a young child.

Lymphatic malformations PMID: 24157637

MALIGNANT CONNECTIVE TISSUE TUMOURS

Sarcomas of virtually any type can affect the oral soft tissues, but most are rare. Sarcomas grow rapidly, are invasive, destroy surrounding tissues and metastasise by the bloodstream. Most present as destructive masses that cannot be distinguished clinically. Occasional sarcomas are complications of therapeutic irradiation.

Osteosarcomas and chondrosarcomas are described in Chapter 12 and lymphomas in Chapter 27.

General review PMID: 19216845

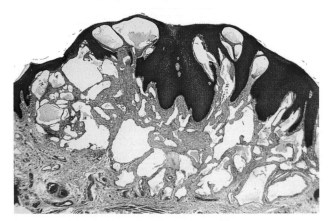

Fig. 25.12 Lymphangioma. There is a localised aggregation of cavernous lymphatics which form a pale superficial swelling. Bleeding into these lesions causes them suddenly to become purple or almost black.

Rhabdomyosarcoma

Rhabdomyosarcomas show striated muscle differentiation and are the most common oral sarcomas in children or adolescents. They form rapidly growing soft swellings, usually centred around the maxilla or in the orbit. Two main forms affect the head and neck, alveolar and embryonal.

Embryonal rhabdomyosarcomas consists of cells of variable shape and size, often strap- or tadpole-shaped, like rhabdomyoblasts in the early embryo. Sometimes muscle cross-striations can be seen in their cytoplasm to indicate their muscle nature.

Alveolar rhabdomyosarcomas consist of slit-like spaces into which hang tear-shaped, darkly staining cells attached to the walls. These alveoli are separated by a fibrous stroma. Muscle-like cells are not seen.

Diagnosis of both types can be difficult and relies on immunostaining for markers of muscle differentiation such as desmin or myogenin and on molecular analysis. The alveolar type has a characteristic chromosomal translocation t(2;13).

Treatment is by excision and combination chemotherapy, but the prognosis is poor.

In children PMID: 26231745

Mixed case series PMID: 12001077

Sarcomas of fibroblasts

Fibrosarcomas and myofibroblastic sarcomas are the second commonest sarcomas in the head and neck after rhabdomyosarcoma, but are still rare. Some are cellular, others contain collagen and others are myxoid; several different types are recognised. In general, treatment is by radical excision. Local recurrence and spread are common, but metastasis is rare. These sarcomas may follow radiotherapy to the head and neck after an interval of 10 years or so.

Kaposi's sarcoma → Summary chart 26.1 p. 390

Kaposi's sarcoma is a low-grade and relatively indolent malignant multifocal tumour of lymphatics or blood vessels caused by infection with human herpesvirus 8 (HHV-8). Its status as a true malignant neoplasm is unclear as it shows a range of behaviours.

Most patients are immunosuppressed. Therapeutic immunosuppression with ciclosporin and tacrolimus can be associated with Kaposi's sarcoma, but by far the main predisposing condition is HIV infection, and almost all oral Kaposi's sarcoma is in HIV-infected patients. Among HIV-infected patients, Kaposi's sarcoma affects mainly men who have sex with men. Antiretroviral therapy for HIV has greatly reduced the incidence of Kaposi's sarcoma, but it remains the most common type of intraoral sarcoma.

The HHV8 virus is endemic in sub-Saharan Africa, common around the Mediterranean and rare elsewhere. In endemic regions it is transmitted vertically and elsewhere sexually, through saliva. After infection the virus remains latent under control of the immune system, probably for life. While latent, HHV8 inhibits the p53 and retinoblastoma tumour suppressor genes causing cell proliferation, although the full mechanism of sarcomagenesis is still unclear. The same virus also causes some lymphomas and types of Castleman's disease.

Within the mouth, the palate and gingiva are the most frequent sites, and the tumour appears initially as a flat purplish area and enlarges rapidly into a nodular mass that may ulcerate and bleed readily (Fig. 25.13). The clinical

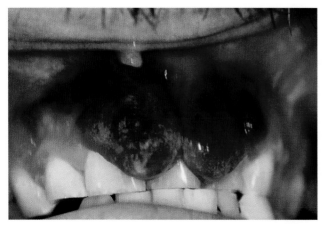

Fig. 25.13 Kaposi's sarcoma. Lesions are red, maroon or bluish and highly vascular. They may be flat or form tumour masses, and the gingivae or palate are characteristic sites. *(Courtesy of Prof WH Binnie.)*

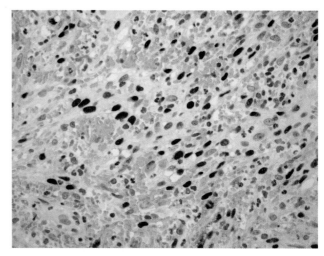

Fig. 25.15 Kaposi's sarcoma. Immunocytochemistry for human herpesvirus 8 reveals numerous infected cell nuclei (*dark brown stain*) confirming the diagnosis.

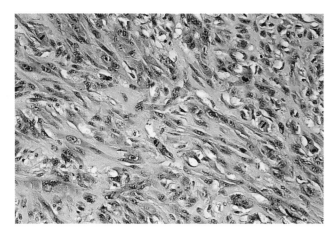

Fig. 25.14 Kaposi's sarcoma. The tumour is composed of spindle and plump cells with cytological atypia and frequent mitoses. Many of the small holes visible are the result of formation of capillaries by the tumour cells.

> **Box 25.1 Kaposi's sarcoma: key features**
> - The most common type of oral sarcoma
> - Most common in HIV-infected men who have sex with men
> - Due to herpesvirus 8
> - Appears clinically as a flat or nodular purplish area
> - Consists histologically of minute, proliferating blood vessels
> - Good response to highly active antiretroviral treatment, but long-term control is difficult
> - Multifocal and often widespread when oral lesions appear
> - Death more frequently from associated opportunistic infections
> - Endemic form in sub-Saharan Africa and in countries around the Mediterranean

differential diagnosis is from oral purpura, bacillary angiomatosis and pyogenic granulomas, from which it can be distinguished by microscopy. The colour is usually maroon or purple, rather than the bright red of haemangiomas or pyogenic granulomas. Associated HIV infection is usually suggested by other clinical and oral manifestations, notably candidosis.

Histologically, Kaposi's sarcoma is a proliferation of endothelial cells and poorly organised vessels. In the early stages these are capillary-size blood vessels and resemble granulation tissue, particularly in the mouth where traumatised superficial lesions become secondarily inflamed. Later, the vessels are slit shaped and compressed in a densely cellular mass of spindle cells that show mitotic activity and ultimately dominate the picture (Fig. 25.14). Leakage of blood from the poorly formed vessels results in haemosiderin pigment that contributes to the colour seen clinically. Diagnosis is aided by immunostaining for podoplanin, a lymphatic endothelial cell marker, and confirmed by immunohistochemical staining for the HHV-8 virus (Fig. 25.15).

Management

Any patient with such a presentation must have Kaposi's sarcoma excluded since, in the absence of immunosuppressive treatment, it is pathognomonic of AIDS. Kaposi's sarcoma is occasionally the presenting complaint in HIV infection, although other less symptomatic or visible lesions may also be present such as candidosis or hairy leukoplakia.

Many Kaposi sarcomas are relatively indolent and may not require aggressive treatment, but this depends on extent. Localised oral lesions may be amenable to excision. However, disease is always multifocal, and chemotherapy is required for more widespread involvement. Radiation is widely used in other parts of the body, but is usually avoided in the mouth because of adverse effects. Currently, the most effective chemotherapy regimens are interferon alpha with didanosine for slowly progressing disease or doxorubicin and paclitaxel with antiretroviral treatment. Antiretroviral treatment alone will induce remission in approximately one-half of cases. With other treatments, remission can usually be induced in 90% of cases, but Kaposi's sarcoma remains a disease that is controlled rather than cured.

Oral Kaposi sarcoma PMID: 3059252

Histological diversity PMID: 23312917

General review and treatment PMID: 25843728

Classical and endemic forms

The original description of Kaposi's sarcoma among elderly persons of Mediterranean or Jewish origin in Central Europe was in 1872, long predating HIV infection. This classical or sporadic form affects the skin, mainly the lower extremities and hardly ever the head and neck. Kaposi's sarcoma with broadly similar characteristics is also common as an endemic form in Africa, particularly in Zaire, where it formed approximately 12% of all malignant tumours in the pre-AIDS era.

Key features of Kaposi's sarcoma are summarised in Box 25.1.

Oral pigmented lesions

26

There are many causes of colour change in the mucosa, but the significant causes are melanin, superficial blood vessels, haemorrhage and blood pigments, and extrinsic agents (Box 26.1).

Review oral pigmentation PMCID: PMC3775277

Box 26.1   Oral pigmented lesions

Usually brown or black

Melanin pigmentation

- Physiological pigmentation
- Melanotic macules
- Melanoacanthoma
- Naevi
- Lichen planus (Ch. 16)
- Malignant melanoma
- Addison's disease (Ch. 36)
- HIV infection (Ch. 29)
- Peutz–Jeghers and other syndromes
- Melanotic neuroectodermal tumour (Ch. 12)
- Heavy smoking

Extrinsic agents

- Amalgam tattoo
- Black hairy tongue (Ch.17)
- Chlorhexidine staining
- Minocycline staining of bone
- Some drugs
- Heavy metal poisoning

Usually purple or red

Superficial, enlarged or numerous blood vessels

- Erythroplasia (Ch. 19)
- Haemangiomas (Ch. 25)
- Kaposi's sarcoma (Ch. 25)
- Telangiectases and lingual varices (Chs 28 & 1)
- Pyogenic granuloma (Ch. 24)
- Pregnancy epulis (Ch. 24)

Haemorrhage or blood pigments

- Purpura (Ch. 28)
- Other blood blisters
- Giant-cell epulis (Ch. 24)

Inflammation

- Geographical tongue (Ch. 17)
- Erythematous candidosis (Ch. 15)
- Median rhomboid glossitis (Ch. 15)

DIFFUSE MUCOSAL PIGMENTATION

→ Summary chart 26.1 p. 390

Addison's disease is the most important cause of diffuse pigmentation (Ch. 36), but it is rare and a sign of late disease in an obviously debilitated patient.

Drugs, including non-steroidal anti-inflammatory drugs, phenothiazines and antimalarials, may increase melanin formation (Fig. 26.1) and also deposit in skin and less densely in mucosa. Chlorhexidine, bismuth and iron salts stain the mucosa. Hydroxychloroquine causes pigmentation particularly of the palate.

Remote carcinomas can occasionally cause diffuse oral pigmentation, usually around the soft palate, as a paraneoplastic syndrome.

Heavy smoking is probably the commonest cause, increasing pigmentation and causing melanin 'drop out' into the connective tissue.

General review pigmentary disorders PMID: 16631966

LOCALISED MELANIN PIGMENTATION

→ Summary chart 26.1 p. 390

Melanin in epidermis functions as a protective sunshade for the DNA of basal cells. The oral mucosa contains equivalent numbers of melanocytes to the skin, but they are usually inactive, and melanin in the mouth has no function. However, it is synthesised by oral melanocytes and passed to adjacent keratinocytes by phagocytosis in exactly the same way as in the skin. Increased melanin pigmentation can arise from increased synthesis or by increase in the number of melanocytes.

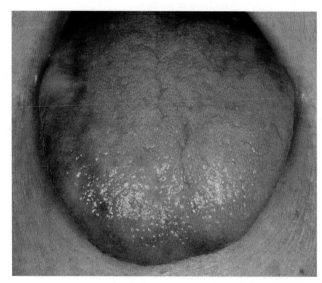

Fig. 26.1   Drug-induced melanin pigmentation. This example was caused by chemotherapy. *(From Alawi, F. 2013. Pigmented lesions of the oral cavity. Dent Clin North Am, 57, pp. 699-710.)*

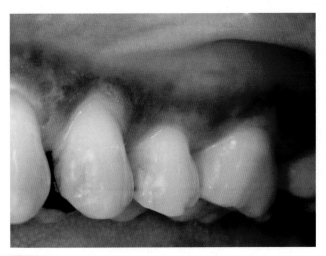

Fig. 26.2 Physiological or racial pigmentation. The distribution of melanotic mucosa around the gingival margin is characteristic.

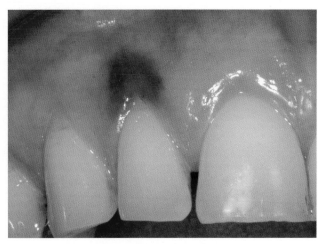

Fig. 26.3 Melanotic macule. This pigmented patch on the gingiva has no specific clinical features to aid diagnosis, other than that is unchanged for many years. *(Courtesy of Mr R Saravanamuttu.)*

The colour of melanin varies with its depth in the mucosa. When superficial, it appears black or brown, and when deeply sited, it can appear dark blue.

Light-skinned individuals have an average of 30 cutaneous local pigmented lesions of various types, and occasionally one will be present in the mouth.

Physiological pigmentation

This is the most common cause of oral pigmentation. The gingivae are particularly affected (Fig. 26.2). The inner aspect of the lips is typically spared. Intraoral pigmentation is commoner in those with a dark skin and is often called *racial pigmentation*. Although pigmentation may be widespread, it is in well-defined symmetrical zones. Melanocyte numbers are normal, and activity is increased.

Physiological pigmentation PMCID: PMC3994327

Melanotic macules

These are well-defined flat brown or black pigmented patches a few millimetres in diameter caused by increased melanocyte activity. They are unusual, but still the commonest intraoral melanotic lesions.

Gingiva, buccal mucosa and palate are the favoured sites (Fig. 26.3). The lesions are completely benign. However, as the appearance is indistinguishable from early melanoma and because they are infrequent, they are usually excised for confirmation of diagnosis unless a long history is obtained.

Case series review PMID: 8351123

Oral melanotic macules associated with HIV infection

Oral and labial melanotic macules may develop in as many as 6% of patients with HIV infection, approximately twice the frequency seen in HIV-negative persons. Oral melanotic macules may appear before infection is recognised and become more numerous while HIV infection advances.

Histologically, the patches are the same as conventional melanotic macules.

Excision biopsy of melanotic macules is necessary for diagnosis. Unlike those in HIV-negative persons, these macules are more likely to enlarge and to recur after excision, giving a clue to the HIV infection.

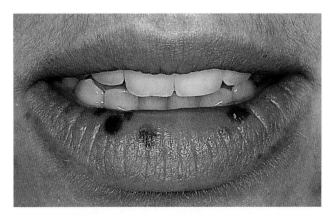

Fig. 26.4 Melanocytic naevi. These flat, pigmented patches are occasionally found on the lip and intraorally.

Case series and review PMCID: PMC4783540 and PMID: 2175872

Oral melanocytic naevi → Summary chart 26.1
p. 390

Acquired melanocytic naevi are otherwise known as moles. These are common developmental conditions in which melanocytes proliferate and form a mass between the epithelium and connective tissue (melanocytes outside the epithelium are called *naevus cells*). Moles appear in childhood, grow until adolescence and then regress until the age of approximately 30 years. While they regress, the naevus cells produce less melanin and migrate deeper into the underlying tissue and become inactive. Intraoral lesions are unusual and form circumscribed brown to black patches, usually flat, approximately 5 or 6 mm across (Fig. 26.4). Palate and gingiva are favoured sites.

Histologically, the cluster of naevus cells is seen below the epithelium (Fig. 26.5).

Blue naevus is a deeply sited cluster of pigmented naevus cells, hence the blue colour. They are almost always on the palate of children or young adults. A focus of spindle-shaped pigmented melanocytes lies deeply.

Congenital naevi cannot be distinguished from acquired naevi when they arise in the mouth.

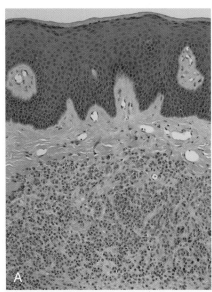

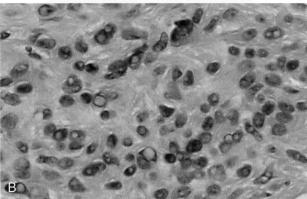

Fig. 26.5   Intramucosal naevus. In this late lesion (A), the naevus cells have migrated down into the underlying tissue and are separated from the epithelium by a band of fibrous tissue, the intramucosal stage of development. The naevus cells at higher power (B) are pale staining, often have vacuoles in their nuclei and occasionally form a small amount of dark melanin pigment, as in the cell near the top.

All these naevi are asymptomatic but, unless in children or having a long unchanged course, should be excised and sent for microscopy to exclude early malignant melanoma.

Case series PMID: 2359037

Melanoacanthoma

Oral melanoacanthoma is rare lesion, poorly understood and considered to be a reaction to an unknown insult. Those affected are almost always of African descent and of middle age.

Buccal mucosa is the common site, but any intraoral site may be involved. The lesions are asymptomatic flat or domed brown-black patches with an ill-defined periphery (Fig. 26.6). They enlarge during several weeks, remain stable for a variable period and then slowly regress. The rapid growth usually triggers a biopsy to exclude melanoma or excision of the whole lesion if small.

Histologically, there is an increase in melanocytes, increased melanin production and the melanocytes migrate up from the basal layers to all levels in the epithelium (Fig. 26.7).

Case series PMID: 12544093

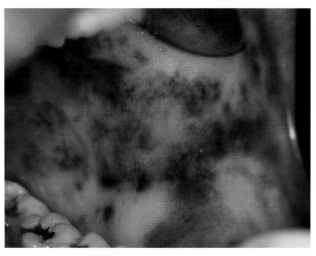

Fig. 26.6   Melanoacanthoma. An extensive example of this benign condition that would raise the concern of melanoma. *(From Alawi, F. 2013. Pigmented lesions of the oral cavity. Dent Clin North Am, 57, pp. 699-710.)*

Post-inflammatory pigmentation

Inflammation interferes with both melanin synthesis by melanocytes and its transfer to keratinocytes. Melanosomes can escape from the epithelium into the underlying connective tissue where they are taken up by macrophages, a process known as melanin 'drop out'. Accumulation of this subepithelial melanin gives rise to post-inflammatory pigmentation. The process is commoner in dark-skinned races.

Intraorally, the most common inflammatory condition to become pigmented is lichen planus (Fig. 26.8), and it can become very dark. Pigmentation may also develop in other inflamed sites and scars. This type of pigmentation is also seen diffusely through the mouth of heavy cigarette smokers.

Case series PMID: 20526252

Syndromes with oral pigmentation

→ Summary chart 26.1 p. 390

Peutz–Jeghers syndrome

Peutz–Jeghers syndrome is a rare disease characterised by multiple mucocutaneous pigmented macules and intestinal polyposis. The cause is mutation or inactivation of the STK11 gene that encodes a signalling kinase.

The pigmented patches typically develop during the first decade of life and can be widespread, affecting the hands and feet and perioral skin, as well as the oral mucosa. Cutaneous patches usually fade after puberty, but the oral macules persist. The oral patches resemble melanotic macules and affect the lips, buccal mucosa, tongue and palate (Figs 26.9 and 26.10). They are often the first feature.

The intestinal polyps affect mainly the small intestine, are regarded as hamartomatous and rarely undergo malignant change, but can cause obstruction and recurrent pain. However, patients are at risk of pancreatic, breast, ovarian and other cancers. This includes bowel cancers, even though they do not arise in the polyps.

Histologically, the oral lesions show slight acanthosis and increased numbers of melanocytes in the basal layer, so these lesions are lentigos and not melanotic macules (which have normal melanocyte numbers).

No treatment is required, but patients should be referred for genetic diagnosis and follow-up.

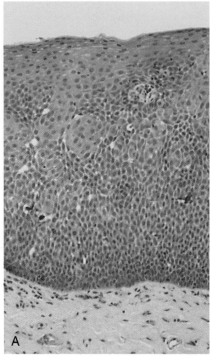

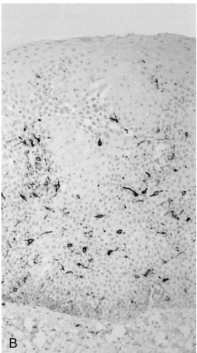

Fig. 26.7   Melanoacanthoma. In routine stains the increased number of melanocytes is difficult to see. A few contain melanin and appear brown, but many are seen as clear spaces (A). An immunohistochemical stain for melanocytes reveals very many and shows them throughout the prickle cell layer (B). Normally, melanocyte cell bodies are limited to the basal cell layer.

Web URL 26.1 Genetics and description: http://omim.org/entry/175200

Review and treatment PMID: 20581245

Other syndromes with pigmentation

Several rare syndromes include oral lentigos, including LEOPARD and Laugier–Hunziker syndromes,

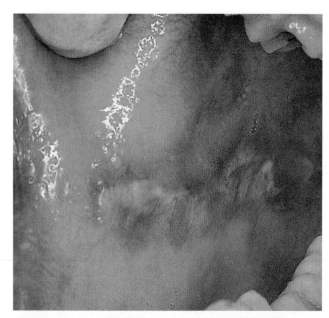

Fig. 26.8   Post-inflammatory pigmentation in lichen planus. Inflammatory conditions may become pigmented, especially in dark-skinned races. Here, melanin delineates mucosa affected by lichen planus.

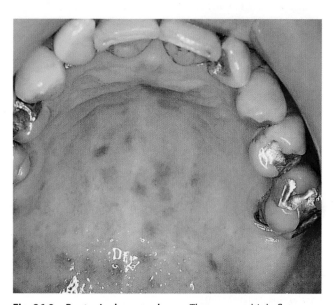

Fig. 26.9   Peutz–Jeghers syndrome. There are multiple flat, pigmented patches on the palate. Those on the lips are most characteristic but fade with age.

neurofibromatosis type I, Albright's syndrome and Carney complex.

Laugier-Hunziker case and review PMID: 23562360

OTHER LOCALISED PIGMENTED LESIONS

→ Summary chart 26.1 p. 390

Amalgam and other tattoos

Fragments of amalgam frequently become embedded in the oral mucosa and form the most common intraoral pigmented patches. Amalgam is usually traumatically implanted close to the dental arch, and tattoos are typically 5 mm or more across and dark grey or bluish (Fig. 26.11).

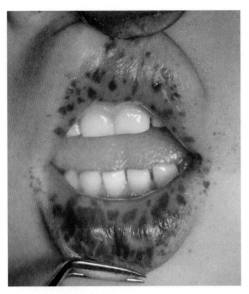

Fig. 26.10   Peutz–Jeghers syndrome. Typical multiple pigmented patches on the labial mucosa. *(From Alawi, F. 2013. Pigmented lesions of the oral cavity. Dent Clin North Am, 57, pp. 699–710.)*

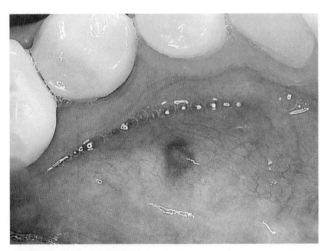

Fig. 26.11   Amalgam tattoo. Typical appearance and site; however, the lower second premolar, from which the amalgam probably originated, has been crowned.

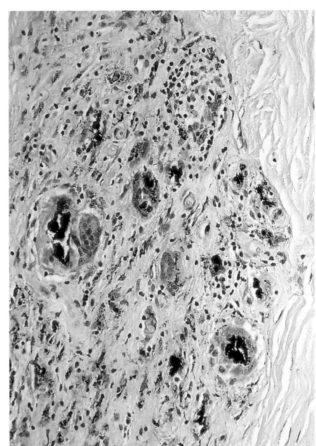

Fig. 26.12   Amalgam tattoo. There are large fragments of amalgam surrounded by foreign body giant cells and macrophages and smaller particles dispersed in fibrous tissue. Silver leaching from the smaller fragments has stained the adjacent collagen brown.

Fate of implanted amalgam PMID: 6752362

Case series PMID: 6928285

Lead line and heavy metal poisoning

Heavy metals such as mercury, bismuth and lead can cause black or brown deposits in the gingival sulcus. The metals pass in solution from serum into the crevice, where they are reduced to sulphides by bacterial products and are visible through the thin gingival margin as a dark line running along the floor of the crevice or pocket (Burton's line). The blue line caused by lead ('lead line') may be particularly prominent and sharply defined and is a good indicator of chronic exposure and still an important sign for diagnosis (Fig. 26.13).

Mercury and bismuth are no longer used in medicine, and lead is no longer a major industrial hazard. However, platinum released from cisplatin, a cytotoxic drug, can cause a blue line, and unintentional toxicity can develop in hobbyists and others using metals or their salts without sufficient protection. Older houses may still have lead piping, lead can be inhaled during battery recycling and a cluster of cases in Germany was due to contamination of marijuana.

Case report PMID: 108646

Soft tissue pigmentation

Topical antibiotics and antiseptics may cause dark pigmentation, particularly of the dorsum of the tongue, due to

Large dense tattoos may be radiopaque. The amount of implanted amalgam necessary to produce a tattoo is very small. Initially they are sharply defined, but the amalgam becomes dispersed and lesions slowly enlarge and develop irregular outlines, and components dissolve and reprecipitate on nearby collagen. Particles are also dispersed by migrating macrophages.

Early after implantation, there is a foreign body reaction with macrophages or giant cells, but this fades with time. Histologically, amalgam is seen as brown or black granules with fine particles deposited along collagen bundles and around small blood vessels (Fig. 26.12) because of the affinity of silver for collagen. Any free mercury solubilises in a few weeks and is excreted, remaining in the tissues only complexed in amalgam.

If radiographs fail to show metal and there is no record of implantation in the patient's records, excision is often necessary to exclude a melanocytic lesion.

Corundum, other dental materials, traumatically implanted pencil lead fragments (usually in children) and cosmetic tattoos are occasionally seen.

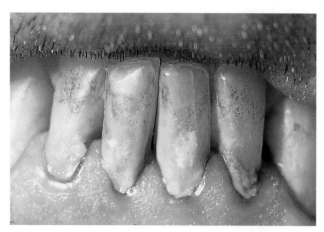

Fig. 26.13   Lead line. The lead line is the bluish grey darkening of the gingival crevice, not the physiological melanin also present on the labial gingiva. *(From Forbes, C., and Jackson, W. 2003. Color atlas and text of clinical medicine. 3rd ed. St Louis: Mosby.)*

Box 26.2   Malignant melanoma: key features

- Peak incidence between 40 and 60 years
- Usually appear as black or brown patches
- Amelanotic melanomas appear red
- Later cause soreness and bleeding
- Biopsy required for diagnosis
- Very variable histological features
- Should be widely excised
- Median survival probably not longer than 2 years

---

overgrowth of pigment-forming bacteria. Chlorhexidine stains the mucosa directly, as does bismuth in antacids.

MELANOMA → Summary chart 26.1 p. 390

Melanomas are malignant neoplasms of melanocytes, and intraoral melanomas are rare but important. They have a long asymptomatic period, are diagnosed late and have an appallingly poor prognosis. As noted previously, many other pigmented lesions cannot be distinguished clinically from melanoma, making biopsy of oral pigmented lesions mandatory in almost all cases.

Ultraviolet light exposure, fair complexion and sun sensitivity cause cutaneous melanoma, but no aetiological factors are known for mucosal melanoma. Very few melanomas are intraoral, 1% in Europe and the United States, but a much higher proportion of 12% in Japan. Mucosal melanomas are also common in India and Africa and in individuals from these areas. The peak age incidence is between 40 and 60 years.

Key features are summarised in Box 26.2.

Clinical

The most frequent sites are the palate and upper alveolar ridge (Fig. 26.14). Early oral melanomas are asymptomatic dark brown or black flat patches. Pigment may be so readily shed that rubbing the surface with gauze stains the latter black or dark brown. Symptoms only develop in the late stages with nodular growth, pain, ulceration, bleeding or loosening of teeth.

Melanomas grow in a predictable fashion. Initially, the malignant melanocytes grow only within the epithelium,

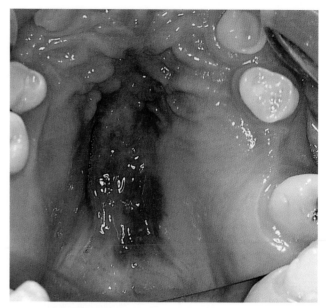

Fig. 26.14   Melanotic patch. There is poorly-demarcated pigmentation of varying density in the palate. All pigmented lesions such as this should be treated with the utmost suspicion and biopsied to exclude melanoma.

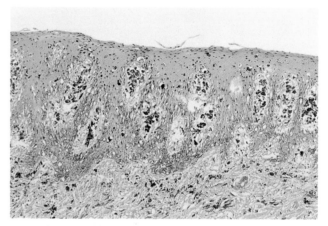

Fig. 26.15   Superficial spreading melanoma. Numerous pigmented and atypical melanocytes form nests and clusters along the basement membrane and are present within the epithelium and superficial connective tissue.

spreading laterally. This preinvasive or in situ stage is called the *radial* or *horizontal growth* phase, and lesions at this stage rarely metastasise. Later, the melanocytes extend out of the epithelium into the connective tissue in the vertical growth phase. This stage is associated with metastases. In the mouth, almost all melanomas are diagnosed late and are invasive on diagnosis. Because of their rapid growth, most oral melanomas are at least a centimetre across before being noticed, and approximately 50% of patients have metastases at presentation, most commonly in cervical lymph nodes. In addition to the regional lymph nodes, metastases can involve the lungs, liver, brain and bones.

Approximately 30% of melanomas are preceded by an area of hyperpigmentation, often by many years. These preceding lesions are either dysplasia of melanocytes or melanoma in the radial growth phase. Early diagnosis by biopsy is essential if there is to be a chance of surgical removal before metastasis.

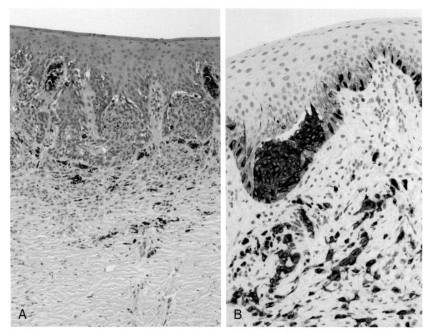

Fig. 26.16   Melanoma. (A) Hematoxylin and eosin–stained melanocytes are seen to form nests along the basement membrane. Invading melanocytes are difficult to see, but melanin is present in the deep connective tissue giving a clue. (B) At slightly higher magnification, immunohistochemistry for a melanocytic marker reveals numerous dispersed melanocytes invading deeply, indicating the vertical growth phase and a poor prognosis.

Pathology

Malignant melanocytes invade both epithelium and connective tissue. In the radial growth phase, they cluster along the basement membrane. In the invasive vertical growth phase, melanoma spreads into the connective tissue. The neoplastic melanocytes range from round to spindle-shaped cells with hyperchromatic and angular nuclei and usually granules of melanin (Figs 26.15 and 26.16). However, melanoma is highly variable and cells can be plasmacytoid, epithelioid or small clear cells, and mitotic activity may or may not be prominent.

Diagnosis is greatly helped by immunohistochemistry, which is often essential for confident diagnosis. The cells are positive for the immunohistological markers S-100, MelanA and SOX10.

Amelanotic melanomas

Approximately 15% of oral melanomas produce so little pigment that they appear red or reddish brown rather than grey, brown or black, causing difficulties in clinical diagnosis. Probably because of greater delay in diagnosis, the prognosis is appreciably worse than for these non-pigmented melanomas. In such cases, the diagnosis is rarely made until a biopsy and immunohistochemistry have been carried out.

Treatment

Oral melanomas are highly invasive, metastasise early and have a high mortality. Early diagnosis is critical to survival so that early biopsy of all oral pigmented lesions is essential.

As many as 50% of oral melanomas involve regional lymph nodes at presentation, and 20% have distant metastasis. Wide excision with, if possible, a 2–5 cm margin (often with a simultaneous neck dissection) followed by radical radiotherapy or chemotherapy or both is recommended.

The 5-year survival for node-negative patients may be 30%, but as low as 10% after metastasis. Many experimental treatments are in trial including chemotherapy, immunotherapy, immunostimulatory antibodies and novel biological agents targeting genes and signalling pathways.

Case series PMID: 7633281

Review PMID: 21540752 and 12744608

Treatment and survival PMID: 22349277

Summary chart 26.1   The common causes of oral pigmented lesions.

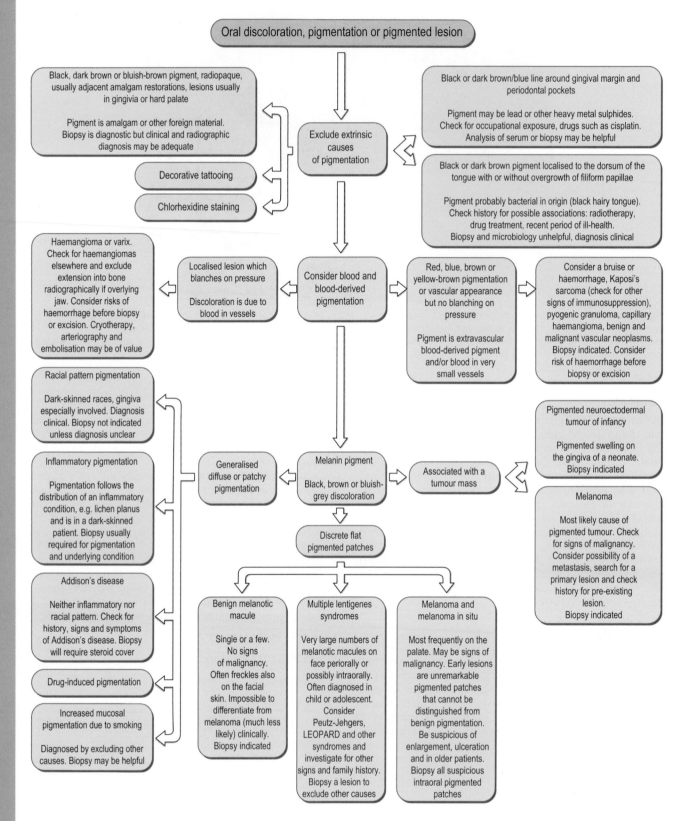

Oral discoloration, pigmentation or pigmented lesion

Black, dark brown or bluish-brown pigment, radiopaque, usually adjacent amalgam restorations, lesions usually in gingivia or hard palate

Pigment is amalgam or other foreign material. Biopsy is diagnostic but clinical and radiographic diagnosis may be adequate

Decorative tattooing

Chlorhexidine staining

Exclude extrinsic causes of pigmentation

Black or dark brown/blue line around gingival margin and periodontal pockets

Pigment may be lead or other heavy metal sulphides. Check for occupational exposure, drugs such as cisplatin. Analysis of serum or biopsy may be helpful

Black or dark brown pigment localised to the dorsum of the tongue with or without overgrowth of filiform papillae

Pigment probably bacterial in origin (black hairy tongue). Check history for possible associations: radiotherapy, drug treatment, recent period of ill-health. Biopsy and microbiology unhelpful, diagnosis clinical

Haemangioma or varix. Check for haemangiomas elsewhere and exclude extension into bone radiographically if overlying jaw. Consider risks of haemorrhage before biopsy or excision. Cryotherapy, arteriography and embolisation may be of value

Localised lesion which blanches on pressure

Discoloration is due to blood in vessels

Consider blood and blood-derived pigmentation

Red, blue, brown or yellow-brown pigmentation or vascular appearance but no blanching on pressure

Pigment is extravascular blood-derived pigment and/or blood in very small vessels

Consider a bruise or haemorrhage, Kaposi's sarcoma (check for other signs of immunosuppression), pyogenic granuloma, capillary haemangioma, benign and malignant vascular neoplasms. Biopsy indicated. Consider risk of haemorrhage before biopsy or excision

Racial pattern pigmentation

Dark-skinned races, gingiva especially involved. Diagnosis clinical. Biopsy not indicated unless diagnosis unclear

Inflammatory pigmentation

Pigmentation follows the distribution of an inflammatory condition, e.g. lichen planus and is in a dark-skinned patient. Biopsy usually required for pigmentation and underlying condition

Addison's disease

Neither inflammatory nor racial pattern. Check for history, signs and symptoms of Addison's disease. Biopsy will require steroid cover

Drug-induced pigmentation

Increased mucosal pigmentation due to smoking

Diagnosed by excluding other causes. Biopsy may be helpful

Generalised diffuse or patchy pigmentation

Melanin pigment

Black, brown or bluish-grey discoloration

Associated with a tumour mass

Pigmented neuroectodermal tumour of infancy

Pigmented swelling on the gingiva of a neonate. Biopsy indicated

Melanoma

Most likely cause of pigmented tumour. Check for signs of malignancy. Consider possibility of a metastasis, search for a primary lesion and check history for pre-existing lesion. Biopsy indicated

Discrete flat pigmented patches

Benign melanotic macule

Single or a few. No signs of malignancy. Often freckles also on the facial skin. Impossible to differentiate from melanoma (much less likely) clinically. Biopsy indicated

Multiple lentigenes syndromes

Very large numbers of melanotic macules on face periorally or possibly intraorally. Often diagnosed in child or adolescent. Consider Peutz-Jehgers, LEOPARD and other syndromes and investigate for other signs and family history. Biopsy a lesion to exclude other causes

Melanoma and melanoma in situ

Most frequently on the palate. May be signs of malignancy. Early lesions are unremarkable pigmented patches that cannot be distinguished from benign pigmentation. Be suspicious of enlargement, ulceration and in older patients. Biopsy all suspicious intraoral pigmented patches

Anaemias, leukaemias and lymphomas | 27

Haematological disease is common and can cause serious complications or oral symptoms (Box 27.1).

ANAEMIA

Causes and important types are summarised in Table 27.1.

Haemoglobin estimation and routine indices should be carried out when any patient has signs suspicious of anaemia in the mouth or has to undergo oral surgery.

Iron deficiency (microcytic) anaemia is the most common type and usually results from chronic menstrual blood loss. Males are more likely to have a cause such as peptic ulcer, haemorrhoids or bowel carcinoma.

Pernicious anaemia chiefly affects women of middle age or over and is the main cause of macrocytic anaemia. Unlike other anaemias, it can cause neurological disease.

Folate deficiency also causes a macrocytic anaemia, often in younger patients, particularly in pregnancy. It must be accurately differentiated from pernicious anaemia because administration of folate to the latter can worsen neurological disease.

Leukaemia is an uncommon cause of anaemia, but should be suspected in an anaemic child.

Sickle cell anaemia and trait are most common in those of African descent.

Thalassaemia is mainly seen in those from the Mediterranean area.

Clinical features

The skin complexion is a poor indicator of anaemia. The conjunctiva of the lower eyelid, the nail beds and, sometimes, the oral mucosa, are more reliable.

Anaemia, irrespective of cause, produces essentially the same clinical features (Box 27.2), particularly if severe, but some anaemias have distinctive features.

Glossitis and oral diseases (Box 27.3) can be the earliest signs.

Mucosal disease

Glossitis

Anaemia is the most important, though not the most common, cause of a sore tongue. It is discussed in detail in Chapter 17. Soreness *can precede a fall in haemoglobin*

Box 27.1   Important effects of haematological diseases

- Anaesthetic complications
- Oral infections
- Prolonged bleeding
- Mucosal lesions

Table 27.1   Types and features of important anaemias

Type of anaemia	Causes or effects
1. Iron deficiency (microcytic, hypochromic anaemia)	Usually due to chronic blood loss
2. Folate deficiency (macrocytic)	Pregnancy, malabsorption, alcohol*, phenytoin-induced, etc.
3. Vitamin B_{12} deficiency (macrocytic anaemia)	Usually due to pernicious anaemia, occasionally to malabsorption
4. Leukaemia and aplastic anaemia (normochromic normocytic)	Reduced erythrocyte synthesis, susceptibility to infection and bleeding tendency often associated
5. Sickle cell disease (normocytic anaemia)	Genetic. Haemolytic anaemia. Sickle cells seen in special preparations
6. Beta-thalassaemia (hypochromic, microcytic)	Genetic. Haemolytic anaemia. Many misshapen red cells
7. Chronic inflammatory disease (normochromic, normocytic)	Rheumatoid arthritis is a common cause
8. Liver disease (usually normocytic)	Haemorrhagic tendency may be associated

*Alcoholism should always be excluded when macrocytosis in the absence of anaemia is found – it is a characteristic sign of alcoholism.

Box 27.2   General clinical features of anaemia

- Pallor
- Fatigue and lassitude
- Breathlessness
- Tachycardia and palpitations

Box 27.3   Features of anaemia important in dentistry

Mucosal disease

- Glossitis
- Angular stomatitis
- Recurrent aphthae
- Infection, particularly candidosis

Risks from general anaesthesia

- Shortage of oxygen can be dangerous

Lowered resistance to infection

- Apart from candidosis, this is seen only in severe anaemia or when due to leukaemia

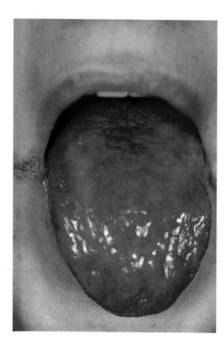

Fig. 27.1 Iron deficiency anaemia causing glossitis. See also Chapter 17.

levels, particularly when resulting from vitamin B$_{12}$ or folate deficiency, and can be their first sign. Later, there may be lingual atrophy (Fig. 27.1). Sore tongue always requires careful haematological investigation, by means of haemoglobin indices, serum iron, ferritin and folate levels. If any deficiency is found, the underlying cause must be investigated.

General nutritional deficiency PMID: 2693058 and 19735964

Pain and iron deficiency PMID: 10555095

Subclinical B12 deficiency PMID: 8600284

Recurrent aphthae

Aphthae are sometimes worsened by haematological deficiency, as discussed in Chapter 16.

Candidosis and angular stomatitis

Iron deficiency, in particular, is a predisposing factor for candidosis (Ch. 15). Angular stomatitis is also a classical sign of iron deficiency anaemia.

Dangers of general anaesthesia

Reduction of oxygenation in severe anaemia can precipitate brain damage or myocardial infarction. General anaesthesia, particularly in sickle cell disease, requires special precautions.

Lowered resistance to infection

Oral candidosis is the main example. Osteomyelitis can follow extractions in severe anaemia. Sickle cell disease is most important in this context.

SICKLE CELL DISEASE AND SICKLE CELL TRAIT

Sickle cell anaemia, caused by mutations in the HBB gene encoding beta-globin, mainly affects people of African,

---

Box 27.4   Factors that can precipitate sickling crises
- Hypoxia, particularly during anaesthesia
- Dehydration
- Infections (including dental)
- Acidosis and fever

Box 27.5   The main types of sickling crises
- Painful crises
- Aplastic crises
- Sequestration crises

Afro-Caribbean, Indian, Mediterranean or Middle Eastern origin. Approximately 13,000 persons in Britain are estimated to have sickle cell disease (homozygous mutation), and 250,000 sickle cell trait (heterozygous mutation). In sickle cell disease, abnormal haemoglobin (HbS) causes haemolysis, anaemia and other effects. In heterozygotes, sufficient normal haemoglobin (HbA) is formed to allow normal life.

Sickle cell disease

Deoxygenated HbS is less soluble than HbA and precipitates into long polymeric fibres that deform the red cells into sickle shapes* and make them vulnerable to haemolysis. Chronic haemolysis causes anaemia. Periodic exacerbation of sickling raises blood viscosity, causing blocking of capillaries and tissue ischaemia, called *sickling crises* (Boxes 27.4 and 27.5).

Patients, under normal circumstances, typically feel well but are predisposed to infection, particularly pneumococcal or meningococcal, and osteomyelitis.

Painful crises are caused by blockage of blood vessels and bone marrow infarcts. Painful crises can affect the jaws, particularly the mandible, and mimic acute osteomyelitis clinically and radiographically. The infarcted tissue forms a focus susceptible to infection,

Sequestration crises result from sickle cells pooling in the spleen, liver or lungs. Spleen infarction requires splenectomy, and this renders the patients prone to infection with encapsulated organisms for life; *Salmonella* osteomyelitis in bone infarcts is a recognised hazard.

Managing infection PMID: 26018640

Web URL 27.1 Description and genetics: http://omim.org/entry/603903

General review PMID: 15474138

Dental aspects

Enquiries should be made about family members with sickle trait when anyone in a predisposed genetic group requires anaesthesia or sedation. If the haemoglobin is less than 10 g/dL, the patient probably has sickle cell disease. Rapid screening tests show erythrocyte deformation when a reducing agent is added to blood, and haemoglobin electrophoresis confirms the diagnosis.

---

*Sickling was first identified in 1910 in the blood of a dental student from Grenada.

Sedation and general anaesthesia must be carried out with haemoglobin over 10g/dL, full oxygenation and hydration.

Radiographic changes were discussed in Chapter 13.

Occasionally, crises may be precipitated by dental infections such as acute pericoronitis. Prompt antibiotic treatment is therefore important, and facial cellulitis should prompt hospital referral for those with sickle cell disease.

Painful bone infarcts should be treated with non-steroidal anti-inflammatory analgesics, and fluid intake should be increased, with hospital admission if unresponsive.

Rigorous dental prevention is necessary because of the susceptibility to infection. Prophylactic antibiotics for dental interventions are not recommended.

Sedation relevance PMID: 22046909

Treatment, complications, review PMID: 7676364

Oral complications PMID: 8863314

THE THALASSAEMIAS

Alpha-thalassaemias mainly affect those of Asian or African descent, whereas beta-thalassaemias mainly affect those from Mediterranean countries. Diminished synthesis of one or more of the globin chains of haemoglobin causes the other alpha or beta globin chains to precipitate in erythrocytes. Haemolysis can result.

The severity of the disease depends on the numbers of alpha or beta globin genes affected. *Thalassaemia minor or trait* (in heterozygotes) causes mild but persistent microcytic anaemia but is otherwise asymptomatic apart, sometimes, from splenomegaly. Anaemia in mild alpha thalassaemia is easily mistaken for iron deficiency.

Thalassaemia major (usually homozygous beta-thalassaemia) causes severe hypochromic, microcytic anaemia, great enlargement of liver and spleen and skeletal abnormalities (Ch. 13). Regular blood transfusions are life-saving and prevent the development of bony deformities. However, progressive iron deposition in the tissues leads to dysfunction of glands and other organs, including salivary glands, causing xerostomia.

Frequent blood transfusions carry a risk of blood-borne virus infection if these have been performed in countries without blood screening. Sedation and anaesthetic management is as for sickle cell disease.

Craniofacial features PMID: 26219152

Dental implications PMID: 9161189

LEUKAEMIA

These malignant neoplasms of bone marrow overproduce one type of white cell and expand to replace the normal marrow, suppressing production of normal cells and platelets (Box 27.6). The excess white cells circulate in the blood (leukaemia means *white blood*). There are approximately 9000 cases each year in the UK.

Acute leukaemia → Summary chart 24.2 p. 373

Acute lymphoblastic leukaemia is the most common leukaemia in children (usually between 3 and 5 years old), whereas acute myeloblastic anaemia is the most common type in adults. Diagnosis depends on the peripheral blood picture and marrow biopsy. The following signs should raise suspicion of acute leukaemia (Table 27.2).

Box 27.6   Major effects of acute leukaemia

- Anaemia due to suppression of erythrocyte production
- Raised susceptibility to infection due to deficiency or abnormalities of granulocytes
- Bleeding tendency (purpura) due to suppression of platelet production
- Organ failure due to infiltration by leukaemic cells

Table 27.2   Features and causes for clinical features of leukaemias

Sign	Notes
Lymphadenopathy	Usually present, particularly in lymphocytic leukaemia, but may also be secondary to many infections
Anaemia	Mucosal pallor is an important sign in children, among whom anaemia is otherwise uncommon
Abnormal gingival bleeding	In a child, without other cause, strongly suggests acute leukaemia. Caused by thrombocytopaenia. Worse with poor oral hygiene
Gingival swelling	The gingivae become packed and swollen with leukaemic cells, particularly in acute myelogenous leukaemia in adults. Worse when oral hygiene is poor. The gingivae are often purplish and may become necrotic and ulcerate (Figs 27.2 and 27.3)
Leukaemic deposits	Tumour-like masses of leukaemic cells which may occasionally form in the mouth or salivary glands (Fig. 27.4)
Mucosal ulceration	Immunodeficiency caused by leukaemia predisposes to herpetic infections and thrush commonly but ulceration may be caused by a variety of other diseases. Also caused by cytotoxic drugs given for leukaemia
Purpura	Purplish mucosal patches, blood blisters, or prolonged bleeding after surgery result from thrombocytopaenia
Delayed healing	Caused by lack of normal white cells and leukaemic infiltration of the wound. Extraction sockets may be affected and acute osteomyelitis can result (Fig. 27.5)

Management

Being suspicious about features in Table 27.2 is key for early diagnosis. Gingival swelling unresponsive to conventional treatment requires a biopsy.

Any patient having cytotoxic treatment requires dental review and preventive treatment. Meticulous oral and dental hygiene control the bacterial population and prevent infectious complications (see Fig. 7.34).

During treatment, chlorhexidine mouthwash will often control severe gingival changes and superficial infections. Mucosal ulceration by Gram-negative bacilli or anaerobes may need specific antibiotic therapy. Oral ulceration caused by methotrexate may be controlled by folinic acid. Extractions and oral surgery must be deferred until remission, other than in an emergency, because of the risks of severe infections and bleeding.

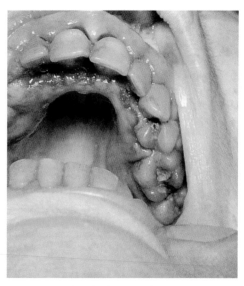

Fig. 27.2 Acute myeloid leukaemia. The gingiva are grossly swollen and purplish, and there is ulceration of the palatal aspect of the anterior teeth.

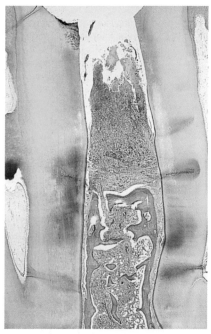

Fig. 27.3 Acute leukaemia. The gingiva, bone marrow and interdental bone contain a confluent infiltrate of leukaemic cells.

Chronic leukaemia

Chronic lymphocytic leukaemia is a slowly progressive disease of adults, can be asymptomatic and may not shorten life. Conversely, myeloid leukaemia becomes acute after a few years and necessitates chemotherapy or bone marrow transplantation.

Oral manifestations (Box 27.7) are relatively uncommon or mild.

Management

Routine dentistry can usually be carried out with normal care. If there is significant anaemia, bleeding tendency or susceptibility to infection, similar precautions need to be taken to those for acute leukaemia.

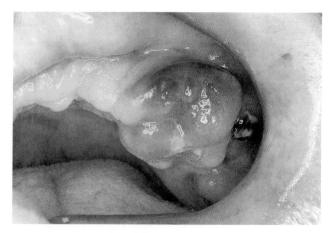

Fig. 27.4 Myeloid leukaemia. An ulcerated tumour mass formed by leukaemic cells emigrating into tissues and proliferating there.

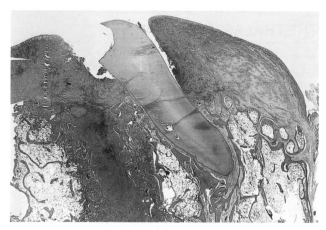

Fig. 27.5 Acute myeloid leukaemia. To the left of the remaining tooth root is a recent extraction socket. Leukaemic cells have densely infiltrated the gingiva and extraction socket, which has been prevented from healing.

Box 27.7 Possible oral effects of chronic leukaemia

- Mucosal pallor
- Gingival or palatal swelling in myeloid leukaemia
- Purpura
- Oral ulceration (ulceration may be due to infection or cytotoxic drugs or both)

Paediatric leukaemia dental considerations PMID: 1831649 and 10895145

Dental manifestations children PMID: 9177429

Dental management adults PMID: 25784937 and 25189149

LYMPHOMAS

Lymphomas are malignant neoplasms of lymphocytes that remain localised in bone marrow, lymph nodes and other organs. Classification is complex; only common and key types are discussed here.

Lymphomas often present with enlarged cervical lymph nodes but are rare in the mouth except those in HIV infection (Ch. 29). Most lymphomas in the head and neck arise from B lymphocytes. Their inappropriate cytokine secretion

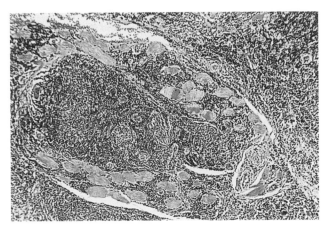

Fig. 27.6 High-grade non-Hodgkin lymphoma. Small darkly staining lymphoma cells infiltrating diffusely through muscle and destroying it.

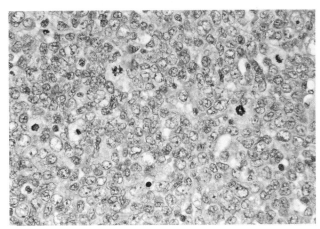

Fig. 27.7 High-grade non-Hodgkin lymphoma. Neoplastic lymphocytes with large vesicular nuclei are packed in a confluent sheet. Mitotic figures are numerous.

causes 'B symptoms', which are common features of Hodgkin's lymphoma and many B-cell lymphomas: intermittent fever, severe night sweats and weight loss.

The risk of developing a lymphoma is raised in the following conditions:

1. some of the primary immunodeficiency diseases
2. cytotoxic immunosuppressive treatment
3. HIV infection
4. connective tissue diseases, especially rheumatoid arthritis and Sjögren's syndrome
5. obesity

Review head and neck lymphoma PMID: 20374502

Hodgkin's lymphoma

Patients are either adolescents or young adults, or elderly. Three-quarters of patients present with, or have, enlarged cervical lymph nodes. Nodes are rubbery and mobile and often very large. The mouth is almost never involved.

Diagnosis is made on fine needle aspiration or node biopsy. Excision of cervical nodes is best avoided because of scarring.

Permanent cure of some types is possible, and the overall 5-year survival rate is 90% using irradiation and chemotherapy. Those treated with radiotherapy when young are at increased risk of thyroid and salivary gland tumours in later life.

Non-Hodgkin lymphomas

Adults are predominantly affected and, within the mouth, lymphomas form non-descript, usually soft, painless swellings, which may ulcerate and resorb adjacent bone. Many patients present with enlarged cervical lymph nodes as in Hodgkin's lymphoma.

There are many types classified by histology, expression of various lymphocyte cell surface marker proteins, proliferation rate and genetic changes.

The tissues contain sheets of diffusely infiltrative atypical lymphocytes (Fig. 27.6), sometimes with a follicular pattern like normal lymph nodes. The presence of necrosis, high mitotic activity and cytological atypia indicate high-grade lymphomas with a poorer prognosis (Fig. 27.7).

Lymphoma diagnosis is aided by immunohistochemistry (Ch. 1) revealing production of kappa or lambda light chains

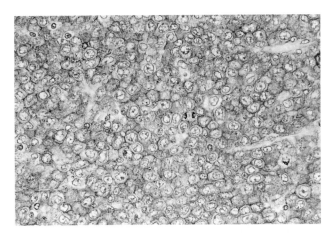

Fig. 27.8 High-grade lymphoma. Immunohistochemistry for a B-cell marker produces a ring of positive brown stain around the membrane of virtually every tumour cell, indicating their B-cell origin.

only, indicating the infiltrate to be monoclonal and markers to identify the type of lymphocyte (Fig. 27.8).

In general, localised disease is treated by irradiation, whereas disseminated disease (the majority of patients) is treated by combination chemotherapy. Oral ulceration and infection are common complications.

Burkitt's lymphoma

Burkitt's lymphoma is a B-cell lymphoma caused, in almost all cases, by Epstein–Barr virus infection in an immunocompromised host. It may be endemic, sporadic (rare) or immunodeficiency-associated. All are caused by chromosomal translocations that deregulate the c-myc transcription factor controlling cell proliferation and apoptosis.

In its endemic form, onset is in childhood, and incidence is high across a belt of tropical Africa, paralleling the incidence of malaria. Immunodeficiency-associated lymphoma usually arises in HIV infection or the immunosuppressed after transplants, an older age group.

Burkitt's lymphoma is predominantly extranodal. In the endemic form, the jaw is the single most common initial site and spread to the parotid glands is common.

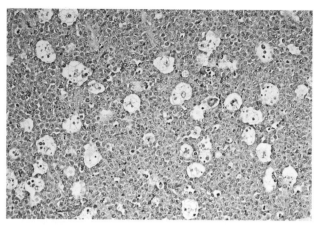

Fig. 27.9 Burkitt's lymphoma. Small darkly staining neoplastic lymphocytes form a sheet in which macrophages containing cellular debris form round pale holes, producing the 'starry sky' appearance.

Histologically, Burkitt's lymphoma comprises sheets of small lymphocytes containing scattered pale macrophages, which produce a so-called *starry sky* appearance (Fig. 27.9).

More than 95% of endemic cases respond completely to single-dose chemotherapy. Immunosuppression-associated cases have a poorer prognosis.

MALT lymphoma

MALT (mucosa-associated lymphoid tissue) lymphomas, or extranodal marginal zone lymphoma of MALT, develop from the marginal zone B lymphocytes that circulate through tonsils, Peyer's patches and other gut-associated lymphoid tissue to generate mucosal immune responses. Thus, these lymphomas usually arise in the stomach and small intestine rather than in lymph nodes. MALT lymphomas account for 10% of all non-Hodgkin lymphomas.

MALT lymphomas are unusual. They are mostly low grade and indolent, and survival is excellent even in disseminated disease. Some are associated with infectious causes. MALT lymphomas of the stomach are triggered by *Helicobacter pylori* infection, and elimination of infection can lead to regression of the lymphoma.

MALT lymphomas also arise in autoimmune diseases as a result of continuous antigenic stimulation, in the thyroid in Hashimoto thyroiditis and in salivary glands as a complication of Sjögren's syndrome.

Salivary MALT lymphoma usually presents as persistent painless swelling, sometimes with enlarged lymph nodes. MALT lymphoma complicates primary rather than secondary Sjögren's syndrome, and most patients are 50–65 years old at diagnosis.

Histologically, the salivary gland is replaced by sheets of small lymphocytes, many of which appear like monocytes and have a rim of clear cytoplasm. These neoplastic cells destroy the gland and infiltrate the residual ducts, which proliferate in response to form much larger epithelial islands. The islands of epithelium containing numerous lymphocytes are called *lymphoepithelial* ('epimyoepithelial') lesions. The MALT lymphoma is centred on these islands, but the remainder of the gland is replaced by non-neoplastic lymphocytes and lymphoid follicles, so that the gland comes to resemble a huge lymph node histologically.

Management

Any patient with primary Sjögren's syndrome and persistently swollen glands must be followed up and investigated with MALT lymphoma in mind.

Diagnosis is difficult, as Sjögren's syndrome itself causes replacement of the gland by lymphocytes. A biopsy of the tail of parotid is usual because fine needle aspiration cannot be used for diagnosis of low-grade lymphomas. Even histologically, the diagnosis is not always obvious and definitive diagnosis requires molecular analysis. Polymerase chain reaction analysis of the immunoglobulin chain gene rearrangements can identify that the lymphocytes are a clonal population. However, clones of cells can also develop in Sjögren's syndrome, as in all autoimmune diseases. Identifying early MALT lymphoma with certainty remains difficult.

The management of MALT lymphoma is also highly controversial. Patients tend to be treated by radiotherapy or chemotherapy, even though evidence suggests that the low-grade lymphomas progress very slowly. Some untreated patients have remained well for 30 years after diagnosis. Despite this indolent behaviour, MALT lymphoma can spread to other mucosal sites and can progress to high-grade lymphoma. All patients require long-term follow-up because high-grade transformation requires much more aggressive treatment.

Key features are shown in Box 27.8.

Lymphoma in Sjögren's syndrome PMID: 25316606

Salivary MALT lymphoma PMID: 26268740

Nasopharyngeal extranodal NK/T-cell lymphoma

These rare and very aggressive lymphomas start in the upper respiratory tract. They are commoner in those of Asian and South American origin and are strongly associated with, and probably caused by, Epstein–Barr virus infection. Presentation is usually after the age of 50 years.

The malignant cells may be natural killer or cytotoxic T cells, and they cluster around and within blood vessels in a dense mixed inflammatory infiltrate with many eosinophils. Obliteration of blood vessels leads to extensive ischaemic necrosis of tissues of the nasal wall, septum, sinuses, base of skull and palate, sometimes perforating the palate (Fig. 27.10). Symptoms are minimal initially, perhaps only stuffiness or epistaxis, but it is not unusual to discover a very large bony defect on imaging at presentation (see midfacial destructive lesions, Ch. 33).

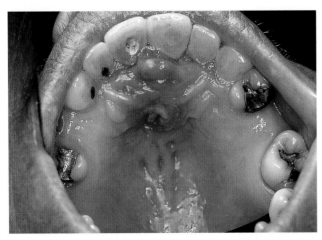

Fig. 27.10 **Natural killer/T cell angiocentric or nasopharyngeal type lymphoma.** Typical ulcer with minimal swelling in the midline of the palate caused by perforation through from the nasal cavity, where these lymphomas usually originate.

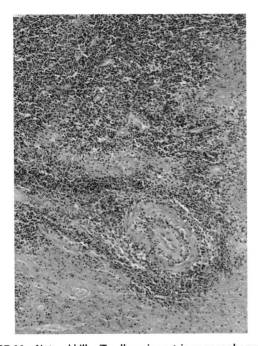

Fig. 27.11 **Natural killer/T cell angiocentric or nasopharyngeal type lymphoma.** A dense infiltrate of lymphocytes, within which are smaller numbers of the neoplastic cytotoxic T cells or natural killer cells, has infiltrated a vessel wall causing thrombosis and thus tissue necrosis, seen along the lower and right edges.

In their early stages, they can be indistinguishable clinically from Wegener's granulomatosis. However, they are anti-neutrophil cytoplasmic autoantibody-negative.

Diagnosis requires biopsy and immunohistochemical stains to identify the relatively small numbers of malignant cells present. Histological diagnosis is difficult because of the extensive necrosis, and several biopsies may be required to find affected vessels (Fig. 27.11).

Treatment is with radiotherapy combined with chemotherapy, and initial response rates are good, but the lymphoma eventually recurs and disseminates. Median survival

may only be 1 year, and only a third of patients are disease free at 2 years, and many of them relapse later.

Key features are shown in Box 27.9.

Oral presentations PMID: 9049909

Other types of lymphoma

Myeloma affects primarily bone and is discussed in Chapter 12.

Treatment in survivors PMID: 20059589

Non-Hodgkins treatment review PMID: 19101479

Oral Manifestations Hodgkin lymphoma PMID: 11885430

Oral complications Hodgkin lymphoma PMID: 10687450

LEUCOPENIA AND AGRANULOCYTOSIS

Leucopenia is a deficiency of white cells (fewer than 5000/μL) with many possible causes (Box 27.10). It is a peripheral blood manifestation of actual or incipient immunodeficiency and may result from destruction of bone marrow or loss of either the myeloid or lymphoid stem cells. Leukopenia requires adjustments to dental management (Box 27.11). Agranulocytosis typically presents with oropharyngeal ulceration.

Aplastic anaemia

Aplastic anaemia is rare, a failure of production of all bone
marrow cells (pancytopenia). The systemic and oral effects
are not unlike those of acute leukaemia (purpura, anaemia
and susceptibility to infection). Aplastic anaemia may be
autoimmune, viral or an effect of drugs.

Patients suffer anaemia, infections from lack of neutrophils and bleeding from lack of platelets. Without successful marrow stimulation, treatment of the cause or a
bone marrow transplant, approximately 50% of patients die
within 6 months, usually from infection or haemorrhage.

Agranulocytosis

Agranulocytosis is lack of granulocytes (neutrophils, eosinophils and basophils). Severe neutropenia causes fever,
prostration and mucosal ulceration, particularly of the gingivae and pharynx, and bacterial infections. Periodontitis is
accelerated; candidosis is frequent.

Cyclic neutropenia

In cyclic neutropenia, there is a fall in the number of circulating neutrophils at regular intervals of 3–4 weeks. This is
a rare disease; undue emphasis has been placed on the fact
that cyclic neutropenia occasionally, but not necessarily,
causes oral ulceration or rapidly progressive periodontitis.

Haemorrhagic disorders

PREOPERATIVE INVESTIGATION

When a patient gives a history of excessive bleeding, a careful history (Box 28.1) is absolutely essential.

The most common causes of bleeding for up to 24 hours after an extraction are local and should be manageable by local measures.

The majority of patients with more prolonged bleeding have acquired medical conditions, most are not severe and the medical history will normally reveal a cause. Conversely, the severe haemorrhagic diseases are mostly hereditary, and the cause also needs to be sought in the family history.

Prolonged bleeding is significant. Even a *mild* haemophiliac can bleed for weeks after a simple extraction, and minor oral surgery is often the first sign of these diseases.

Signs of anaemia and purpura should be looked for. Any extractions should be carried out at a single operation and radiographs taken to anticipate possible difficulties.

Laboratory investigations

Details of investigations are decided by the haematologists, but summarised in Box 28.2.

Box 28.1   Information required about haemorrhagic tendencies

- Results of previous dental operations? Have simple extractions led to prolonged bleeding?
- Has bleeding persisted for more than 24 hours?
- Has admission to hospital ever been necessary for dental bleeding?
- Have other operations or injuries caused prolonged bleeding?
- Is there a family history of prolonged bleeding?
- Are anticoagulants or other drugs being taken?
- Is there any medical cause such as leukaemia or liver disease?
- Does the patient carry a warning card or hospital letter about bleeding tendencies?

Box 28.2   Important investigations in haemophilia

- Haemoglobin level
- Cell and platelet counts
- Assessment of haemostatic function, particularly the
  - Bleeding time
  - Prothrombin time (expressed as the International Normalised Ratio)
  - Activated partial thromboplastin time (APTT)
  - Thrombin time
- Blood grouping and cross-matching

It is essential to look for anaemia. It is a result of repeated bleeding, increases the risks of general anaesthesia and is a feature of some haemorrhagic diseases.

Blood grouping is required in case transfusion is needed during or after operation, if blood loss is severe.

MANAGEMENT OF PROLONGED DENTAL BLEEDING

Some oozing is to be expected for 24 hours after extraction. Patients returning with prolonged bleeding from an extraction socket are a relatively common problem. It is not usually a real emergency, except to patients and accompanying friends or relatives. A small amount of blood diluted with saliva can appear significant and engender worry in patients and onlookers.

Bleeding starting a few hours after surgery is probably secondary to vasoconstriction wearing off. If no clot ever formed, and bleeding has been continuous, a coagulation defect is likely. Onset after a few days is likely to indicate infection.

If bleeding stopped and has restarted, do not waste time reapplying pressure, which is unlikely to be a definitive treatment. After local anaesthetic, clean the mouth and identify the source of bleeding, usually soft tissue. Any rough edges of the socket should be tidied up, the margins squeezed together and the soft tissue neatly sutured over it. A small piece of Surgicel, fibrin gauze or other proprietary haemostatic agent can be put in the socket mouth beforehand, but suturing is the essential measure, compressing the soft tissue. Soft tissue bleeding may also be reduced with electrocautery, laser or tranexamic acid if other methods fail. If there is a bleeding point in bone, it can be crushed with an instrument first. If this fails, a socket pack is required.

Take the pulse and blood pressure and, if significant blood loss is suspected, assess for shock.

Once this is done, enquiry should be made about the information in Box 28.1.

The patient should be kept under observation to ensure that bleeding has been completely controlled. Continued oozing of blood suggests some haemorrhagic disease and this, or a family history of this, is an indication for referring the patient to hospital, because prolonged dental bleeding is a recognised way in which haemophilia is sometimes first identified.

Post-extraction bleeding PMID: 24930250

BLOOD VESSEL ABNORMALITIES

Hereditary haemorrhagic telangiectasia

This is an uncommon autosomal dominant disorder caused by different mutations that weaken the walls of small blood vessels. Superficial telangiectases develop, particularly around the lips and in the nose and mouth and on the hands

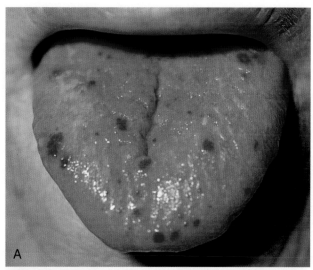

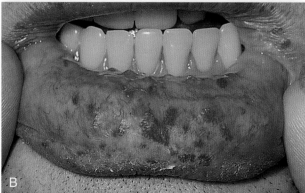

Fig. 28.1   Hereditary haemorrhagic telangiectasia. Two patients with multiple telangiectasias on tongue and lips. The distribution can vary between patients, not all have lip or perioral lesions. *(From Textbook of Physical Diagnosis: History and Examination, 'The Oral Cavity and Pharynx', 2006)*

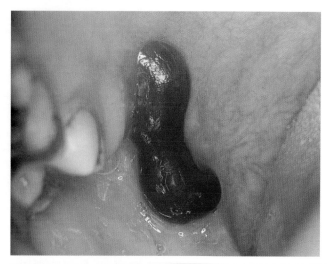

Fig. 28.2   Angina bullosa haemorrhagica. An intact blood blister on the soft palate and fauces.

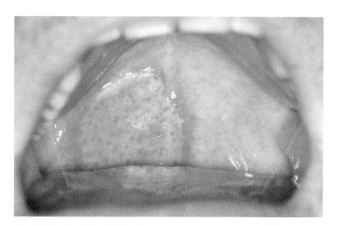

Fig. 28.3   Angina bullosa haemorrhagica. A ruptured blood blister has formed a large ulcer on the soft palate.

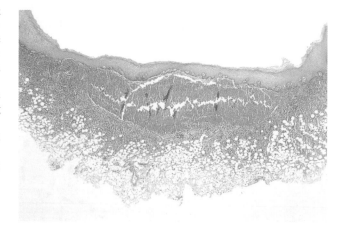

Fig. 28.4   Angina bullosa haemorrhagica. A blood-filled space lies immediately below the epithelium in this intact bulla.

(Fig. 28.1). Significant haemorrhage is rarely a problem, but intracranial or visceral bleeding can be dangerous, and intestinal bleeding causes anaemia. Nosebleeds are often the presenting sign. Cerebral abscesses may result from circulatory shunting, compromising bacterial clearance in bacteriaemias.

Oral surgery is generally safe, but regional anaesthetic blocks should be avoided because of the risk of deep bleeding into the soft tissues.

Cryosurgery or laser can obliterate superficial vessels that have bled significantly.

Similar mucosal changes may be present in patients with CREST syndrome (page 225).

Genetics and diagnosis PMCID: PMC4306304

Dental relevance PMID: 18230376

Angina bullosa haemorrhagica

Angina bullosa haemorrhagica* causes apparently spontaneous blood blisters in the oral mucosa, probably after minor trauma, but there is no haemostatic defect. Rupture of the blood blisters leaves an ulcer that heals without scarring (Figs 28.2–28.4). Older adults are affected, and blisters

are usually on the soft palate. They last a few hours or 2 days; patients often burst them to be rid of the discomfort. The condition has been linked to diabetes and steroid inhaler use, but the majority of cases remain unexplained.

The condition can be confused clinically with an immunobullous disease, usually pemphigoid.

Case series PMID: 25386327

---

*The name comes from the fact that blisters may form in the throat and cause a choking sensation. Angina originally meant choking or pain in the throat.

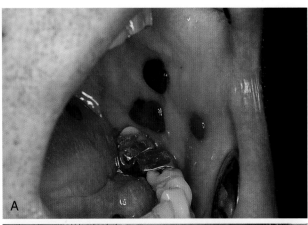

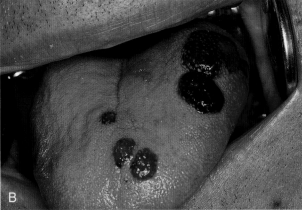

Box 28.3   Causes of purpura

Platelet disorders

- Idiopathic thrombocytopaenic purpura
- Conditions with splenomegaly
- Antiphospholipid syndrome
- Connective-tissue diseases (especially lupus erythematosus)
- Acute leukaemias
- Drug-associated
- HIV infection

Vascular disorders

- Von Willebrand's disease
- Corticosteroid treatment
- Ehlers–Danlos syndrome
- Infective
- Nutritional
- Hereditary haemorrhagic telangiectasia
- Scurvy
- Vasculitis, often allergic types

Ehlers–Danlos syndrome

The vascular presentation of this syndrome is noted in Chapter 14.

PURPURA AND PLATELET DISORDERS

Purpura is typically the result of platelet disorders (Box 28.3) and relatively rarely caused by vascular defects. As well as platelet aggregation, platelets contribute to coagulation.

General features of purpura

Purpura is bleeding into the skin or mucous membranes, causing petechiae or ecchymoses. It predicts prolonged bleeding after injury or surgery. Unlike haemophilia, haemorrhage immediately follows the trauma but, usually, bleeding in purpura ultimately stops spontaneously as a result of normal coagulation.

The bleeding time is prolonged and is the most informative test; clotting is normal. Platelet function tests and counts are a second step. Thrombocytopenia is defined as fewer platelets than 100,000/mm³, but spontaneous bleeding is uncommon until the count falls below 50,000/mm³.

Purpura forms at any site subjected to minor trauma, and the gingival margin is the most common site for bleeding (Fig. 28.5).

Management

For urgent operative treatment, platelet numbers frequently increase after systemic corticosteroids. Transfusion of platelet concentrate is usually reserved for emergency situations and those with very low counts, below 30,000/mm³. At levels between 50,000/mm³ and 100,000/mm³ oral surgery is safe, and local haemostatic measures alone are usually sufficient, although hospital-based care is prudent. Block analgesia carries risks at platelet levels below 50,000/mm³ and must be avoided below 30,000/mm³.

Tranexamic acid 5% mouthwash, four times per day, started just before surgery and continued for 2 days, is effective for most oral surgery.

As with other platelet disorders, aspirin and other anti-inflammatory analgesics should be avoided.

Fig. 28.5   Systemic purpura. (A) The lesions are due to spontaneous bleeding into the tissues and often form at sites of trauma. (B) Lesions on the tongue.

Causes of purpura

Idiopathic thrombocytopaenic purpura The cause is autoimmune destruction of platelets. Both children and middle-aged adults are predominantly affected. The first sign is usually purpura on the skin but may be profuse gingival bleeding or post-extraction haemorrhage.

Some cases resolve spontaneously, with thrombopoietin receptor agonist drugs Eltrombopag or Romiplostim that stimulate platelet production, or with splenectomy, which reduces platelet destruction.

AIDS-associated purpura Autoimmune thrombocytopenia can complicate HIV infection and can be an early sign. Purpuric patches in the mouth need to be distinguished from oral Kaposi's sarcoma by tests of haemostasis and, if necessary, biopsy.

Drug-associated purpura Many drugs, particularly aspirin, interfere with platelet function (Box 28.4). Others act as haptens and cause immune destruction of platelets or suppress marrow function causing aplastic anaemia, of which purpura is typically an early sign.

Fibrinolytic drugs, such as streptokinase, used in the acute treatment of myocardial infarction, are potential causes of bleeding tendencies, so dental surgery is possibly hazardous.

If purpura develops, the drug should be stopped but, in the case of aplastic anaemia, the process may be irreversible and fatal.

Tropical haemorrhagic fevers These rare diseases – Ebola, Lassa, Marburg and other fevers – are highly infectious,

Box 28.4   Some drugs causing thrombocytopenia or reduced platelet function*

- Aspirin
- Clopidogrel and the ADP receptor inhibitors
- Dipyridamole
- Glycoprotein inhibitors
- Non-steroidal anti-inflammatory drugs
- Loop and thiazide diuretics
- Colloidal gold
- Penicillins
- Quinine and quinidine
- Chemotherapy agents

*These usually do not result in purpura but extend the bleeding time. They should not be stopped for dental treatment.

Box 28.5   Important causes of coagulation defects

Heritable deficiencies of plasma factors

- Haemophilia A (by far the most important cause)
- Haemophilia B
- Von Willebrand's disease with low factor VIII levels

Acquired clotting defects

- Liver disease
- Vitamin K deficiency
- Therapeutic anticoagulation
- Disseminated intravascular clotting

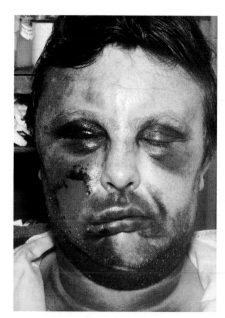

Fig. 28.6   Haemophilia. This was a mild and unsuspected haemophiliac who had never had any previous serious bleeding episodes. This enormous haematoma developed after a submucous injection for extirpation of an incisor pulp. *(By kind permission of Mr AJ Bridge.)*

Clinical features

Severity varies with the level and function of any factor VIII produced. Some patients have bleeding into muscles or joints after minor injuries in childhood. Others are asymptomatic and unrecognised until an injury, surgery or a dental extraction in adult life.

Typically, bleeding starts after a short delay as a result of normal platelet and vascular constriction, which provide the initial phase of haemostasis. There is then persistent bleeding which, if untreated, can continue for weeks or until the patient dies. Pressure packs, suturing, or local applications of haemostatics are ineffective.

Haemarthroses are well-recognised complications of uncontrolled haemophilia.

Frequent use of blood and blood products place haemophiliacs at risk of blood borne viral infections if the donations have not been screened. Formation of antibodies to factor VIII is another complication, and it reduces the effectiveness of treatment.

Principles of management

Patients must be identified by their history. Inheritance is an X-linked recessive trait, thus affecting mostly males. However, a third of cases are spontaneous mutations and have no family history. Severity in females is less than in males. A positive family history is always significant. By contrast, a patient who has had extractions without serious bleeding is not haemophiliac.

Patients require aggressive prevention and carefully planned treatment to minimise the number of admissions to hospital and episodes of factor VIII replacement. Treatment plans must emphasise prevention to minimise the risk of emergency treatment being required.

Severe and prolonged bleeding can follow local anaesthetic injections. Inferior dental blocks are most dangerous because of the rich plexus of veins in this area from which blood can lead down to the glottis. Even a submucous infiltration can occasionally have severe consequences (Fig. 28.6).

frequently fatal and a risk to healthcare workers. Extensive bleeding from orifices and internally is caused by infection of vessels causing their lysis. Guidance to healthcare workers is provided during outbreaks.

Scurvy is now of little more than historical interest. Defective collagen synthesis weakens blood vessels, and platelet function is impaired.

Extractions in thrombocytopaena PMID: 23932116

Dental treatment bleeding in HIV PMID: 18841624

Dentistry and antiplatelet drugs PMID: 12513936

Web URL 28.1 Guideline antiplatelet drugs: http://www.sdcep.org.uk/ and then enter 'anticoagulants' into search box.

CLOTTING DISORDERS

Important causes are shown in Box 28.5.

Haemophilia A

Haemophilia is the most common and severe clotting disorder. Haemophilia A (factor VIII deficiency) affects approximately 1 in 5000 males and is approximately 10 times as common as haemophilia B (Christmas disease, factor IX deficiency). In the past, extractions in haemophiliac patients have been fatal.

Box 28.6 Principles of dental management of haemophilia

- History
- Laboratory findings
  - Prolonged activated partial thromboplastin time
  - Normal prothrombin time
  - Normal bleeding time
  - Low factor VIII levels
- Liaison with patient's haemophilia centre
- Regular meticulous dental care to avoid the need for extractions
- Preoperative planning of unavoidable extractions or other surgery
- Preoperative replacement therapy
- Post-operative precautions

Box 28.7 Important acquired clotting disorders

- Vitamin K deficiency
- Anticoagulants
  - Coumarins
  - Dabigatran
  - Rivaroxaban and apixaban
  - Heparin
- Liver disease

Box 28.8 Current United Kingdom recommendations for treatment of patients on warfarin

- If the International Normalised Ratio (INR) is normally stable, check it 72 hours before surgery; if not stable, within 24 hours.
- Patients with INR <4.0 should not adjust dose for dental treatment.
- Minor oral surgery and scaling can be carried out in primary care if the INR is stable and below 4.0.
- Local haemostatic measures are sufficient.
- Follow surgical or periodontal procedures with 5% tranexamic acid mouthwashes four times per day for 2 days.
- Do not prescribe aspirin or non-steroidal anti-inflammatory drugs.
- Avoid inferior dental nerve blocks if the INR exceeds 3 and inject slowly in patients with INR less than 3.0. Use other local anaesthetic techniques where possible.
- Only a few teeth should be extracted at one session, usually no more than three at a time; avoid excessive trauma.

Intraligamentary analgesia is without risk. Gingival bleeding in periodontitis is increased, but must not inhibit tooth brushing.

Patients with mild (5%–40% factor VIII level) or moderate haemophilia (2%–5% level) can be managed routinely in dental practice. Extractions or treatment requiring inferior dental or lingual block analgesia or subgingival scaling of 6 mm pockets require factor VIII supplementation. The timing can be adjusted to be at the same time as any prophylactic cover given routinely, or patients may self-administer from their own stock. Severe haemophilia (less than 1% level) or those with antibodies or inhibitors require hospital care. Tranexamic acid mouthwash can be used but must be prescribed in hospital; a 7–10 day regime is recommended for haemophilia A. Desmopressin can be used to release body stores of factor VIII, reducing the requirement for supplementation.

As in all bleeding disorders, local measures must be followed, and aspirin and related analgesics should be avoided.

Principles for management in dentistry are shown in Box 28.6.

Christmas disease (haemophilia B)

Christmas disease is autosomal and has equal sex incidence. The bleeding disorder is clinically similar to haemophilia A, but milder. Factor IX fraction, fresh frozen plasma, tranexamic acid and desmopressin are all used, depending on severity, which is unpredictable from serum factor level.

Factor IX remains active in the blood for more than 2 days; replacement therapy can be given at longer intervals than for haemophilia A. Otherwise, management is similar.

Inherited defects dental management PMID: 24279214 and 24264665

ACQUIRED CLOTTING DEFECTS

Overall, these are more common than the inherited defects (Box 28.7).

Dental management anticoagulation PMID: 24120910

Web URL 28.2 UK guidelines: http://www.b-s-h.org.uk/ then enter 'anticoagulant dental surgery' into search box

Web URL 28.3 Scottish guidance: http://www.sdcep.org.uk/ and then enter 'anticoagulants' into search box.

Web URL 28.4 NICE guide and drug information: http://cks.nice.org.uk/anticoagulation-oral

Coumarin anticoagulant treatment

Coumarin anticoagulants, such as warfarin, are used to prevent thromboembolic disease in atrial fibrillation, for deep vein thrombosis, pulmonary embolism and prosthetic heart valves. The underlying condition may therefore influence dental management more than the treatment.

Anticoagulation is checked regularly to maintain the prothrombin time, and the patient should have a record card of the results. Many patients now self-test at home, and some adjust their own drug dose. If a practice has its own machine, it must follow a quality assurance scheme to ensure the accuracy of results.

The INR (International Normalised Ratio) prothrombin test is not highly reproducible to decimal places, and the overall trends and level of anticoagulation are more important than small changes in decimal places of the result. INR is maintained at 2–3 in most cases, but at 3–4 for those with prosthetic valves or recurrent embolism. Dental extractions can usually be carried out safely with an INR of 2–3, but the INR alone is not a completely reliable guide to haemostatic function. Adjusting the INR downward for treatment carries significant risks of thrombosis.

Current recommendations for treatment are shown in Box 28.8.

If serious bleeding starts, tranexamic acid can be given but, if otherwise incontrollable, vitamin K may be needed or fresh frozen plasma, depending on the INR.

Drugs prescribed in dentistry can enhance warfarin anticoagulation, notably antibiotics (erythromycin, metronidazole, ciprofloxacin) and azole antifungals. Significant increased anticoagulation has been reported following use of miconazole gel on a denture surface.

Novel anticoagulants

Dabigatran is a direct thrombin inhibitor. **Rivaroxaban** and **Apixaban** are inhibitors of factor Xa. These new agents are rapidly acting, have a short half-life and are used for similar indications as warfarin. They do not require close monitoring and regular dose adjustment like warfarin and are not subject to fluctuations in coagulation caused by vitamin K intake, bowel flora changes and drug interactions.

Little evidence base yet exists for oral surgery or dentistry for these agents. Being short-lived, the possibility of dose adjustment before surgery exists but would require advice from a haematologist. The INR cannot be used to monitor these drugs' effects, and no other test is effective. Until recently they were not reversible, but new antagonists are in trial, although they are unlikely to be used in a dental environment.

Routine treatment in primary care is unaffected, including extractions of up to three teeth and scaling, using precautions as for warfarin.

Novel anticoagulants and dentistry PMID: 26386350

Heparin

Short-term anticoagulation with heparin is given before renal dialysis and is effective only for about 6 hours. Extractions or other surgery can therefore be delayed for 12–24 hours after the last dose, when the benefits of dialysis are also maximal. Patients with renal failure also have mild anticoagulation and platelet defects as a result of their disease.

Otherwise heparin will have been prescribed because of a high risk of thrombosis and dental treatment is best avoided until anticoagulation is stabilised on another drug.

Liver disease

Viral hepatitis, alcoholism and obstructive jaundice are important causes of liver failure that result in inability to absorb and metabolise vitamin K, inhibiting synthesis of most clotting factors. Thrombopoietin production also reduces, leading to reduced platelet production. Haemorrhage can be severe and difficult to control. In severe cases vitamin K is valueless, but tranexamic acid and fresh plasma infusions may control bleeding.

A clotting screen is required in any patient with a history of alcoholism or liver failure. Those with jaundice may require vitamin K. Local measures should always be used.

Vitamin K deficiency

Causes include obstructive jaundice (usually from hepatitis, gallstones or carcinoma of the pancreas) or, less commonly, malabsorption. Long-term antibiotics can reduce the bowel flora, a significant source of vitamin K.

Extractions or other surgery should preferably be delayed until haemostasis recovers. Oral supplementation is effective, provided there is not significant liver disease.

COMBINED BLEEDING DISORDERS

Von Willebrand's disease

Von Willebrand's disease is a complex group of inherited disorders with both a prolonged bleeding time and deficiency of factor VIII. It is usually inherited as an autosomal dominant: both males and females are therefore affected. Many patients are asymptomatic until revealed by dental extraction.

Von Willebrand factor circulates bound to factor VIII, which it protects from degradation. It also binds to activated platelets, enhancing aggregation and activation. Lack of von Willebrand factor causes primarily a platelet functional defect, so that purpura and nosebleeds are the more common manifestations. Some patients have factor VIII levels low enough to cause a significant clotting defect.

Desmopressin nasal spray is effective but cannot be used in some rare types. Tranexamic acid and factor VIII may be required depending on severity and medical advice.

Diagnosis and management PMID: 25113304

Review PMID: 24762277

Disseminated intravascular coagulation

This disorder, also known as consumption coagulopathy, is an uncommon and complex acute disorder of haemostasis triggered by incompatible blood transfusions, severe sepsis, burns and trauma. The chronic form is usually seen in patients with cancer or large aortic aneurysms, and no clinical features may be evident.

Clotting in capillaries can damage the kidneys, liver, adrenal glands and brain in particular.

Consumption of platelets and clotting factors in the circulation, and activation of the fibrinolytic system, result in purpura and internal bleeding.

Complication of extraction PMID: 15772592

PLASMINOGEN DEFICIENCY

This rare autosomal recessive condition is not a haemorrhagic disorder but causes excessive and abnormal fibrin exudation at sites of inflammation or trauma. Mutations in the plasminogen gene reduce levels of plasmin formed to break down fibrin, control clot formation and allow maturation of the clot. Excess fibrin oozes from sites of chronic inflammation, particularly mucous membranes, forming large masses and also accumulates within the tissues.

In the mouth, the gingival margin is the usual site (Fig. 28.7). Apparently ulcerated masses of soft tissue originate at the gingival margin. Excision is associated with rapid recurrence. The eye is also frequently affected, and the fibrin here, and deposited in other mucosae, becomes hard, producing the condition of ligneous conjunctivitis. Other mucosal surfaces affected include nose, larynx, bronchi and vagina and cervix.

Histologically, the nodules comprise fibrin clot, often with hyperplastic strands of degenerate epithelium partly covering the surface. Fibrin leaks into the tissues and forms a deposit that resembles amyloid. Fresh frozen plasma can be used to supplement plasmin to cover surgical removal and prevent recurrence, but treatment is often unsatisfactory.

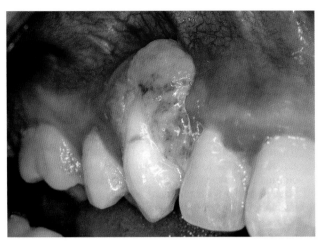

Fig. 28.7 Plasminogen deficiency. Fibrin exudation at the gingival margin.

The disease is sometimes called *ligneous gingivitis*, but this is a misnomer, as the deposits are not woody in consistency, as they are in the eye.

Many patients are of Turkish origin.

Review and treatment PMID: 18996031

Case report PMID: 19302964

Nature of lesions PMID: 21993334

IgA deficiency may facilitate absorption of allergens. There is predisposition to allergy, particularly asthma and eczema, and autoimmune disease, notably idiopathic thrombocytopaenic purpura and juvenile arthritis. Salivary and serum IgA deficiency appears to have no effect on dental caries or periodontal disease.

General review PMID: 24157629

C1 ESTERASE INHIBITOR DEFICIENCY

The familial form of this disease, hereditary angio-oedema, is, pedantically speaking, an immunodeficiency, but there is no abnormal susceptibility to infection. It is discussed in Chapter 30.

LEUKOPENIA AND AGRANULOCYTOSIS

Deficiency of circulating leucocytes is one cause of immunodeficiency. Causes and effects are discussed in Chapter 27.

IMMUNOSUPPRESSIVE TREATMENT

Bone marrow transplantation

Two main types of bone marrow transplantation are used. For congenital immunodeficiency a related donor is required (allogenic transplant). In some leukaemias, lymphomas and myeloma the patient's own stem cells can be harvested while the disease is in remission and reimplanted (autologous stem cell transplant). In this second type, the stem cells are harvested from blood after treatment to induce them to emigrate from the marrow.

During the transplant procedure there is total immunosuppression as the marrow is ablated by cytotoxic chemotherapy. An intensive preventive treatment is required while the immune system recovers during a few weeks or months after autologous transplantation or as long as a year in allogenic transplants.

Preoperatively, oral sources of infection should be eliminated and the mouth brought to as near perfect health as possible. Elimination of periodontal disease has a significant effect on lessening post-transplant complications.

Possible complications after transplantation are numerous (Box 29.4), particularly during the initial intensive phase of immunosuppression.

The main dental considerations are maintenance of meticulous oral hygiene, fluorides to control caries and prompt treatment of infections. Any oral surgery should be avoided during engraftment.

Box 29.4 Possible complications of bone marrow transplantation

- Oral complications
  - Mucositis, mucosal ulceration, haemorrhage, dry mouth, parotitis
  - Candidosis and bacterial infection
  - Gingival hyperplasia if ciclosporin is used
  - In children, dental hypoplastic defects may develop (chronological hypoplasia)
- Graft-versus-host disease
- Systemic infections (sometimes by oral bacteria)
- Tumours such as Kaposi's sarcoma or lymphomas

Oral effects stem cell transplant PMID: 24817792

Graft-versus-host disease

This is caused by transplanted immunocompetent cells mounting an immune response against tissues in their immunosuppressed host. It is, in effect, a graft rejection reaction in reverse. It most frequently follows bone marrow transplantation, both because of the deep immunosuppression and because of the many immunologically active cells produced by the implanted marrow.

The oral effects of graft-versus-host disease are a lichen planus-like disease, a Sjögren's-like syndrome with xerostomia, and a condition resembling systemic sclerosis with limited oral opening.

Graft-versus-host disease can be acute and self-limiting or chronic. Treatment is unpredictable.

Review oral lesions PMID: 9167093

OTHER ORGAN TRANSPLANTS

Transplantation of other organs, most frequently kidneys, is associated with similar complications to those of bone marrow transplantation. The main differences are that immunosuppression is less complete but has to be maintained indefinitely to prevent rejection. Initial suppression is with antibodies against T cells (basiliximab or daclizumab) followed by long-term ciclosporin, tacrolimus or mycophenolate.

The chief problems are therefore the enhanced susceptibility to infections and the greater risk of lymphomas. Gingival hyperplasia due to cyclosporin may be difficult to control, particularly after renal transplant when nifedipine is commonly given in addition.

HIV INFECTION AND AIDS

The most marked acquired immunodeficiency is AIDS caused by HIV infection. Oral features are important for diagnosis and staging.

AIDS/HIV infection was first recognised in 1981. It rapidly became a global pandemic that peaked in incidence around 1997 and is now in very slow decline (Fig. 29.2). It has become a disease of two populations.

The vast majority of new infections are in developing countries, particularly sub-Saharan Africa, which accounts for two-thirds of cases. There, limited healthcare and lack of education and understanding are associated with high infection rates and high mortality, although mortality has

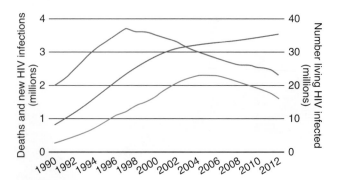

Fig. 29.2 The changing nature of the AIDS epidemic worldwide. Total new infections (*green*), deaths (*red*) and those living infected by HIV (*blue*).

reduced in some countries with access to antiretroviral treatment. In the richer nations of the developed world, HIV infection has become almost a treatable chronic disease, but there is evidence of a worrying resurgence in individuals who put themselves at high risk. The highest incidence areas are now sub-Saharan Africa, Russia, Eastern Europe and Southeast Asia. In some areas of Africa, nearly a third of the population is infected. Portugal has the highest incidence in Western Europe.

In 2013, there were just more than 100,000 individuals infected in the UK, 90% of whom were receiving antiretroviral treatment. Widespread access to testing may account for part of the fall in incidence, but approximately half of cases are still diagnosed in late disease, potentially having transmitted the infection for a prolonged period. It is hoped that the UK epidemic will continue to decline. The main barriers to this are discrimination, stigma and lack of knowledge. Although new infections overall are reducing, the number of individuals with HIV infection continues to increase because treatment increases their lifespan. Effective treatment also means that HIV infection now affects all age groups in the UK.

The main populations at risk in the UK are those of African descent and men who have sex with men. Drug users are now a very small risk group. Unfortunately, between 10%–25% of infected patients are unaware of their status, the percentage varying in different risk populations. A worrying rise in infection in men who have sex with men has just produced more than 3000 new cases in a year, the highest ever recorded. Just less than half of cases in the UK are transmitted heterosexually, and half of those are transmitted within the UK.

Web URL 29.1 Global epidemiology: http://www.who.int/gho/hiv/en/

Web URL 29.2 HIV in the UK: https://www.gov.uk/government/collections/hiv-surveillance-data-and-management

Web URL 29.3 HIV in the United States: http://www.cdc.gov/hiv/statistics/overview/

Aetiology

The HIV retrovirus is an RNA virus. Originally a pathogen of primates, it has successfully jumped species barriers several times and first infected humans early in the 20th century. The HIV-1 species is more virulent and accounts for most of the pandemic; HIV-2 is more or less limited to West Africa, is less infectious and causes less deep immunosuppression.

The chief mode of transmission is sexual. The risk of sexual transmission is higher in developing countries, probably because of the high incidence of other urogenital infections, particularly those that cause mucosal ulceration.

Direct spread to the baby occurs during pregnancy via the placenta, during birth and afterward by breast feeding. The risk of vertical transmission is approximately 30%, and this accounts for almost all cases of HIV infection in children.

Saliva is not infectious, unless contaminated with blood.

Life cycle

HIV directly infects cells, using its gp120 surface protein to bind to the cell CD4+ surface protein and chemokine co-receptors. Viral RNA is released into the cytoplasm of the cell, and viral reverse transcriptase generates viral DNA using the host cell synthetic pathways. The viral DNA integrates into the host genome and synthesises viral

components that assemble into new virus particles and are released from the surface coated in host cell plasma membrane.

Initially it is thought that dendritic antigen–presenting cells are infected in the mucosa and lymph nodes. These infect lymphocytes and macrophages by cell-to-cell contact during the process of antigen presentation. Free virus is also shed into the blood, but direct cell-to-cell transfer is much more efficient in spreading the infection through the body.

Each virus particle contains two RNA strands of slightly different sequence, and during reverse transcription the sequences are recombined to generate virus with a novel sequence. Mistakes in transcription are frequent. These mechanisms generate genetic variation while the virus replicates, and each patient becomes infected with multiple genetic variants of the virus. This genetic variability is important in generating resistance to antiretroviral drugs.

Only a minority of infected cells produce new virus; the majority die through a process called *pyroptosis*. This is a variant of apoptosis, in which the cells detect that their DNA has been damaged and undergo apoptosis mediated by the enzyme caspase 1, rather than the usual apoptotic pathway mediated by caspase 3. Unlike conventional apoptosis, in which the dying cell debris is cleanly disposed of, pyroptosis causes cell lysis and inflammation, attracting further lymphocytes and macrophages that become infected. This cycle of infection and destruction of CD4+ cells slowly reduces the helper T-cell count and reverses the ratio of helper to suppressor lymphocytes.

The effect of depletion of T-helper cells is depression of cell-mediated immunity and progressive immunodeficiency.

The humoral immune system is also affected. Apparently paradoxically, there is polyclonal B-lymphocyte activation resulting in hypergammaglobulinaemia and autoantibody production. Antibody is produced in response to the virus but is not protective initially. After several years, some mildly protective antibodies may develop and slow progression, but antibodies indicate only that a patient is infected.

The human immunodeficiency virus also attacks the central nervous system. Virus is carried to the brain in infected macrophages and infects glial cells, which carry receptors for the virus.

Basic biology of HIV PMID: 24162027

Diagnosis of HIV infection

Testing for HIV infection has been surrounded by stigma and previously required formal counselling before testing. However, current practice in the UK is to offer testing as widely as possible in an effort to reduce late diagnosis. The majority of patients who die of AIDS have been diagnosed late.

The UK national testing action plan suggests that 'opt-in' testing schemes should be replaced with 'opt-out' schemes in which patients are offered HIV testing alongside other routine medical tests and must actively refuse the test. This has proved extremely successful in antenatal testing and is also recommended for all new general medical practice registrations, all surgical hospital admissions, drug dependency schemes and services for those with blood-borne viral infection, TB or lymphoma. HIV testing needs to become routine.

A range of tests are available. Antibodies appear approximately 6–8 weeks after infection and persist for life. Tests may detect antibody or viral RNA/DNA. Detection of antibody alone by enzyme-linked immunosorbent assay

Table 29.1   HIV disease stage for adults*

Stage	CD4+ cells/μL	% total lymphocytes CD4+
1	≥500	≥26
2	200–499	14–25
3 (AIDS)	<200	<14

*CD4+ absolute counts take precedence over percentage of lymphocytes. Patients must also be positive for HIV infection.

Box 29.5   In an adult patient with a positive HIV test, the following indicate stage 3 HIV infection*

- Bacterial infections, multiple or recurrent
- Candidosis of bronchi, trachea, or lungs
- Candidosis of oesophagus
- Cervical cancer, invasive
- Coccidioidomycosis, disseminated or extrapulmonary
- Cryptococcosis, extrapulmonary
- Cryptosporidiosis, chronic intestinal
- Cytomegalovirus disease (other than liver, spleen, or nodes)
- Cytomegalovirus retinitis (with loss of vision)
- Encephalopathy attributed to HIV
- Herpes simplex: chronic ulcers (>1 month's duration)
- Histoplasmosis, disseminated or extrapulmonary
- Isosporiasis, chronic intestinal (>1 month's duration)
- Kaposi sarcoma
- Lymphoma, Burkitt or immunoblastic
- Lymphoma, primary, of brain
- Atypical mycobacterium infection, disseminated or extrapulmonary
- Mycobacterium tuberculosis of any site, pulmonary, disseminated, or extrapulmonary
- *Pneumocystis jirovecii* (*Pneumocystis carinii*) pneumonia
- Pneumonia, recurrent
- Progressive multifocal leukoencephalopathy
- Salmonella septicemia, recurrent
- Toxoplasmosis of brain
- Wasting syndrome attributed to HIV

*Simplified Centers for Disease Control criteria. Several of these AIDS-defining illnesses can be detected in the mouth.

(ELISA)-based tests requires confirmation by Western blotting or immunofluorescence. Viral load testing to monitor treatment and progression is performed by measuring viral nucleic acids.

Caution is required in use of some rapid screening techniques and home testing kits based on blood or saliva as these have worrying false-negative rates.

HIV staging and diagnosis of AIDS

AIDS is the symptomatic period of HIV infection. In developing countries it is defined clinically by the presence of opportunistic infections alone; developed countries use the Centers for Disease Control system based on laboratory tests (Table 29.1) and infections (Box 29.5). Staging of HIV infection is important for selecting patients for treatment and assessing prognosis and for epidemiological studies. AIDS is equivalent to HIV infection stage 3.

In children, HIV infection is staged N (non-symptomatic infection) or A to C based on specific infections.

CDC AIDS definition PMID: 24717910

Clinical course

After HIV infection there is a short incubation period, followed by an acute disseminated infection and then a long latent period until opportunistic infections arise.

Approximately half of patients develop an acute glandular fever-like illness 2–4 weeks after exposure with fever and headache, tender lymphadenopathy, throat inflammation and a rash. The features are non-specific and easily misdiagnosed or ignored. Symptoms last 1–2 weeks, and those whose illness lasts longer than 14 days progress more rapidly to stage 3. The patient is highly infectious during the acute illness. Antibodies develop, and virus is detectable during the acute phase (also known as 'seroconversion illness').

This is followed by a prolonged latent period during which CD4+ lymphocyte numbers slowly decline but immune responses are sufficient to prevent opportunistic infection. Approximately two-thirds of patients develop persistent lymphadenopathy during this period. Note that the term *latent period* relates to *clinical* latency, and that the patient is infectious during the latent phase. This is different from viral latency, as seen in herpes viruses, during which the patient is not infectious.

The latent phase lasts on average approximately 8 years but is very variable in duration. Some patients, termed *long-term non-progressors*, may remain in the latent phase for 25 years or longer as a result of polymorphisms or mutations in viral receptors or by producing weakly protective antibody. Only approximately 1 in 300 infected individuals are long-term non-progressors; the vast majority of infected patients progress to symptomatic infection, otherwise known as stage 3 or AIDS.

AIDS is characterised by multiple infections by bacteria, fungi, parasites and viruses. These tend to become symptomatic when the CD4+ cell count falls below 300 cells/μL. Many of these infections, such as *Pneumocystis* pneumonia, are opportunistic and almost unknown in immunocompetent persons. Almost any commensal or pathogenic species can cause infections, including species normally considered environmental organisms. The infections are more severe and more difficult to treat than in the immunocompetent and often in unusual body sites. Non-specific fever, diarrhoea and weight loss are common.

Though infections are the main cause of death, there is also a greatly raised incidence of tumours, particularly Kaposi's sarcoma and lymphomas because these are caused by infectious agents, notably Epstein–Barr virus. Plasmablastic lymphoma has a predilection for the oral cavity and is virtually only seen in HIV infection.

Neuropsychiatric disease in AIDS can range from depression to dementia and death.

A lesser manifestation of AIDS in some patients is autoimmune disease, particularly thrombocytopenic purpura or, less frequently, a lupus erythematosus-like disease.

Once AIDS has developed, the outcome *without treatment* is death within 2 years, approximately 10 years after initial infection.

The outcomes are summarised in Fig. 29.3.

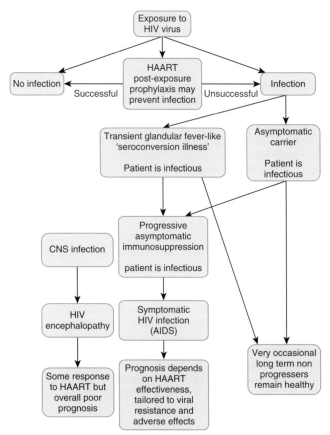

Fig. 29.3 Outcomes of HIV infection.

> **Box 29.6   Antiretroviral drugs used for highly active antiretroviral treatment and some oral adverse effects**
>
> **Entry inhibitors**
> - Maraviroc
> - Enfuvirtide
>
> **Nucleoside/nucleoside reverse transcriptase inhibitors**
> - Abacavir (Stevens–Johnson syndrome)
> - Lamivudine
> - Zidovudine
> - Emtricitabine
> - Tenofovir
>
> **Non-nucleoside reverse transcriptase inhibitors**
> - Nevirapine (Stevens–Johnson syndrome)
> - Efavirenz (Stevens–Johnson syndrome)
> - Etravirine
> - Rilpivirine
>
> **Protease inhibitors**
> - Indinavir (dry mouth, taste disturbance)
> - Nelfinavir
> - Ritonavir (taste disturbance, circumoral paraesthesia)
> - Saquinavir (oral ulceration)
> - Darunavir
> - Atazanavir
>
> **Integrase inhibitors**
> - Raltegravir
> - Elvitegravir
> - Dolutegravir

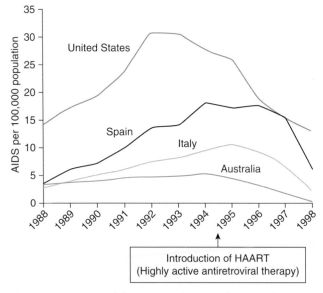

Fig. 29.4   Progress of the AIDS epidemic. Before and after highly active antiretroviral treatment in developed nations.

Treatment

Effective treatment of HIV infection is provided by highly active anti-retroviral treatment (HAART), regimes of combinations of antiretroviral drugs with different modes of action. These have changed prevention and treatment dramatically since their introduction (Fig. 29.4).

A plethora of antiretroviral drugs is available. They fall into five main classes, and some important oral adverse effects from the drugs mentioned in Box 29.6 are indicated in brackets. New drugs are constantly being introduced.

Treatment should start as early as possible because this is more effective and also reduces transmission of infection to others. The drugs must be changed repeatedly because the high viral mutation rate constantly produces resistant strains. Treatment cannot be stopped without risking emergence of highly resistant strains, which can infect others, and the drugs are best continued for life. The exact combination of drugs used varies from country to country.

Problems with these drugs include many adverse effects that can limit patient tolerance. HAART can never cure the infection, it only suppresses viral replication and delays onset of immunosuppression. The virus remains integrated into the host cells and currently cannot be eradicated.

Provided the viral load can be suppressed, patients with HIV can expect to avoid death from AIDS and live a normal life span, but are at risk of adverse drug effects, neurological effects and increased rates of hypertension, heart disease and diabetes. HIV infection is now a medically managed chronic disease.

Key features of AIDS are summarised in Box 29.7.

ORAL LESIONS IN HIV INFECTION

More than 75% of patients with AIDS have orofacial disease (Box 29.8).

Since the introduction and improvements in HAART, the frequency of HIV-related oral lesions is declining.

Box 29.7   AIDS: key features

- Caused by a retrovirus – usually HIV-1
- Transmitted sexually, during pregnancy, at birth or in breast milk
- Acute seroconversion disease like glandular fever
- Long clinical latent period
- Progressive deterioration mainly of cell-mediated immunity
- Immunodeficiency leads to opportunistic infections
- Common oral lesions include candidosis and hairy leukoplakia
- Kaposi's sarcoma and lymphomas, often in oral regions
- Neurological and psychological disorders
- Effectively treated with highly active antiretroviral treatment

Box 29.8   Oral disease in HIV infection (EC Clearinghouse 1993)

Lesions strongly associated with HIV infection

- Candidosis, erythematous and pseudomembranous
- Hairy leukoplakia
- Kaposi sarcoma
- Non-Hodgkin's lymphoma
- Periodontal disease
- Linear gingival erythema
- Necrotising (ulcerative) gingivitis and periodontitis

Lesions less commonly associated with HIV infection

- Mycobacterial infections
- Melanin pigmentation
- Necrotising (ulcerative) stomatitis
- Xerostomia
- HIV salivary cystic disease
- Thrombocytopenic purpura
- Ulceration, non-specific
- Viral infections
- Herpes simplex
- Condyloma acuminatum
- Multifocal epithelial hyperplasia
- Papillomas
- Varicella zoster infections

Lesions seen in HIV infection

- Bacterial infections
  - Actinomyces israelii
  - Escherichia coli
  - Klebsiella pneumoniae
- Cat scratch disease
- Drug reactions
- Bacillary angiomatosis
- Other fungal infections
- Facial palsy
- Trigeminal neuralgia
- Recurrent aphthous stomatitis
- Cytomegalovirus infection
- Molluscum contagiosum

However, many patients on HAART still develop oral manifestations.

Undiagnosed HIV disease still presents with oral signs, and it is possible to diagnose HIV infection on the basis of oral signs. These same signs are also seen in those in late disease with treatment failure.

The accepted list of oral conditions associated with HIV infection is now old but remains a useful categorisation for clinical use. The conditions strongly associated with HIV infection remain significant. A third of those on HAART still have oral lesions, mostly oral candidosis. Ulcers affect approximately 5%, and Kaposi's sarcoma and hairy leukoplakia each affect approximately 1%–5% of those on HAART. In the developing world, oral manifestations appear to be more common.

Oral manifestations are likely when the circulating CD4$^+$ lymphocyte count falls below 200/mm^3, the viral load exceeds 3000 copies/mL or the patient also has other predisposing factors such as dry mouth. Although oral lesions should be a good marker of the failure of HAART, no definite predictors are known. However, it would be prudent to report any increase in, or new, oral manifestations (other than papillomas, see later) to the patient's HIV physician. Onset of signs such as recurrent candidosis or hairy leukoplakia often coincides with a rise in circulating viral copy number as the disease progression accelerates. For a patient on HAART, this indicates emergence of a new genetic variant and a need to consider changing drugs to regain control of viral replication.

Oral manifestations PMID: 8229864

Oral Manifestations controversies PMID: 23517181

Since HAART PMID: 12656429

Candidosis

Thrush or other forms of oral candidosis may be seen in more than 50% of patients at some stage, regardless of HAART, and candidosis is often the first oral sign. With HAART, candidosis is now usually chronic or erythematous in type (Fig. 29.5). Decline in incidence of thrush may be partly an effect of antiretroviral protease inhibitors on the fungi, as well as improved immune status.

Erythematous infections respond to topical antifungals. It has recently been suggested that HIV-infected patients require no longer courses of antifungals than non-HIV

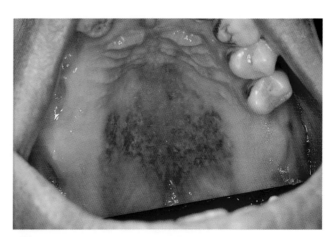

Fig. 29.5   Erythematous candidosis. An extensive red patch on the palate without white flecks which appears as denture stomatitis but without any denture being worn. Such a presentation is characteristic of immunodeficiency.

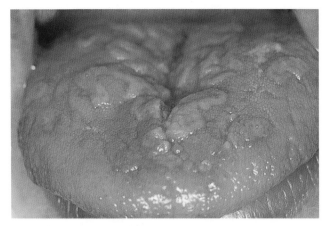

Fig. 29.6 Herpes simplex ulceration in immunodeficiency. There is extensive ulceration along the midline of the dorsal tongue and separate ulcers toward the lateral margins. In immunodeficiency, the ulcers may be chronic and their clinical appearance may not suggest viral infection. Biopsy may be required for diagnosis.

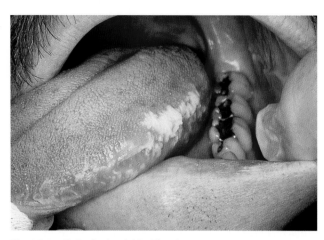

Fig. 29.8 Hairy leukoplakia. The characteristic appearance on the lateral margin of the tongue. Posteriorly, the vertical ridging pattern of the lateral tongue is enhanced. *(By kind permission of Professor WH Binnie.)*

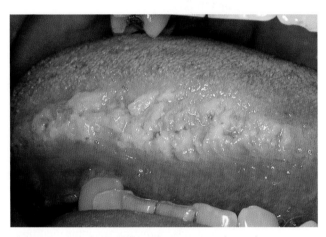

Fig. 29.7 Hairy leukoplakia. Close-up view shows the corrugated surface and suggests the soft texture of the lesion.

infected patients. A single dose of 750 mg fluconazole may be effective, but other factors such as smoking, dry mouth or denture wearing may need to be taken into account.

Linear gingival erythema, previously thought a bacterial infection or type of gingivitis, is now thought to be candidosis (later in this chapter).

Viral mucosal infections

Herpetic stomatitis is less common than might be expected and causes chronic ulceration unlike the typical infection (Fig. 29.6). Those with HIV are at greater risk of intraoral secondary herpes infection. Severe orofacial zoster indicates disease progression and a poor prognosis.

The Epstein–Barr virus (EBV) is the cause of hairy leukoplakia which is highly characteristic of HIV infection (Figs 29.7 and 29.8).

HIV-infected patients have an increased risk of papillomas. Counterintuitively, treatment with HAART causes a much higher risk of oral warts of all types, verruca vulgaris, condyloma acuminatum and focal epithelial hyperplasia. This appears to be an adverse effect of immune reconstitution. After HAART, papillomas can be very numerous or form large confluent patches that are very difficult to

eradicate. Repeated excisions, cryosurgery or laser ablation may only keep them under control.

Oral hairy leukoplakia is discussed in Chapter 18.

Bacterial infections

Infections by bacteria that otherwise rarely involve the oral tissues, such as *Klebsiella pneumoniae*, *Enterobacter cloacae* and *Escherichia coli*, can develop. In the later stages, there may be ulcers secondary to systemic infections, particularly mycobacterial.

Bacillary angiomatosis is a vascular proliferative disease caused by *Bartonella henselae* and should respond to antimicrobial therapy. However, it can mimic Kaposi's sarcoma clinically and, to some extent, histologically. It affects the skin more frequently than the oral cavity.

Systemic mycoses

Histoplasmosis or cryptococcosis can give rise to proliferative or ulcerative lesions. Histoplasmosis most frequently affects the palate, gingivae and oropharynx.

Malignant neoplasms

Kaposi's sarcoma → Summary chart 26.1 p. 390

This is mainly seen in men who have sex with men. Despite reduced incidence following introduction of HAART, this is still the commonest oral malignant neoplasm in HIV infection.

Kaposi sarcoma is also very occasionally seen in HIV-negative immunosuppressed organ transplant patients, but one in the mouth of a young or middle-aged male is virtually pathognomonic of HIV infection. It is usually associated with a CD4$^+$ lymphocyte count of less than 200/μl and frequently associated with other effects of HIV infection such as candidosis, hairy leukoplakia or HIV-associated gingivitis.

Although oral Kaposi's sarcoma may be the presenting complaint, the tumour is usually multifocal, with lesions affecting skin, lymph nodes and viscera.

Head and neck sites are typically oropharyngeal, cutaneous or in the cervical lymph nodes. Within the mouth, the palate is the most frequently affected site and the tumour produces a flat or nodular purplish lesion. The clinical differential diagnosis is from oral purpura, bacillary angiomatosis and pyogenic granulomas, from which it can be distinguished by biopsy (Ch. 25).

Lymphomas

These develop in intraoral sites or salivary glands far more frequently than in HIV-negative persons. Typical sites within the mouth are the palate or gingiva, causing soft painless swellings that ulcerate when traumatised.

Most lymphomas in AIDS are high-grade B-cell lymphomas of large cell or immunoblastic type, and many are caused by EBV infection. Lymphomas are increasingly the first presenting sign of HIV infection but are overall are rarer since HAART.

Burkitt's lymphoma is the second commonest lymphoma in HIV-positive persons and carries a poor prognosis.

Plasmablastic lymphoma is seen virtually only in HIV-positive persons and has a strong predilection for the oral cavity. It is caused by coinfection with HIV and EBV and, unlike other lymphomas, has increased since HAART was introduced.

Lymphomas combined with immunosuppression used to have a dire prognosis, but with HAART they have much the same prognosis as in the non-HIV population.

Plasmablastic lymphoma PMID: 21783402

Lymphadenopathy

Lymphadenopathy is characteristic of AIDS and its prodrome. Cervical lymphadenopathy is probably the most common head and neck manifestation of HIV infection.

The nodes have reduced T-helper cells in the paracortical region and greater numbers of T-suppressor cells there and in the follicles. The nodes are enlarged initially because of hyperplasia but later undergo involution and contain dendritic antigen-presenting cells infected with HIV virus. Untreated, the lymph nodes become virtually or entirely functionless.

Enlarged cervical lymph nodes can also be due to lymphomas.

Autoimmune disease

The most common autoimmune phenomenon in AIDS is thrombocytopenic purpura (Fig. 29.9). This can give rise to oral purple patches that may be mistaken for Kaposi's sarcoma, petechiae or blood blisters. Other autoimmune diseases reported in AIDS are lupus erythematosus and a Sjögren's-like salivary gland disease.

Gingivitis and periodontitis

HIV-related periodontal disease includes necrotising gingivitis and periodontitis and accelerated periodontitis (Ch. 7). Necrotising ulcerative periodontitis (NUP) indicates marked immunosuppression and a poor prognosis. The causative organisms are as in immunocompetent patients, and there is marked pain with local bone loss, tooth mobility, ulceration and bleeding (Fig. 29.10). Systemic metronidazole or penicillin with topical povidone iodine or chlorhexidine are rapidly effective.

Linear gingival erythema is a controversial entity currently considered a manifestation of candidosis in the gingival crevice and attached gingiva. Scaling, improved oral hygiene and chlorhexidine is usually effective, but antifungals may be required. Linear gingival erythema usually affects the anterior region. Whether candidal infection accounts for all cases is unclear as the diagnostic criteria are not very specific.

Types of gingivitis and periodontitis seen in HIV infection are summarised in Summary chart 29.1.

Review PMID: 22909108 and 23755999

Salivary gland disease

Chronic parotitis in children, possibly due to EBV or cytomegalovirus, is almost pathognomonic of HIV infection.

A Sjögren's-like syndrome with xerostomia, but lacking the characteristic autoantibodies (particularly SS-A and SS-B), can affect adults.

HIV-associated salivary gland disease

→ Summary chart 22.2 p. 354

This disease affects primarily children and young adults with HIV infection, causing chronic soft parotid enlargement of one or both glands, sometimes painful. Additionally, xerostomia is seen in adults. As many as 20% of HIV-positive children are affected. The disease has increased

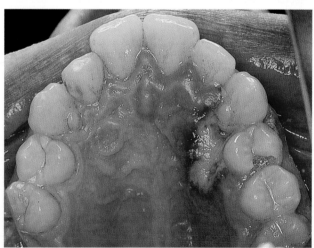

Fig. 29.10 HIV-associated necrotising periodontitis. Soft tissue and bone are lost virtually simultaneously, and tissue destruction of the degree shown here can take only a few months. A low CD4$^+$ count and a poor prognosis are typically associated.

(By kind permission of Professor WH Binnie.)

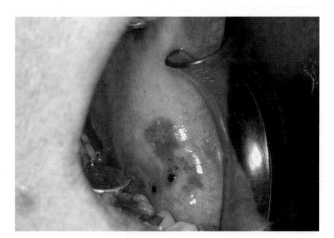

Fig. 29.9 Purpura. Patches such as these in AIDS can be mistaken for Kaposi's sarcoma.

Summary chart 29.1   Types of gingivitis and periodontitis seen in HIV infection.

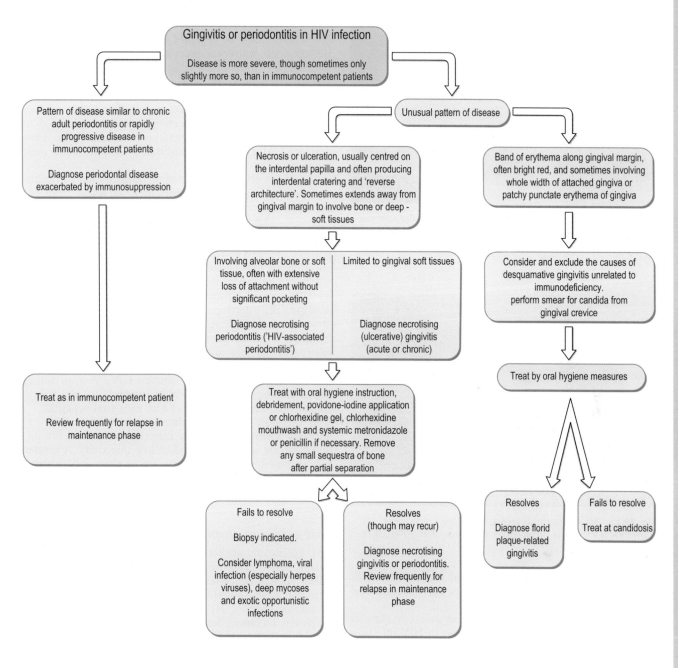

in incidence since antiretroviral therapy was introduced, suggesting it is an infection, and the BK virus has been implicated.

The glands are infiltrated by CD8+ T cells, mostly memory T cells, an HIV effect called *diffuse CD8+ lymphocytosis syndrome* that affects many organs. The T cells localise around ducts, kill and replace the acini and cause fibrosis in a similar manner to Sjögren's syndrome. In addition, there is hyperplasia of the intraparotid lymph nodes and development of new lymphoid tissue with lymphoid follicles in the gland. The ducts enlarge to form numerous cysts. Salivary secretion is reduced.

Ultrasound scans and the clinical presentation are usually sufficient for diagnosis, but if HIV infection is not suspected, biopsy shows the typical features and HIV p24 protein can be identified by immunohistochemistry in the lymphoid follicles.

Lymphoma is a risk, developing in 1% of patients.

Review PMID: 23614399

Cases PMID: 9619675

Diffuse CD8+ lymphocytosis syndrome PMID: 25660200

Miscellaneous oral lesions
Mucosal ulcers

Major aphthae (Figs. 29.11 and 29.12) can be troublesome, interfere with eating and accelerate deterioration of health. They become more frequent and severe with declining

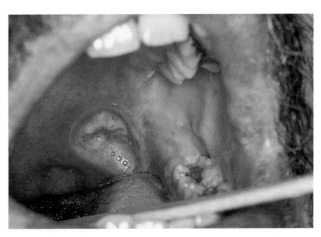

Fig. 29.11 HIV-associated aphthous stomatitis. Major aphthae typically become more frequent and severe while immune function deteriorates and can add considerably to the patient's disabilities. Note the deep ulceration.

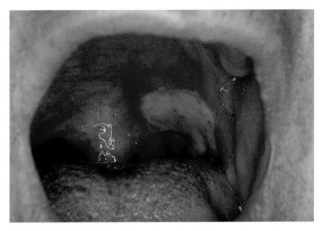

Fig. 29.12 Major aphthous ulcers. A shallower ulcer with surrounding erythema , in an earlier stage than that in Fig. 29.11.

immune function. Necrotising oral ulceration of an ill-defined nature and aphthae-like ulcers are common oral signs.

Persistent ulcers that might be left to assess healing in a non-HIV infected person require biopsy in HIV infection to assess them for possible infectious causes: herpesvirus, cytomegalovirus or mycobacteria, and also for lymphoma.

Major aphthae usually respond dramatically to thalidomide, but this should only be used when other possible causes of ulcers have been excluded.

Diagnosis and treatment PMID: 14507229

Oral hyperpigmentation → Summary chart 26.1
p. 390

Pigmentation in HIV infection is of unknown cause. It may also be a complication of treatment with zidovudine (see Ch. 26).

Oral adverse effects of HAART

Most of the protease inhibitors can cause xerostomia, disturbed taste sensation and perioral paraesthesia. Many of these and other components of HAART can also cause erythema multiforme.

RISKS OF TRANSMISSION OF HIV INFECTION TO HEALTHCARE WORKERS

All patients must be regarded as potentially infective and treated with universal precautions. These are effective against HIV transmission, so infection in a healthcare setting is very rare. The usual cause has been a needle-stick injury causing accidental injection of a significant amount of infected blood. By contrast, many other needle injuries in which little blood has been transferred have failed to transmit the virus. Most healthcare workers who have developed AIDS have not acquired it as a result of their occupation.

Almost all documented cases of transmission to healthcare workers in the United States occurred before 1995. No cases have been confirmed since 2000.

General aspects of dental management

Possible oral and systemic features of this disease that may affect dental management have been discussed previously.

It would be unethical and unprofessional to refuse to treat an HIV-infected patient regardless of the possibilities of acquiring the infection or transmitting it to other patients. However, strict adherence to universal infection control measures must be implemented, and the operator should take particular care to avoid accidental self-injury with an instrument that may have been contaminated with serum or blood. The possibility of transmitting HIV infection during dental treatment inevitably causes anxiety, but the risk is considerably lower than that of acquiring viral hepatitis.

At the time of writing, there are more than 100,000 antibody-positive, potentially infective persons in Britain, but most are on HAART and of low infectivity. A greater risk is posed by patients unaware of their HIV-positive status.

References for infection control are with hepatitis in Chapter 34.

Post-exposure prophylaxis and sharps injury

Any healthcare worker suffering a needle-stick or other sharps injury exposure to potentially HIV infected body fluids should be assessed to determine whether anti-retroviral drugs should be prescribed. This reduces the risk of transmission of HIV. All UK national health service employers including dental practices are required to have a procedure in place that allows post-exposure prophylaxis to be given within 24 hours. After that time the effectiveness is much reduced.

Whether or not post-exposure prophylaxis with HAART is appropriate depends on the risk of transmission as assessed by the type of injury and infectivity of the patient. If required, the drugs are selected to take into account any drug-resistant HIV strains known in the donor. The adverse effects of post-exposure prophylaxis are significant, and treatment is usually continued for 4 weeks.

The immediate action for any injury potentially contaminated with infectious body fluids is to wash liberally with soap and water and encourage free bleeding. Wounds should not be sucked or scrubbed. Splashes to the mucous membranes, including conjunctivae, should be irrigated copiously with water. This should be done before and after removal of contact lenses. Saliva is considered infectious in the context of a dental surgery because it is almost certainly contaminated with small amounts of blood.

HIV infection is transmitted by 0.3% of medical sharps injuries and 0.6% of exposures to mucous membranes, including the eye. Post-exposure prophylaxis is considered more than 90% effective in preventing transmission, but these data come from sexual transmission, and it may be even more effective in healthcare exposure for a variety of reasons. Pregnancy is not a contraindication. Prophylaxis is not recommended for bite injuries.

RISKS OF TRANSMISSION OF HIV TO PATIENTS

Although transmission to healthcare workers is exceedingly rare, transmission to patients has occurred. A dentist in Florida infected six patients, and three other healthcare workers have been documented to have infected a single patient each. However, all these cases occurred many years ago in the early years of the epidemic, before HAART. There has been no documented case of transmission to a patient in the UK.

Current regulations require that dental clinicians who have become or think that they have become infected by HIV, hepatitis or other blood-borne viruses should seek appropriate medical supervision.

HIV-positive dentists, who are receiving effective treatment, have a viral load less than 200 copies/mL and are regularly monitored, are now allowed to undertake exposure-prone procedures. The decision on fitness to practice is made by the patient's HIV consultant physician, and the dentist will need to be listed on a confidential register. Individuals may be subject to restrictions on a case-by-case basis.

Web URL 29.4 UK guidance for HIV dentists: https://www.gov.uk/government/groups/uk-advisory-panel-for-healthcare-workers-infected-with-bloodborne-viruses

Allergy, autoimmune and autoinflammatory disease

30

Abnormal immune reactions against environmental antigens (allergy) and self-antigens (autoimmunity) are common (Box 30.1). They cause specific diseases, adverse drug reactions and can affect dental management.

Box 30.1 Important immunologically-mediated diseases

Atopic disease and related allergies (reactions to exogenous antigens)

- Asthma; eczema; hay fever; urticaria
- Food allergies: nuts, wheat, shellfish, milk, eggs
- Insect stings
- Latex
- Some drug reactions, especially penicillins
- Anaphylaxis and acute allergic angio-oedema
- Contact dermatitis
- Exercise-induced/food anaphylaxis

Autoimmune diseases (reactions to self-antigens)

Autoimmune connective tissue diseases

- Rheumatoid arthritis
- Sjögren's syndrome*
- Lupus erythematosus*
- Systemic sclerosis*

Autoimmune diseases with specific autoantibodies

- Pernicious anaemia (chronic atrophic gastritis)*
- Idiopathic and drug-associated thrombocytopenic purpura*
- Drug-associated leucopenia*
- Autoimmune haemolytic anaemia
- Addison's disease*
- Hashimoto's thyroiditis
- Hyperthyroidism
- Idiopathic hypoparathyroidism*
- Pemphigus vulgaris*
- Mucous membrane pemphigoid*

Autoinflammatory diseases (triggered by abnormal inflammatory response)

- Crohn's disease*
- Orofacial granulomatosis*
- Sarcoidosis *
- PFAPA (**P**eriodic **F**ever, **A**phthous stomatitis, **P**haryngitis, and cervical **A**denitis) syndrome
- Possibly Behçet's disease

*Can give rise to characteristic oral changes

ALLERGIC OR HYPERSENSITIVITY REACTIONS

Atopy

Atopy is a genetic predisposition to multiple allergic responses, usually of the IgE mediated or type 1 reaction type. Patients who are atopic may have several of the conditions listed in this chapter and usually have more pronounced responses than those with a single allergy. The main atopic diseases are atopic dermatitis (eczema), hay fever and asthma. Incidence of atopic disease rose dramatically in Western countries after the 1960s but has now peaked; it continues to increase in prevalence in developing countries.

The cause(s) of atopy are unknown. Mutations in the filaggrin protein that contributes to the epithelial permeability barriers are very frequent.

Atopy presents in the first year of life with dermatitis; asthma and hay fever develop in later childhood or adolescence. In late adulthood the severity wanes.

There are no oral manifestations of atopic disease itself, and there is no such entity as oral eczema. Food allergies affect 30% of atopic individuals, usually to cow's milk, wheat, soya or fruits, and those with hay fever may also suffer oral reactions in the pollen-food syndrome (discussed later). Atopic individuals are more likely to develop latex allergy, and atopic dentists need to take extra precautions against hand eczema. Contrary to previous belief, atopy does not predispose to penicillin allergy, but atopics tend to have more severe reactions if they do develop this allergy.

Drugs (Box 30.2) used to treat atopic diseases may complicate dental treatment.

Contact dermatitis

Contact dermatitis resembles eczema clinically but is a cell-mediated (type 4) reaction. It affects only where the allergen contacted the skin, appears after 24–72 hours and persists for several weeks after exposure. It causes an erythematous rash, with blisters in severe cases. Nickel is the most common cause. The oral counterpart to contact dermatitis is, however, exceedingly rare (Figs 30.1 and 30.2).

Box 30.2 Effects of drugs used for atopic disease

- Antihistamines (for minor allergies)
  - Drowsiness
  - Potentiation of sedating drugs
  - Dry mouth
- Corticosteroid inhalers
  - Oropharyngeal thrush and chronic candidosis
- Systemic corticosteroids for severe asthma (Ch. 42)
- Oral reactions to sublingual desensitising agents

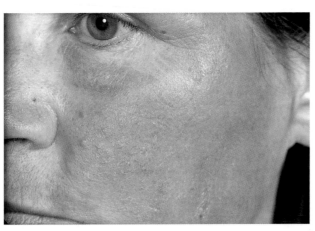

Fig. 30.1 Allergic rash triggered by impression material. There is generalised facial erythema and slight oedema.

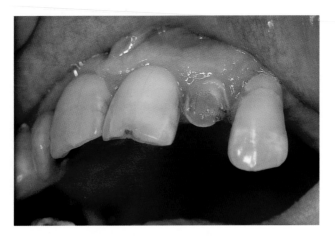

Fig. 30.2 Hypersensitivity to impression material. The same patient as in Fig. 30.1, showing the site of the impression photographed at the same time. No allergic response is evident intraorally.

Contact dermatitis is an occupational hazard in dentistry. Nurses and technicians are at higher risk than dentists. Latex, soaps and detergents and the aromatics they contain, and methyl methacrylate are the most common allergens. X-ray processing chemicals were potent sensitisers, but now are little used. Chlorhexidine has recently become a more frequent cause of contact allergy.

The UK dentist has a legal obligation to protect the dental team against contact dermatitis (Box 30.3).

Chlorhexidine reactions PMID: 23222325

Oral contact reactions PMID: 23010830

Occupational risks PMID: 15884321

Latex allergy

Latex allergy is the main allergic occupational disease affecting healthcare workers.

The necessity for gloving for all clinical work resulted in a dramatic rise in latex allergy in medicine and dentistry since 1980. In one dental school, the prevalence of latex allergy was 9%, whereas 22% complained of chronic glove dermatitis. Powdered latex gloves were particularly dangerous because the starch powder spread latex proteins into the environment.

> **Box 30.3 Summary of United Kingdom Health and Safety executive guidance on work-related contact dermatitis in dentistry**
>
> **Advice for employees**
> - Use machinery and tools provided rather than hands (e.g. equipment cleaning machines).
> - During handwashing, rinse off residual soap/hand cleanser thoroughly.
> - Dry hands thoroughly before continuing work.
> - Use emollient creams regularly, especially after finishing work. Cover all parts of the hands.
> - Check your skin for early signs and report concerns to your 'responsible person'.
>
> **Advice for employers**
> Carry out a practice risk assessment and manage the risks:
> - Consider using less hazardous alternatives, including automation (e.g. an equipment washing machine).
> - Consider use of less hazardous products.
> - Provide hand hygiene products that are effective and minimise the risk.
> - Train employees in use of equipment and gloves, correct hand cleaning and skin care measures (e.g. regular use of moisturisers).
> - Display relevant posters and educational material.
> - Provide good hand-drying facilities (e.g. good-quality, soft paper towels).
> - Provide emollients in suitable dispensers to prevent cross-contamination.

There is no completely satisfactory alternative to latex gloves. Low protein content ('low NRL') latex gloves are available, and these are recommended when a latex glove is considered best, but they cannot be used if there is a risk of triggering asthma in the workplace. Otherwise, alternatives must be available, and in many centres, latex gloves are being phased out.

Once latex allergy to gloves has been acquired, there are reactions to all rubber products such as rubber tubing, anaesthetic masks, catheters and tourniquets, prophylaxis cups and alginate mixing bowls.

Latex allergy is important because it most frequently manifests as a type 1 urticarial contact reaction. In dentistry, this has the potential to put the airway at risk. Rarely, reactions to latex can be severe and have been fatal. Latex also triggers contact dermatitis. Different patients and dental team members have different risks and require different avoidance strategies and treatment.

It is not always obvious that a medical or dental device may contain rubber. For instance, bungs in local anaesthetic cartridges may contain latex. Even covered latex, such as a sphygmomanometer cuff, can shed latex proteins and trigger a reaction. For severe cases, it may be necessary to refer patients to a centre with a latex-free surgery. Premedication with antihistamines or steroids to prevent reactions remains controversial. This may reduce the severity of a reaction but does not prevent it. Avoidance is a better preventive strategy.

Prevention requires identifying those at risk (Box 30.4). Patients allergic to latex often have cross reactions with foods including banana, pineapple, kiwi fruit, avocado, chestnut and mango that contain related latex-type

Box 30.4 Individuals at risk of latex allergy

- Healthcare professionals
- Atopic patients
- Patients with spina bifida
- Patients with urogenital anomalies
- Latex industry workers
- Those subject to multiple surgical procedures before the age of 7 years

molecules. Food allergy must always be included when taking a medical history. Patients may report lip swelling on blowing up balloons.

Each dental practice should have a policy for latex allergy, its management and the safe treatment of allergic patients. The majority of allergic patients can be safely treated in general practice with suitable precautions.

General review PMID: 14616859

Dental implications review PMID: 9927072

Latex-free anaesthetics PMID: 23094572

Allergy to local anaesthetic

Allergic reactions to local anaesthetics are rare but possible, affecting 1% or less of those patients who claim to be affected. The vast majority of patients referred for testing have suffered other recognised complications of analgesia, either expected pharmacological reactions to high doses of the analgesic or vasoconstrictor, intravascular injection, intraparotid injection, intraneural injection or similar adverse events. These are normally readily recognised by their clinical signs and symptoms (Table 30.1).

True allergic reactions may be to latex in the cartridge (unlikely), analgesic agent or other components such as preservative (metabisulphite antioxidant in adrenaline containing preparations), or to some unrelated dental material to which the patient was exposed at the same time. Amide agents used in dentistry are the less likely type to cause allergy. Unfortunately, determining the exact cause of a reaction is not always possible with confidence. Nevertheless, it is important to investigate potential reactions as genuine allergy could cause a medical emergency. The dentist should be able to screen out the non-allergic reactions listed in Table 30.1 by questioning the patient and, if necessary, contacting the dentist who administered the analgesic to check which agent was given.

Features suggesting a true allergy are facial swelling or other peripheral oedema, hypotension and itchy erythematous or urticarial rash, which indicate a possible type 1 reaction. A few patients suffer delayed reactions, usually with a rash and sometimes delayed oedema. Reactive patients are also likely to have multiple allergies or atopy.

The more common allergens appear to be metabisulphite preservative and bupivacaine, much more rarely lidocaine. Prilocaine causes more reactions, but these are rarely allergic. Referral for testing is indicated when no definite alternative explanation is found or multiple reactions have developed.

Testing is difficult because a definitive result requires a challenge injection and thus carries some, albeit small, risk. Skin patch tests may reveal a delayed reaction but are of little value. Skin scratch tests, allowing a minute amount of various solutions to penetrate to the dermis, are usually

Table 30.1 Some reactions to local analgesics in dentistry

Reaction	Cause
Failed analgesia	Usually poor technique
Pain on injection	Poor technique
Persistent anaesthesia or paraesthesia	Direct toxic effect of agent on nerve, not necessarily following intraneural injection Commonest with Articaine, possible with Lidocaine
Post-operative trismus	Injection into medial pterygoid muscle, resulting in inflammation or haematoma, haematoma from venous plexus distal to nerve. Trismus for several days
Syncope	Stress of injection, anxiety. By far the commonest adverse reaction. See Box 43.3.
Diplopia, blanching of skin of face, loss of vision, ptosis	Intra-arterial injection or venous injection with retrograde flow. Effects mostly related to vasoconstrictor
Facial palsy or weakness	Intraparotid injection
Neuralgic pain on injection, prolonged analgesia	Intraneural injection or injection close to nerve
Methaemoglobinaemia. Cyanosis, tachycardia and, at high dose, sedative effect 1–3 hours after administration	Pharmacological effect of prilocaine metabolite, non-allergic. Recommended dose exceeded. Increased risk in glucose-6-phosphatase deficiency
Muscle twitching and tremors With increasing dose, epileptiform seizures. At high doses central nervous system depression drowsiness, tinnitus, respiratory depression, bradycardia and arrhythmias	Lidocaine toxicity Recommended dose exceeded. Also some effects specific to particular agents
Angio-oedema	Could be non-allergic angio-oedema, but consider allergic reaction first.
Oedema, urticarial or erythematous rash and itching	Likely allergic reaction.

performed, followed by a small intradermal (very superficially placed) injection of those agents that produce no reaction on a scratch test. Control saline injections are required to identify patients with an exaggerated inflammatory response that might be misconstrued as allergy. If allergy appears likely, the solutions may be diluted to reduce the challenge. A positive reaction is identified by a wheal and erythematous flare around the agent, but not the control. A negative result makes allergy extremely unlikely, but a full-dose injection is required to exclude other types of pharmacological or idiosyncratic reaction. The whole procedure must be performed in an environment equipped to deal with a severe anaphylactic reaction, even though this is extremely unlikely.

> **Box 30.5   Typical features of autoimmune disease**
>
> - Significantly more common in women
> - Onset often in middle age
> - Levels of immunoglobulins usually raised
> - Family history frequently positive
> - Circulating autoantibodies frequently also detectable in unaffected family members
> - Multiple circulating autoantibodies to several different and possibly unrelated antigens
> - Often a higher risk of developing a second autoimmune disease
> - Immunoglobulin and/or complement often detectable at sites of tissue damage (e.g. pemphigus vulgaris)
> - Often associated with human leukocyte antigen-B8 and DR3
> - Immunosuppressive or anti-inflammatory treatment frequently limits tissue damage

> **Box 30.6   Types and examples of autoimmune disease**
>
> **Organ or cell-specific autoantibodies**
>
> - Hashimoto's thyroiditis
> - Chronic atrophic gastritis (pernicious anaemia)
> - Addison's disease
> - Idiopathic hypoparathyroidism
> - Pemphigus
> - Pemphigoid
> - Idiopathic thrombocytopenic purpura
> - Autoimmune haemolytic anaemia
> - Myasthenia gravis
>
> **Non-organ-specific autoantibodies (the connective tissue diseases)**
>
> - Lupus erythematosus
> - Rheumatoid arthritis
> - Sjögren's syndrome
> - Systemic sclerosis
> - Primary biliary cirrhosis
> - Dermatomyositis
> - Mixed connective tissue disease

> **Box 30.7   Features of rheumatoid arthritis of importance in dentistry**
>
> - Association with Sjögren's syndrome
> - Chronic anaemia and its sequelae (Ch. 27)
> - Fatigue
> - Reduced manual dexterity, difficulty with oral hygiene
> - Access to dental care may be problematic
> - Reduced mobility, difficulty lying supine, or still for long periods
> - Atlantoaxial weakness in severe cases
> - Joint replacement (currently not thought to merit antibiotic cover for dentistry)
> - Drug treatment
>   - Aspirin (bleeding, anaemia)
>   - Non-steroidal anti-inflammatory drugs (bleeding, anaemia, lichenoid reactions)
>   - Corticosteroids (adrenal suppression, immunosuppression, infections)
>   - Antimalarials, gold (lichenoid reactions, oral and skin pigmentation)
>   - Penicillamine (lichenoid reactions, taste loss)
>   - Methotrexate (poor healing, oral ulcers, folate deficiency)

components such as collagen, proteoglycan and elastin. In reality the targets and mechanisms of immune damage are unclear. The main examples are rheumatoid arthritis, lupus erythematosus, systemic sclerosis, primary biliary cirrhosis and Sjögren's syndrome. The last can be associated with any of them or develop in isolation. Many patients have mixed connective tissue disease or overlap diseases.

Rheumatoid arthritis

Rheumatoid arthritis is by far the most common connective tissue disorder and affects at least 1% of the population and is three times more common in women than men. The general features of arthritis and temporomandibular joint involvement are discussed in Chapter 14.

The implications of rheumatoid arthritis for dentistry are shown in Box 30.7.

Sjögren's syndrome

See Chapter 22.

Systemic lupus erythematosus

Systemic lupus erythematosus (SLE) is an autoimmune disease caused by autoantibodies against DNA and its associated proteins. Antibodies against double-stranded DNA are almost diagnostic of SLE. There are also genetic predispositions affecting genes involved in non-specific immune mechanisms and complement. Circulating autoantibody-antigen complexes lodge in small vessels where they trigger complement and activate neutrophils and macrophages, damaging the tissue. This happens particularly in the kidney.

SLE affects approximately 0.05% of the UK population. Those of Asian or African descent are prone, and females are eight times more frequently affected than men. It is a disease of early adulthood and middle age. SLE can affect almost any body system, and the features vary according to the main organ systems affected (Table 30.2).

plasma immunoglobulin concentration. This explains why these diseases often have an increase in many different autoantibodies, for example, anti-thyroid antibodies are common in Sjögren's syndrome despite having no apparent connection to salivary glands. Similarly, rheumatoid factor, an autoantibody against immunoglobulin Fc is found in many autoimmune and connective tissue diseases.

The autoimmune diseases have many features in common (Box 30.5). By no means are all of their mechanisms are clearly understood (Box 30.6). Those with particular dental relevance have been discussed in other chapters, and only the connective tissue diseases are described here.

Oral manifestations autoimmunity PMID: 23040353

The connective tissue diseases

The connective tissue diseases used to be thought of as autoimmune diseases directed against connective tissue

Table 30.2 Organs and tissues affected in systemic lupus erythematosus

Organ/tissue	Clinical feature
Joints	Joint pains and arthritis
Skin	Rashes, erythema nodosum
Mouth	Stomatitis, Sjögren's syndrome
Serous membranes	Pleurisy, pericarditis
Heart	Endocarditis, myocarditis, pericarditis Libman-Sacks endocarditis of valves
Lungs	Pneumonitis
Kidneys	Nephritic syndrome, kidney failure
Central nervous system	Neuroses, psychoses, strokes, cranial nerve palsies
Eyes	Conjunctivitis, retinal damage
Gastrointestinal tract	Hepatomegaly, pancreatitis
Blood	Anaemia, purpura

Box 30.8 Features of lupus erythematosus of importance in dentistry

- Association with Sjögren's syndrome
- Painful oral lichen-planus-like lesions
- Chronic anaemia and its sequelae (Ch. 27)
- Bleeding tendencies (antiplatelet antibodies or anticoagulants)
- Cardiac disease and risk of endocarditis
- Lower lip vermillion border involvement is potentially malignant
- Drug treatment
  - Non-steroidal anti-inflammatory drugs (bleeding, anaemia, lichenoid reactions)
  - Corticosteroids (adrenal suppression, immunosuppression, infections)
  - Antimalarials (lichenoid reactions, oral and skin pigmentation)
  - Methotrexate (poor healing, oral ulcers, folate deficiency)
  - Belimumab (anti-B cell cytokine, immunosuppressant)

Clinically, joint pains and rashes are the most common manifestations, but the 'classical' picture of a young woman with a butterfly rash across the midface is uncommon and not peculiar to SLE. Some patients have mild disease affecting only the skin; in others severe and debilitating disease can be fatal.

Approximately 20% of patients with SLE develop oral lesions. These somewhat resemble lichen planus (Ch. 16) but are more difficult to treat. The discoid form that affects the skin is also associated with oral lesions. Otherwise, it is the individual manifestations rather than the disease process itself that affect dental management (Box 30.8).

Oral manifestations PMID: 15567365

Systemic sclerosis (scleroderma)

Systemic sclerosis is rare but has a poor prognosis. Clinically, the most common early signs are Raynaud's phenomenon and joint pains. Later, the skin becomes thinned, stiff

and pigmented and the facial features become smoothed-out and mask-like. Opening of the mouth may become limited. This condition is discussed in detail in Chapter 14.

AUTOINFLAMMATORY DISEASES

A recent concept is that some diseases are autoinflammatory, caused by defects in genes that enhance inflammation and thus damage the host.

The majority of such diseases recognised to date, such as familial Mediterranean fever, have little significance to dentistry, but others such as Crohn's disease (Ch. 34) and sarcoidosis have oral lesions. PFAPA (**P**eriodic **F**ever, **Aph**thous stomatitis, **P**haryngitis, and cervical **A**denitis) syndrome (Ch. 16) may also be an example.

Autoimmune and autoinflammatory diseases are proposed to form a spectrum, with conditions such as Behçet's disease and ankylosing spondylitis being diseases caused by both autoimmune and autoinflammatory mechanisms.

Sarcoidosis → Summary charts 22.2, 24.2 and 34.1 pp. 354, 373, 459

Sarcoidosis is probably an autoinflammatory disease. A number of genes are linked, and there is sometimes a familial predisposition. Mutations in the NOD2 gene, that regulates recognition of bacterial peptidoglycan and induces inflammation, are known to cause childhood sarcoidosis. This gene is also linked to Crohn's disease, a similar granulomatous disease.

Inflammation is enhanced, and immune reactions are suppressed. An extrinsic trigger remains suspected but unknown. Micro-organisms, pollens and environmental antigens have all been proposed, but this is not a traditional hypersensitivity reaction.

The disease is more frequent in those of African descent and those from Scandinavia, and the age of onset is usually 20–40 years. Almost any tissue can be affected. Common effects include fever, loss of weight, fatigue, breathlessness, cough and arthralgia. Erythema nodosum is the most common skin lesion. Hypercalcaemia can lead to nephrocalcinosis.

Pathology

Affected tissues contain numerous small non-caseating granulomas that often contain multinucleate giant cells and are surrounded by lymphocytes (Fig. 30.4). Granulomas and the fibrosis they induce around them expand to destroy the tissues. Cells in the granulomas produce vitamin D3, causing hypercalcaemia, and angiotensin converting enzyme. The granulomas are not distinguishable from those of other diseases. Tuberculosis and other granulomatous diseases must therefore be excluded by specific investigations (Box 30.9).

Lung and lymph node involvement

Sarcoidosis is primarily a disease of lungs and lymph nodes. Over 90% of patients have lung damage, but only in a minority is there diffuse fibrosis and a risk of death. Most patients have a dry cough and a few have breathlessness on exertion.

Lymphadenopathy is usually hilar or mediastinal, bilateral and associated with lung lesions (Fig. 30.5). Other sites are involved in 40% of patients, including cervical lymph nodes (Ch. 31).

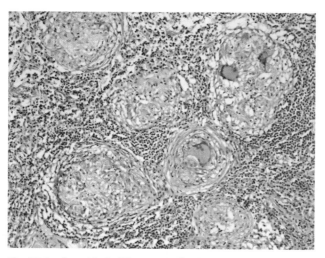

Fig. 30.4   Sarcoidosis. Microscopically, the granulomas are small and round with occasional small multinucleate cells and no caseation. Microscopically, sarcoidosis can be difficult to distinguish from tuberculosis and additional tests are usually performed.

Box 30.9   Important granulomatous diseases

Infections

- Tuberculosis and atypical mycobacterial infections
- Systemic mycoses
- Cat-scratch disease
- Toxoplasmosis
- Syphilis

Reactive

- Foreign body reactions

Unknown causes

- Sarcoidosis
- Crohn's disease
- Melkersson–Rosenthal syndrome
- Orofacial granulomatosis
- Wegener's granulomatosis

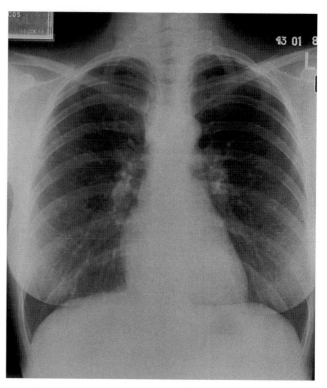

Fig. 30.5   Sarcoidosis. Prominent hilar lymphadenopathy is the main radiological finding, though granuloma formation may be widespread.

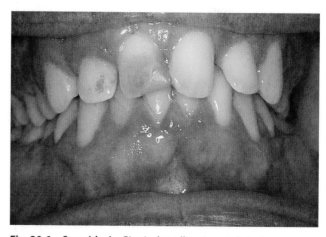

Fig. 30.6   Sarcoidosis. Gingival swelling is not clinically distinguishable from several other possible causes, and in this case is relatively mild and easily overlooked, but biopsy showed granuloma formation.

Oral involvement

The most frequently affected oral sites are the gingivae (Fig. 30.6) and lips, followed by palate and buccal mucosa. Gingival involvement produces a lumpy multifocal or diffuse gingival enlargement identical to that in Crohn's disease or orofacial granulomatosis. Granulomas are present on biopsy.

Other lesions include ulcers and swellings. Although they are uncommon overall, oral lesions frequently precede other manifestations and are the presenting sign in two-thirds of patients.

Salivary gland involvement

Sarcoidosis causes bilateral diffuse swelling of major salivary glands, almost always parotid glands (Figs 30.7 and 30.8). This is uncommon but can occasionally be the first manifestation of sarcoidosis. The disease also affects minor glands, and in more than 50% of patients with bilateral hilar lymphadenopathy, biopsy of a labial salivary gland shows typical granulomas and is a valuable, minimally invasive diagnostic aid. Concurrent lacrimal gland involvement produces a Sjögren's syndrome-like clinical presentation.

Heerfordt's syndrome is the combination of parotid swelling, xerostomia, uveitis and, often, facial palsy due to sarcoidosis in salivary gland, eye and facial nerve.

Diagnosis and management

Diagnosis depends on chest radiography (Fig. 30.5) and biopsy of affected tissue. In the active stages of the disease, plasma levels of angiotensin-converting enzyme (ACE) and calcium are frequently raised. Tuberculosis must be excluded.

The great majority of patients require no treatment. When required, non-steroidal anti-inflammatory drugs are usually sufficient and spontaneous resolution follows in a

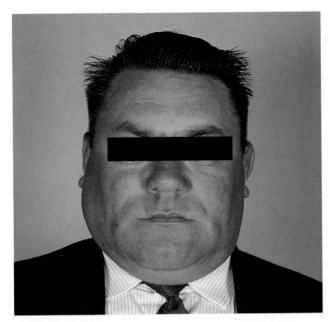

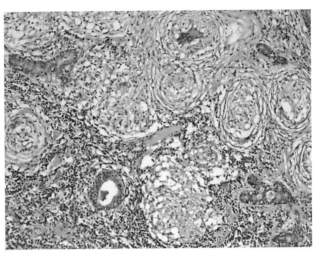

Fig. 30.8 **Sarcoidosis of salivary gland.** The acinar cells are completely effaced, and only a few ducts remain, surrounded by fibrosis and pale staining rounded granulomas of loosely cohesive macrophages. The granuloma near the top centre contains a small multinucleate cell.

Fig. 30.7 Bilateral parotid swelling in a case of sarcoidosis.

few years. However, those with extrapulmonary or extensive lung involvement may be given corticosteroids, methotrexate or azathioprine, other immunosuppressants or tumour necrosis factor-alpha antagonists. Many novel targeted agents are in trial.

The mortality rate is 5%, usually from lung or central nervous system disease. Lung transplants may be used in severe cases. Sarcoidosis carries a risk of lung cancer and leukaemia in later life.

General review PMID: 24090799

Orofacial manifestations PMID: 18953304

Literature review PMID: 15888103

Cervical lymphadenopathy

31

There are so many potential causes of enlargement of the cervical lymph nodes that differential diagnosis is complex and requires knowledge of many diseases. Dental causes are common (Fig. 31.1), and the primary role of the dentist is to exclude them. Cervical lymphadenopathy without an obvious local cause is a warning sign that must not be ignored, and no dental examination is complete without an examination of the cervical lymph nodes.

Important causes of cervical lymphadenopathy are summarised in Box 31.1. Many have been discussed in other chapters.

Investigation

Lymphadenopathy of acute onset and with tender or painful nodes bilaterally is the easiest type to diagnose. The causes are mostly acute viral or bacterial infections, and spontaneous resolution follows. It is persistent enlargement without such a history that causes diagnostic problems. Various clinical features provide important guides as to the likely cause of lymphadenopathy (Box 31.2), but there is no simple algorithm for diagnosis; the diseases are simply too diverse and individually variable.

A soft lymph node in an otherwise healthy child is unlikely to be of great significance. It is usually due to a recent viral infection and typically resolves spontaneously after a month or so.

Cervical lymphadenopathy associated with generalised lymphadenopathy in a child or young adult with a sore throat and fever is likely to be due to infectious mononucleosis as discussed later in this chapter. By contrast, persistent lymphadenopathy raises the possibility of leukaemia.

In the older patient with a hard lymph node, a carcinoma must be suspected. Thyroid carcinomas and human papillomavirus (HPV)-associated oropharyngeal and base of tongue carcinomas often present with lymph node metastases before the primary is evident. Conversely, oral carcinomas are usually obvious by the time they metastasise.

Various patterns of involvement of cervical lymph nodes can be produced by spread of carcinoma of the mouth (Ch. 20).

Box 31.1   Some important causes of cervical lymphadenopathy

Infections

- Bacterial
  - Dental
    - apical abscess
    - cellulitis
    - periodontitis
    - pericoronitis
  - Tonsil, face or scalp infections
  - Tuberculosis
  - Syphilis
  - Cat-scratch disease
  - Lyme disease
- Viral
  - Herpetic stomatitis
  - Infectious mononucleosis
  - HIV infection
  - Childhood fevers
- Parasitic
  - Toxoplasmosis
- Possibly infective
  - Mucocutaneous lymph node syndrome (Kawasaki's disease)

Neoplasms

- Primary
  - Hodgkin's disease
  - Non-Hodgkin lymphoma
  - Leukaemia – especially lymphocytic
- Secondary
  - Carcinoma – oral, salivary gland, thyroid, oro- or nasopharyngeal
  - Malignant melanoma
  - Metastases from gastric and abdominal cancers

Miscellaneous

- Sarcoidosis
- Drug reactions
- Connective tissue diseases
- Recent surgery to mouth or face
- 'Normal' enlarged nodes in children

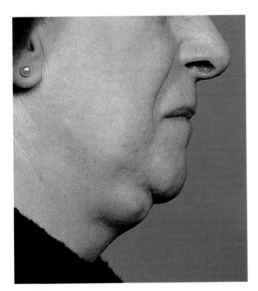

Fig. 31.1   Enlarged submandibular lymph node with incipient drainage to the skin resulting from a dental abscess.

In a patient with Sjögren's syndrome, enlargement of cervical lymph nodes may be due to infection secondary to the dry mouth, but may alternatively be due to the development of lymphoma – a recognised hazard of this disease.

Investigations for cervical lymphadenopathy where the cause is not obvious are summarised in Box 31.3. The first-line investigation should always be fine needle aspiration (FNA). This will provide an accurate diagnosis of most

lymphomas, metastases, and many infections including tuberculosis. Inadequate specimens or failed diagnosis should trigger a re-aspiration in the first instance.

In difficult cases or when FNA fails, biopsy provides the most reliable diagnosis. Biopsy is only justified if all other investigations have proved inadequate and must be done by an expert. Biopsy may spill infectious material or malignant cells into the neck and produce unsightly scarring. Needle core biopsy is usually preferred, but surgical excision of a node may be required depending on the likely diagnosis.

Approach to lymphadenopathy in dentistry PMID: 15954248

TUBERCULOUS CERVICAL LYMPHADENOPATHY

One-third of the world's population is infected by *Mycobacterium tuberculosis*, but only 10% will develop clinical disease. In the UK, infection rates for tuberculosis (TB) can reach 1% in high incidence areas, and incidence is increasing. This is mostly accounted for by latent disease that has been contracted outside the UK, or is in low socioeconomic or marginalised social groups.

Cervical lymph node enlargement indicates spread beyond the lungs. Extrapulmonary spread is seen in 10% of cases with active disease and is much more likely in the immunosuppressed, particularly HIV infection. In 5% of cases, the cervical nodes are the presenting sign.

Cervical node infection by *Mycobacterium tuberculosis* accounts for 95% of cases. Patients are mostly adults, in the risk groups noted previously. Non-tuberculous ('atypical') mycobacteria account for the remaining 5%. The clinical features are summarised in Box 31.4.

Cervical disease always accompanies pulmonary disease, and other sites may be involved. Treatment with antituberculous drugs remains highly effective in developed countries, but multiple drug-resistant strains are becoming widespread, especially in Southeast Asia.

Pathology

A tuberculin skin test (Mantoux test) or interferon gamma release assay will usually be positive, unless the patient is immunosuppressed. However, these measure the immune response to the organisms, not active disease. It is usually easier, faster and more specific to perform fine needle aspiration to detect granulomas in the node (Fig. 31.3) and provide material for culture or polymerase chain reaction (PCR)–based detection. Ideally, mycobacteria should be demonstrable by Ziehl–Neelsen or other staining techniques, but the organisms are sparse and often not found. Similarly, positive cultures are often not obtained, and patients must be treated regardless if granulomas are found, the clinical picture fits and sarcoidosis and other granulomatous disease is excluded. Open biopsy and incision of a cold abscess must be avoided at all costs as this would spread the infection widely.

Affected tissues contain numerous well-organised non-caseating granulomas with frequent Langhans-type giant cells in a background of fibrosis. After many years, fibrotic nodes may calcify and be seen radiographically (Fig 31.2).

ATYPICAL MYCOBACTERIAL INFECTION

Non-tuberculous ('atypical') mycobacteria, particularly *Mycobacterium avium intracellulare* or *Mycobacterium scrofulaceum*, account for only 5% of mycobacterial cervical lymphadenitis in adults but 95% in children (Fig. 31.4).

This infection is very different from TB, and the organisms are environmental or spread from pets such as birds and not spread person to person. It is thought that children contract these infections through oral contact, developing the equivalent of a tuberculous primary infection. A further difference is that the treatment for this disease is often surgical. Features are shown in Box 31.5.

Case series PMID: 18312877

SARCOIDOSIS

Multiple cervical lymph nodes are firm, and the hilar nodes and lung are affected, producing a picture like that of tuberculosis, but with numerous small granulomas and no caseation. Sarcoidosis is discussed in detail in Chapter 30.

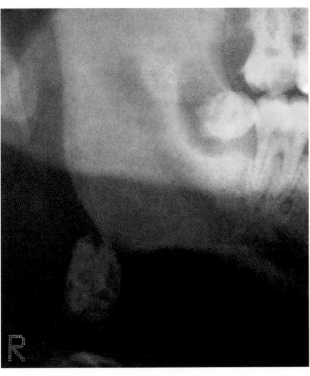

Fig. 31.2 Tuberculosis. Calcified cervical lymph node seen in a panoramic tomogram. Calcified nodes are often multiple and indicate past rather than active infection. *(By kind permission of Mr EJ Whaites.)*

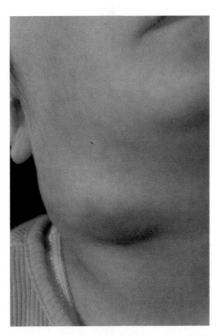

Fig. 31.4 Atypical mycobacterial infection in a child. Typical single large node, slightly tender and with mild erythema of the overlying skin. *(From Hambleton, L., Sussens, J., Hewitt, M., 2016. Lymphadenopathy in Children and Young People. Paediatr. Child Health 26, 63–67.)*

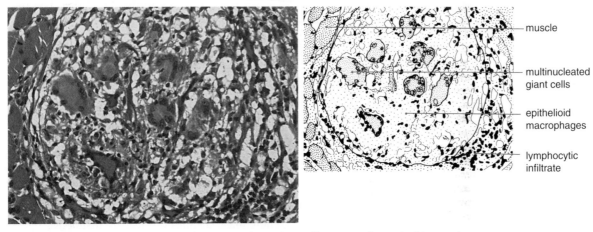

- muscle
- multinucleated giant cells
- epithelioid macrophages
- lymphocytic infiltrate

Fig. 31.3 Tuberculosis. Numerous multinucleate Langerhans giant cells are conspicuous in this granuloma.

Box 31.6   Typical features of cat-scratch disease

- Children frequently affected
- Frequently a history of a scratch by a cat or other animal
- Formation of papule, which may suppurate, at the site of inoculation
- Mild fever, malaise and regional lymphadenitis 1–3 weeks after exposure
- Lymph nodes soften and typically suppurate
- Conjunctivitis may be associated
- Encephalitis is a rare complication

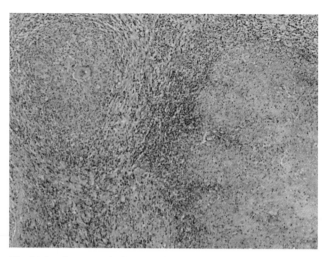

Fig. 31.5   Cat-scratch disease. There is a large area of necrosis on the bottom right, surrounded my macrophages, and a separate granuloma with a giant cell top left.

Box 31.7   Typical features of Lyme disease

- A rash spreading outwards from the insect bite
- Enlarged regional lymph nodes
- Fever, malaise, other systemic symptoms
- Arthritis (the main chronic effect) particularly of the knees, rarely of the temporomandibular joints
- Neurological complications (in about 15% of patients) include facial palsy or other cranial nerve lesions
- Diagnosis by serological tests for antibody or polymerase chain reaction reaction for the organism

SYPHILIS

The cervical lymph nodes are enlarged, soft and rubbery when the primary chancre is in the mouth or on the lip. Cervical nodes are also involved in the widespread lymphadenopathy of the secondary stage. Features are discussed in Chapter 15.

CAT-SCRATCH DISEASE

This infection is common in the United States and is increasingly frequently found in Britain. Ticks spread the causative organism *Bartonella henselae*, a small Gram-negative bacillus, among cats, and cats transmit the infection to humans through scratches or saliva. However, it may also be spread by dogs, rabbits, guinea pigs and probably other pets.

Typical features are summarised in Box 31.6.

Pathology

Adults and the immunocompetent usually clear the infection without signs. Young adults and children develop signs and symptoms 1–3 weeks after infection and eventually clear the infection in a month or two. An ulcer or nodule forms at the site of infection. In the immunosuppressed, the infection may spread to cause bacillary angiomatosis, a nodular infection of blood vessels that presents like Kaposi sarcoma but is unrelated to it.

If infection persists, the site of infection usually heals but infection persists in lymph nodes. There is destruction of lymph node architecture, necrosis and lymphocytic infiltration, formation of histiocytic granulomas and central suppuration (Fig. 31.5). The organisms may be seen on silver (Warthin–Starry) stain, but immunohistochemistry or PCR are more reliable, and serological tests also aid diagnosis.

Review PMID: 23654065

LYME DISEASE

Lyme disease is caused by a spirochaete, *Borrelia burgdorferi*, which is transmitted by insects, particularly deer ticks. The disease is found in the temperate northern hemisphere but is far more common in the United States than in the UK. However, the disease is underrecognised in the UK and likely to increase with global warming.

Diagnosis is by the history and clinical picture. It is confirmed serologically or, sometimes, by demonstration of the spirochaete by silver staining of a skin biopsy. Antibiotics are effective. However, joint pains may recur or destructive arthritis may develop later, apparently an immunologically mediated reaction to the treated infection. Note that erythema migrans in Lyme disease is a rash, unrelated to lingual erythema migrans.

Typical features are summarised in Box 31.7.

Review PMID: 21903253

INFECTIOUS MONONUCLEOSIS

The Epstein–Barr virus (EBV) is the main cause of this self-limiting lymphoproliferative disease. Infection is by saliva, but with relatively low infectivity. The virus replicates in pharyngeal epithelium and tonsils, from where it disseminates by infection of B lymphocytes. By early adulthood, almost all individuals are immune through subclinical infection.

The clinical features are usually distinctive but, rarely, there is more persistent lymphadenopathy that may mimic

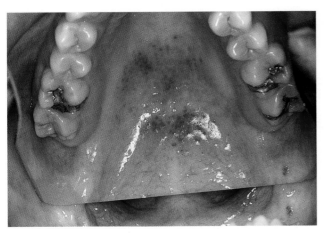

Fig. 31.6 Petechiae on the palate are frequently seen in infectious mononucleosis.

> **Box 31.8   Typical features of infectious mononucleosis**
>
> - In children especially
>   - Generalised lymphadenopathy, typically with conspicuous enlargement of the cervical nodes
>   - Sore throat
>   - Fever
> - In adolescents
>   - Lymphadenopathy often less conspicuous
>   - Vague illness with fever
>   - Fatigue
> - In adults
>   - Greater risk of complications: anaemia, jaundice, encephalitis

a lymphoma both clinically and histologically. Patients with severe sore throat, palatal petechiae (Fig. 31.6), enlarged tonsils with exudate and pharyngeal oedema are said to have the anginose form, which may compromise the airway.

Typical features are summarised in Box 31.8.

General review PMID: 20505178

Oral manifestations PMID: 5255344

Management

The diagnosis is confirmed by a peripheral blood picture showing the atypical (monocyte-like) lymphocytes. A heterophil antibody (Paul-Bunnell) test and, if necessary, demonstration of a raised titre of EBV antibodies are confirmatory. If these tests are negative in an otherwise typical case, cytomegalovirus infection, toxoplasmosis and acute HIV infection (seroconversion disease) should be considered.

There is no specific treatment, but infection is self-limiting.

Ampicillin or amoxicillin should be avoided during the disease as they cause irritating non-allergic macular rashes.

THE ACQUIRED IMMUNE DEFICIENCY SYNDROME

Lymphadenopathy is one of the most frequent manifestations of HIV infection and is discussed in detail in Chapter

> **Box 31.9   Possible effects of toxoplasmal infection**
>
> **Acute toxoplasmosis in normal children or adults**
> - Cervical lymphadenopathy in a disease resembling infectious mononucleosis
> - Atypical lymphocytes present in the blood but heterophil (Paul Bunnell) antibody production is absent
> - Infection usually self-limiting
>
> **Toxoplasmosis in immunodeficient patients**
> - Disseminated disease
> - Risk of complications including encephalitis
>
> **In pregnant women**
> - Transmission across placenta, an important cause of foetal abnormalities

29. Soon after infection there may be a transient glandular fever-like illness. Later, there may be widespread and persistent lymphadenopathy. Lymphadenopathy in AIDS may also be due to lymphomas.

TOXOPLASMOSIS

Toxoplasma gondii is a common intestinal parasite of many domestic animals, particularly cats. *T. gondii* is a low-grade pathogen in humans but can affect previously healthy persons, particularly young women. Infection is acquired by ingestion of parasites in poorly cooked foods or contact with cat litter, and three main types of disease can result (Box 31.9). Chorioretinitis is a complication that can lead to loss of sight and more often follows congenital infection.

Acute toxoplasmosis produces enlarged lymph nodes, often asymptomatic, but usually with mild malaise and fatigue. In adults only a single node may be enlarged; in children they are usually multiple. Node enlargement gradually resolves during several months, often 6 months. In immunosuppression, toxoplasmosis can be a severe infection with spread to the brain.

The diagnosis is confirmed serologically by a high or rising titre of antibodies or by other immunological methods. The enlarged lymph nodes are reactive to the infection and contain small granulomas that contain the parasites around and within the germinal centres (Fig. 31.7). If the diagnosis is not suspected or confirmed, a node may be removed for diagnosis.

Antimicrobial treatment is required only for severe infections.

Toxoplasma lymphadenopathy PMID: 3326123

MUCOCUTANEOUS LYMPH NODE SYNDROME (KAWASAKI'S DISEASE)

Kawasaki's disease is discussed in detail in Chapter 16. It causes an acute disease with fever, malaise, stomatitis, a characteristic rash and lymphadenopathy. Vasculitis of coronary arteries is a common feature. The disease is usually in a child younger than 5 years.

The lymphadenopathy is seen in three-quarters of cases and can be the main presenting feature. There is either a single large node or cluster of adjacent nodes. They are soft asymptomatic or minimally tender and usually unilateral. There may be erythema of the overlying skin.

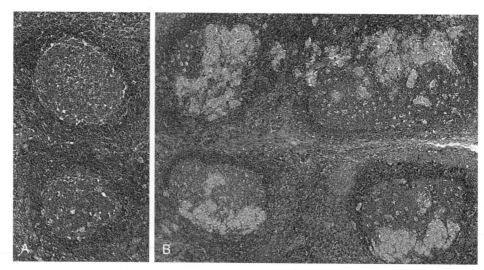

Fig. 31.7 **Toxoplasmosis.** *(A)* Two normal lymphoid follicles from a normal reactive node for comparison, showing the paler germinal centres surrounded by the dark mantle zones of immature lymphocytes. *(B)* Four lymphoid follicles from a lymph node in toxoplasmosis showing granulomas formed by pale clustered macrophages around the edges of, and within, the germinal centres.

Fine needle aspiration of nodes may show necrosis but is not diagnostic. Diagnosis is based on multiple features; there are no specific tests.

LANGERHANS CELL HISTIOCYTOSIS

Cervical lymph nodes can be enlarged, sometimes massively, in multisystem types of Langerhans cell histiocytosis, which is discussed in detail in Chapter 12. Occasionally lymphadenopathy is the presenting or only feature, and then the neck is the usual site. Fine needle aspiration is usually diagnostic, otherwise node excision or biopsy of another involved body site may be required.

SINUS HISTIOCYTOSIS WITH MASSIVE LYMPHADENOPATHY

This condition, also known as Rosai-Dorfman disease, is rare and causes extensive grossly enlarged lymph nodes, almost always cervical nodes bilaterally. It may also develop in the salivary glands, soft tissues and the respiratory sinuses. The name comes from the sinuses of the lymph nodes that are packed with large macrophages or histiocytes containing cell debris, not the respiratory sinuses. The cause is unknown.

Key features are shown in Box 31.10.

In cervical nodes PMID: 24412136 and 16618918

CASTLEMAN'S DISEASE

This uncommon disease is also known as angiofollicular lymph node hyperplasia and occurs in two forms, unicentric and multicentric.

Viral infection, either by human herpes virus 8 (Kaposi-sarcoma associated virus) or HIV infection, accounts for half of cases. The remainder are probably unknown viral infections.

Adolescents or young adults are most frequently affected, rarely children. The extent of lymphadenopathy is very variable.

Review both types PMID: 25310208

Box 31.10   Features of sinus histiocytosis with massive lymphadenopathy

- Most cases in children in first decade
- Occasional young adults affected
- Markedly enlarged cervical nodes bilaterally
- May be very high levels of circulating immunoglobulin
- Skin sometimes involved
- Cause unknown
- Lymph node biopsy or fine needle aspiration diagnostic
- Most cases resolve spontaneously
- Otherwise treatment by steroids, methotrexate or chemotherapy, rarely surgery

---

Unicentric Castleman's disease

This is the most common type, causing enlargement of a group of nodes, often in the mediastinum or neck, and consisting of a single large mass of nodes. Occasionally parotid nodes are involved, mimicking a parotid gland enlargement. Many cases are asymptomatic, but some develop the systemic features of the multicentric form. The prognosis is excellent. Surgical removal is curative, but if not possible, steroids control symptoms and the mass may remain for many years without progression or remission.

Multicentric Castleman's disease

In this type, nodes at many sites are affected and there are systemic features including fever, night sweats, weight loss and rash. Most cases are associated with human herpesvirus (HHV)-8 or HIV infection. HHV-8 encodes a homologue of interleukin 6 (vIL6) which mediates some of the systemic features. These features mimic lymphoma closely.

Multicentric disease is aggressive. In cases not caused by these viruses, treatment with monoclonal antibodies directed against IL-6 or its receptor are effective. When HIV or HHV8 infection are present, treatment is by antiretroviral treatment for HIV and ganciclovir for HHV8 in conjunction with chemotherapy. Treatment is complex, evolving and not always successful. Death can result from a number

Box 31.11 Complications and disease associations of multicentric Castleman's disease

- Anaemia
- Lymphoma of Hodgkin's and non-Hodgkin's types
- Kaposi sarcoma in human herpesvirus 8–positive disease
- Paraneoplastic pemphigus
- Autoimmune and connective tissue diseases
- Infection due to neutropaenia or immunsuppression
- Amyloidosis
- POEMS syndrome*
- Other complications of HIV disease if HIV positive

*POEMS, **P**olyneuropathy, **O**rganomegaly, **E**ndocrinopathy, **M**onoclonal gammopathy and **S**kin abnormalities syndrome.

Box 31.12 Drugs that can cause lymphadenopathy

- Phenytoin
- Carbamazepine
- Allopurinol
- Sulphasalazine
- Phenobarbital
- Lamotrigine
- Nevirapine
- Isoniazid
- Iodine
- Penicillin
- Captopril
- Tetracycline
- Atenolol

of complications. Only 30% of HIV and HHV8-positive patients survive 3 years versus 75% of HIV-negative patients.

Complications of multicentric Castleman's disease are shown in Box 31.11.

Pathology

The node is enlarged by proliferation of either plasma cells or lymphocytes. In the plasma cell type the lymphoid follicles are active and enlarged. In the lymphocyte-rich type (hyaline vascular type) the follicles are atrophic and shrunken leaving prominent epithelioid blood vessels and proliferating dendritic cells, surrounded by concentric rings of lymphocytes (Fig. 31.8). This latter type accounts for almost all cases in the head and neck. Diagnosis is usually based on lymph node biopsy, and the specimen can be tested for HHV8 by immunohistochemistry.

DRUG-ASSOCIATED LYMPHADENOPATHY

Lymphadenopathy is an occasional adverse effect of long-term treatment with the antiepileptic drug phenytoin. Phenytoin lymphadenopathy is not associated with systemic symptoms and frequently first affects the neck before becoming widespread. Substitution of phenytoin with an alternative usually leads to resolution.

Other drugs that can cause lymphadenopathy (Box 31.12) do so very rarely. Lymphadenopathy caused by these drugs is typically associated with fever, rashes, eosinophilia and joint pains, and they are thought to be drug hypersensitivity reactions. Other organ damage may be associated, making these potentially fatal drug reactions. Cervical nodes are the most frequently affected.

VIRCHOW'S NODE

A single firm or hard node in the lower left side of the neck immediately above the medial end of the clavicle should raise suspicion of a Virchow's node presentation*.

*Rudolf Virchow, a German pathologist (1821–1902) from what is now Poland, described this sign. Contrary to some reports he did not actually suffer it himself. Although renowned as the father of modern pathology and cellular theories of disease, he is perhaps more widely remembered for choosing sausages as a duelling weapon when challenged by Bismarck, the first Chancellor of Germany.

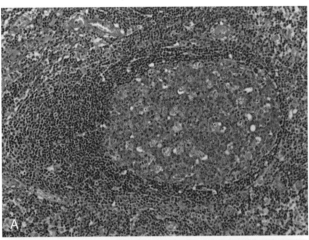

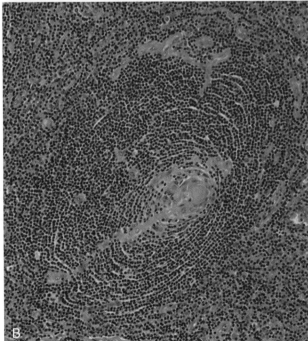

Fig. 31.8 Castleman's disease. Hyaline vascular-type disease. *(A)* A normal lymphoid follicle, with a germinal centre surrounded by a mantle of small dark lymphocytes. *(B)* Atrophic follicle with a prominent swollen vessel entering the follicle from lower left. The vessel is surrounded by concentric rings of lymphocytes, resembling the mantle zone of the normal follicle.

Lymphatic drainage from the chest, abdomen and pelvis flowing in the thoracic duct regularly flows in a retrograde manner into the lymphatics of the lower neck because of their low pressure or variations in lymphatic and venous anatomy. Cells from cancers in the thorax and abdomen can thus seed a metastasis in a lymph node low in the neck.

The left side is more frequently the site of metastases, and these usually originate from the stomach, abdomen and pelvis. Although classically described on the left, the right side may develop metastases from the oesophagus, chest and lungs.

DELPHIAN NODE

A Delphian node is a single midline level VI lymph node (Fig. 20.17) anterior to the cricothyroid membrane of the larynx that is often the first involved by carcinoma of the larynx or thyroid. It is named after the mythical oracle of Delphi, because historically enlargement was known to predict that cancer would subsequently become apparent at one of these sites.

Cardiovascular disease

32

Cardiovascular disease is commonly encountered in dental practice. Heart disease becomes more frequent and severe in later life and is the most frequent single cause of death in Britain in males, with only dementia slightly more common in females. Younger patients can also be affected. Infective endocarditis is one of the few ways in which dental treatment could lead to death of a patient.

The nature of the relationships among periodontitis, atheroma and diabetes remain unclear, although these conditions are often associated.

Acute angina and myocardial infarction are discussed with medical emergencies (Ch. 43).

In terms of dental management, patients with cardiac problems provide no significant barriers to treatment. Patients in ASA groups 3 and 4 (American Society of Anaesthesiologists Physical Status score) for cardiac reasons can still be managed with intravenous sedation, provided the treatment is individually assessed and provided by a person with specialist training and in a specialist centre. It is important to be aware of each patient's disease type, medication (Table 32.1) and severity to assess the likelihood of a cardiac emergency, but the main risks are for general anaesthesia.

General review PMID: 11060950

Table 32.1 Some dental implications or adverse effects of drugs used for heart disease

Drugs	Implications for dental management
Diuretics	Dry mouth sometimes
Angiotensin-converting enzyme (ACE) inhibitors, captopril, perindopril, etc.	Burning mouth symptoms, lichenoid reactions, angio-oedema
Angiotensin II receptor blockers, losartan, disopyramide, etc.	Taste disturbance, dry mouth
Calcium channel blockers, amlodipine, diltiazem, etc.	Gingival overgrowth (especially with diltiazem and nifedipine – Fig. 32.1)
Beta-adrenergic blockers, labetalol, propranolol, etc.	Dry mouth, lichenoid reactions, theoretical interaction with epinephrine
Antihypertensives (as above)	Potentiated by general anaesthetics
Anticoagulants	Risk of prolonged post-operative bleeding
Warfarin	Risk of prolonged post-operative bleeding
Antianginal drugs Nicorandil Digoxin	Oral ulceration (Ch.16)

GENERAL ASPECTS OF MANAGEMENT

Patients at risk of cardiac events are usually severe hypertensives, those with severe angina or those who have had a previous myocardial infarct. Anxiety or pain can precipitate a dangerous increase in cardiac load and dysrhythmias through the action of epinephrine. To die of fright may be a figure of speech but can sometimes result from severe dysrhythmia. The first essential element for these patients is therefore to ensure painless dentistry and to alleviate anxiety.

Consideration may be given to providing an anxiolytic before treatment (a benzodiazepine at low dose on the preceding night and again before treatment) in very anxious patients. If sedation is required, inhalational sedation is safe because nitrous oxide has no cardiorespiratory depressant effects and is more controllable, but it should be administered by an expert and not given within 3 months of a heart attack or angina attack requiring hospitalisation.

Patients with severe or longstanding hypertension are at risk from ischaemic heart disease. Medical advice should be sought before treating those with a resting systolic blood pressure over 160 or a diastolic over 95 mmHg.

Lingual varices and hypertension PMCID: PMC4499223

Treatment in heart failure PMID: 23444163

Dentistry in heart disease PMID: 20527501

Local analgesia

Over many decades, different precautions have been recommended for combinations of local analgesics and vasoconstrictors with various drugs. Concern often arose with what were newly introduced classes of drugs at the time. None of these theoretical interactions have ever proved significant in a dental setting with normal doses of drugs. Patients with

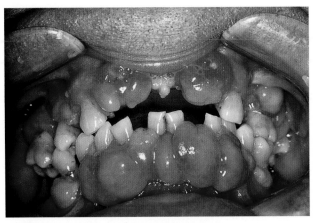

Fig. 32.1 Drug-induced gingival hyperplasia resulting from treatment of hypertension with nifedipine. These swellings are centred on the interdental papillae.

cardiovascular disease need to be treated with care, but the risks of adverse reactions are very low indeed.

The most effective analgesic agent is 2% lidocaine with epinephrine and, after half a century of use, no local anaesthetic has been shown to be safer. The epinephrine content can *theoretically* cause a hypertensive reaction in patients receiving beta-blocker antihypertensives, because of an unopposed alpha-adrenergic effect. This interaction is only likely if doses of epinephrine are considerably larger than normally used in dentistry.

In view of the risk of dysrhythmias, it is important to reduce anxiety and achieve good analgesia. Doses of local anaesthetics should be kept to the minimum necessary and treatment split into several sessions if extensive. Good injection technique is essential. If larger doses have to be given, for example for multiple extractions, then continuous cardiac monitoring is prudent and hospital treatment probably wise.

If general anaesthesia is unavoidable, it must be given by a specialist anaesthetist in hospital, especially as some of the drugs used for cardiovascular disease increase the risks. Cardiovascular disease is the chief cause of sudden death under anaesthesia.

Cardiac effects LA PMID: 19893562

Vasoconstrictor safety review PMID: 10332135

Adrenaline effects PMID: 19330241

Anxious patient PMID: 19023307

Cardiac transplant PMID: 11863154

INFECTIVE ENDOCARDITIS

If there is a cardiac defect that can be colonised by circulating organisms, infective endocarditis can develop. Patients at risk are mainly those with congenital anomalies, such as valve or septal defects, or who have prosthetic heart valve replacements and often with an additional risk factor (Box 32.1). The majority of these patients have no symptoms and some valve defects, such as a bicuspid aortic valve, cause no symptoms to signal their presence.

Damaged valves are infected by bacteria passing through the lumen of the large vessels, when turbulent flow around a damaged valve brings bacteria in contact with the endothelium.

There are many causes of bacteraemia. Bacteria can spread into the blood from tissue infections, during surgery, colonoscopy and, particularly, from infection of peripherally inserted central catheters ('PICC' lines), cannulae and traditional central lines. Intravenous drug users risk bacteraemia by using contaminated needles. Mucosal surfaces are potent sources of bacteraemia because they are heavily colonised by bacteria, as in the bowel. Oral organisms are responsible for 30%–40% of all cases of infective endocarditis.

Bacteraemias can be detected in more than 80% of persons after tooth extraction and even after tooth brushing or chewing, but the numbers of bacteria released by the latter are much lower. Although a large number of bacteria in the circulation appear to pose the higher risk, it is unclear whether chronic low-grade bacteraemia may be as dangerous as a short high-level bacteraemia.

Normally, bacteria entering the bloodstream are rapidly cleared by the phagocytic cells lining the sinusoids in the liver or spleen, or by circulating leucocytes, aided by complement. These are largely non-specific mechanisms that do not depend on an immune response or the virulence of the organism. Almost all circulating bacteria are cleared within a few minutes to an hour, and even in a patient with a heart lesion, infective endocarditis does not necessarily follow.

The main sources of oral bacteria causing bacteraemia are the gingival crevice and periodontal pockets. The risk is high when oral hygiene is poor. At these sites, large numbers of bacteria are in close contact with inflamed tissue containing dilated, thin-walled blood vessels (Fig. 32.2). The chance of bacteria entering vessels is increased by movement of teeth, even just during mastication. When teeth are mobile, movement repeatedly compresses and stretches the periodontium so that bacteria can be pumped into the tissues, and possibly the bloodstream.

Either an acute or subacute endocarditis can follow infection of cardiac valves. Acute endocarditis is not linked to bacteraemia of dental origin and is usually associated with species of high virulence such as *Staphylococcus aureus*, fungi or unusual organisms.

Bacteraemias of oral organisms are associated with subacute infective endocarditis and are of low virulence organisms such as viridans streptococci. These bacteria adhere to the valve using fibronectin and other carbohydrate receptors to bind to platelets and fibrin on the damaged surface, similar to the mechanisms by which they adhere to plaque matrix. The more virulent obligate anaerobes of the periodontal pocket cannot survive long enough in the blood to cause endocarditis.

Attributing infective endocarditis to a bacteraemia caused by dental procedures is difficult. Fewer than 15% of cases of infective endocarditis can be related to (but not necessarily caused by) dental operations. When dental procedures are linked to endocarditis, the most common likely precipitating factor is dental extraction, found in more than 95% of cases.

Box 32.1 Additional non-cardiac risk factors for infective endocarditis

- Age
- Prior severe kidney disease
- Diabetes mellitus
- Poor oral hygiene (although the relative risk is very low)

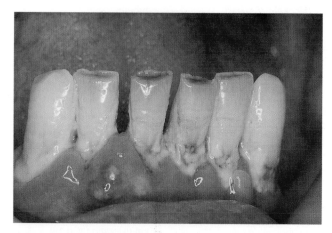

Fig. 32.2 Poor oral hygiene and severe pocketing such as this constitutes a risk to life, particularly in an elderly patient with a cardiac valve defect.

More than 2000 cases arise each year in the UK, and a quarter of patients die within 1 year.

Once bacteria adhere to the damaged valve, platelets and fibrin deposit over them. Lumpy 'vegetations' of bacteria and fibrin form on the free edges of the valves, which are progressively destroyed by inflammation and immune response against the bacteria, rendering the valves incompetent. Cardiac failure is the main cause of death, but infective emboli and bacteria released into the bloodstream can also cause renal or cerebral damage.

General review PMID: 26341945

Clinical features

It is important to appreciate that the onset of subacute infective endocarditis is typically very insidious. Symptoms are vague, variable among patients and may not be related to the heart valve damage itself. The descriptions that follow relate to subacute bacterial endocarditis caused by oral organisms, almost always streptococci, and not to acute or other types of endocarditis in intravenous drug users or other groups at risk.

The mitral valve is most frequently affected, but surprisingly congestive heart failure due to valvular insufficiency is a very infrequent presenting sign.

The most common signs and symptoms are all non-specific: fever, malaise, headache, night sweats, shortness of breath, joint pains and, over the longer term, anorexia and weight loss. Although association with a dental procedure is rarely if ever proven, when it appears likely, the onset is usually between 2 weeks and 2 months later.

The valve vegetations shed small emboli into the systemic circulation. Classically, these cause distant effects such as splinter haemorrhages and damage to various organs. These embolic phenomena are rare in oral streptococcal endocarditis, but nevertheless a range of rare complications such as stroke, osteomyelitis, meningitis and renal infarcts may be seen. Similar complications can arise from sterile deposition of immune complexes in the kidney and joints.

These variable and non-specific symptoms make it important that patients at risk understand that they should report any mild, unexplained, febrile illness within 3 months of dental treatment. Delay in diagnosis is the main factor affecting survival in infective endocarditis.

PREVENTION OF ENDOCARDITIS

Principles of antibiotic prophylaxis

The principle of antibiotic prophylaxis is that high doses of antibiotic given before a dental or medical intervention will achieve a sufficiently high blood level to kill any bacteria that enter the circulation before they have the opportunity to adhere to the heart valves. In the past, patients at risk would be given antibiotics such as amoxicillin or clindamycin as a single dose before any procedure that was considered likely to trigger a significant bacteraemia.

This approach remains sound and antibiotic prophylaxis is used before procedures such as colonoscopy or barium enema that displace large numbers of bacteria into the circulation.

However, it has never been possible to prove that the previously recommended prophylactic measures used for dentistry were effective. It was estimated that in the UK, in a year, no fewer than 670,000 at-risk patients may have been undergoing high-risk dental procedures without antibiotic prophylaxis. Despite this, only a tiny minority of all cases of endocarditis might have been associated with dentistry. The incidence of infective endocarditis does not appear to have been significantly reduced by the introduction of antibiotic prophylaxis.

It has always been accepted that there is little evidence that prophylaxis is effective. It is known that infective endocarditis may develop despite appropriate prophylaxis, and also that bacteraemia from mastication and tooth brushing may constitute a significant risk because of the frequency with which it occurs.

In the absence of clear evidence, antibiotic prophylaxis has previously been provided on the precautionary principle.

Current guidance on antibiotic prophylaxis

The evidence on antibiotic prophylaxis has been reviewed by several groups in different countries, including the European Cardiac Society and the American Heart Association. All, apart from the UK group, consider that antibiotic prophylaxis should be provided, although over the years the complexity of prophylaxis and the number of patients considered at risk have reduced.

In the UK, the definitive guidance is that of The National Institute for Health and Care Excellence (NICE) and published in the British National Formulary. The guidance was issued in 2008, updated in 2015 and 2016 and remains current at time of publication. It states that antibiotic prophylaxis is 'not recommended routinely' for dental procedures. The use of chlorhexidine around teeth before extraction is also not recommended.

Instead, prevention of endocarditis should rely on a high standard of oral health, the responsibility of both patient and professionals.

This decision is based primarily on the lack of evidence to support prophylaxis for dental procedures balanced against the risks. If the benefit is small, the risk of anaphylaxis and antibiotic resistance become more significant. It has been estimated that death from anaphylaxis to penicillin cover is approximately five times more likely than death from endocarditis.

Review PMID: 26794105

Web URL 32.1 NICE guidance: https://www.nice.org.uk/guidance/cg64

Previous UK guideline PMID: 16624872

IE increasing UK PMID: 25467569

European Soc Cardiol Guidelines PMID: 26320109

Dental IE in Taiwan PMID: 26512586

US guidelines PMID: 9431393

Case reports PMID: 26992086

Web URL 32.2 UK medicolegal advice: http://www.dentalprotection.org/uk/ and enter 'antibiotic prophylaxis' into search box

After the discontinuation of antibiotic prophylaxis in 2008, the number of cases of infective endocarditis in the UK rose by a statistically significant number (Fig. 32.3). This has caused some consternation, but review of this additional evidence by NICE did not change the guidance in 2016. This type of epidemiological evidence cannot make a causative link between the increasing incidence and discontinuation of antibiotic prophylaxis, although the temporal association is striking. No other cause for the rise

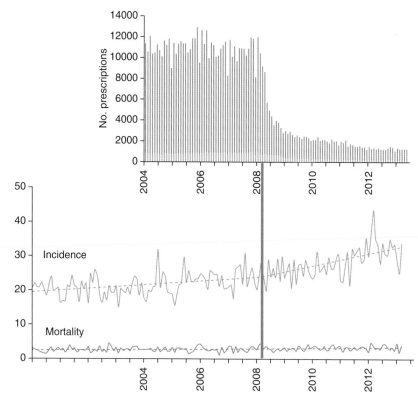

Fig. 32.3 Reduction in antibiotic prophylaxis since 2008 NICE guidance and incidence and mortality of endocarditis in England plotted on the same timescale. The upper graph shows the number of prescriptions for antibiotic cover given by dentists (*brown*) and doctors (*blue*). The vertical brown line indicates the introduction of the 2008 NICE guidance in March 2008. The lower graph shows the incidence (*blue*) and mortality (*brown*) from all cases of endocarditis over the same period. *(From Dayar, M., Jones, S., Prendergast, B., et al., 2015. Incidence of infective endocarditis in England 2000-2013: a secular trend, interrupted time-series analysis. Lancet 385 (9974), 1219–1228.)*

could be detected, although increasing incidence is expected with the ageing population, increasing use of artificial valves and implanted cardiac devices, and increase in predisposing conditions such as diabetes mellitus and renal dialysis.

A randomised controlled trial to define the benefit of routine prophylaxis is unlikely to be performed, and the low level evidence used to support the guidance is open to different interpretations. It is noteworthy that anaphylactic reactions against amoxicillin used for prophylaxis in dentistry are vanishingly rare because the allergy history is known, most patients will have received previous doses and there is time to confirm any suspected allergy before administration. Single-dose amoxicillin prophylaxis has not caused a single fatal reaction in the UK for several decades, and its adverse effects may have been overestimated.

Although the NICE recommendations are clear, some feel that antibiotic prophylaxis should still be given to the highest risk patients. The 2016 amendment, stating that prophylaxis is 'not recommended routinely' (as opposed to 'not recommended' in the 2008 and 2015 versions) does leave open the possibility that prophylaxis may be given for certain patients. However, the guidance does not provide any help to determine when prophylaxis might be of benefit, which patients are at highest risk or which dental procedures carry a risk.

Prevention

It is critical to understand that the discontinuation of antibiotic prophylaxis does not absolve the dentist from responsibility for preventing and detecting endocarditis.

The first step is to identify patients at risk through their medical history (Box 32.2) and, if necessary, by consulting

> **Box 32.2**
>
> Patients at risk of infective endocarditis have:
>
> - structural congenital heart disease, including surgically corrected or palliated structural conditions, but excluding isolated atrial septal defect, fully repaired ventricular septal defect or fully repaired patent ductus arteriosus, and closure devices that are judged to be endothelialised
> - acquired valvular heart disease with stenosis or regurgitation
> - hypertrophic cardiomyopathy
> - previous infective endocarditis
> - valve replacement
> - cardiac surgery with implanted prosthetic materials

the relevant medical consultant. It must also be recognised that occasionally patients without valve damage can contract endocarditis, though this is rarely caused by oral organisms.

Patients who have become accustomed to receive antibiotic prophylaxis may not always feel happy to do without it, given the emphasis that was previously placed on its administration. Guidance therefore includes an important element of patient education. The recommendations are that dentists should offer patients at risk 'clear and consistent information about prevention, including the benefits and risks of antibiotic prophylaxis, and an explanation of why antibiotic prophylaxis is no longer routinely recommended'.

Those at risk must also be educated in the importance of maintaining good oral health and returning immediately should they suffer any symptoms suggesting that they have developed infective endocarditis. Patient advice could also include general health advice such as the risks of undergoing other medical invasive procedures, body piercing or tattooing. Ensuring patients are informed and involved in any decision is paramount. Medicolegally they must be advised of potential adverse effects of treatment.

Any foci of oral infection should be addressed and eliminated promptly. Current guidance refers to infection, but this should be taken to include any foci of periodontitis or gingivitis, as well as overt tissue infection. There needs to be a good preventive regime in place to prevent development of caries and odontogenic infection, as well as of gingival inflammation. All patients at risk must maintain the highest standards of oral health.

Some patients will continue to demand antibiotic prophylaxis. Similarly, some cardiologists will request prophylaxis for certain high-risk groups. The recommendations are guidance rather than mandatory so that clinical judgement may allow a different course of action provided it can be justified.

The dentist should always contact the relevant medical consultant about any high-risk patient to ask whether cover is recommended or when a patients requests cover. Those at particularly high risk are those who have had previous infective endocarditis, those with prosthetic heart valves or prosthetic surgical heart repair and those with congenital cyanotic cardiac defects. In the absence of national recommendations, there is no guidance on prophylaxis, but the cover regime most likely to be recommended is either 2g or 3g amoxicillin 30–60 minutes preoperatively before extractions or similar significant interventions. For those allergic, clindamycin, 600 mg, remains the safest alternative. Even among those who believe that prophylaxis is useful, there is a tendency to restrict it to high-risk dental procedures including extraction, scaling, root canal treatment and other surgical procedures. These suggestions are in line with the European Society of Cardiology guidelines (Appendix 32.1). Inclusion of these guidelines is not to suggest that they are better than current UK guidance. They are given only as a reasonable alternative to follow in the absence of UK guidance on what to do when cover *is* requested by a cardiologist or patient. Guidance changes continually, and the current version must always be consulted.

Whether or not cover is given, all patients at risk need to be reminded of the signs and symptoms and the need to return if unwell, after all types of dental treatment.

Web URL 32.3 Patient advice leaflet/warning card: https://www.bhf.org.uk/publications/heart-conditions/m26a-endocarditis-card

IMPLANTED CARDIAC DEVICES

Increasing numbers of patients have either pacemakers or implantable cardioverter defibrillators to treat bradycardia, arrhythmias, tachycardia, fibrillation and heart block.

Some types of ultrasonic scalers (the magneto-constrictive and not the piezoelectric type) and electrosurgical equipment produce a magnetic field that potentially interferes with their function, and use should be avoided as a precautionary measure even though the risk appears largely theoretical. Pulp testers and apex locators are safe. In the absence of a good evidence base, seeking advice from the manufacturer seems sensible and use of the magnetic type of ultrasonic scaler should be avoided for these patients.

There is no indication for antibiotic prophylaxis.

Case report PMID: 21439866

Published European guideline PMID: 26320109

Appendix 32.1

European Society of Cardiology guidelines for the management of infective endocarditis

Antibiotic prophylaxis should only be considered for patients at highest risk for endocarditis, as described in Table 1 below, undergoing at-risk dental procedures listed in Table 2 below, and is not recommended in other situations. The main targets for antibiotic prophylaxis in these patients are oral streptococci. Table 3, below, summarises the main regimens of antibiotic prophylaxis recommended before dental procedures.

Table 1
Antibiotic prophylaxis should be considered for patients at highest risk of infective endocarditis:
1. Patients with any prosthetic valve, including a transcatheter valve, or those in whom any prosthetic material was used for cardiac valve repair
2. Patients with a previous episode of infective endocarditis
3. Patients with any type of cyanotic congenital heart disease or any type of congenital heart disease repaired with a prosthetic material, whether placed surgically or by percutaneous techniques, as long as 6 months after the procedure or lifelong if residual shunt or valvular regurgitation remains.
Antibiotic prophylaxis is not recommended in other forms of valvular or congenital heart disease

Table 2
Antibiotic prophylaxis should only be considered for dental procedures requiring manipulation of gingival or periapical region of the teeth or perforation of the oral mucosa.

Table 3

Situation	Antibiotic	Single-dose 30–60 minutes before procedure	
		Adults	Children
No allergy to penicillin or ampicillin	Amoxicillin or ampicillin	2 g orally or i.v.	50 mg/kg orally or i.v.
Allergy to penicillin or ampicillin	Clindamycin	600 mg orally or i.v.	20 mg/kg orally or i.v.

Note that either 2g or 3g amoxicillin may be used, 3g the more readily available preparation in the UK.
Clindamycin has a significant rate of adverse effects and should only be used for high risk patients.
It is no longer necessary to avoid Amoxicillin if the patient has already been exposed it in the previous month.
From 2015 ESC Guidelines for the management of infective endocarditis: The Task Force for the Management of Infective Endocarditis of the European Society of Cardiology (ESC) Endorsed by: European Association for Cardio-Thoracic Surgery (EACTS), the European Association of Nuclear Medicine (EANM). Habib, G., Lancellotti, P., Antunes, M.J., et al., 2015. Eur. Heart J. 36 (44), 3075-30128.

Respiratory tract disease

33

ACUTE SINUSITIS → Summary chart 38.1, p. 486

Acute maxillary sinusitis is a very common condition that often presents with pain suggesting a dental cause. However, almost all acute sinusitis is a sequela of viral infection in the nasal passages and sinuses. Inflammation inhibits mucociliary clearance, and oedema restricts sinus drainage by narrowing the ostium, raising the internal pressure.

Clinical features

Onset almost always follows a respiratory viral illness. Infection of the lining mucosa is by the same virus that caused the respiratory infection and usually resolves with the main infection in 7–10 days. Symptoms lasting longer probably indicate bacterial infection.

There is sudden onset of pain from the sinus, often poorly localised, with tenderness of the overlying skin. Teeth with roots in or close to the antrum are painful on pressure. There are also nasal congestion, weakened sense of smell and sometimes referred pain to the ear. Fluid will often discharge into the nose on tilting the head or lying down and movement of the head worsens pain. Involvement of ethmoid or sphenoid sinuses is often perceived by patients as headache.

Diagnosis and management

The diagnosis may usually be made on the history and examination. Radiography of the sinuses provides little additional information in acute sinusitis. Computerised tomography is the method of choice if radiographs are required (Fig. 33.1), mainly to detect polyps after repeated attacks and not for diagnosis.

Acute sinusitis is self-limiting. No active treatment may be required, but nasal decongestants aid drainage, speed recovery and provide symptomatic relief. Many patients manage well with non-prescription steam inhalations containing menthol or eucalyptus oils. More severe cases benefit from ephedrine or oxymetazoline nose drops, but these should not be continued for more than 7 days.

Even when bacterial infection is present, antibiotic treatment is not indicated, at least initially. Persistence or worsening of symptoms after 10 days or presence of pus suggest bacterial infection, and the usual organisms are aerobes such as *Streptococcus pneumoniae*, *Haemophilus influenzae* and beta-haemolytic streptococci. *Staphylococcus aureus* is a more frequent isolate from the sphenoid sinus. These pathogens are beta-lactamase positive in half of cases, and either high-dose amoxicillin or amoxicillin with clavulanic acid are appropriate empirical first-line drugs. If these fail, a pus sample for sensitivity testing must be obtained by puncture of the sinus.

Dental causes need to be excluded but are present in only 5% of cases, being much more likely to be identified in chronic sinusitis (see later).

Although most cases resolve, sinusitis may become recurrent or chronic.

US guideline PMID: 22438350

European guideline PMID: 22764607

UK guideline PMID: 18167126

Web URL 33.1 NICE guidance: http://cks.nice.org.uk/sinusitis

CHRONIC SINUSITIS

→ Summary chart 38.1, p. 486

Chronic sinusitis may develop with or without a preceding acute sinusitis.

The clinical features are those of the acute disease but milder and without the generalised symptoms of upper respiratory tract viral infection. When pain is poorly localised, radiographic examination of the sinuses may reveal mucosal thickening, mucosal polyps or a fluid level. Computerised tomography is the examination of choice (Fig. 33.2), but the maxillary antrum is well visualised on panoramic tomography or occipitomental view.

Chronic sinusitis in some patients produces nasal polyps, oedematous thickenings and pedunculated polyps of the mucosa. These can fill the lumen, block drainage and cause persistence of sinusitis.

Management

When no dental cause is present, the bacteria are initially those found in acute sinusitis, but the flora gradually shifts to an anaerobic population after 3 months and *S. aureus* is often present.

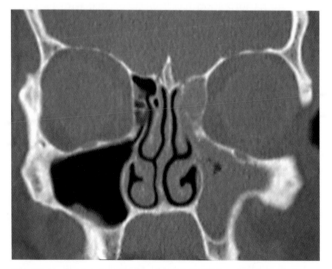

Fig. 33.1   Acute sinusitis involving maxillary antrum and ethmoid sinuses unilaterally. The sinuses are completely filled by oedematous sinus lining mucosa and inflammatory exudate, seen radiographically as opacified sinuses. *(Courtesy of Mr EJ Whaites.)*

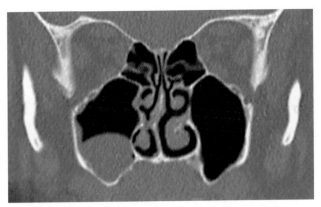

Fig. 33.2 Chronic sinusitis with an antral polyp, a localised area of mucosal oedema and thickening. Mucosal thickening or polyps on the floor of the antrum indicate a need to exclude dental and periodontal causes. (See also Fig. 33.5.) *(Courtesy of Dr S Connor.)*

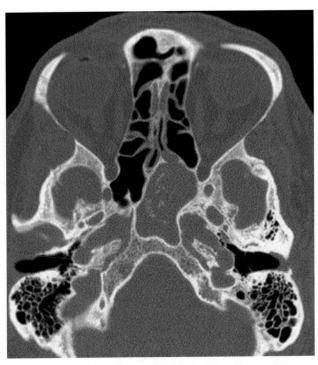

Fig. 33.3 A fungus ball or mycetoma in the sphenoid sinus. The sinus is opacified and faint spotty mineralisation can be seen in the centre of the fungus ball, which has grown to expand and distort the sinus. Maxillary sinus lesions appear identical.

Patients with chronic sinusitis without a dental cause must be referred to a specialist. Polyps, allergic and fungal causes must be excluded by endoscopy. Antibiotic treatment alone usually fails and a combined approach with improving drainage, saline irrigation, reducing inflammation with topical steroids and tackling infection is required. It is suggested that in chronic sinusitis the bacteria exist in a biofilm, resistant to antimicrobials and the host response. Endoscopic sinus surgery may be required if there is no improvement in a few weeks.

US guideline PMID: 22438350

European guideline PMID: 22764607

UK guideline PMID: 18167126

Web URL 33.1 NICE guidance: http://cks.nice.org.uk/sinusitis

Odontogenic sinusitis

Potential dental causes are relatively frequent in chronic sinusitis but may not necessarily be the primary cause. Dental contributing factors are often poorly diagnosed in medical management and the role of the dentist in identifying and treating possible causes is important for success of treatment. Odontogenic sinusitis is usually unilateral.

The roots of the maxillary molar teeth lie close to or within the antrum. In some patients, the root apex perforates the cortex so that only mucous membrane covers it. The commonest dental causes of sinus inflammation are therefore periapical periodontitis from a non-vital molar, extraction, root treatment or severe periodontal disease. A new cause is excessive sinus lift graft material placed for implants. These causes are best identified by vitality testing, clinical examination and dental radiography, particularly cone beam computed tomography (CT).

When dental infection is a factor, additional anaerobic oral bacteria such as *Prevotella* spp. and *Fusobacterium* spp. are found. Antibiotic treatment is only effective in conjunction with removal of the cause. Appropriate regimens are amoxicillin with clavulanic acid or a penicillin with metronidazole or as guided by culture and sensitivity, but integrated with the timing of medical and endoscopic treatments.

Odontogenic sinusitis PMID: 26662929, 26319958 and 25732329

Fungal sinusitis

Fungal sinusitis results from inhalation and germination of air-borne fungal spores that are not cleared by mucociliary transport, usually because of pre-existing sinus inflammation. The causative fungi originate in soil and their spores are widespread in the environment.

The commonest type is a 'fungus ball' or mycetoma, a tangled mass of fungal hyphae bound together with mucus and inflammatory exudate. The ball may grow to fill the sinus and is commonly *Aspergillus* spp. Radiographic diagnosis is aided by the frequent presence of spotty mineralisation in the fungus ball (Figs. 33.3 and 33.4).

Mycetoma formation has been associated with particles of zinc-containing root filling material. These presumably enter the sinus after root treatment and may sometimes be seen on radiographs. Inflammation from apical periodontitis would prevent clearance of spores from the sinus and zinc encourages fungal growth.

Mycetomas are treated by surgical removal of the fungus followed by irrigation and sometimes topical or systemic antifungal treatment.

Sinus mycetoma PMID: 17361410

Allergic fungal sinusitis

Some patients mount a florid type 1 hypersensitivity reaction to fungus in the sinuses. Serum immunoglobulin (Ig) E is usually raised. The inflammatory reaction produces thick putty-like masses of dense mucin containing numerous eosinophils and a few fungal hyphae. Mucosal polyps are usually present.

Some studies have suggested that almost all cases of chronic sinusitis refractory to treatment are caused by these fungi. Many species are identified, usually environmental species such as *Alternaria sp., Aspergillus sp.* or *Bipolaris sp.*

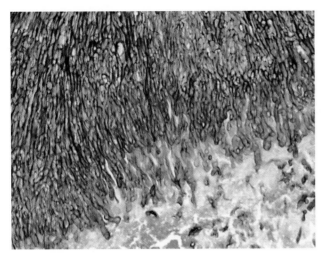

Fig. 33.4 A fungus ball or mycetoma from the maxillary sinus. Grocott stain has a green background and stains the cell walls of the fungal hyphae black. At the top the hyphae are densely packed together in a single huge colony, and at the edge individual hyphae can be seen growing outwards.

Allergic fungal sinusitis requires surgical removal of the thick 'allergic mucin'. Antifungal drugs are sometimes used but of limited value.

Allergic fungal sinusitis can produce worrying signs radiographically. The chronic inflammation may cause resorption of the sinus wall, mimicking a malignant neoplasm.

Allergic fungal sinusitis PMID: 14515093 and 19330659

Invasive fungal sinusitis

In the immunocompromised, the fungi may invade the sinus wall, cause rapid extensive destruction and often a fatal outcome. Such cases are caused by more virulent environmental fungi such as *Mucor sp*. and require aggressive surgical and antifungal treatment (Ch. 9).

SURGICAL DAMAGE TO THE MAXILLARY ANTRUM

The floor of the antrum may be damaged during dental extractions that cause an oroantral communication. If the antrum is opened during an extraction, a displaced root or bacteria from the mouth can introduce infection. There is also damage to the ciliated lining and loss of normal muco-ciliary transport, which carries foreign material out of the cavity. If sinusitis becomes established and the fistula has not been closed, the walls of the passage may become epithelialised, polyps develop in the sinus mucosa and the opening becomes a permanent fistula.

Displacement of a root or tooth into the maxillary antrum

A tooth or root can be driven into the antrum if excessive force has been used during extraction or in attempting to elevate fragments, particularly when a thin antral floor extends down into the alveolar ridge.

Displacement of a tooth or root into the antrum can give rise to signs (Box 33.1), partly depending on the size of the opening.

> **Box 33.1   Signs suggesting a tooth or root displaced into the antrum**
>
> - The root or tooth suddenly disappears during the extraction
> - Blowing the nose may force air into the mouth or cause frothing of blood from the socket
> - The patient may notice air entering the mouth during swallowing, or fluid from the mouth escapes into the nose
> - Bleeding from the nose on the affected side, occasionally
> - Later, a salty taste or unpleasant discharge
> - Facial pain if acute sinusitis develops
> - Rarely, antral lining or polyps may prolapse into the mouth

> **Box 33.2   Principles of management of a root displaced into the antrum**
>
> - Explain to the patient how the accident has happened and give the necessary reassurance
> - Do not to try to retrieve the lost root immediately by digging through the socket opening and damaging the antral floor and lining further
> - If a root or tooth has been displaced into the antrum, it should be removed by elective surgery (see later)
> - If the tip of a root causes a minimal antral reaction or lies between the bony floor and the mucosal lining, removal may not be essential but there is a risk of infection later

Management

The position of the root or tooth should be confirmed. Sometimes it is still within the alveolar process or between the mucosal lining and bony floor. If the fragment is not visible on a periapical radiograph and occlusal view, cone beam CT provides the best localisation. Plain films taken with the head in two different positions will reveal whether the tooth is mobile.

A root displaced into the antrum usually causes sinusitis, but it may cause no more than mucosal thickening. Severe sinusitis is less common. The root should be removed from the antrum as soon as possible and any oroantral opening closed. Several measures are important (Box 33.2).

After any acute sinusitis has been treated, the surgical approach depends on the position of the root and whether there is a wide oroantral opening. The classical method is to reflect a mucoperiosteal flap in the labiobuccal sulcus, open the antrum in the canine fossa (Caldwell–Luc approach) and find the root by direct vision or endoscopy. The tooth or fragment may then be removable on a sucker nozzle. A more conservative approach without the need for wide external surgical access is by functional endoscopic sinus surgery, which preserves the sinus ciliary transport, improves drainage after the operation and causes less morbidity.

Oroantral communication

The usual test for communication is to ask the patient to blow gently against pinched nostrils. Air (detectable with a tuft of cotton wool held in tweezers), blood, pus or mucus will then be expelled from the opening into the mouth.

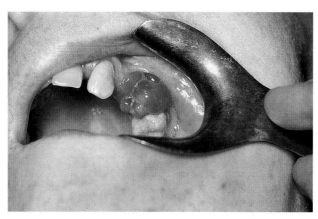

Fig. 33.5　Antral polyp. A polyp of inflamed antral mucosa has prolapsed through an oroantral fistula left untreated after the extraction of an upper first permanent molar.

Box 33.3　Principles of management of an oroantral communication

The communication (non-epithelialised)

- If small or only suspected, treat conservatively by socket pack and suturing
- Or, reflect a mucoperiosteal flap and suture it to give an air-tight seal over the opening

Post-operatively

- Give penicillin for 5 days and a 10-day course of decongestant nose drops and inhalations
- Warn the patient against blowing the nose

The established fistula (epithelialised communication) with infection

- Control chronic sinusitis by removal of any polyps, usually via a Caldwell–Luc approach, or through the oral opening if the fistula is sufficiently large
- Excise the entire epithelialised fistula
- Close the opening by reflecting a mucoperiosteal flap over it

---

However, if the communication is small, or only suspected, this can cause more damage or even produce a communication. In such cases it is better to pack and suture the socket and allow a period of healing during which the patient must avoid nose blowing and use nasal decongestants and antibiotics. Definite or large communications are best closed immediately surgically.

Unrepaired communications undergo epithelialisation to form a fistula, which is thereby prevented from healing spontaneously. Usually, a large oroantral fistula gives adequate drainage, but a pinhole fistula is often associated with recurrent attacks of sinusitis. If the patient is not seen until late after the accident, there is typically chronic antral infection, persistent discharge and proliferation of granulation tissue or sinus polyps.

Occasionally, the opening may be blocked by prolapsed oedematous sinus lining or antral polyp which is purplish red (Fig. 33.5). If the opening is large enough, these may sometimes be pushed gently back into the antrum to confirm their origin, but need to be removed surgically.

Principles of management are summarised in Box 33.3.

Review PMID: 20591776

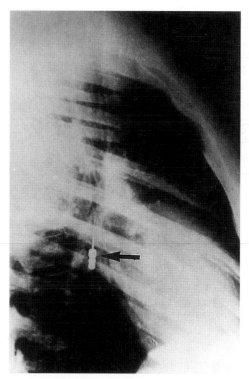

Fig. 33.6　Radiograph of the chest used to localise an inhaled reamer.

ASPIRATION OF A TOOTH, ROOT OR INSTRUMENT

A tooth or root that slips from extraction forceps is more frequently swallowed than inhaled. Small instruments such as reamers can also occasionally be inhaled if rubber dam is not used (Fig. 33.6). The patient should be reassured but should be sent for a chest radiograph and, if necessary, bronchoscopy.

If left, a tooth in a bronchus can cause collapse of the related lobe and a lung abscess. Prevention by good technique is key.

TUBERCULOSIS

Dentists and dental personnel in the UK previously all received a BCG (Bacillus Calmette–Guérin) vaccination, but routine vaccination of healthcare workers has now ceased, although all students and dentists should be offered vaccination. Prevention now relies on screening patients and contacts using newer sensitive indicators of infection such as the interferon gamma release assay. An individual decision on the need for vaccination is made and may vary depending on practice in a high incidence area, with high-risk patients or the dentist's origin in a high incidence area.

BCG vaccination reduces only slightly the risk of infection but prevents progression to active tuberculosis in 70% of those immunised in the UK. Protection rates are lower in tropical countries. Infection control and other precautions must therefore be maintained, particularly while the incidence of tuberculosis is rising.

Tuberculous cervical lymphadenopathy is discussed in Chapter 31 and oral tuberculous ulcers in Chapter 15.

CHRONIC OBSTRUCTIVE AIRWAYS DISEASE

Chronic obstructive airways disease (COAD) is typically caused by smoking and recurrent respiratory infections, environmental pollution or genetic α1-antitrypsin deficiency. Patients are hypoxic and may be cyanotic. COAD is a contraindication to intravenous sedation because of its respiratory depressant effect and to general anaesthesia except in hospital. Dental treatment must often be provided in an upright position, and severely affected patients may be taking corticosteroids.

Dental significance PMID: 25213520

ASTHMA

Asthma is a common respiratory disease characterised by paroxysmal wheezing on expiration due to intermittent bronchospasm. Cough and variable degrees of dyspnoea may be associated. Many cases are mild with only minor wheezing but, at the opposite extreme, it can be a lethal disease.

Asthma is common in atopy (Ch. 30), but only so-called *extrinsic asthma* is a response to allergens such as house-dust mites, feathers or animal dander and is IgE mediated. Intrinsic asthma is non-allergic and is a result of mast cell degranulation and a hyperresponsive airway. Attacks of either type of asthma can be triggered by inhaled irritants such as tobacco smoke, respiratory infections, exercise and food additives. Emotional stress can also precipitate episodes.

Management is by identification and avoidance of allergens and respiratory irritants. The medical history should include specific questions about triggers and allergies. Many patients respond well to beta-2 agonists such as salbutamol by inhaler. Longer-term control may require steroid inhalers such as beclomethasone, leukotriene receptor antagonists or mast cell stabilisers, such as cromoglycate.

The mortality from asthma is mainly due to under treatment, and use of anti-asthmatic drugs is increasing.

Dental aspects of asthma are shown in Box 33.4.

Dental treatment asthmatic children PMID: 27012346

Review and dental relevance PMID: 11709681

Box 33.4 Dental significance of asthma

- Steroid inhalers predispose to candidosis
- Potential triggers of attack in dental surgery: acrylic, colophony, aspirin, stress
- Dry mouth
- Adverse effects of systemic steroid therapy, adrenal suppression and infection
- Status asthmaticus is a medical emergency
- Increased frequency of allergy to a variety of drugs
- Some antibiotics interact with theophylline
- Some patients have difficulty lying supine
- Ensure patients bring inhalers to appointments in case of attack

---

MIDFACIAL DESTRUCTIVE LESIONS

This is not a group of diseases, rather a list of diseases with a common presentation: variable degrees of destruction of the central facial tissues. Improved diagnosis and treatment have made the previous term 'midline lethal granuloma' inappropriate.

All these conditions start in the upper respiratory tract, sinuses, skin around the nose or oral cavity, and they are not clinically distinguishable in their early stages. All cause extensive necrosis, and this makes diagnosis by biopsy difficult. The commonest and most important in the UK are Wegener's granulomatosis, nasopharyngeal T/natural killer (NK)-cell lymphoma (Ch. 27) and mucormycosis (Ch. 9).

Causes of midfacial destructive lesions are shown in Box 33.5.

Wegener's granulomatosis

→ Summary chart 24.2, p. 373

Wegener's granulomatosis, or granulomatosis with polyangiitis, is a potentially lethal and uncommon systemic vasculitis with a predilection to present in the nose and sinuses. It is thought that the vasculitis is an anomalous, probably cross-reacting, immune reaction to an infection or environmental agent. There is a strong genetic association with genes that modulate immune responses. All ages are affected.

Circulating antibodies ('antineutrophil cytoplasmic antibodies' or ANCA) against the neutrophil granule proteinase, proteinase 3, bind to the enzyme when it is secreted onto the surface of neutrophils in an inflammatory focus or during emigration through vessel walls. Binding activates the neutrophil and triggers a positive feedback loop of acute inflammation. ANCA-producing autoreactive B cells migrate into granulomas in the lesion and produce the antibody locally to further sustain the inflammation.

Damage to small arterioles causes kidney damage, focal lung lesions, a rash and characteristic nasal lesions.

Biopsy of affected tissue shows a dense inflammatory infiltrate, small dispersed granulomas and collections of

---

Box 33.5 Causes of necrotic midfacial destructive lesions

Infectious

- Rhinoscleroma, bacterial infection by *Klebsiella* sp.
- Mucormycosis and similar deep mycoses
- Noma/cancrum oris
- Gumma of tertiary syphilis

Inflammatory disease

- Wegener's granulomatosis
- Systemic lupus erythematosus

Malignant neoplasms

- Nasopharyngeal natural killer/T cell lymphoma
- Poorly differentiated and undifferentiated carcinoma
- Carcinoma associated with NUT gene rearrangements
- Adenoid cystic carcinoma
- Rhabdomyosarcoma

Other

- Cocaine abuse

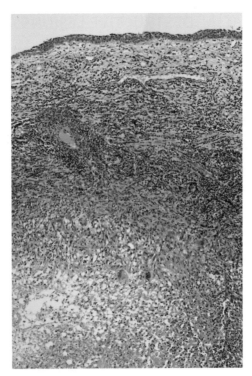

Fig. 33.7   Wegener's granulomatosis. In the deepest tissues there is necrosis with a few small multinucleate giant cells at the periphery. Superficially there is intense inflammation with numerous eosinophils (not visible at this magnification) around a blood vessel, a focus of vasculitis.

Box 33.6   Wegener's granulomatosis: key features
- Granulomatous inflammation of nasal tract
- Vasculitis, small vessel destruction and tissue necrosis
- Potentially fatal glomerulonephritis
- Proliferative gingivitis occasionally
- Oral mucosal ulceration occasionally
- Antineutrophil cytoplasmic antibodies (ANCAs)
- Biopsy diagnosis often difficult, may require several biopsies

giant cells (Fig. 33.7). In deeper tissues, vasculitis with destruction of small arteries is seen. Circulating ANCA antibodies are present in approximately 85% of cases and aid diagnosis but are not completely specific. Autoantibodies directed against proteinase 3 (PR3) are highly specific.

The features are summarised in Box 33.6.

General review PMID: 25149391

Oral and nasal lesions

In the nose, granulomatous inflammation with discharge is typically the first sign. Untreated, necrosis will destroy the nasal septum producing a saddle nose deformity and may perforate the palate, appearing as a large ulcer. Signs and symptoms are very similar to NK/T cell lymphoma.

In the mouth, a characteristic proliferative gingivitis is the first sign in a minority of patients. The changes initially resemble pregnancy gingivitis, but the gingivae become swollen with a granular surface and dusky or bright red colour ('strawberry gums' – Fig. 33.8). The changes can be widespread or patchy (Fig. 33.9). Alternatively, superficial

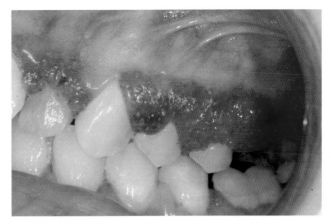

Fig. 33.8   Wegener's granulomatosis. In this florid presentation, the typical stippled appearance is well shown. *(From Staines, K.S., Higgins, B., 2009. Recurrence of Wegener's granulomatosis with de novo intraoral presentation treated successfully with rituximab. Oral Surg. Oral Med. Oral Pathol. Oral Radiol. Endod. 108, 76–80.)*

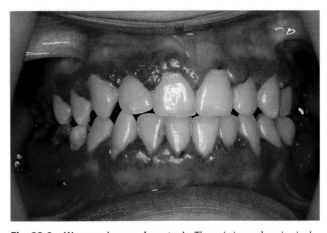

Fig. 33.9   Wegener's granulomatosis. There is irregular gingival hyperplasia affecting a few teeth and redness extending the full depth of the attached gingiva. The distribution is not related to plaque.

mucosal ulceration can be widespread but appears at a later stage.

Parotitis is an uncommon but early manifestation of Wegener's granulomatosis.

Oral features PMID: 1995819 and 17332039

Management

The diagnosis must be established by biopsy at the earliest possible moment to initiate treatment and prevent renal damage. Haematuria suggests glomerulonephritis and a poor prognosis. Treatment is frequently with cyclophosphamide and corticosteroids, switching to azathioprine or methotrexate for long-term control. On these drugs, 80% of patients survive 5 years; without treatment almost all die in a few months. Immunosuppressive monoclonal antibodies such as infliximab are also used.

Those patients with oral and nasal lesions but no systemic signs have a much better prognosis.

CARCINOMA OF THE ANTRUM

Carcinoma of the maxillary antrum is rare. Pain is not an early symptom, and a large size can be attained before

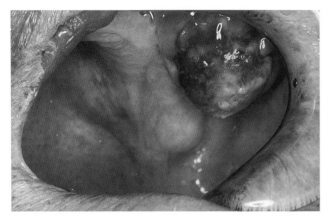

Fig. 33.10 **Antral carcinoma.** Occasionally, an antral carcinoma will present intraorally, either after eroding the maxilla or through an extraction socket.

presentation. Later, pain and anaesthesia in the distribution of adjacent nerves develop. Most are squamous and often poorly differentiated; some are adenoid cystic carcinomas arising in the mucosal glands. Spread to vital structures around the base of the skull is often present on diagnosis.

Oral and dental symptoms from carcinoma of the antrum result from involvement of its floor. This may cause pain in the teeth or under a denture. As the disease advances, teeth may become loose and a swelling becomes obvious (Fig. 33.10).

Any dental radiograph from a person older than 40 years showing an opaque maxillary antrum or erosion of the antral wall without obvious underlying dental or nasal disease indicates a need for further investigation.

CYSTIC FIBROSIS (MUCOVISCIDOSIS)

In this autosomal recessive disease caused by mutation in the CFTR gene, there is failure of water and chloride transport across epithelium in exocrine glands. Saliva and sputum are viscid, airways become blocked and recurrent respiratory infections develop in childhood.

There is reduced growth and malabsorption from pancreatic failure. Eruption of the teeth may be delayed, and repeated infections and other sequelae cause chronological hypoplastic defects.

Salivary gland swelling is frequent, but mild and significant salivary obstruction is surprisingly rare. The saliva is high in sodium and calcium, and slightly reduced in amount, but this seems to be a problem only rarely, though it probably predisposes to stones.

Chronic sinusitis and sinonasal polyps are present in most patients.

Dental surgical treatment PMID: 18201621

SLEEP APNOEA SYNDROME

In sleep apnoea syndrome, there is recurrent spontaneous obstruction of the airway during sleep. Approximately 2%–4% of the middle-aged population are affected, particularly obese males. Fragmented sleep patterns and poor quality sleep cause daytime drowsiness and difficulty in concentrating, with a consequently raised risk of impaired work performance and of road traffic accidents for drivers. Depression and irritability may be associated. In the longer

term, there is a significantly raised risk of hypertension, ischaemic heart disease and stroke.

During sleep there are snoring and breathing pauses. The cause is recurrent occlusion or partial occlusion at the back of the throat, partly due to relaxation of the palatoglossus and genioglossus which, during wakefulness, maintain the patency of the airway. Most patients have several areas of narrowing in their airway, and a deviated nasal septum, a high arched palate, large tonsils or long soft palate are among other contributing factors. The apnoea causes lowered oxygen saturation and risk of dysrhythmias.

Snoring does not itself indicate sleep apnoea.

General review PMCID: PMC3909558

Management

Medical treatment involves weight loss, forcing sleeping on one side and avoiding evening alcohol and sedatives.

The primary medical treatment is positive pressure ventilation using a mask. This is highly effective.

Alternatively, intraoral appliances that hold the mandible 2–5 mm anteriorly can be worn at night. These increase the size of the airway by pulling the soft palate forward; long-term compliance is good, and they are highly effective in mild obstructive sleep apnoea. Alternative designs can be used that are intended to hold the tongue forward. Compliance with use of these large and uncomfortable appliances is surprisingly good, but they may trigger temporomandibular joint pain-dysfunction or occasionally worsen apnoea in some patients. Use of appliances is preferred if patients do not tolerate ventilation, or if it fails to improve sleep.

Trials have found that oral appliances can be as effective for improving oxygenation as continuous positive pressure ventilation, but only the latter has been shown to improve mortality in the long term.

In the event that the mandible cannot be held sufficiently forward with an appliance and pressure ventilation fails, surgery may be required. Several different operations are available depending on the site of airway narrowing. This may seem drastic, but failure to control symptoms in severe cases may necessitate a tracheostomy, which can bring other complications.

Dental treatment for snoring or apnoea in the UK falls outside the practice of dentistry because a full medical assessment and diagnosis are required before any treatment by a dentist, who should work in a multidisciplinary team with an integrated treatment plan.

Dental appliances US guideline PMID: 26094920

Dental appliances Australia guideline PMID: 24320895

Web URL 33.2 UK guideline: http://cks.nice.org.uk/obstructive-sleep-apnoea-syndrome

BRONCHOGENIC CARCINOMA

With reduction in smoking, lung cancer has been in decline for 40 years but is still the second commonest cancer in the UK, after breast carcinoma. There is now almost equal incidence in males and females.

Clinically, recurrent cough is the most common feature and often ignored as 'smoker's cough'. Later manifestations include haemoptysis, chest pain and dyspnoea. Loss of weight and anorexia may also develop. The diagnosis is confirmed by radiography, CT and magnetic resonance imaging, sputum cytology, bronchoscopy and endoscopic biopsy.

Only approximately 25% of patients present at a stage suitable for surgery. Treatment is frequently therefore by radiotherapy. The overall 5-year survival rate is 10% and has changed little in decades.

Dental aspects

Management depends greatly upon the stage of the cancer when the patient is seen. In the early stages, dental treat-ment can be carried out as usual, but conscious sedation should preferably be avoided.

Metastases to the jaw or cervical lymph nodes are usually a late manifestation, and an uncommon manifestation is diffuse pigmentation of the soft palate.

Patients with lung carcinoma are at risk of a second primary carcinoma in the upper aerodigestive tract and must be screened for potentially malignant changes in the oral mucosa.

Gastrointestinal and liver disease 34

GASTRO-OESOPHAGEAL REFLUX AND GASTRIC REGURGITATION

Gastro-oesophageal reflux and consequent oesophagitis are a common cause of the symptoms of dyspepsia and 'heart burn'. Smoking, excessive alcohol consumption, obesity, frequent stooping and overlarge meals are frequent precipitating factors. If persistent, the oesophageal lining may undergo metaplasia to a more resistant gastric-type mucosa (Barrett's oesophagus). Acid rarely reaches the mouth in any quantities and, unless severe, reflux alone is not a potent cause of dental erosion, though it may contribute. Inhibition of acid secretion by protein pump inhibitors, such as omeprazole, is highly effective in controlling it.

By contrast, chronic vomiting or regurgitation of gastric acid contents, due to such causes as hypertrophic pyloric stenosis or in bulimia, can lead to marked dental erosion, often, but not always, worse on the palatal and occlusal aspects of the anterior teeth (Fig. 34.1).

Erosion intrinsic causes PMID: 24993266

COELIAC DISEASE

Coeliac disease is a common and important cause of malabsorption affecting 1% of the population. The cause is hypersensitivity to gluten in wheat and other cereal products. Almost all patients have the predisposing human leukocyte antigen (HLA) DQ2. Specific degradation products of gluten trigger ileal mucosal inflammation, with loss of villi causing failure of absorption.

The disease is frequently asymptomatic, and it may not be recognised until adult life as a result of its complications. It can also have a great variety of effects. Malabsorption, stunting of growth, fatty diarrhoea and abdominal pain or discomfort are typical consequences. The malabsorption

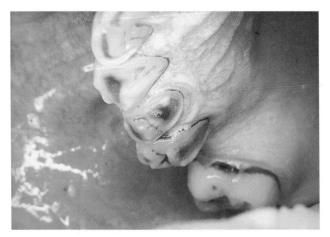

Fig. 34.1   Erosion of the palatal surfaces of the upper teeth due to repeated vomiting.

can lead to vitamin and mineral deficiencies resulting in anaemia or bleeding tendencies.

Dental aspects

Anaemia can have a variety of oral effects such as glossitis or recurrent aphthae as discussed in Chapter 27. As many as 5% of patients with coeliac disease may have recurrent aphthae, even in the absence of anaemia.

Enamel hypoplasia is common in coeliac disease, seen as spotty hypoplastic mottling, localised opacities, chronological banding, pitting or discolouration. These probably result from malabsorption and are not specific to the disease. Usually only permanent teeth are affected.

Hypoplasia in a child of short stature and with bowel symptoms should raise suspicion of coeliac disease, recognising that many cases are diagnosed late.

General and oral review PMID: 23496382

CROHN'S DISEASE

→ Summary chart 34.1 and 24.2, p. 459, 373

Crohn's disease is an inflammatory bowel disease of unknown aetiology. However, it shares many features with the autoinflammatory diseases, and some cases are known to be associated with mutations in the gene NOD2 that controls inflammatory responses to bacteria. Mutations cause failure of the formation of the mucin and antimicrobial barrier lining the bowel and may also inhibit degradation of bacteria. Changes in bowel flora are probably also important.

Granulomatous inflammation affects the ileocaecal region, causing thickening and ulceration. Symptoms vary with the severity of the disease, but effects can include abdominal pain, variable constipation or diarrhoea and, sometimes, obstruction and malabsorption. Repeated bowel resections may ultimately be needed. Many other sites can be affected including any part of the bowel, joints and skin.

Treatment controls symptoms but is not curative. Dietary adjustment, corticosteroids, antibiotics, sulfasalazine or mesalazine, immunosuppressants and tumour necrosis factor (TNF)-alpha blockers (e.g. infliximab) are used.

General review PMID: 22914295

Oral effects

Most patients have no oral signs, although aphthous ulcers and candidosis may be associated with anaemia.

When the disease process itself affects the mouth, the signs and symptoms are the same as those in orofacial granulomatosis (discussed later).

Non-caseating granulomas resembling those in the intestine develop in the oral mucosa. The common sites of involvement are lips and buccal mucosa. These show prominent oedema with folds tethered to the underlying deeper tissues, producing the characteristic cobblestone mucosa appearance (Figs 34.2–34.3). Linear ulcers often run along

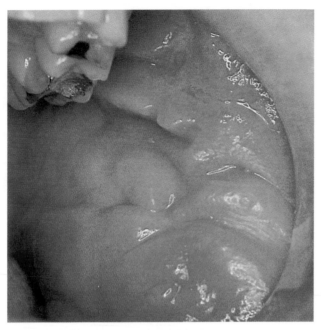

Fig. 34.2 **Crohn's disease.** Soft nodular thickening of the oral mucosa is a typical feature and, in this case, was associated with facial swelling and intermittent diarrhoea.

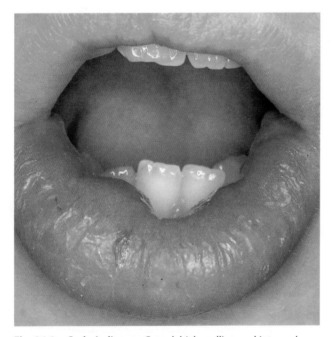

Fig. 34.3 **Crohn's disease.** Gross labial swelling and intraoral mucosal oedema with typical histological changes led to the finding of extensive intestinal involvement.

the buccal sulci, particularly the lower sulci, and have hyperplastic folds of inflamed mucosa along their margins. The gingiva (Fig. 34.4) show an erythematous nodular gingivitis with hyperplastic tags.

The granulomas are typically small, loose and contain few multinucleate giant cells and are often sited deeply in underlying muscle. They may be few in number, and a biopsy needs to extend unusually deeply to increase the chance of finding them because only by identifying granulomas can the diagnosis be made (Figs 34.5–34.6). The granulomas are associated with vascular dilatation and tissue swelling in

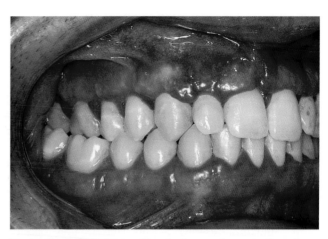

Fig. 34.4 **Crohn's disease.** The gingivae are hyperplastic and irregular and erythematous. These changes are obvious, but more subtle signs are easily missed. The appearances are identical to those in sarcoidosis in the gingivae.

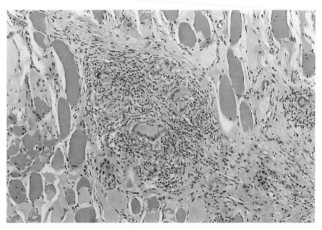

Fig. 34.5 **Crohn's disease.** The granulomas are frequently deep in the mucosa and widely dispersed. Here granulomas are present in muscle, showing the importance of adequate biopsy depth.

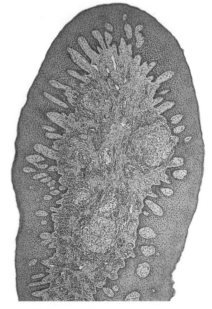

Fig. 34.6 **Crohn's disease.** A hyperplastic tag of gingiva contains several large round granulomas.

Box 34.1 Typical orofacial features of Crohn's disease

- Diffuse soft or tense swelling of the lips, or mucosal thickening
- Cobblestone thickening of the buccal mucosa, with fissuring and hyperplastic folds
- Gingivae may be erythematous and swollen
- Sometimes, painful mucosal ulcers, linear in sulci or resembling aphthae
- Mucosal tags in sulcuses
- Glossitis due to iron, folate or vitamin B$_{12}$ deficiency can result from malabsorption
- Orofacial granulomatosis shares many features

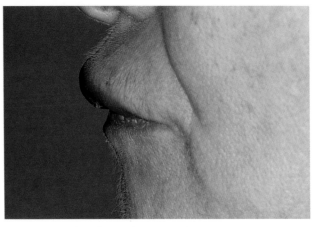

Fig. 34.7 Orofacial granulomatosis. There is conspicuous swelling of the upper lip with eversion of the vermilion border. The lip is thickened and tense.

early disease. Later, there is dense fibrosis that fixes the tissues in their distorted shape.

These features can be the presenting features of Crohn's disease, and occasionally oral lesions precede gastrointestinal symptoms by a long period. Oral disease is much more likely to progress to bowel disease in children than when diagnosed in an adult.

Oral lesions may lessen in severity with treatment of systemic disease. Aggressive treatment is merited in the early stages to prevent fibrosis and permanent disfigurement. The same drugs as are used for bowel disease are required, together with steroid injections of swollen mucosa.

Key features are shown in Box 34.1.

Oral features PMID: 2007740

Treatment PMID: 26593695

OROFACIAL GRANULOMATOSIS

→ Summary chart 34.1 and 24.2, p. 459, 373

Orofacial granulomatosis is used to describe oral mucosal granulomatous inflammation without an identifiable cause. The clinical features are very similar to oral lesions of Crohn's disease, but this is probably a distinct disease. However, distinguishing these conditions is difficult, and some patients considered to have orofacial granulomatosis will subsequently prove to have Crohn's disease after several years. The chances of eventually developing Crohn's disease are higher if orofacial granulomatosis is diagnosed in childhood.

Orofacial granulomatosis presents mainly in young adults, and lip and buccal mucosa are the main sites involved (Fig. 34.7), with marked oedema and a cobblestone appearance. Linear sulcus ulcers and gingival lesions are less frequent than in Crohn's disease. Diagnosis requires biopsy and, as in Crohn's disease, a deep biopsy is required to give the best chance of finding granulomas (Figs 34.8 and 34.9).

The cause of orofacial granulomatosis is related to food allergy. The patients often have subclinical bowel disease, a higher than average risk of allergy to a range of common allergens and react to common food additives such as cinnamon, benzoates and phenolic compounds. Both type 1 and type 4 hypersensitivity mechanisms are implicated.

Treatment is initially by exclusion diet, and nearly two-thirds of patients respond. Intralesional steroid injections, immunosuppressants such as tacrolimus or ciclosporin, methotrexate or tumour necrosis factor (TNF)-alpha inhibitors (infliximab) may be used depending on severity.

Differences from Crohn's PMID: 21910172

Treatment by diet PMID: 23574355 and 21815899

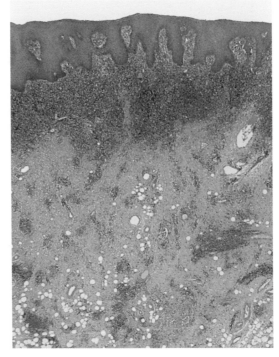

Fig. 34.8 Orofacial granulomatosis. Low power showing the dense inflammation and scarring extending deeply into fat. These changes are common to both Crohn's disease and orofacial granulomatosis.

MALABSORPTION SYNDROMES

Malabsorption syndromes (Box 34.2) can cause haematological deficiencies that can contribute to development or exacerbation of recurrent aphthae, glossitis, candidosis or other symptoms.

ULCERATIVE COLITIS

Ulcerative colitis is an inflammatory disease of the large intestine causing ulceration and fibrosis. Patients are typically between 15 and 50 years. The main effect is intractable diarrhoea with blood and mucus in the stools. Abdominal pain, fever, anorexia and weight loss are seen in severe cases.

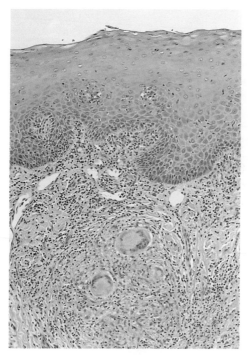

Fig. 34.9   Orofacial granulomatosis. Below the epithelium is a patchy inflammatory infiltrate and scattered granulomas containing large multinucleate giant cells.

Box 34.2   Important causes of malabsorption syndrome

- Coeliac disease and other allergies
- Crohn's disease
- Resection of stomach or ileum
- Pancreatic insufficiency
- Liver disease (failure of bile secretion into the gut)
- Some parasitic and other chronic gut infections

Oral aspects

Anaemia can have its usual effects on the oral mucosa (Ch. 27).

There is no direct oral involvement, but the oral condition of pyostomatitis vegetans is closely associated. This is a rare disease, with diffuse mucosal oedema and erythema on which there are slightly raised multiple tiny pustules just below the surface (Fig. 34.10). Histologically, the epithelium contains clusters of neutrophils and eosinophils. The lesions often resolve with treatment of the bowel disease or with steroids, but occasionally they are the presenting sign of unsuspected bowel disease.

Oral signs inflammatory bowel disease PMID: 25917394

Pyostomatitis vegetans review PMID: 14723710 and 17236948

INTESTINAL POLYPOSIS SYNDROMES

Gardner's syndrome with polyposis of the colon, multiple osteomas of the jaws and a high malignant potential in the colon is discussed in Chapter 12.

Peutz-Jeghers syndrome of intestinal polyposis with skin pigmentation is discussed in Chapter 26.

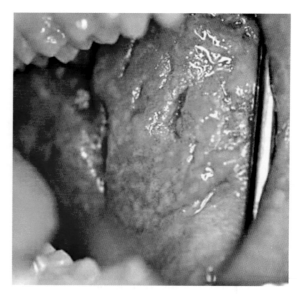

Fig. 34.10   Pyostomatitis vegetans. Diffuse erythema with multiple pinpoint abscesses or ulcers. *(From Markiewicz, M., Suresh, L., Margarone, J. 3rd, et al., 2007. Pyostomatitis vegetans: a clinical marker of silent ulcerative colitis. J. Oral Maxillofac Surg. 65, 346–348.)*

ANTIBIOTIC-ASSOCIATED COLITIS

Mild diarrhoea following prolonged antibiotic treatment follows disturbance of the bowel flora and is often self-limiting.

Pseudomembranous colitis is more severe, with passage of blood and mucus in the stools and sometimes fragments of necrotic bowel mucosa (pseudomembrane). It is typically a complication of prolonged antibiotic therapy, particularly with clindamycin or lincomycin and due to proliferation of *Clostridium difficile* resistant to these antibiotics. Pseudomembranous colitis is treated with metronidazole but can be fatal in the elderly and debilitated.

Antibiotics prescribed for dental reasons must be used for the shortest courses that are effective and selected according to guidelines or culture and sensitivity and not repeated unnecessarily to avoid such adverse effects.

Pseudomembranous colitis general review PMID: 25875259

Dental prescribing and pseudomembranous colitis PMID: 26404991

Case report in dentistry PMID: 11209501

Clindamycin in dentistry PMID: 16003416

LIVER DISEASE

Common types of liver disease are infections (particularly viral hepatitis), obstructive jaundice, cirrhosis (often due to alcohol) and tumours. There are various aspects of liver disease that are relevant to dentistry (Box 34.3).

Impaired drug metabolism

Most drugs are metabolised in the liver, and no drugs should be given to patients with liver disease without first consulting the British National Formulary or drug datasheet. Drugs of dental relevance metabolised by the liver include local anaesthetics, aspirin, diazepam and intravenous sedatives, penicillins and metronidazole.

Causes of parenchymal liver disease and liver failure are shown in Box 34.4. Cirrhosis is frequently the result of alcoholism but often of unknown cause.

VIRAL HEPATITIS

The main types of hepatitis, relevant here, are B, C and D. Hepatitis B is the chief risk to dental personnel, but hepatitis C can also be transmitted during dentistry. The hepatitis B virus can also carry within it the delta agent that can cause a particularly virulent combined infection (hepatitis D).

All types in dentistry PMID: 10203901

Hepatitis A

Hepatitis A is the common form of infectious hepatitis. It is frequently acquired from contaminated food or water during a holiday abroad in a hot developing country. The incubation period is 2–6 weeks, jaundice is usually mild and spontaneous recovery takes 3 months or so. Long-term complications are extremely rare. A vaccine is available.

Hepatitis E

Hepatitis E transmission is also by the faecal–oral route, but the reservoir of infection is in animals. Infection is endemic in hot developing countries, particularly India, but the risk to travellers abroad is small. Spontaneous recovery is usual. A vaccine has recently become available.

Hepatitis B

Hepatitis B is usually spread vertically at birth or horizontally in families in endemic areas. Where prevalence is low, as in developed countries, transmission is by sexual contact or through infected blood. Before effective vaccination, this was the greatest infective hazard to dental staff (Box 34.5), and there are still risks from blood transfusions and medical procedures in parts of the world. The effects of hepatitis B infection vary widely (Box 34.6).

Hepatitis B general review PMID: 24954675

Clinical aspects

The incubation period is at least 2–6 months. The virus replicates in hepatocytes, and the immune response to the virus eventually clears the infection, damaging the liver in the process. The majority of infections are subclinical (anicteric), but 5%–10% of patients, particularly those who have had no overt illness, become persistent carriers and can transmit the infection. A minority develop acute hepatitis with loss of appetite, muscle pains, fever, jaundice and often a swollen, painful liver. The illness is often severe and debilitating but usually followed by complete recovery and long-lasting immunity. Overall mortality from clinical infection is probably approximately 1%. Occasionally, it has been as high as 30%, probably as a result of co-infection by the delta agent.

Biochemical markers of infection are raised serum levels of liver enzymes, bilirubin and often of alkaline phosphatase. However, confirmation of the diagnosis is by serology (Fig. 34.11 and Table 34.1).

Serological markers of hepatitis B

The hepatitis B virus (HBV) is a DNA virus termed the *Dane particle*. The Dane particle consists of a central core and an outer shell. The core contains DNA, an enzyme (DNA polymerase – DNA-P) and the hepatitis B core antigen (HBcAg). The protein shell contains the hepatitis B surface antigen (HBsAg). The e antigen is related to the HBcAg but is only expressed by some strains and is only produced during viral replication by alternative transcription. Immune responses to these antigens can be used to track the progression of disease, recovery and infectivity.

Web URL 34.1 Hepatitis B tests: http://emedicine.medscape.com/article/2109144

The carrier state and complications

Most patients with acute hepatitis B recover completely within a few weeks. Approximately 5%–10% fail to clear the

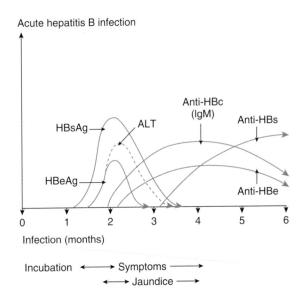

Acute hepatitis B infection

ALT

HBsAg

Anti-HBc
(IgM)

Anti-HBs

HBeAg

Anti-HBe

0   1   2   3   4   5   6

Infection (months)

Incubation ⟷ Symptoms ⟶

⟷ Jaundice ⟶

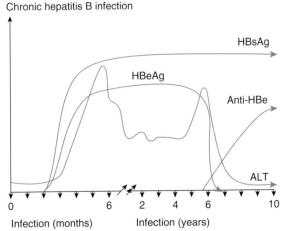

Chronic hepatitis B infection

HBsAg

HBeAg

Anti-HBe

ALT

0   6   2   4   6   10

Infection (months)   Infection (years)

Fig. 34.11 Serological markers of hepatitis B infection. ALT, serum alanine aminotransferase; HBc, hepatitis B core; HBs, hepatitis B surface; HBe, e antigen; Ag, antigen; anti, antibody against. *(From Crash course: gastrointestinal system. 2012. In: Kumar, P., Clarke, M. Clinical Medicine. third ed. Saunders, London, pp. 99–133.)*

virus within 6–9 months and develop chronic infection and become chronic carriers.

Chronic carriage of HBsAg alone indicates a low risk of severe liver damage. Persistent carriage of both HBsAg and HBeAg is associated with chronic active hepatitis and infectivity. These patients have biochemical evidence of liver damage. They are chronically ill and at special risk from cirrhosis and, possibly, carcinoma of the liver as a result of continued viral replication and damage mediated by the immune response.

Chronic active hepatitis with persistent malaise, and sometimes mild jaundice, is particularly likely to develop in the very young, the old and the immunosuppressed.

Risks to dental staff

The carriage rate of hepatitis B virus in the general population of Britain is 0.3%. The rate in British dentists used to be double that in the general population, though this should fall now that dentists are vaccinated. There are also high-risk groups (Box 34.7).

In endemic areas in Asia and Africa, carriage rates may be 20% and dental staff there are potentially at high risk.

Transmission of hepatitis B

Blood and blood products can transmit infection in as little as 0.000 000 1 mL fluid, particularly when containing the e antigen. Many cases have followed needle-stick injuries, injections and blood transfusions. Saliva can also contain hepatitis B antigens and, experimentally, can transmit the virus. Saliva is frequently also contaminated with blood and, when splashed on to the conjunctiva, might transmit infection to a dentist.

Hepatitis B can also be transmitted sexually, and carriage rates are high in sex workers and those with HIV infection.

The degree of infectivity is indicated by the serological markers (Fig. 34.11). Infective carriers can only be suspected if they have a history of jaundice or are in a high-risk group. Nevertheless, it must be emphasised that only 1 in 4 carriers gives a positive medical history. Many infectious patients, as in the case of HIV carriers, will therefore be treated unknowingly.

Table 34.1 Serological markers of hepatitis B and their significance

Serological marker	Relation to infection	Significance
The surface antigen (HBsAg)	HBsAg particles detectable in late incubation period and during acute and chronic infections	HBsAg carriage indicates past infection, but confers little risk of transmitting infection, unless HBeAg is also present
Antibody to HB surface antigen (HBsAb)	Begins to appear when recovery starts but HBsAg may briefly disappear before anti-HBs becomes detectable. Both serological tests then become negative	During recovery, anti-HBs usually appears and rises in titre; it usually implies persistent immunity Anti-HBs also appears after hepatitis B immunisation
Hepatitis B core antigen (HBcAg)	Found only in liver cells, not serum	
Antibody to HB core antigen (HBcAb)	Anti-HBc appears at onset of disease Quickly rises in titre and persists for many years	One of the most sensitive indicators of past infection
Hepatitis B e antigen (HBeAg)	Appears in the serum simultaneously with HBsAg but disappears earlier if there is full recovery	Indicator of high infectivity
Antibody to e antigen (anti-HBe, HBeAb)*	Usually appears in the serum soon after the e antigen and heralds recovery	Failure of development of anti-HBe indicates high infectivity
DNA polymerase (DNA-P)		Indicates high infectivity

*Carriers of both HBsAg and HBeAg but who lack anti-HBe are more likely to develop chronic active hepatitis and serious complications, and to transmit the infection.

Box 34.7 Patients with higher risk of being hepatitis B carriers

In the UK vaccination is now offered to:

- Intravenous drug users and their partners
- Men who have sex with men
- Those with frequent changes of sexual partners
- Babies, family and partners of those infected
- Anyone with chronic liver or renal disease
- Those who need regular blood transfusions
- Male and female sex workers
- Travellers to endemic areas
- Prison staff and prisoners
- Healthcare staff, including dentists
- Families adopting children from endemic areas

And these are also at risk:

- Patients and staff of institutions for the handicapped
- Immunosuppressed or immunodeficient patients
- Patients who have received unscreened blood or blood products
- Patients who have had acupuncture or tattooing, especially in tropical countries

Box 34.8 Important differences between hepatitis C and B

Hepatitis C:

- is less widespread
- is less readily transmitted by needle-stick injuries
- is more vulnerable to disinfection
- is rarely transmitted during dentistry
- acute hepatitis is uncommon and usually mild

But

- no protective vaccine is as yet available
- infection persists in 80%
- infection more frequently leads to chronic active hepatitis
- there is a higher risk of cirrhosis and liver cancer

Transmission in dentistry PMID: 23539395

Occupational infection risk dentistry PMCID: PMC3375115

Patient to patient transmission PMID: 17397000

Prevention and management of hepatitis B

It is *essential* for dentists to have active immunisation. It is effective, safe and protects against both hepatitis B and delta infection. The vaccine is the HBsAg engineered in yeast and thus contains no complete virus. Three injections should be given at intervals into the deltoid muscle (the vaccine is less effective injected into fatty tissue), but adequate protection may not develop until after 6 months. Side effects are mild and rare, but a few (particularly the obese) do not produce adequate antibody levels after a normal course of vaccination and may need it to be repeated.

It is technically possible to measure the resulting antibody levels, but this is no longer considered necessary, either to measure effectiveness or the need for a booster vaccination. Immunity does not depend on the circulating antibody level, rather on the cell-mediated response and memory B lymphocytes primed to respond when needed. Although booster doses are no longer recommended in the UK, they are in other countries. The effectiveness of the current vaccines exceeds 95% but is not complete.

Vaccine review PMID: 26978406 and 1971874

Booster vaccination PMID: 10683019

Hepatitis D: the delta agent

The delta agent is a defective RNA virus that can only infect and replicate in the presence of HBsAg, which it uses to bind to hepatocyte receptors. Delta infection is, therefore, only transmitted with hepatitis B or to a person already infected by it. It is endemic in the Middle East, Africa and parts of South America, but in the UK and developed countries it is usually spread by intravenous drug users, by blood or blood products. Only 100 patients per year test positive for hepatitis D in the UK, and approximately 2% of patients in the UK with hepatitis B carry the delta agent.

Delta infection causes acute hepatitis, and this rarely resolves but causes progressive liver disease with a high mortality rate. Carriage rates are in decline because immunisation against hepatitis B also protects against the delta agent.

Delta agent review PMCID: PMC4641224

Hepatitis C

The hepatitis C virus (HCV) is now more important than the B virus in dentistry because no vaccination is available. It is also a more severe infection and more frequently fatal.

After infection, only approximately 15% of patients have signs or symptoms of hepatitis. Few patients, perhaps 20%, clear the infection despite their immune response. This is because the virus has an extremely high rate of genetic variability (even higher than HIV virus) and each patient becomes infected with many newly generated genetic variants. Most patients become chronically infected without realising it.

Almost all transmission is via blood, not transfusion products (which are tested in the UK), but primarily through needle sharing by drug users or tattooing. Unfortunately, blood is not screened in most developing countries, and the highest incidences are in China, Africa and parts of South America. Only approximately 150,000 patients are chronically infected in the United Kingdom, but 2% of the population in the United States and 3% worldwide are infected. Many HIV-positive patients are also positive for hepatitis C.

Once infected, 85% of patients progress to chronic hepatitis, potentially causing cirrhosis and liver failure.

Hepatitis C and B are similar in most respects but have some important differences (Box 34.8).

In some high-incidence countries, particularly in Italy, an association between hepatitis C infection and lichen planus is reported. This has not been confirmed in Britain or the United States, and a plausible pathological link between the two diseases does not yet exist, although infection is associated with other autoimmune diseases.

Hepatitis C review PMID: 25687730

Hepatitis C in dentistry PMID: 24666473 and 24282263

Management

HCV is detected serologically by anti-viral antibodies, and polymerase chain reaction (PCR) reaction for viral RNA is used to monitor treatment. Liver damage can be assessed by circulating liver enzymes and confirmed by biopsy.

Treatment is improving, and success depends on the strain of virus. Interferon and various hepatitis C specific antiviral drugs such as ledipasvir can prevent chronic hepatitis in over three-quarters of patients. However, hepatitis C remains the commonest cause requiring a liver transplant, though even this is not guaranteed to remove the infection as the virus can also replicate in lymphocytes. Those that do not respond to treatment have a high mortality from liver failure, liver carcinoma and a range of unusual extrahepatic complications including encephalopathy, myocarditis or the complications of cirrhosis such as oesophageal varices.

Hepatocellular carcinoma will develop in approximately 2% of patients after 30 years. This complication continues to appear in those who contracted the disease before screening tests for blood and blood products were available.

Universal infection control is more than adequate to prevent transmission, and sharps injury is the main risk to dentists.

Control of transmission of viral hepatitis

The principles of standard precautions (or 'universal' precautions) should be well understood. Although hepatitis B vaccination and improved infection control have much reduced occupational transmission, the risk remains. There is as yet no vaccine against hepatitis C. Hepatitis B vaccination is not completely effective, immunity may fade with age and it is less effective when given to older individuals. Immunisation is not a substitute for good infection control.

Gloves, masks and eye shields provide only partial protection and must be used correctly. Many infected patients will be treated unknowingly, and hepatitis B can be transmitted by saliva.

In the event of a sharps injury, follow local guidelines. Knowing the patient's medical history may be important in assessing the risk. The average UK dentist gives themselves 2–3 sharps injuries a year, and nurses are at higher risk while clearing away and cleaning instruments.

Standard precautions are summarised in Box 34.9.

Hepatitis B virus is more resistant than HCV, but sterilisation and disinfection measures (Box 34.10) apply to both.

Restrictions on dentists who are infected by any blood-borne virus change from time to time. In the UK, advice is available from the UK Advisory Panel for Healthcare Workers Infected with Bloodborne Viruses (UKAP) and working restrictions from the General Dental Council UK, both of which are available on their websites. Almost all dentistry constitutes 'exposure prone procedures', and any potential infection risk to a patient will probably require restriction of practice. Note that it is the *infectivity* of the dentist that is key, not simple serological positivity.

Box 34.9 Standard precautions against transmission of viral hepatitis

- Take a good medical history, following a sharps injury you may need details from it
- Treat all patients as infectious ('universal precautions')
- Wear gloves for all clinical dental work and cover exposed skin and abrasions
- Take special care to avoid sharps injuries
- Use safety syringes or needle retraction devices
- Wear goggles for eye protection
- Consider use or rubber dam for more procedures
- Zone work areas, disinfect them and follow good working practice with zoning
- Follow hand hygiene protocols
- Use disposable instruments and autoclave all others
- Clean and prepare instruments for sterilisation without risking injury
- Handle saliva contaminated impressions and patient samples as though infected
- Clean saliva and blood contaminated spillages correctly and quickly
- Be immunised against hepatitis B
- Be aware of guidelines for dealing with possible exposure and follow them
- Be aware of legal responsibilities under the Health and Safety at Work Act 1974 and the Control of Substances Hazardous to Health Regulations 1999 (COSHH).
- Take precautions with waste disposal

Box 34.10 Sterilisation and disinfection for hepatitis B and C

Sterilisation

- Autoclaving at 134°C for 3 minutes or
- Hot air at 160°C for 1 hour (effective but automatic control necessary; not used in UK)

Disinfectants

- Sodium hypochlorite, 1% of freshly diluted stock solution (0.1% with detergent for surface disinfection) (hepatitis C virus is also susceptible to solvent detergents)

Web URL 34.2 Infection control NICE guidance CG139 primary care: https://www.nice.org.uk/ and enter cg139 into search box

Evidence-based guidelines infection control PMID: 24330862

Book: infection control for dental team ISBN: 978-1-85097-132-0

Web URL 34.3 US Infection prevention guidance: http://www.cdc.gov/ and enter 'infection prevention dental settings' into search box

Summary chart 34.1   Causes and treatment of diffuse swelling of the lips and mucosa.

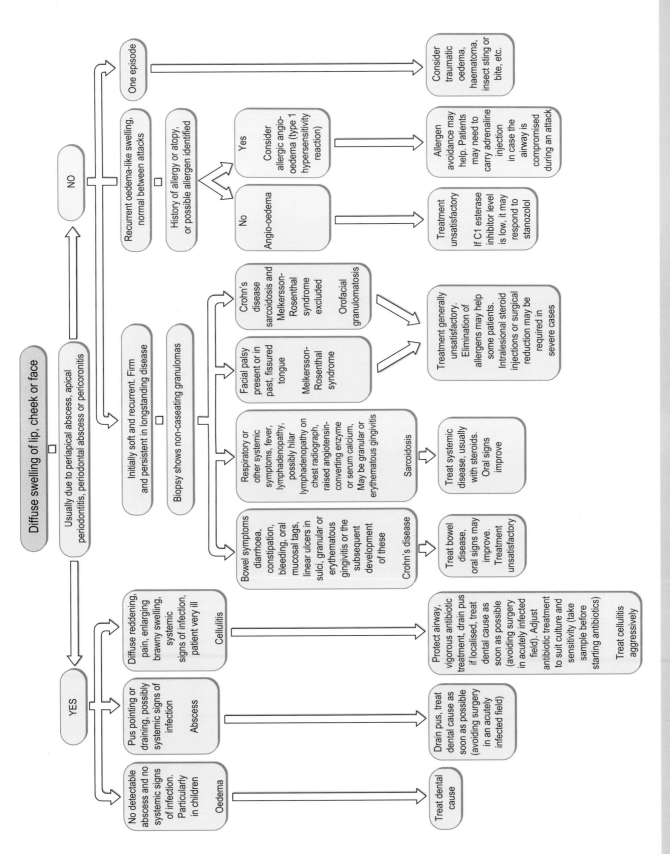

Nutritional deficiencies

35

Despite the UK population living on an unhealthy diet high in fat, sugar and salt, nutritional deficiencies are rarely seen in Britain. Susceptible patients are the elderly living on a scanty diet, severe alcoholics living on a grossly unbalanced diet and those following diets or food fads. On average, dietary intakes of all vitamins are adequate, apart from vitamin D. Intake of some B vitamins is too low in young and elderly females

Malabsorption syndromes (Ch. 34) are a rare cause of deficiency.

Although several oral conditions are linked to vitamin deficiencies, patients are generally found to be otherwise healthy and well fed with only a borderline deficiency. Prescribing vitamin preparations brings benefit largely to the multibillion pound vitamin industry.

VITAMIN DEFICIENCIES

The effects of specific deficiencies are summarised in Table 35.1.

Vitamin A deficiency

Vitamin A has a role in epithelial maturation and retinoids, more potent analogues, have been tried in conditions with abnormal keratinisation such as leukoplakia. Lycopene and β-carotenes, vitamin A precursors, have also been tried. Changes in keratinisation are reported but are not reproducible, and whether this might reduce the risk of carcinoma is unclear. Adverse effects are significant. Deficiency has no oral significance.

Table 35.1 Effects of specific vitamin deficiencies

Deficiency	Systemic effects	Oral effects
Vitamin A	Night-blindness xerophthalmia	None
Thiamin (B$_1$)	Neuritis and cardiac failure	None
Riboflavin (B$_2$)	Dermatitis	Angular stomatitis and glossitis
Nicotinamide	Dermatitis, central nervous system disease, diarrhoea	Glossitis, stomatitis and gingivitis
Vitamin B$_{12}$	Pernicious anaemia	Glossitis, aphthae
Folic acid	Macrocytic anaemia	Glossitis, aphthae
Vitamin C	Scurvy (purpura, delayed wound healing, bone lesions in children)	Gingival swelling and bleeding
Vitamin D	Rickets	Hypocalcification of teeth (severe rickets only)

Riboflavin (B$_2$) deficiency

Riboflavin deficiency can occasionally result from a malabsorption syndrome. In severe cases, there is typically angular stomatitis, with painful red fissures at the angles of the mouth, and shiny redness of the mucous membranes. The tongue is commonly sore. A peculiar form of glossitis in which the tongue becomes magenta in colour and granular or pebbly in appearance, due to flattening and mushrooming of the papillae, may be seen but is uncommon. The gingivae are not affected. Resolution follows within days when riboflavin (5 mg, three times per day) is given.

Riboflavin is ineffective for the commonly seen cases of glossitis and angular stomatitis, which are rarely due to vitamin deficiency.

Recently, riboflavin has been used to cross-link dentine collagen in an attempt to toughen dentine for adhesion of restorations. This is because it absorbs blue light and not for any nutritional reasons.

Nicotinamide deficiency (pellagra)

Pellagra, which affects the skin, gastrointestinal tract and nervous system, is rare in Britain but may occasionally result from malabsorption or alcoholism. Weakness, loss of appetite and changes in mood or personality are followed by glossitis or stomatitis and dermatitis. The tip and lateral margins of the tongue become red, swollen and, in severe cases, deeply ulcerated. The dorsum of the tongue becomes coated with a thick, greyish fur which is often heavily infected. The gingival margins also become red, swollen and ulcerated, and generalised stomatitis may develop.

A combination of nicotinamide and tetracycline is sometimes used to treat oral pemphigoid, particularly in the United States, but there is no convincing mechanism of action and no good evidence base.

Vitamin B$_{12}$ deficiency

This disease has many oral effects (see Ch. 17).

Folic acid deficiency

Deficiency can result from malnutrition but is more often seen in pregnancy, or as a result of malabsorption or drug treatment (particularly with phenytoin) (Ch. 17). Women are advised to take folic acid supplements preconceptually with the aim of reducing the risk of neural tube defects. It also appears that multivitamin preparations containing folic acid may reduce the risk of orofacial clefts.

Vitamin C deficiency

Scurvy, once common among crews of sailing ships, is now exceedingly rare. In Britain, scurvy may very occasionally be seen among elderly people with an inadequate diet or eccentric diet or the homeless. The main features of scurvy are dermatitis and purpura and, in advanced cases, anaemia and delayed healing of wounds. In the young, bone growth is delayed by poor collagen synthesis (Fig. 35.1).

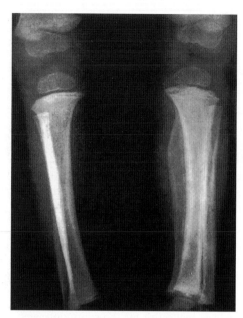

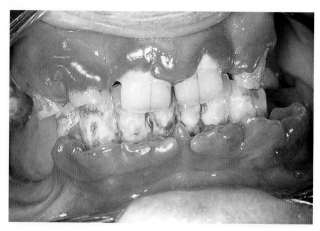

Fig. 35.2 **Scurvy.** There is gross periodontal destruction with deep pocketing and mobility of several teeth resulting from the combination of poor oral hygiene and deficiency of vitamin C.

Fig. 35.1 **Scurvy.** In contrast to rickets, calcification is unimpeded and there is a thick layer of calcified cartilage at the end of the bone. Osteoid formation, on the other hand, is poor, so little bone can be formed. The attachment of the periosteum to the bone is weak, so it is easily separated; haemorrhage beneath it (as here) is due to scorbutic purpura, and this becomes calcified.

Grossly swollen bleeding gums may develop (Fig. 35.2). The gingival swelling is due to a combination of chronic inflammation and an exaggeration of the inflammatory congestion due to purpura. In children, severe scurvy causes early tooth loss. The diagnosis should only be made on clear evidence of dietary deficiency and of purpura. In these cases, treatment with vitamin C and adequate oral hygiene relieves the gingival condition. There is no evidence that deficiency of vitamin C plays any part in periodontal disease except in frank scurvy.

Scurvy review PMID: 11838878

Case reports PMID: 16301149 and 21462768

Vitamin D deficiency

Deficiency of vitamin D during skeletal development causes rickets (Ch. 13). Dental hypocalcification is a feature only of exceptionally severe rickets (Ch. 2).

In sunlight, vitamin D is synthesised in the skin, and this is the main source, even in the UK. A few foods, notably, fish liver oils, eggs and butter contain significant amounts. In Britain, fat spreads are fortified with vitamins A and D, but not milk as in many other countries.

As much as 15% of the UK population is deficient, mostly the elderly and very young. Serum levels are lower in winter when as many as 40% of children become temporarily deficient. Requirements are small except during bone growth or pregnancy, and a small reserve is stored in fat.

Rickets is now rare, but immigrants in the North of Britain are at risk. Contributory factors are lack of sunlight, a high-carbohydrate diet and possibly also the use of wholemeal flour (as in chupattis) containing factors that impair calcium absorption.

There is no basis for the idea that dental caries is due to poor calcification of the teeth. Giving vitamin D and calcium for dental caries is valueless and dangerous. Hypervitaminosis D causes hypercalcaemia and renal calcinosis.

Mild osteoporosis has been considered to predispose to periodontitis.

Rickets general review PMID: 24412049

Vitamin D and periodontitis PMID: 23574464

Endocrine disorders and pregnancy | 36

Endocrine disorders, apart from diabetes mellitus and thyroid disease, are uncommon. They are rare causes of oral disease but, occasionally, oral changes can lead to their diagnosis. Patients with Addison's disease, diabetes mellitus and thyrotoxicosis, in particular, may also need special care for dental surgery.

PITUITARY GIGANTISM AND ACROMEGALY

Overproduction of growth hormone by the anterior pituitary during skeletal growth causes overgrowth of the skeleton and soft tissues to produce gigantism.

Acromegaly arises from excess hormone in middle age, after the epiphyses have fused. The hormone then only increases growth of the hands and feet, membranous bones of the skull and jaws, and soft tissues. Growth is slow, and diagnosis is often delayed.

The condylar growth centre becomes reactivated and the mandible enlarged and protrusive (Fig. 36.1). Radiographically, the whole jaw is lengthened and the angle becomes more oblique (Fig. 36.2). The jaw and other bones are also made thicker by subperiosteal bone deposition, producing frontal bossing. The teeth become spaced or, if the patient is edentulous, dentures cease to fit the growing jaw. The hands and feet become spade-like (Fig. 36.1). Overgrowth of soft tissues causes thickening and enlargement of the facial features, particularly the lips and nose. The tongue, lips, nose and ears enlarge, and vocal cord thickening causes a deep voice.

The cause is usually an adenoma of growth hormone–secreting cells in the pituitary. Expansion of this tumour commonly causes headaches and visual disturbances. Blindness may result from pressure on the optic chiasma. Occasionally ectopic hormone production by a neoplasm of the pancreas or adrenal is the cause. Diabetes results from insulin resistance caused by growth hormone. Hypertension is common and may be associated with cardiomyopathy and dysrhythmias.

Treatment is with octreotide, a somatostatin analogue that inhibits hormone secretion or pegvisomant, a growth hormone receptor blocker. Irradiation or resection of the pituitary tumour may also be required. Established growth changes do not resolve.

Rarely, a growth hormone–producing pituitary tumour is part of type 1 multiple endocrine neoplasia syndrome (MEN1), as described later. In such patients, gingival papules have also been described.

Acromegaly case report PMID: 21467827

Dental considerations

Orthognathic surgery may be considered to improve the appearance. There is a risk of post-operative airway

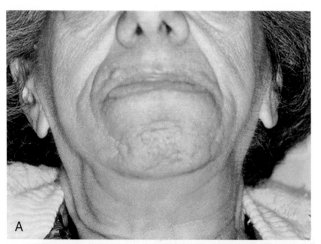

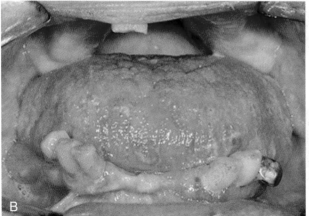

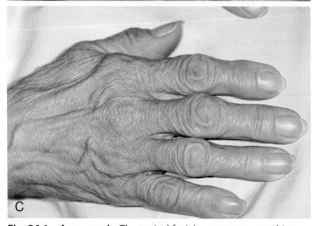

Fig. 36.1 Acromegaly. The typical facial appearance, resulting from excessive mandibular growth and thickened skin (A), tongue enlargement (B) and consequent playing of teeth and broad 'spade-like' hands (C). *(From Regezi, J.A., Sciubba, J.J., Jordan, R.C.K. 2003. Oral pathology: clinical pathological correlations, fourth ed. WB Saunders, Philadelphia.)*

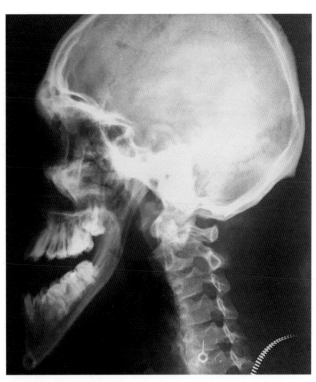

Fig. 36.2 Acromegaly. The mandible is enlarged with an elongated ramus and increased obliquity of the angle. The pituitary fossa is also enlarged due to the tumour causing the disease.

obstruction because of the large tongue and narrowing of the glottis. Hypertension and diabetes can also affect dental management. Otherwise, there is no special risk from treatment, local analgesia or sedation.

THYROID DISEASE

Hyperthyroidism

Hyperthyroidism is most common in young adults, particularly women. Causes include diffuse thyroid enlargement (goitre), a hypersecreting nodule or adenoma in the gland, and autoimmune thyroiditis caused by stimulatory autoantibodies (Graves' disease).

Clinical features are shown in Box 36.1. Graves' disease has additional exophthalmos and pretibial myxoedema caused by autoimmune inflammation.

Treatment of hyperthyroidism is by drugs such as carbimazole, iodine[131], or surgical removal of part of the gland. All may cause hypothyroidism. Beta-blockers may be used for symptom control.

Thyrotoxicosis general review PMID: 22394559

Dental considerations

Dental treatment of untreated hyperthyroid patients risks the medical emergency of thyrotoxic crisis, so recognition of signs and symptoms is key. Treatment must be deferred until thyrotoxicosis is controlled and any emergency treatment performed in hospital.

Dental treatment in treated disease is affected by several factors (Box 36.2), particularly excitability and anxiety. Excessive cardiac excitability is only a theoretical contraindication to lidocaine with epinephrine, and no other local

anaesthetic has been shown to be safer. Conscious sedation (nitrous oxide and oxygen) is frequently helpful.

Periodontal adverse effects treatment PMID: 25577420

Dental treatment in thyroid disease PMID: 12148678

Hypothyroidism

Cretinism

Cretinism results from deficient thyroid activity from birth, usually in areas of iodine deficiency or occasionally as a result of thyroid developmental anomalies.

The main features are particularly short stature and intellectual impairment, but dental abnormalities are frequently associated (Box 36.3). In the untreated patient, sedatives and tranquillisers such as benzodiazepines can precipitate myxoedemic coma and should generally be avoided. Conscious sedation with nitrous oxide and oxygen can be given.

Thyroid hormone treatment must begin early to allow normal physical and mental development.

Adult hypothyroidism

Hypothyroidism in the UK is most frequently due to Hashimoto autoimmune thyroiditis but can follow radioiodine, drug or surgical treatment for hyperthyroidism. In most of the world, iodine deficiency is the main cause.

Features are shown in Box 36.4 and aspects of dental management summarised in Box 36.5.

Lingual thyroid

The thyroglossal tract and cysts arising from it are discussed in Chapter 10.

Failure of normal development of the thyroid gland is almost always caused by failure of the embryonic thyroid anlage to descend into the neck. The patient's thyroid gland then lies somewhere along the path of the thyroglossal tract

- Skeletal development and dental eruption greatly delayed
- Impaired mental development
- Broad, rather flat face partly due to defective growth of the skull and facial bones
- Overlarge, protrusive tongue
- Dull facial expression, dry thick skin
- Short stocky build and, often, umbilical hernia
- Sensitivity to cold
- Bradycardia and hypotension

Box 36.4   Typical features of adult hypothyroidism. Signs are often mild and easily missed.

- Weight gain
- Slowed activity and thought, fatigue
- Myxoedema and hoarse voice
- Bradycardia
- Dry skin and hair loss
- Intolerance of cold
- Susceptibility to ischaemic heart disease

Box 36.5   Dental management of hypothyroidism

- Avoid sedatives including diazepam, opioid analgesics and general anaesthetics because of the risk of myxoedemic coma
- Anaemia or ischaemic heart disease may require modification of dental treatment
- Local anaesthesia always preferable
- Nitrous oxide/oxygen sedation acceptable
- Iodine containing agents such as radiographic contrast for sialograms or povidone iodine may disturb thyroid function
- Sjögren's syndrome occasionally associated with autoimmune thyroiditis

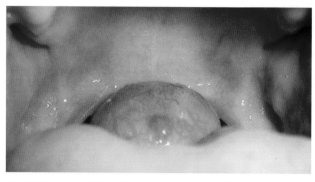

Fig. 36.3   Lingual thyroid. A large lingual thyroid at the typical site. *(From Amr, B., Monib, S., 2011. Lingual thyroid: A case report. Int. J. Surg. Case Rep. 2, 313–315.)*

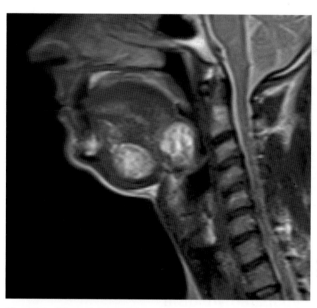

Fig. 36.4   Lingual thyroid tissue. Magnetic resonance imaging scan showing two rounded masses of thyroid tissue in the posterior and inferior parts of the tongue.

PARATHYROID DISEASE

→ Summary chart 12.2 p. 203

Hyperparathyroidism

The causes of hyperparathyroidism and its effects on bone are discussed in Chapter 13. The usual cause is an adenoma of a parathyroid gland, very occasionally a parathyroid carcinoma.

The commonest type is secondary hyperparathyroidism, a reaction to low serum calcium levels caused by chronic renal failure or prolonged dialysis. It may also be an effect of lithium treatment.

High levels of calcium cause weakness, fatigue, constipation and kidney stones and features summarised in Box 36.6. However, such florid presentations are now rare, and most cases are asymptomatic and discovered by chance because of a high serum calcium or when patients are seen with a renal stone.

Hyperparathyroidism is the presenting sign of the uncommon disease, type 1 multiple endocrine neoplasia syndrome (see the following section). There are also other familial forms. The hyperparathyroidism-jaw tumour syndrome is a rare autosomal dominant disease whose features include parathyroid adenomas or carcinomas, renal cysts

but is usually on the dorsum of the tongue at the site of the foramen caecum (Fig. 36.3), within the tongue or near the hyoid bone (Fig. 36.4). Females are mainly affected.

Clinically a lingual thyroid is an asymptomatic midline, purplish soft swelling and may cause dysphagia. Presentation is often at puberty or in pregnancy, when the thyroid normally enlarges. Lingual thyroid may not be recognised as such clinically, and biopsy may cause considerable bleeding. Otherwise, the nature of the swelling may be determined by fine needle aspiration. Patients with lingual thyroid are often hypothyroid.

Lingual thyroid tissue must not be removed before confirming that a thyroid gland is present in the neck by ultrasound scanning. If not, I^{131} or MRI scanning should be used to detect more deeply placed thyroid tissue. If no other thyroid tissue is present, removal would precipitate hypothyroidism and life-long thyroxine supplementation would be required. Malignant change in lingual thyroid is rare and more frequent in males.

Review PMID: 25439547

Box 36.6   Typical features of hyperparathyroidism

- General malaise
- Peptic ulceration
- Bone resorption
- Renal stones or nephrocalcinosis
- Polyuria

Box 36.7   Effects of hypoparathyroidism on calcified tissues

- Retarded new bone formation and diminished resorption are usually in equilibrium so that skeletal changes are rare
- Aplasia or hypoplasia of developing enamel*, which becomes deeply grooved
- Dentine may be incompletely mineralised but lamina dura may be thickened
- Short roots to teeth (Ch. 2)

*Results from associated ectodermal defects in developmental conditions, not lack of calcium.

Box 36.8   Typical clinical features of Addison's disease

- Lassitude, anorexia, weakness and fatigue
- Abnormal oral and cutaneous pigmentation
- Gastrointestinal disturbances, diarrhoea, nausea, vomiting
- Craving for salt (caused by lack of aldosterone)
- Loss of weight
- Low blood pressure
- Susceptibility to hypotensive crises
- Associated with chronic mucocutaneous candidosis in polyendocrinopathy syndrome (Ch.15)

and fibro-osseous jaw lesions, as discussed in Chapter 11. Brown tumours of hyperparathyroidism are discussed in Chapter 13.

Bone lesions case report PMID: 25398922

Hypoparathyroidism

The most common cause of hypoparathyroidism by far is thyroidectomy, when parathyroid glands are excised with the thyroid. Despite the fact that residual parathyroid tissue undergoes compensatory hyperplasia, 20% of patients are affected.

Early-onset hypoparathyroidism is rare and developmental in origin, sometimes part of autoimmune polyendocrinopathy or other syndromes.

Hypocalcaemia from any of these causes presents as mental changes or heightened neuromuscular excitability and tetany. These are controlled by giving the vitamin D analogue cholecalciferol (D_3) and calcium orally, with dietary adjustment to avoid phosphorus. Recombinant parathormone (PTH residues 1-34 (teriparatide) or PTH1-84) is now available.

Effects on calcified tissues are summarised in Box 36.7. See also Fig. 2.36.

Early onset hypoparathyroidism case PMID: 19201623

Tetany

In mild cases, tetany is latent but can be triggered by tapping on the skin over the facial nerve; this causes the facial muscles to contract (Chvostek's sign). In more severe cases, muscle cramps and tonic contractions of the muscles may progress to generalised convulsions. An early symptom of tetany is paraesthesia of the lip and extremities.

Tetany in the dental surgery more frequently results from overbreathing due to anxiety, producing the same signs.

Pseudohypoparathyroidism

This rare genetic condition is caused by mutations in genes that affect the PTH receptor cell activation pathway, including the GNAS gene associated with Albright's syndrome. Clinical features vary with the defect, but most patients are short, with a round face, hypocalcaemic, and have missing teeth, teeth with large pulps and enamel hypoplasia.

Pseudohypoparathyroidism case report PMID: 1881816

ADRENOCORTICAL DISEASES

Adrenocortical insufficiency is rarely primary (Addison's disease) and more frequently secondary to corticosteroid therapy.

Adrenocortical hypofunction or Addison's disease

Addison's disease results from failure of secretion of cortisol and aldosterone. The disease is usually autoimmune with organ-specific circulating autoantibodies. Tuberculous or fungal adrenal destruction are rare causes, sometimes secondary to HIV infection. Addison's disease is also the most frequent feature of the rare polyglandular autoimmune syndromes and is then associated with chronic mucocutaneous candidosis as described later.

The result is a severe disorder of electrolyte and fluid balance and serious clinical effects (Box 36.8).

Pigmentation results from compensatory adrenocorticotropic hormone (ACTH) secretion as this peptide hormone has a similar amino acid sequence to melanocyte-stimulating hormone. Pigmentation is often an early sign and, in the mouth, is patchily distributed on gingivae, buccal mucosa and lips (Figs 36.5 and 36.6). It is brown or almost black. The skin pigmentation looks similar to suntan but with a sallow appearance due to underlying pallor. Exposed and normally pigmented areas are most severely affected.

Addison's disease is an exceptionally rare cause of oral pigmentation but, if there is recent onset with general weakness and lassitude, the diagnosis should be considered.

Long-term treatment of Addison's disease is usually by oral hydrocortisone and fludrocortisone, with salt supplementation if necessary. The dose of steroid needs to be adjusted to provide additional steroid support in times of stress, infection, other illness, surgery or exercise. Failure to provide sufficient steroid, or untreated disease, may lead to Addisonian crisis.

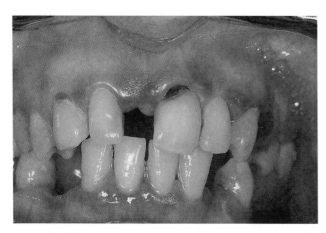

Fig. 36.5 Addison's disease. A close-up shows the characteristic distribution of pigment rather patchily along the attached gingivae. It is a brownish-black in colour.

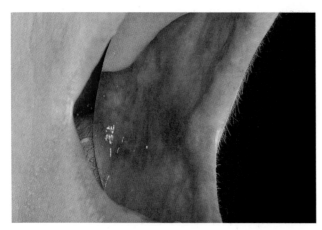

Fig. 36.6 Addison's disease. Deep pigmentation of the buccal mucosa.

In an Addisonian or adrenal crisis (Ch. 43), there is a rapid fall in blood pressure, circulatory collapse (shock: pale, cold, clammy skin, sweating, rapid, shallow breathing, dizziness) and vomiting. These may be associated with dehydration, headache, drowsiness or loss of consciousness. These crises may be fatal, and they require immediate treatment with intravenous hydrocortisone (several 100 mg) and fluid replacement.

Patients may also suffer adverse effects of excess therapeutic corticosteroids (Table 42.1).

Oral pigmentation in Addison's PMID: 16209154

Adrenocortical hyperfunction

Cushing's disease is usually due to an adrenocorticotrophic hormone-secreting pituitary adenoma that causes adrenocortical hyperplasia. Cushing's syndrome refers to the same features caused by ectopic ACTH production by another neoplasm, or corticosteroid treatment, the last being by far the commonest cause. The effects (Box 36.9) are rarely dentally important.

Cushing's review for dentistry PMID: 23094575

Box 36.9 Important features of Cushing's disease

- Obesity of trunk and face
- Bruisability and haematomas on trauma
- Hirsutism
- Headaches
- Hypertension
- Osteoporosis, especially of the skull
- Glycosuria, hyperglycaemia and thirst

Table 36.1 Polyendocrinopathy syndromes

	Percentage of patients affected by the different syndrome components	
	Type 1	Type 2
Addison's disease	100	100
Hypoparathyroidism	76	–
Chronic mucocutaneous candidosis	73	–
Pernicious anaemia	13	0.5
Alopecia	32	0.5
Malabsorption syndromes	22	–
Gonadal failure	17	3.6
Chronic active hepatitis	13	–
Insulin-dependent diabetes	4	52
Autoimmune thyroiditis	11	69
Female:male ratio	1.5:1	1.8:1

AUTOIMMUNE POLYENDOCRINE SYNDROMES

These three diseases are also known as *polyglandular autoimmune disease* (or APECED). They have different inheritance patterns, and several genes are responsible but all feature autoimmune attack on multiple endocrine glands. The two more common types both have Addison's disease as an invariable feature, and there are several other components of significance to dental treatment, notably chronic mucocutaneous candidosis in type 1 (Table 36.1). Candidosis is an early and common presenting feature. Dental defects can also result from hypoparathyroidism in the type 1 syndrome (Fig. 2.36) and as many as 10% of patients with Type 1 disease develop oral or oesophageal carcinoma.

General review PMID: 24055063

Case report PMID: 1407992

Case report with carcinoma PMID: 20304522

DISEASES OF THE ADRENAL MEDULLA

Phaeochromocytoma

Phaeochromocytoma is a catecholamine-producing tumour of the adrenal medulla. The main effect is potentially lethal hypertension, tachycardia and dysrhythmias. A third of

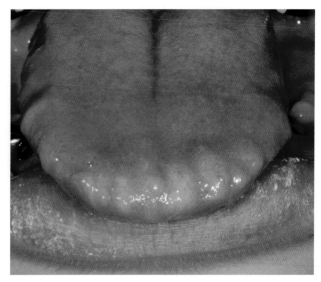

Fig. 36.7   Mucosal neuromas in MEN2b. These slightly firm pale nodules along the border and dorsum of the tongue are tangled masses of nerves. *(By kind permission of Professor D Emmanouil.)*

cases have a genetic predisposition. It may be part of the multiple endocrine adenoma syndrome type IIb, when it is associated with oral mucosal neuromas (Box 36.10). Alternatively, it may be associated with neurofibromatosis, von Hippel-Lindau or other inherited diseases.

When an oral neuroma is found, the possibility of a phaeochromocytoma should be considered, especially if the patient is hypertensive.

Dental treatment must be delayed in any patient with a phaeochromocytoma. A stressful event may precipitate a hypertensive crisis.

MULTIPLE ENDOCRINE NEOPLASIA SYNDROMES

Multiple endocrine neoplasia (multiple endocrine adenomatosis) syndromes (MEN) are autosomal dominant disorders with a prevalence of approximately 1 in 20,000 that cause gland hyperplasia and benign and malignant neoplasms.

MEN1 is caused by mutation in the tumour suppressor gene *MEN1*, which encodes a nuclear transcription factor. Parathyroid, pancreas and pituitary are affected, and presentation is in the second and third decades. Hyperparathyroidism develops in 95%. Enteropancreatic tumours develop in more than 40% and pituitary tumours in more than 30%. Also described are gingival papules and nodular lesions on the vermilion border.

In MEN2, the mutated gene is the RET proto-oncogene, a growth factor receptor that affects cell cycle and also the development of autonomic nerves. In this disease, medullary carcinoma of the thyroid is present in 95%, phaeochromocytoma in 50% and hyperparathyroidism in 15% of cases. Two forms are recognised, 2a and 2b (the latter sometimes called *type 3*).

A striking oral feature of MEN2b is mucosal neuromas, particularly along the lateral borders of the tongue (Fig. 36.7). These are neither neurofibromas nor schwannomas, but developmental anomalies of tangles of enlarged nerves. Large neuromas enlarge the tongue, lips and other sites. Small ones produce small mucosal nodules or a papillary mucosa. These are often the first sign and can be diagnosed in infancy or childhood. Diagnosis following

dental examination is not unusual. Screening for MEN2 is relatively readily carried out by identifying the RET mutation. Confirmed cases will be offered total thyroidectomy in infancy to avoid developing medullary carcinoma, which can develop in the very young.

Features of multiple endocrine neoplasia syndromes are summarised in Box 36.10. Note that several features individually may be parts of other syndromes or familial diseases.

General review all types PMID: 26363542

Case report MEN2b: 25454714 and 1351093

DIABETES MELLITUS

Diabetes mellitus results from relative or absolute deficiency of insulin, causing persistently raised blood glucose. UK prevalence has doubled in 20 years, and 5% of the population are affected, but probably at least 50% of diabetics with mild or early disease pass unrecognised. By 2025 the UK incidence will be 8%, a level already attained in the United States. World incidence is rising as populations become urbanised, eat a more Western diet and become obese.

There are two main clinical types.

Type 1 diabetes ('insulin-dependent') accounts for 10% of cases. Symptoms typically appear before the age of 25, and the disease is usually severe with thirst, polyuria, hunger, loss of weight and susceptibility to infection. The cause is failure of secretion of insulin after autoimmune destruction of the pancreatic islets and insulin replacement is the treatment.

Type 2 ('maturity onset') accounts for 90% of cases. Patients are typically older than middle age and obese. The onset is insidious, often with deterioration of vision or pruritus or, sometimes, thirst, polyuria and fatigue. However, many cases are asymptomatic. The cause is end organ resistance to insulin, and the disease can be controlled by dietary restriction and, if necessary, oral hypoglycaemic drugs. The current epidemic of childhood obesity seems likely to lead to the onset of this variety of diabetes early in life.

In practice the division between these two types is somewhat blurred.

> **Box 36.11   Complications of diabetes mellitus that can affect dental management**
>
> - Susceptibility to infection, particularly candidosis, also mucormycosis
> - Hypoglycaemic coma
> - Diabetic coma
> - Ischaemic heart disease
> - Acceleration of periodontal disease if control is poor
> - Dry mouth secondary to polyuria and dehydration
> - Oral lichenoid reactions due to oral hypoglycaemic drugs
> - Delayed healing
> - Sialadenosis

> **Box 36.12   Principles of dental management of diabetics**
>
> - Time treatment to avoid disturbance of routine insulin administration or meals
> - Use local anaesthesia for routine dentistry – the amount of adrenaline (epinephrine) in local anaesthetic solutions has no significant effect on the blood sugar
> - Sedation can be given if required
> - Deal with any diabetic complications (Box 36.11)
> - Manage hypoglycaemic coma as described in Chapter 43
> - General anaesthesia requires special precautions

> **Box 36.13   Pregnancy: oral effects and management considerations**
>
> **Effect on the mother**
>
> - Aggravated gingivitis and epulis formation
> - Variable effect on recurrent aphthae
> - Increased intensity of pigmentation, face and sometimes oral
> - Risk of hypotension when laid supine
> - Possible hypertension of pregnancy
> - Hypersensitive gag reflex and vomiting
> - Possible iron or folate deficiency, especially if anaemic before pregnancy
>
> **Risks to the fetus**
>
> - X-rays hazardous, especially in first trimester
> - Respiratory depression due to sedatives, including benzodiazepines
> - Tooth discolouration due to tetracycline
> - Prilocaine may rarely cause methaemoglobinaemia
> - Theoretical risk of uterine contraction caused by felypressin
> - Aspirin may cause neonatal haemorrhage
> - Theoretical risk of depressed vitamin B_{12} metabolism by nitrous oxide
> - Teratogenic risks of thalidomide, retinoids, azathioprine and possibly other drugs

In terms of dental management, it is usually said that the greatest problems are with 'uncontrolled' diabetes. However, 'uncontrolled' applies to several diabetic states. At one extreme, there is the mild, unrecognised, and therefore untreated, diabetic. At the other, there is the treated diabetic whose disease is difficult to control ('brittle diabetes') or has been mismanaged. This last group is the one most likely to have oral complications and present difficulties in dental management (Box 36.11).

Dental aspects

The main oral manifestations of diabetes are usually due to the lowered resistance to infection, particularly to fungi as a result of impaired neutrophil function. Oral candidosis is frequent, and severe deep mycoses such as mucormycosis are a risk, albeit small.

Rapidly destructive periodontal disease occurs, and severity is proportional to blood glucose levels. Severe periodontitis also seems to complicate insulin control and treatment appears to improve diabetic markers of disease severity. Diabetics with more severe periodontitis are at higher risk of diabetic complications such as nephropathy and ischaemic heart disease.

The relationship between diabetes and dental caries is unclear. Many patients have low caries susceptibility, probably as a result of the sugar-free diet. However, poorly controlled childhood patients have higher caries rates.

The principles of dental management are summarised in Box 36.12.

Type 2 diabetics with good dietary or oral hypoglycaemic drug control can be treated as a non-diabetic patient.

In type 1 diabetes, well-controlled patients are similarly very low risk. However, hypoglycaemic coma may be precipitated by dental treatment that delays a normal meal or unbalances food intake and insulin. This can cause an emergency in the dental surgery (Ch. 43). Treatment should therefore be so timed as to avoid these risks – ideally, soon after the patient's breakfast. Many patients now have their own glucose monitors and can check the level immediately before treatment and when signs suggest onset of hypoglycaemia.

Diabetic (hyperglycaemic) coma is a complication of poorly controlled diabetes mellitus and much less likely to be seen.

Patients with recurrent candidosis or severe periodontitis without cause can be relatively easily tested in a dental setting using urine dipsticks to detect glycosuria, enabling confident referral to their medical practitioner.

Management in dentistry PMID: 17376713, 17000275 and 15188524

Oral features review PMID: 15196139

Oral health type 2 diabetes PMID: 23531957 and 18302671

PREGNANCY

Pregnancy is a physiological process and should not deter dental treatment; this is an important time to establish good oral health for mother and child. Nevertheless, the changes of pregnancy do impact on dental care in three main ways: hormonal influences on the oral cavity, risks to the fetus and adjustments required for medication (Box 36.13).

Fetal considerations

The main risks of fetal abnormalities are from drugs and radiation; the hazard is greatest during organogenesis in the first trimester.

Few drugs are known to be teratogenic for humans and, in many cases, the risk is no more than theoretical or results only from prolonged, high dosage. For example, no teratogenic risk from metronidazole for humans has ever been substantiated though effects in animals have led to the avoidance of metronidazole during pregnancy.

The risks from dental radiography are small, but only essential radiographs should be taken, the minimal radiation exposure should be given and radiography delayed if possible. An abdominal dose of radiation, particularly in the first trimester, risks congenital abnormality, learning disorder and malignant neoplasms. Because the risk period is likely to be before the patient will know she is pregnant, precautions must be taken for all women of child-bearing age. In the UK this does not require routine use of lead aprons as the beam in dental radiography will not be directed toward the abdomen. Routine collimation, fast films or digital capture, and good technique are more important in reducing dose. Nevertheless, during pregnancy, the patient may be offered a lead apron because the topic is so emotive, but routine radiation protection measures are safe. In some countries, a lead apron is required.

Non-steroidal anti-inflammatory drugs in high dosage may cause premature closure of the ductus arteriosus and fetal pulmonary hypertension. Aspirin may also increase the risk of neonatal haemorrhage and paracetamol is the only safe analgesic. Systemic corticosteroids can cause fetal adrenosuppression. However, the only drugs known to be teratogenic are thalidomide (used occasionally for major aphthae), etretinate (used experimentally for leukoplakia) and possibly azathioprine (used for Behçet's syndrome and autoimmune diseases). Systemic antifungals and antiviral agents are considered safe, with adverse effects limited to animal studies. For details of drug usage in pregnancy, see the current British National Formulary.

Maternal considerations

Pregnant patients should be fully evaluated as early as possible so that any treatment necessary can be planned for the second trimester and emergency dental care avoided. Temporary restorations and stabilisation may be required when oral health is poor. An intensive preventive regime of oral hygiene and diet control will benefit both the mother and future child. Prenatal fluoride supplementation provides no benefit to the child.

The chief oral effects of pregnancy are aggravation of gingivitis (Fig. 36.8) and possible development of a pregnancy epulis (Fig. 36.9; Ch. 24). Initiation of a high standard of dental care and dental education at the earliest opportunity is essential. These complications usually affect those with pre-existing gingivitis and start around the second month.

Occasionally, recurrent aphthae remit during pregnancy but may worsen due to any iron or folate deficiency.

A few women in the third trimester of pregnancy become hypotensive when laid supine, when the enlarged uterus impedes venous return. Respiratory reserve is diminished, and there is a risk of fetal hypoxia. It is easiest to treat all late pregnant patients in a sitting position and in short appointments, as this is more comfortable.

Neonatal respiration is further depressed by drugs such as general anaesthetics and sedatives, especially barbiturates, diazepam and opioids, all of which cross the placenta and are contraindicated in pregnancy.

There is no evidence of risks from local anaesthesia, and pain is likely to cause greater adverse consequences. Felypressin is an oxytocin analogue and in theory could induce

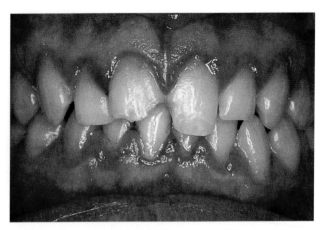

Fig. 36.8 Pregnancy gingivitis. Marginal gingivitis despite relatively good oral hygiene during the first trimester of pregnancy.

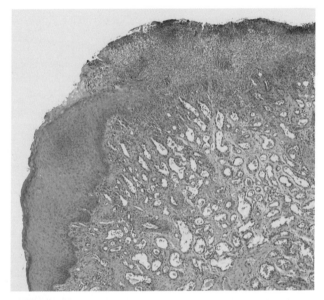

Fig. 36.9 Pregnancy epulis. These are usually detected and removed during growth and so are often ulcerated and highly vascular.

uterine contractions and fetal methaemoglobinaemia. These are not considered risks at dental doses, but lignocaine and epinephrine is generally taken to be preferable as it is more effective. As noted earlier, the risks from benzodiazepines such as midazolam for sedation are such that intravenous sedation is contraindicated. Nitrous oxide sedation carries a risk of interference with B_{12} and folate metabolism after very prolonged administration (weeks), but there is no evidence that it is teratogenic and it is safe after the first trimester used with 50% oxygen. Exposure should be limited to 30 minutes and repeated exposure avoided.

The myth that mothers lose a tooth for every pregnancy reflects poor oral health in past decades and is nothing to do with increased calcium requirements during pregnancy; this calcium is provided from bone and diet, not teeth.

Oral Surgery during pregnancy PMID: 18088879

Dental treatment during pregnancy PMID: 23570802

Oral health and pregnancy PMID: 15042797

Prescribing considerations in dentistry PMID: 9766109

Renal disease

37

Renal disease has become important in dentistry because of the growing number of patients who, as a result of renal dialysis or transplantation, survive renal failure. In the UK, nearly 2 million patients have renal failure and a further million at least are undiagnosed. Aspects of renal disease relevant to dentistry are summarised in Box 37.1.

CHRONIC RENAL FAILURE AND DIALYSIS

The common causes are diabetes, hypertension or glomerulonephritis. Some patients are unsuitable for, or unable to obtain, dialysis or a transplant. They can suffer a variety of oral effects (Box 37.2). Prolonged dialysis or renal failure are now the most common causes of hyperparathyroidism. The jaws may be first affected (Ch. 13). In severe uraemia, urea may crystallise on the skin and oral mucosa ('urea frost').

Dental management of patients with renal disease, but particularly chronic renal failure, may be affected by many factors (Box 37.3).

Patients in renal failure may receive regular dialysis while awaiting a transplant, but remain otherwise in reasonably good general health. Approximately 70% can return to full-time work.

Peritoneal dialysis has no implications for dental treatment, but haemodialysis does. Patients are heparinised before haemodialysis, and haemostasis is impaired for 6–12 hours. Dental treatment should be delayed until the next day.

These patients' permanent venous fistulas for the dialysis lines are susceptible to infection, and antibiotic cover may be considered for dental surgical procedures. Drugs, including sedation, should not be given intravenously because of the risk of damage to superficial veins, which are patients' lifelines. A blood pressure cuff must never be placed on the arm with the shunt. Dialysis patients also have a greater incidence of cardiovascular and cerebrovascular disease.

Patients under dialysis will still have a uraemic oral odour and bad taste, xerostomia and sore mouth with increased calculus

Oral findings in haemodialysis PMID: 17577325, 23597063 and 15723858

Periodontitis and renal disease PMID: 18173441

Dental treatment in renal disease PMID: 17378316

Prescribing considerations in dentistry PMID: 21037190

RENAL TRANSPLANTATION

Normal renal function and health can be restored by transplantation, but it is associated with the complications of prolonged immunosuppressive treatment, particularly susceptibility to infections or lymphomas.

Ciclosporin, which is widely used to help control graft rejection, can cause persistent gingival overgrowth, and patients are often taking a calcium channel blocker, such as nifedipine, for hypertension, enhancing the effect (Ch. 7).

Hairy leukoplakia can rarely develop in HIV-negative renal transplant patients as a complication of immunosuppression.

Complications of graft rejection, such as bone lesions due to secondary hyperparathyroidism, may be seen (Ch. 13).

Box 37.1   Aspects of renal disease affecting dental management

- Heparinisation before dialysis
- Possible hepatitis B or C carriage after chronic dialysis
- Permanent venous fistulae susceptible to infection
- Increased risk of endocarditis
- Secondary hyperparathyroidism
- Immunosuppressive treatment for nephrotic syndrome or transplant patients
- Oral lesions due to drugs, particularly for immunosuppression
- Reduced excretion of some drugs
- Oral lesions of chronic renal failure (Box 37.2)

Box 37.2   Oral changes in uraemia of renal failure

- Mucosal pallor (anaemia)
- Xerostomia
- Purpura
- Mucosal ulceration
- Thrush or bacterial plaques
- White epithelial plaques (Ch. 18)
- Brown tumours of the jaws (secondary hyperparathyroidism)

Box 37.3   Factors potentially affecting dental management of patients with renal disease

- Corticosteroid and other immunosuppressive treatment
- Haemorrhagic tendencies
- Anaemia
- Impaired drug excretion
- Hypertension
- Hepatitis B or C carriage
- Underlying causes (e.g. diabetes mellitus, hypertension or connective tissue disease)

Prescribing in renal failure depends on its severity. Local analgesics cause no problems, and the usual antibiotics for dental infections are safe except in severe disease. Dose reduction according to the glomerular filtration rate is usually sufficient precaution for most dental prescribing, but medical advice should be sought. However, tetracyclines, itraconazole and systemic antivirals should be avoided.

Children with renal failure may have chronological enamel hypoplasia and dysplastic dentine with delayed eruption of teeth.

Drugs and gingival overgrowth PMID: 25680368

Management gingival overgrowth PMID: 16677333

Gingival overgrowth children PMID: 16238650

Pain and neurological disorders

38

Pain is the most common symptom for which patients seek help. Pain has strong emotional associations which, in turn, may be determined to a varying degree by patients' preconceptions. Emotional disturbance itself can also produce the symptom of pain.

There are many causes of oral or maxillofacial pain (Box 38.1). Pulpitis and periapical periodontitis as sequels of dental caries are by far the most common causes. The source of such pain is usually obvious on examination. However, some sources of dental pain can be exceedingly difficult to identify (Box 38.2) and may only become apparent after a period of time.

Approximately 8% of the British population reported a toothache in the last 12 months. A key role of the dentist is to exclude dental and mucosal causes of pain before further medical investigation and to be able to formulate a differential diagnosis, but the expected role of the dentist in non-dental pain varies among countries.

Principles of taking a pain history and diagnosis are discussed in Chapter 1. Transmission of information when referring is critical for efficient diagnosis in secondary care. Table 38.1 provides a reminder of the types and mechanisms of pain.

Review orofacial pain in dentistry PMID: 16444222

Classification and assessment orofacial pain PMID: 26058224 and 26062258

Team management chronic facial pain PMID: 25899741

How to refer PMID: 27056518

Incidence chronic pain types in dentistry PMID: 25338483

Diagnosis review and management guidelines PMID: 23794651

Prescribing for pain (US perspective) PMID: 22329011

DENTAL AND PERIODONTAL PAIN

Pulpitis

Pulpitis is usually the cause when hot or cold food or drinks trigger the pain. It is also the main cause of spasmodic, poorly localised attacks of pain, which may be mistakenly ascribed to a variety of other possible causes. The pain of acute pulpitis is of a sharp lancinating character peculiar to itself, impossible to describe but unforgettable once experienced. Recurrent attacks of less severe, subacute or chronic pain, often apparently spontaneous, suggest a diseased or dying pulp.

One key feature of pulpitis is poor localisation. All tooth pain fibres converge in the trigeminal nerve and trigeminal sensory complex, which also receives pain and sensation from other nerves and extends into the upper spinal cord. The complex pathway means that the sensation is sometimes perceived and recognised as a toothache but cannot be localised. Patients often cannot localise pulpitic pain even to one quadrant. Although left and right are accurately distinguished, upper and lower arches often cannot be. Thus, investigation for pulpitis may require checking many teeth.

The only non-dental condition that is indistinguishable from pulp pain by the patient is the pain of early herpes zoster. If no local cause can be found after the most careful search, it is important to look for early signs of the characteristic rash and ask about contact with chicken pox and zoster (Ch. 15). Herpes zoster is an uncommon cause of toothache-like pain but has been the cause of unnecessary dental extractions and pulp extirpations.

Apical periodontitis

→ Summary chart 38.1 p. 486

Unlike pulpitis, pain from periapical periodontitis is readily identifiable and precisely localised as the nerves have accurate spatial representation in the cortex, being critical for mastication. There is tenderness of the tooth in its socket on percussion or pressure.

Radiographs are of little value in the early stages but useful after inflammation causes loss of definition of the periapical lamina dura. Later, a chronic apical periodontitis will produce a rounded area of radiolucency as a periapical granuloma develops. Most of these are asymptomatic (Ch. 5).

Acute maxillary sinusitis can rarely cause similar tenderness of a group of teeth, particularly upper molars, as discussed in Chapter 33.

Box 38.1   Types of pain felt in the oral tissues

- Disease of teeth and/or supporting tissues
- Oral mucosal diseases
- Diseases of the jaw
- Pain in the edentulous patient
- Post-operative pain
- Pain triggered by mastication
- Referred pain
- Neurological diseases
- Psychogenic pain

Box 38.2   Causes of pain from the teeth or supporting tissues

- Pulpitis
- Dentine hypersensitivity, cracked tooth or cracked cusp syndrome
- Periapical periodontitis
- Lateral (periodontal) abscess
- Acute necrotising ulcerative gingivitis
- HIV-associated periodontitis
- Pericoronitis

Table 38.1   Types and mechanisms of pain

Source of pain	Example	Mediators
Peripheral nerve stimulation (nociceptive pain)	Pulpitis and apical periodontitis	Inflammatory mediators and products of tissue damage, some bacterial factors bradykinin, histamine, serotonin, prostaglandin E2
Nerve damage	Herpes zoster infection, infiltration of nerve by malignant tumour	Unclear, inflammatory mediators, direct damage to pain fibres
Central or neuropathic pain	Possibly burning mouth disorder	Probably mediated by glial receptors, immune mediators and/or psychoimmunological mechanisms in brain and spinal cord. Glial cells can perform macrophage-like functions. Persistent activation leads to functional changes in pain pathways and thresholds.
Psychogenic pain	Usually no specific pattern	Unclear, possibly generated by failure to suppress low-level pain or emotional overlay mediated by psychoimmunological mechanisms

Periodontal abscess and pericoronitis

The tooth is tender in its socket, and there is a deep localised pocket, either swollen or draining pus. The tooth is normally vital unless there are other reasons for loss of vitality, although involvement of the furcation by the abscess or periodontitis may devitalise molar teeth.

Occasionally, a periodontal abscess may be precipitated by endodontic root perforation on the side of the root, or a 'perioendo' lesion may result from drainage of an apical infection through a pocket, triggering a periodontal abscess.

Pericoronitis is similar to a periodontal abscess in terms of pain, but with added elements of pain on biting on the swollen operculum.

Cracked teeth

The pain of a cracked tooth is distinctive, sharp, excruciating, lasting only a second or two and experienced only when occlusion or mastication opens the crack. However, identifying which cusp is cracked can be difficult as the pain, like pulpitis, is poorly localised. The best approach is to identify the crack by oblique pressure or instilling a dye such as disclosing solution.

Acute necrotising ulcerative gingivitis

Acute ulcerative gingivitis usually causes soreness, but when it extends deeply and rapidly, as in HIV infection, destroying the underlying bone, there may be severe aching pain (Ch. 7).

Odontogenic pain review PMID: 26630860

Acute orofacial pain PMID: 26964446

PAIN IN EDENTULOUS PATIENTS

Dental causes can be excluded, and pain is usually caused by dentures or to some condition of the mucosa or jaws on which a denture is pressing (Box 38.3).

Traumatic ulcers, usually the consequence of overextension, often cause trouble with a new denture. After the denture has been relieved, these ulcers heal within 24–48 hours. Persistent ulceration after relief of an otherwise adequate denture is likely to be due to some more serious cause, and a biopsy is then essential. Later, dentures cause traumatic pain when alveolar bone has become severely resorbed, allowing the denture to bear on the mylohyoid ridge or genial tubercles.

Lack of freeway space due to excessive vertical dimension of the dentures prevents the mandible and masticatory

> **Box 38.3   Important causes of pain in edentulous patients**
> - Denture trauma
> - Excessive vertical dimension
> - Mucosal diseases of the denture-bearing mucosa
> - Diseases of the jaws (Box 38.4)
> - Teeth or roots erupting under a denture

muscles from reaching their natural rest position. This causes the teeth to be held permanently in contact. Aching pain is usually felt in the fatigued masticatory muscles, but the excessive stress imposed on the denture-bearing area sometimes causes pain in this region. There may be interference with speech or swallowing if the vertical discrepancy is large.

The best investigation to determine whether pain is caused by the dentures themselves is for the patient to cease wearing them.

Few painful mucosal diseases affect the denture-bearing area. Denture stomatitis is common but painless. Lichen planus can extend to the sulcus and impinge on the margin of the denture-bearing area and mucous membrane pemphigoid may affect the palate and sulci. The most important conditions to be excluded are neoplasms. As most edentulous patients are elderly, persistent lesions, whether ulcerated or not, developing beneath or at the margins of dentures, must be biopsied without hesitation. A carcinoma can persist for a long time with minimal symptoms, and the patient may notice no more than the fact that the fit of the denture has deteriorated.

Jaw lesions causing pain in the edentulous patient may be associated with a swelling or an area of radiolucency. A painful swelling of the jaw in the edentulous patient is probably most often due to an infected residual cyst. Metastatic malignant neoplasms are very much less common but must be considered and intraosseous lesions evaluated for a biopsy.

Osteomyelitis of the jaws in edentulous patients must be considered in those who have had radiotherapy, bisphosphonates or similar drugs (Ch. 8).

Late eruption of buried teeth, retained root fragments and exfoliation of small sequestra following extraction may all cause pain beneath a denture as the mucosa is pinched between them and the denture. In a very atrophic mandible, fracture may need to be considered.

Box 38.4   Causes of pain in the jaws
- Fractures
- Osteomyelitis
- Infected cysts
- Malignant neoplasms
- Sickle cell infarcts
- Referred pain of angina and myocardial infarction

Box 38.5   Post-operative pain
- Alveolar osteitis (dry socket)
- Fracture of the jaw
- Damage to the temporomandibular joint
- Osteomyelitis
- Damage to the nerve trunks or involvement of nerves in scar tissue

Box 38.6   Pain induced by mastication
- Disease of teeth and supporting tissues
- Cracked tooth
- Pain dysfunction syndrome
- Diseases of the temporomandibular joint
- Temporal arteritis
- Trigeminal neuralgia (rarely)
- Salivary calculi

Finally, even well-constructed dentures can be disliked intensely, and pain may become a surrogate complaint for discomfort or appearance. Occasionally, dentures may become the focus of a psychogenic pain (Ch. 40).

PAINFUL MUCOSAL LESIONS

Ulcers generally cause soreness rather than pain, but deep ulceration may cause severe aching pain. Carcinoma, in particular, causes severe pain once nerve fibres become involved. It is important to emphasise again that early carcinoma is painless; pain is a late symptom.

PAIN IN THE JAWS

Pain from inside the mandible is usually felt as dull boring pain, unless related to teeth or fracture, in which cases periodontal ligament or mucosal receptors are involved.

Important causes are listed in Box 38.4. Chronic and low-grade osteomyelitis are particularly difficult causes of pain to diagnose because of their non-specific radiological and clinical features. With the exception of fractures and acute osteomyelitis, diagnosis of identifiable lesions depends on biopsy.

Referred cardiac pain PMID: 22322488

POSTSURGICAL PAIN AND NERVE DAMAGE

Important causes of post-operative pain are summarised in Box 38.5. Meticulous investigation of post-operative pain is important as it is a major cause of complaints and medicolegal claims.

Minor surgical procedures such as a simple extraction or soft-tissue biopsy produce mild pain and discomfort after local analgesia wears off. Patients frequently take no analgesics after the first few hours, if at all.

By far the most common cause of significant pain after dental extractions is alveolar osteitis (dry socket; Ch. 8). Fracture of the jaw following operative treatment is rare but can also be readily recognised. Forcible opening of the mouth, particularly under general anaesthesia to remove wisdom teeth, can crush and inflame the temporomandibular joint periarticular tissues, leading to persistent pain on opening or during mastication. Pain from osteomyelitis develops after extraction (Ch. 8).

Iatrogenic nerve injury

The inferior alveolar and lingual nerves are those most frequently damaged during treatment, usually surgical removal of lower third molars. Placement of implants, and endodontic irrigation with hypochlorite are other causes. Lingual nerve injuries particularly follow lower third molar extraction when a lingual flap is raised; a lingually placed elevator does not 'protect' the nerve, but damage it. Prevention is key: avoiding unnecessary extractions, identifying teeth close to nerves and using alternative techniques such as coronectomy when the nerve is at risk.

Local analgesia also causes similar nerve damage, particularly when using Articaine, especially at a concentration of 4%. Lidocaine is the safest agent for block analgesia. Persistent symptoms do not necessarily follow an 'electric shock' pain during injection and do not necessarily result from direct needle trauma to the nerve.

Symptoms following all causes are of paraesthesia and pain in the relevant distribution, if severe, interfering with speech, mastication and drinking. Light touch in areas of paraesthesia can trigger excruciating sharp pain.

More than three-quarters of lingual nerve injuries resolve spontaneously in 2–3 months. Inferior alveolar nerve effects are usually persistent, and surgical exploration should be considered within 3 months for best effect. In the unlikely event that a nerve is completely severed, it must be repaired surgically as soon as possible. Endodontic materials extruded into the inferior dental canal must be removed within 24 hours.

Rarely, damaged nerves in soft tissue proliferate to form a traumatic neuroma which is tender to pressure. Its excision should lead to relief of the pain.

Avoiding nerve injury PMID: 24157759

Management iatrogenic injuries PMID: 22326447

Hypochlorite and endodontic injury PMID: 25809429, 24878709 and 23767399

Guideline hypochlorite extrusion PMID: 25525012

Associated with implants PMID: 25434563

PAIN INDUCED BY MASTICATION

Pain on mastication is usually dental in origin and caused by apical periodontitis, but any condition that raises the tooth in its socket or displaces it into premature occlusion can cause this symptom (Box 38.6). Cracked teeth usually become evident on mastication (see earlier).

Pain associated with dentures was discussed earlier.

Non-dental causes

Pain of temporomandibular dysfunction is discussed in Chapter 14. Dull, aching facial pain may be present during eating, but trismus and muscle spasm cause more interference than pain. The *least* common cause of pain during eating is organic disease of the temporomandibular joint.

Pain of temporal arteritis is usually interpreted by patients as headache but is a particularly important cause of masticatory pain because of the high risk of blindness. The pain is due to ischaemia of the masticatory muscles, caused by the arteritis (Ch. 14).

Mealtime syndrome caused by calculi and other obstructions of the salivary ducts can cause pain when salivation is triggered by eating, or the thought of eating (Ch. 22).

First-bite syndrome is a rare and peculiar complication of surgery to the neck, similar clinically to mealtime syndrome. A very intense, paroxysmal electric shock-like pain, sometimes with muscle cramp is felt around the parotid gland or temporomandibular joint on the operated side. The pain appears on biting, mastication or swallowing of only the first bite of a meal. Subsequent eating triggers no pain, though further attacks may follow after a few minutes' respite. The cause is thought to be loss of sympathetic nerve supply to the parotid gland when cervical sympathetic trunk nerves in the carotid sheath or parapharynx are cut.

PAIN FROM SALIVARY GLANDS

Causes of pain from salivary glands are summarised in Box 38.7. The parotid gland and submandibular glands become painful immediately they are inflamed, as they have little space for expansion or, in the case of the submandibular gland, a tight capsule. Thus, almost any disease of the glands will present with pain.

NEURALGIA AND NEUROPATHY

Neuralgia is pain felt in the distribution of a nerve. Neuropathy is a disease of a nerve. In sensory nerves, neuropathies produces pain, hyperalgesia, paraesthesia or analgesia, burning or altered sensation. In motor nerves they cause palsies, muscle fasciculation and weakness. Important examples are shown in Box 38.8. Neuralgias are more common in the head and neck than in other parts of the body and may affect cranial or spinal nerves.

Cranial neuralgias review PMID: 23809305

Intracranial tumours as cause PMID: 23036798

Box 38.7   Causes of facial and oral pain from extraoral disease (see Chs 22 and 23)

- Mealtime syndrome
- Acute and chronic parotitis
  - Mumps
- Salivary obstruction
  - Calculi
  - Strictures
- Painful conditions of intraparotid lymph nodes
- Any inflammation or inflammatory disease of the parenchyma
- Malignant neoplasms with perineural spread
  - Adenoid cystic carcinoma

Trigeminal neuralgia

→ Summary chart 38.1 p. 486

Trigeminal neuralgia produces a very characteristic pain. Typical features are summarised in Box 38.9.

Patients older than 50 years are affected. Either the second or third division of the trigeminal nerve is usually first affected, but pain usually extends to involve both. The ophthalmic division is rarely involved. The pain is always unilateral. Importantly, there is no disturbance of sensation in the distribution of the pain. The cause is unknown, but currently compression of the trigeminal nerve by an adjacent artery where it enters the pons is the favoured theory.

The pain is excruciatingly severe, paroxysmal, sharp and stabbing in character, but lasts only seconds or 1–2 minutes. It may be described as 'like lightning'. Then there is complete, or almost complete, absence of pain between attacks.

Pain may be triggered by stimuli to an area (trigger zone) within the distribution of the trigeminal nerve. Common triggers are touching, draughts of cold air, shaving, tooth brushing or mastication. Between attacks, touching the trigger zone has no effect for a few minutes, the so-called *refractory period*. Only occasionally are attacks recurrent at short intervals. During an attack, the patient's face is often distorted with anguish, whereas between attacks the patient may appear apprehensive at the thought of recurrence. The severity of the pain may also make the patient depressed.

Typically, the disease undergoes spontaneous remissions, with freedom from pain for weeks or months, making it difficult to decide whether treatment has been effective.

Box 38.8   Neuralgias and neuropathies

Sensory

- Trigeminal neuralgia
- Multiple sclerosis
- Pain of Herpes zoster
- Postherpetic neuralgia
- Migrainous neuralgia
- Intracranial tumours
- Burning mouth syndrome
- Psychogenic pain (atypical facial pain)

Motor

- Bell's palsy
- Stroke
- Epilepsy
- Intracranial tumours

Box 38.9   Typical features of trigeminal neuralgia

- Affects the elderly
- Pain confined to the distribution of one or more divisions of the trigeminal nerve
- Pain is paroxysmal and very severe
- Trigger zones in the area
- No pain between attacks
- Absence of objective sensory loss
- Absence of detectable organic cause

Diagnosis

In typical cases, the diagnosis should be readily made from the features described. Dental disease can mimic trigeminal neuralgia, particularly early irreversible pulpitis. Pulpitis can usually be identified as toothache by most patients, but dental causes must be excluded before referral to the patient's medical practitioner.

In early disease the pain may be less severe and then more readily mistaken for pain of dental origin.

Less typical features of trigeminal neuralgia, which make diagnosis difficult, are more continuous, long-lasting, burning or aching pain or absence of trigger zones. This is called *atypical trigeminal neuralgia* and can be associated with migraine type symptoms and retro-orbital pain.

The most important differential diagnosis is multiple sclerosis (discussed later), and similar symptoms may arise from intracranial tumours compressing the nerve, usually at the cerebello-pontine angle. Any suggestion of atypical features or impairment of sensation or other nerves requires a cranial magnetic resonance imaging (MRI) scan to exclude these possibilities.

Treatment

The most effective drugs are anticonvulsants, particularly carbamazepine. Carbamazepine seems very specific to trigeminal neuralgia. It has no effect on other types of pain and its effect helps confirm the diagnosis. Carbamazepine must be given continuously and long term (essentially prophylactically) to reduce the frequency and severity of attacks, not intermittently as an analgesic. Adverse effects require starting on a low dose and increasing to the full dose, so there may not be any immediate effect. As many as 80% of patients are relieved of pain partly or completely by carbamazepine, but minor side effects are common. Drowsiness, dryness of the mouth, giddiness, diarrhoea and nausea are all, to some extent, dose-related.

A few patients are unresponsive to carbamazepine or cannot tolerate the side effects. Alternatives include phenytoin, gabapentin and lamotrigine. Surgical treatments can be highly effective in three-quarters of patients, but neurosurgical decompression of the trigeminal ganglion is a high-risk procedure with significant complications and a mortality rate of as high as 1%. Other less invasive surgical procedures using radiofrequency ablation or cryotherapy to the nerve may remove the pain but at the cost of anaesthesia in the distribution of the nerve. A newer treatment with minimal morbidity is gamma knife ablation, in which the nerve is destroyed using a fine focused beam of radiation, but with similar effects on sensation.

Review neuropathic pain PMID: 20650402

Trigeminal neuralgia review PMID: 25767102

Early features mimic toothache PMID: 25000161

Dental overtreatment in neuralgia PMID: 25418511

Web URL 38.1 NICE guideline management: http://cks.nice.org.uk/trigeminal-neuralgia

US guideline PMID: 18716236

Trigeminal neuralgia in multiple sclerosis

Between 3% and 4% of patients with apparently typical trigeminal neuralgia have multiple sclerosis as the cause. It is usually a late, rather than a presenting, symptom. The diagnosis usually depends on the presence of multiple deficits, particularly defects of vision, weakness of the limbs and sensory losses. Disturbed sensation in the trigeminal area is likely only seen in patients with advanced disease and muscle weakness.

Demyelination in the spinal trigeminal nucleus is thought to be a likely cause, but patients with multiple sclerosis can also have vascular compression of the nerve as is found in typical disease. Multiple sclerosis is an important differential diagnosis and should be suspected when a patient is younger than normal, has bilateral pain or atypical pain, constant pain and sensory loss. Extension beyond the trigeminal area is particularly suggestive; however, the symptoms may be completely typical and the underlying disease only come to light when other nerves are affected.

Carbamazepine or gabapentin is sometimes effective; otherwise, surgical treatment as for trigeminal neuralgia may be required.

Oral effects multiple sclerosis PMID: 23767394 and 19716502

Pain in multiple sclerosis general review PMID: 22909889

Cranial neuralgias in multiple sclerosis PMID: 22130044

Trigeminal neuropathy

Trigeminal neuropathy causes pain, burning, paraesthesia, anaesthesia or hyperaesthesia of part or all of the skin and mucosal sensory distribution of the trigeminal nerve. The pain is typically burning or stabbing in character, or there may be persistent unilateral pain with sensory loss. In the most severe type, there is continuous pain associated with complete anaesthesia. This can follow nerve ablation as a treatment for trigeminal neuralgia.

Other causes are trauma, intracranial neoplasms and metabolic or inflammatory disorders. Detailed examination is needed, particularly to exclude a neoplastic cause. Unlike trigeminal neuralgia, sensation is affected, there are no trigger zones and pain is usually continuous.

Long-term analgesic nerve blocks, gabapentin or a tricyclic antidepressant may provide some relief.

Benign trigeminal neuropathy consists of transient sensory loss in one or more divisions of the trigeminal nerve. It is sometimes associated with a connective tissue disorder.

Review trigeminal neuropathy PMID: 21628435

General review PMID: 26467754

In Sjögren's syndrome PMID: 15342972

Glossopharyngeal neuralgia

This rare condition causes pain of the same character as trigeminal neuralgia but felt in the distribution of the glossopharyngeal nerve, the base of the tongue, fauces and ear on one side only. The pain, which is sharp, lancinating and transient, is typically triggered by swallowing, chewing or coughing. It may be so severe that patients may be terrified to swallow and try to keep the tongue as completely immobile as possible, to the extent of causing weight loss.

Like trigeminal neuralgia, sometimes a cause of pressure on the nerve such as an intracranial tumour is found. Otherwise, glossopharyngeal neuralgia sometimes responds to carbamazepine but less reliably than trigeminal neuralgia.

Cranial neuralgias review PMID: 23809305

Postherpetic neuralgia

→ Summary chart 38.1 p. 486

As many as 14% of patients who have had trigeminal herpes zoster develop persistent neuralgia and pain that persists more than 1 month after healing. Most cases resolve slowly and only 3% have pain after 1 year. Neuralgia is particularly likely in the elderly, in females and when the infection was severe. Aggressive antiviral treatment of the acute infection reduces the risk of developing postherpetic complications, including neuralgia.

The pain is more variable in character and severity than trigeminal neuralgia. It is typically persistent rather than paroxysmal, but may be burning, itchy or hypersensitivity to touch or temperature change. Pain is limited to the dermatome affected by the zoster attack. The skin in the affected area may have reduced sensitivity to touch. The diagnosis is straightforward if there is a history of facial zoster or if scars from the rash are present.

Unfortunately, postherpetic neuralgia is remarkably resistant to treatment. Nerve or root section are ineffective, and the response to drugs of any type, including carbamazepine, is poor. When pain is severe, large doses of analgesics may give relief. Alternative drugs include amitriptyline and gabapentin. Application of transcutaneous electrical stimulation to the affected area by the patient is sometimes effective. The instrument is applied hourly for 5–10 minutes every day, and persistent bombardment of the sensory pathways by the stimulator may prevent perception of pain centrally.

Longstanding postherpetic neuralgia carries a significant risk of depression.

Post-herpetic neuralgia review PMID: 25317872

Risk factors for post herpetic neuralgia PMCID: PMC4685754

Bell's palsy

As discussed later, facial paralysis is the predominant and most troublesome feature. In approximately 50% of patients, pain, usually in or near the ear but sometimes spreading down the jaw, either precedes or develops at the same time as the facial palsy. Rarely, a patient with early Bell's palsy seeks a dental opinion for the pain felt in the jaw, since this may precede paralysis by several days.

Burning mouth 'syndrome'

Burning mouth is a distressing and troublesome condition that has many features in common with atypical facial pain. However, recent evidence suggests the condition a neuropathic pain because trigeminal nerve function can be demonstrated to be altered. Whether this is cause or effect remains unclear, and no cause for neuropathy has been identified.

There are confusing classifications and terminology. Some use the term *secondary burning mouth* when a physical cause is present. Others exclude organic disease by definition. Alternative names include *burning mouth disorder*, *glossodynia* and *stomatodynia*. Here, burning mouth syndrome is used to describe the condition when no cause can be found; an equivalent term is *primary burning mouth disorder*.

Although the cause is unknown, the anterior tongue is particularly sensitive, supplied by sensory nerves with a low activation threshold and large cortical representation. The sensitivity of the nerve is controlled by complex pathways with multiple inputs.

> **Box 38.10   Features suggestive of 'burning mouth syndrome'**
>
> - Middle-aged or older women are mainly affected
> - No visible abnormality or evidence of organic disease
> - No haematological abnormality
> - No candidal or bacterial infection
> - Pain typically described as 'burning'
> - Persistent and unremitting soreness without aggravating or relieving factors, often of months or years duration; no response to analgesics
> - Bizarre patterns of pain radiation inconsistent with neurological or vascular anatomy
> - Sometimes, bitter or metallic taste associated
> - Associated depression, anxiety or stressful life situation
> - Obsession with symptoms may rule the patient's life
> - Constant search for reassurance and treatment by different practitioners
> - Occasionally, dramatic improvement with antidepressive treatment

Most patients, more than 80%, are female and older than 50 years. Symptoms may affect the whole mouth, or only the tongue may be sore. The floor of mouth is characteristically not involved. The pain is typically described as burning, sometimes as tingling or 'raw', and the sensation is persistent, unremitting and usually of long duration. It is bilateral and has no aggravating or relieving factors. Classically, it is accompanied by a metallic, bitter or unpleasant taste and often a sensation of dryness despite normal salivary flow. Spicy foods and flavoured toothpastes often aggravate the symptoms.

There is a close association with anxiety, depression and other diseases with a psychogenic component (Box 38.10), but whether these are causative or secondary to the pain is unresolved.

Diagnosis, even when the history is typical, requires exclusion of possible causes. The history, examination and investigations must exclude the potential causes listed in Box 38.11, and the mouth should appear normal. Candidal infection at low intensity can cause symptoms in the absence of visible lesions and should be excluded by smears or salivary candidal counts. Several drugs listed cause similar symptoms, but rarely. Lisinopril and captopril appear to be the most frequent. Biopsy plays no role, unless mucosal disease is suspected.

Treatment is difficult. Reassurance and explanation to provide a realistic patient expectation is essential. Although many medications have been tried, antidepressants appear to help most patients, possibly through central effects other than their antidepressant mechanisms. Cognitive behaviour therapy, anxiolytics, topical capsaicin, hormone replacement therapy and topical analgesics can be used, but with little evidence base. Improving understanding of neuroimmunological causes of central pain may soon support treatment with drugs that modulate glial activation and central pain mediators, such as pentoxifylline and fluorocitrate. Follow up for monitoring and support is required.

Epidemiology PMCID: PMC4532369

Review PMID: 23429751, 12907696, 23809306 and 26525572

Treatment PMID: 17379153 and 26745781

- All visible mucosal disease
- Erythema migrans
- Candidal infection
- Iron deficiency anaemia or subclinical deficiency
- Vitamin B12 and folate deficiency
- Xerostomia
- Menopausal symptoms
- Gastro-oesophageal reflux
- Diabetic neuropathy
- Hypothyroidism
- Dental, dentifrice or food irritants
- Multiple sclerosis
- Drugs
  - Angiotensin converting enzyme inhibitors
  - Angiotensin receptor blockers
  - Antiretrovirals nevirapine and efavirenz
  - Antiepileptic topiramate

Box 38.12   Features suggestive of psychogenic
(atypical) facial pain

- Women of middle age or older mainly affected
- Absence of organic signs
- Pain often poorly localised
- Description of pain may be bizarre
- Delusional symptoms occasionally associated
- Lack of response to analgesics
- Unchanging pain persisting for many years
- Lack of any triggering factors
- Sometimes good response to antidepressive treatment

Atypical facial pain (persistent idiopathic facial pain)

Like burning mouth, atypical facial pain is considered a disease with psychogenic and neuralgic elements. Features are shown in (Box 38.12). The evidence of neuralgia is less strong than in burning mouth, and the condition remains controversial, some still considering it primarily a psychogenic disorder.

It must not be confused with atypical trigeminal neuralgia.

A common site for atypical pain is the maxillary region or in relation to the upper teeth, but localisation may not be precise or in a recognisable anatomical pattern. Neurologically impossible distributions, bilateral or crossing dermatomes and moving pains are particularly suggestive. The description of the pain may be vague, bizarre ('drawing', 'gripping' or 'crushing') or exaggerated ('unbearable') or burning, but without obvious effect on the patient's health. A unilateral deep dull ache is common. It is often described as having been continuous, even unremitting, present daily and unchanging for several years.

Pain is usually not provoked by any recognisable stimulus such as hot or cold foods or by mastication. Despite the fact that the pain may be said to be continuous and unbearable, the patient's sleeping or even eating are usually unaffected.

Analgesics are often said to be completely ineffective, but some patients have not even tried them despite the stated severity of the pain. Objective signs of disease are absent. Although teeth have often been extracted and diseased teeth may be present, none of these can be related to the pain. As a consequence, treatment of diseased teeth does not relieve the symptoms.

A history of repeated consultations for the pain, none satisfactory, is typical. This fact may well not be proffered without specific questioning.

Other signs of emotional disturbance are highly variable. Some patients are more or less obviously depressed; some of them mention, in passing, difficulties they have had in their work or relationships. Others may complain how miserable the pain makes them. Others may complain of bizarre (delusional) symptoms such as 'slime' in the mouth or 'powder' coming out of the jaw. It is not uncommon for atypical facial pain to be associated with other diseases linked to anxiety and depression such as taste disturbance, burning mouth, irritable bowel syndrome, back pain or chronic fatigue. Often an unlikely trigger will be identified by a patient, such as a difficult extraction or other medical intervention, or sometimes a patient will be convinced they are suffering a specific medical condition.

Investigation requires a detailed and exhaustive examination of the teeth and mouth. Any potential sources of pain must be dealt with, but there should not be too much expectation of benefit. There must be no objective signs of nerve dysfunction on a clinical examination, such as loss of sensation or paraesthesia. Radiographs are likely to be needed. If many have been taken at multiple previous consultations, obtaining them is important to avoid unnecessary additional X-ray exposure. Computed tomography or MR imaging, depending on the characteristics of the pain, is usually required.

Treatment needs to be tailored to any underlying mental illness or psychological overlay, usually depression or anxiety. Antidepressants are usually moderately effective, possibly through anti-neuralgic actions, but treatment is difficult. The pain may lessen only over years. One recognised anxiety associated with both burning mouth and atypical facial pain is fear of cancer, and this may respond to reassurance.

Chronic neuropathic pain PMID: 26685473 and 24645661

Management PMID: 20426709 and 23764815

Atypical odontalgia

This is a less common variant of atypical facial pain, and the general features described earlier apply. Pain is often precisely localised in one tooth or in a row of teeth, which are said either to ache or to be exquisitely sensitive to heat, cold or pressure. If dental disease is found, treatment has no effect, or if, as a last resort, the tooth is root filled or removed, the pain moves to an adjacent tooth. Early diagnosis is essential to avoid overtreatment and serious dental morbidity as patients can be very insistent on intervention. As with atypical facial pain, there are neuralgic elements to this pain; it is not purely psychosomatic.

Outcome PMID: 23630687

PARAESTHESIA AND ANAESTHESIA OF THE LOWER LIP

Paraesthesia or anaesthesia of the lower lip is usually caused by pressure on, or damage to, the inferior alveolar nerve by inflammation, osteomyelitis or, rarely, neurological disease. The main causes of anaesthesia or paraesthesia of the lip are summarised in Box 38.13. All of the common causes affect the nerve within the mandibular canal.

Lip signs accompanied by involvement of the tongue or skin of the side of the head indicate a more proximal lesion affecting the posterior division of the mandibular nerve. Further proximal lesions involve motor supply to the muscles of mastication.

Prolonged anaesthesia or paraesthesia of the lip can occasionally follow inferior dental blocks and surgical damage on removal of third molars, as discussed in the previous section.

Paraesthesia of the lip can be a complication of fractures of the mandible where the nerve has become stretched, particularly over the sharp edge of the canal. The effect is temporary, but complete recovery may take some months.

The nerve may be compressed by a neoplasm or a malignant tumour may infiltrate and destroy the nerve itself. Malignant neoplasms are more likely to be metastatic than primary, and recovery is unlikely regardless of treatment.

The mental foramen can become exposed by excessive resorption of mandibular bone in an edentulous patient. A denture can then press upon the nerve as it leaves the foramen. Although these changes are common in the very elderly, they rarely cause paraesthesia of the lip, usually causing pain on pressure and then only in those most severely affected. Relieving the denture or implant placement are the best solutions. Nerve repositioning carries a risk of permanent nerve damage.

Postherpetic neuralgia (discussed previously) may occasionally cause persistent paraesthesia in the nerve distribution affected, but very rarely in the lower lip alone.

Tetany is the result of hypocalcaemic states and causes heightened neuromuscular excitability, together with minor disorders of sensation such as paraesthesia of the lips. A significant cause of tetany is overbreathing, usually due to anxiety (hyperventilation syndrome). The paraesthesia is bilateral and also affects extremities, if marked together with carpopedal spasm.

FACIAL PALSY

Important causes of facial palsy are summarised in Box 38.14. As the muscles of the face are supplied by the facial nerve, facial palsy will be caused by damage to either its upper or lower motor neurons.

Review sensation and movement PMID: 23909236

Upper and lower motor neuron lesions

The facial nerve *lower* motor neurons pass from its motor nucleus in the pons to the facial muscles. In lower motor neuron lesions, such as Bell's palsy, there is impairment of contraction of *all* facial muscles. The cause is usually extracranial.

The facial nerve *upper* motor neurons pass from the primary motor cortex in the frontal lobe to the pons, but the muscles of the upper part of the face receive stimuli from both sides of the brain, whereas the muscles of the lower face are only activated by the contralateral cortex. Thus, the upper face is controlled by both sides of the brain, and when there is upper motor neuron damage, for instance from a stroke, the lower face is more affected. Emotional movements of the face, the blink reflex and ability to wrinkle the forehead may remain normal.

Bell's palsy

Bell's palsy is a common cause of facial paralysis. Those between the ages of 20 and 50 years are at highest risk, but all ages can be affected, including children. Between 1 in 60 and 1 in 70 individuals will have an attack of Bell's palsy in their lifetime, and diabetics and pregnant women are at higher risk. Onset may follow an apparently unrelated viral illness.

By definition, Bell's palsy is idiopathic, but the cause is suspected to be inflammation and swelling around the ganglion caused by viral infection, particularly herpes simplex or zoster. Infection and reactivation mechanisms of viral infection are discussed in Chapter 15.

Onset is rapid and frightening for the patient. Pain in the jaw sometimes precedes the paralysis, or there may be numbness in the side of the tongue, but in most patients facial paralysis is the presenting sign.

Function of the facial nerve is tested by asking the patient to perform facial movements. When asked to close the eyes, the lids on the affected side cannot be brought together, but the eyeball rolls up normally since the oculomotor nerves are unaffected. When the patient is asked to smile, the corner of the mouth on the affected side is not pulled upward and the normal lines of expression are absent (Fig. 38.1). The wrinkling round the eyes that accompanies smiling is also not seen on the affected side, and the eye remains staring, indicating a lower motor neurone disorder.

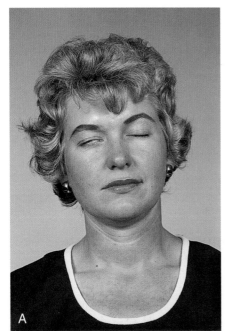

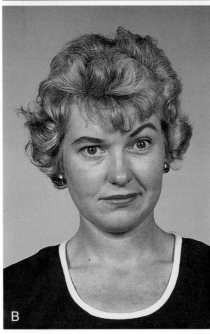

Fig. 38.1 Bell's palsy. (A) When trying to shut the eyes, that on the affected (*right*) side fails to close completely but the eyeball rolls up normally. (B) When trying to smile, the mouth fails to move on the affected side, which remains expressionless, having lost all natural skin folds. The difference is made more striking by covering each side of the picture in turn. This patient, incidentally, complained primarily of facial pain, though was increasingly aware of the facial disability. The severely disfiguring effect of this disorder and the need for early treatment is obvious. In this case, response was complete.

Speech and taste are affected, the latter a result of loss of chorda tympani fibre function in the facial nerve. At rest, saliva may drool from the mouth.

The majority of patients recover fully or partially without treatment, but this can take several months. At least 10% of patients with Bell's palsy are unhappy about the final outcome because of permanent disfigurement or other complications. A guide to the need for treatment is the severity of the paralysis when first seen. Full recovery is usual in patients with an incomplete palsy seen within a week of onset, but more than half of those with a complete lesion fail to recover completely. Prednisolone by mouth may be given for 5–10 days and then tapered off over the following 4 days, and may be effective if given within 24 hours of the onset. The addition of aciclovir, assuming a herpesvirus aetiology, is controversial and of unproven effectiveness. If the eye cannot be closed, it must be protected.

If treatment fails or is not given, persistent facial weakness is disfiguring. The majority of patients with persistent denervation develop muscle atrophy and contracture of the affected side of the face. Watering of the eye (epiphora) due to impaired drainage of tears, or occasionally to excessive and erratic lacrimal secretion, may remain particularly troublesome. An uncommon complication is unilateral lacrimation (crocodile tears) when eating.

It is important to avoid exercises in an attempt to speed recovery. Physiotherapy must be delayed until the acute phase has subsided, to avoid synkinesis, or unwanted facial movement. This complication comprises involuntary facial contractions in association with movement of another part of the face. There may, for example, be twitching of the mouth when the patient blinks.

Treatment PMID: 24685475

Use of antivirals PMID: 22217913

US guideline PMID: 24189771

Outcome PMID: 12482166

Dental aspects

Rarely, as mentioned earlier, pain felt in the jaw may precede paralysis. Paralysis reduces oral clearance of food, and debris can accumulate in the vestibule on the affected side. If treatment fails, sagging of the affected side of the face may be limited by an intraoral prosthesis. Although this disease is uncommon in dental practice, its recognition is important as referral for early treatment may prevent permanent disability and disfigurement.

Melkersson–Rosenthal syndrome

→ Summary chart 34.1 p. 459

Melkersson–Rosenthal syndrome is a rare syndrome of unilateral recurrent facial paralysis, lip or facial swelling, and fissured tongue. Not all these features are present in all patients. Onset is usually in adolescence or young adulthood.

The facial swelling is identical to orofacial granulomatosis (Ch. 34) initially recurrent, soft, painless facial swelling that becomes persistent due to progressive fibrosis. The buccal mucosa may develop a cobblestone pattern and, histologically, granulomas are found. Variants of this disorder include oedema of the eyelids, bilateral facial or rarely multiple cranial nerve palsies, and oedema of the lip. There is a rare familial type. There is probably an immunological or autoinflammatory basis for this disease, and there is sometimes a response to intralesional corticosteroids. Paralysis may become permanent. Treatment is as for orofacial granulomatosis.

Review PMID: 1437063

Case series PMID: 24963969

Oral lesions PMID: 6959055

Other causes of facial palsy

Cerebrovascular accidents (thrombosis or haemorrhage) are a common complication of hypertension in the elderly. Unilateral paralysis (hemiplegia) and often loss of speech (aphasia) are frequent in survivors of the acute episode. Unilateral facial palsy is common but differs from Bell's palsy in that the lower part of the face is mainly affected and spontaneous emotional facial reactions may be retained, as these are upper motor neuron lesions.

Facial palsy is an uncommon but characteristic manifestation of a *malignant parotid tumour* invading the nerve. The many branches of the facial nerve within the parotid gland make it particularly vulnerable to surgical injury, and sometimes the nerve must be sacrificed during a cancer resection. Nerve grafting is moderately successful in avoiding the consequences.

Ramsay Hunt syndrome is severe facial palsy caused by herpes zoster (Ch. 15). It may be differentiated from Bell's palsy by involvement of the ear.

Lyme disease (Ch. 31) causes arthritis, cervical lymphadenopathy and, less commonly, facial nerve paralysis.

Heerfordt's syndrome (Ch. 30) is the rare combination of facial palsy, uveitis and parotid swelling caused by sarcoidosis of cranial nerves and salivary glands.

HEADACHE

Headache diagnosis and management is outside the remit of dentistry, but the lack of a clear definition of headache, as opposed to pains and aches in the face and neck, makes some understanding important. Most patients will differentiate headache from facial and neck pain without difficulty, but there are some conditions that patients find difficult to categorise. Temporal arteritis and migrainous neuralgia are examples.

Primary headaches are conditions such as common tension headaches or migraine without underlying disease. Secondary headaches are caused by a separate disease process, such as an intracranial tumour or haemorrhage.

A number of symptoms identify secondary headaches that are likely to reflect significant underlying disease and merit immediate referral. These are shown in Box 38.15. However, it is primary headaches that may be of dental significance.

Web URL 38.2 Classification of headache: http://www.ichd-3.org

Headache presenting as toothache: PMID 17055919

Dentists often delay diagnosis PMID: 12876249

Migraine

Migraine is a common cause of headache but not of facial pain. It affects as much as 10% of the population, most only occasionally, but a few daily. It is usually readily recognised by the patient. The existence of overlap between migraine, temporomandibular disorders, chronic facial, neck and back pain and their relationship to teeth or occlusion is a controversial area.

Key features are summarised in Box 38.16.

Review for dentistry PMID: 19065884

Mimicking temporomandibular disorder PMID: 18230375

Dental appliance treatment PMID: 8850287 PMCID: PMC2583977

Migrainous neuralgia (cluster headache)

→ Summary chart 38.1 p. 486

Migrainous neuralgia may occasionally be mistaken for trigeminal neuralgia. It is rarely seen in dental practice, but the pain may be mistaken for maxillary toothache. Migrainous neuralgia is thought to be caused by oedema or dilatation of the wall of the internal carotid and probably also the external carotid arteries. It causes severe pain in the region of the eye and maxilla, often associated with facial flushing, nasal congestion and lacrimation. Classically, attacks wake patients at the same time each night for several days in a row, before a period of remission.

Key features are summarised in Box 38.17.

Box 38.16   Typical features of migraine
- Intense throbbing headache, usually unilateral
- Visual disturbances (aura) in classic migraine, not in common migraine
- Photophobia
- Sometimes nausea and vomiting
- Triggers: stress, hunger, certain foods, caffeine, cheese and red wine, menstruation, which vary between patients
- Usually a good response to 5HT agonists such as sumatriptan

---

Box 38.15   Important signs of secondary headache
- Sudden onset
- Onset after age 40
- A new type of headache not experienced before
- Increasing frequency and severity
- Systemic symptoms, fever, weight loss
- Neurological signs or symptoms
- Stiff neck, fever or rash
- Associated disease, HIV, malignancy, infection
- Onset after trauma
- Disorientation, loss of consciousness

Box 38.17   Typical features of migrainous neuralgia
- Commonest in young adult and middle-aged men
- Piercing intense unilateral orbital, retro-orbital or temporal pain
- Conjunctival vessel dilatation and eyelid oedema
- Lacrimation
- Nasal congestion and rhinorrhoea
- Attacks often at the same time each night (or day, 'alarm clock headache')
- Usually attacks recur for several days then remit for many weeks or months
- Triggers: stress, alcohol, organic solvent inhalation
- Early in acute attack, oxygen or sumatriptan highly effective
- Prophylaxis possible with verapamil or ergotamine

An uncommon variant of cluster headache is a chronic variety with attacks confined to the cheek or lower jaw, known as *lower half headache*.

General review PMID: 16139660

Management

MRI may be needed to exclude other causes. Relief of the pain by oxygen inhalations is virtually diagnostic. Otherwise, ipsilateral instillation of 4% intranasal lidocaine can also be effective. Some patients respond to simple analgesics or to ergotamine given an hour before the expected attack by subcutaneous injection or suppository. Alternatively, ergotamine powder can be inhaled from a Spinhaler. Success depends on an accurate idea of the timing of the attacks, and two or three doses a day for the duration of the cluster of attacks may be necessary.

Intracranial tumours

Pain resembling trigeminal neuralgia can rarely be caused by intracranial tumours. Features suggesting an intracranial lesion are associated sensory loss, especially if associated with cranial nerve palsies. Frequently, anatomically related nerves (especially III, IV and VI, causing disordered oculomotor function) are affected.

DISTURBANCES OF TASTE AND SMELL

Dysgeusia is abnormal taste, hypogeusia reduced taste and ageusia, loss of taste. These simple terms cover a range of complaints including one taste being sensed as another and a single abnormal taste being superimposed on normal taste.

Loss of taste is a distressing symptom for many patients, but it is poorly understood and difficult to investigate. The sensation of taste depends heavily on smell, and the two must be considered together. A complaint of loss of taste is frequently explained by loss of smell, which is said to account for 80% of the sensation of taste.

Loss of smell

Anosmia and hyposmia have many causes. Sudden onset of taste loss indicates a likely neurological problem and is a significant sign meriting urgent investigation. A slow onset is usually associated with nasal disease such as hay fever, deviated septum, chronic rhinosinusitis and nasal polyps that either cause mucosal inflammation or prevent air circulating to the olfactory sensors high in the nose. Less common causes include hypothyroidism, Cushing's syndrome, stroke, vitamin B_{12} deficiency and alcohol abuse.

Initial referral to an ear nose and throat specialist in airways disease is a logical first step if nasal disease is suspected. Saline rinses, topical steroid and removal of polyps will often be effective.

Loss of smell carries other risks that are not immediately apparent. Patients should ensure they have smoke alarms fitted in their houses and take care not to suffer food poisoning from eating contaminated food if smell is absent or weak.

Loss of smell in neurological disease PMCID: PMC4399182

Loss of smell with aging PMID: 25968962

Assessing sense of smell PMID: 25761817

Review for dentists PMID: 19732354

Drug effects PMID: 15563912

Loss of taste

The most common cause of taste loss is probably ageing (Box 38.18). This may be compounded by complete dentures that cover taste buds on the palate. Dry mouth prevents transport of soluble taste molecules to the receptors. Ageing causes reduced taste, a more tolerable situation than abnormal taste.

Some drugs that have been associated with taste disturbance are listed in Table 38.2; many more have been reported. Some appear to interfere with detection, whereas others have a strong taste and are secreted into saliva, such as metronidazole. The taste of chlorhexidine is persistent because it binds to the oral mucosa. In most cases, the alterations are reversible, but some drugs can cause permanent taste loss.

Infection may produce a bad taste, particularly when pus is present or in acute ulcerative gingivitis. Candidosis, periodontitis and other infections and mucosal diseases must be excluded as possible causes before referral for further investigation.

Taste is rarely disturbed by sensory nerve lesions because of the large number of nerves that supply taste sensation. However, some neurological conditions such as multiple

---

Box 38.18   Causes of weakened taste sensation

- Ageing (affects smell and taste)
- Loss of smell through nasal disease
- Dry mouth and nose, Sjögren's syndrome
- Parkinson's disease, Alzheimer's disease
- Diabetes mellitus
- Liver disease
- Uraemia, usually from renal disease
- HIV infection
- Halitosis
- Trauma and surgery to nerves, particularly the olfactory nerve
- Radiotherapy and chemotherapy

Table 38.2   Some drugs causing taste disturbance

Drug	Effect
Metronidazole	Bitter metallic taste
Tetracycline	Bitter metallic taste
Tegretol	Taste loss
Biguanide anti-diabetic drugs	Bitter metallic taste
Allopurinol	Bitter metallic taste
Penicillamine	Bitter metallic taste and taste loss
Terbinafine	Taste loss
Many chemotherapy drugs	Abnormal taste and taste loss
Sodium lauryl sulphate (toothpaste detergent)	Loss of subsequent salt and sweet taste
Angiotensin-converting enzyme inhibitors	Weakened taste
Nifedipine	Abnormal taste
Clopidogrel	Taste loss
Beta blockers	Loss of smell

sclerosis can affect taste, and bizarre taste can be experienced in the aura of a migraine or in temporal lobe epilepsy. Bell's palsy causes unilateral taste loss, and this may persist long after the acute attack. Conversely, smell is prone to neurological problems because it depends on a small area of the nasal mucosa and a single cranial nerve.

Taste loss is common following treatment for cancer.

A few patients have a psychogenic complaint of altered taste or smell. The abnormal taste may appear bizarre or limited to a part of the mouth. A complaint of an unremitting bitter taste often accompanies burning mouth syndrome, and a bad taste is often associated with depression. It is rare for an abnormal taste to be a normal taste; they are usually described as metallic or unpleasant.

There is no scientific basis for 'taste maps' suggesting that specific tastes are sensed in different anatomical areas. They cannot be used to investigate taste clinically. Simplistic testing of sweet, sour, salt and bitter in a practice situation is possible using a sugar or a sweetener, citric acid, salt and quinine (in tonic water) and can at least show that normal taste is present. However, testing for taste disturbance is complex and best performed in a specialised centre.

Taste buds review PMID: 26534983

Taste disorders review PMID: 24309062

Drug effects PMID: 15563912

Assessment of taste PMID: 15563906

EPILEPSY

Epilepsy is a common brain disorder causing *recurrent* convulsions or seizures and temporary disturbances of consciousness. Epilepsy affects approximately 1% of the UK population.

Onset is usually in childhood or in the elderly, reflecting different causes. Onset in the elderly is likely to be a sign of a brain lesion such as a cerebral tumour, cerebrovascular disease or senile or Alzheimer's dementia.

The classification is complex, and more than 40 conditions are recognised to cause recurrent convulsions of the epileptic type. Epilepsy is most frequently idiopathic, accounting for three-quarters of cases and assumed to be genetic in origin. This type is common in children and initially causes absence seizures. In the remainder, causes include many known single gene defects, each individually rare, cerebral lesions including strokes, trauma, infections and haemangiomas, and alcohol abuse, Alzheimer's, HIV and other neurodegenerative diseases.

It is easier to understand the seizure types (Box 38.19).

In the classical 'tonic-clonic' (generalised or 'grand mal') seizure, the first event is twitching or jerking of muscles, followed by tonic (constant) contraction of muscles causing neck and limb extension and rigidity. The patient falls to the ground and is at risk of injury. The diaphragm and chest and abdominal muscles are in spasm and the vocal cords contracted, causing a brief cry, after which the patient cannot breathe and may become cyanotic. The contraction then relaxes and develops into a pattern of repeated clonic convulsions (repetitive jerking movements of the whole body). At this stage the bladder and bowels may void. Tongue biting is a risk at this stage, usually of the lateral border, to the extent that it is a useful diagnostic feature for the cause of a seizure. Attempting to prevent this usually fails and risks injury to the helper. After approximately 5 minutes the muscle spasms cease, leaving the patient unconscious for

---

> **Box 38.19   Types of epileptic seizure**
> - Generalised seizures (one-third of all cases)
>   - Tonic-clonic
>   - Absence
>   - Myoclonic
>   - Clonic
>   - Atonic
> - Focal seizures (two-thirds of all cases)
>   - Without impairment of consciousness
>   - With impairment of consciousness
> - Continuous seizure types
>   - Generalised status epilepticus
>   - Focal status epilepticus

15 minutes up to an hour. On waking they will feel exhausted, experience muscle pain, have a headache and be confused. They may sleep for 12 or more hours. Many patients experience a preceding aura (a warning hallucination) that may give warning. In susceptible subjects, fits can be precipitated by fatigue, starvation, acute anxiety, infections, menstruation or rapidly flickering lights.

In the typical 'absence' (petit mal) seizure there is little or no movement apart from blinking or facial spasm, a sudden but brief loss of awareness or activity, without significant loss of postural or muscular control and lasting a few seconds. Consciousness is regained without recollection of the episode. Most patients with petit mal seizures have or develop grand mal epilepsy.

Many patients suffer focal seizures. These usually comprise an aura, loss of speech, clonic movements of one part of the body or automatic apparently purposeful movements such as lip smacking or kicking, and these seizures may not involve loss of consciousness.

Temporal lobe epilepsy is a distinctive cause of focal seizures. Depending on the focus of the seizure in the temporal lobe, the patient may suffer unusual symptoms of *déjà vu*, auditory, olfactory or taste or sensory hallucinations, delusions and emotional disturbances. There may or may not be impaired consciousness. Paranoid or schizophrenic features are often associated.

Status epilepticus is defined as continuous or repeated convulsions lasting more than 30 minutes. 'Convulsive status' is repeated tonic-clonic seizures without recovery of consciousness and is a potentially fatal medical emergency (Ch. 43). All other types of seizure may also be continuous.

General review PMID: 14507951

Management

Dental patients with epilepsy will almost always know their diagnosis and should be under the care of a specialist centre. The main anticonvulsant drugs for major fits are sodium valproate, carbamazepine, lamotrigine or gabapentin. Many drugs are available and have specific indications for different types of seizure. Phenytoin, which causes troublesome drowsiness and many other adverse effects, is largely obsolete. Ethosuximide is the drug of choice for petit mal.

Dental aspects

The risk of a fit in the dental surgery is so disturbing that all precautions should be taken to minimise this hazard. The key is to identify triggers for attacks in the patient

history. Flashing lights are the best-known trigger, but this is relatively rare. Alcohol, tiredness, menstruation and hypoglycaemia are often blamed by individual patients and relatively easily avoided. Unfortunately, stress is a common trigger.

Treatment should be arranged for 'good phases' when attacks are infrequent and within 2–3 hours of medication being taken. Most patients are well-controlled by medication and can be treated as normal. They must be asked to immediately report any symptoms of aura. Those with poor control or frequent fits may benefit from additional medication for treatment and discussion about this with their neurologist is advisable. Some patients carry additional emergency medication, such as midazolam for buccal mucosal application. This can be used only during the premonitory conscious phase.

During treatment, a mouth prop must be kept in place and secured extraorally to prevent displacement into the airway during a fit. This will prevent the patient from biting the tongue, clenching on instruments or the dentist's fingers if an attack develops. As much equipment as possible should be kept out of reach of the patient. Injuries from a major fit include lacerations of the tongue or lips, and injuries due to falling such as maxillofacial damage and fractures to vertebrae or limbs.

Although large doses of intravenous lidocaine given for severe dysrhythmias can occasionally precipitate seizures, there is no evidence of any risk from lidocaine in local anaesthetics.

Severely epileptic patients on high doses of phenytoin or carbamazepine may have a bleeding tendency. Aspirin is contraindicated in those taking valproic acid, as the combination potentiates the anti-platelet effect. Folate deficiency from phenytoin use may exacerbate aphthous stomatitis.

Children and young adults with drug-resistant epilepsy may be treated with an implanted vagal nerve stimulator in the chest wall, connected to the vagus in the neck. This is active continuously but can be further activated on experiencing an aura using a magnet to activate the device. The dentist should be aware how to operate this in case the patient has insufficient warning. Unfortunately, the device lowers pain thresholds and is suspected of causing trigeminal pain. The implanted device does not require antibiotic cover and is not interfered with by ultrasonic scalers, but diathermy must be avoided, as for instance when dealing with gingival overgrowth.

Treatment planning for epileptic patients may require varying degrees of adaptation to their disease and its severity. Good oral hygiene will prevent gingival overgrowth (Ch. 7), and intensive prevention is required to avoid the need for treatment. Tongue biting is common during attacks and

missing teeth, particularly anteriorly, can trap the tongue. Edentulous anterior spaces should be restored, ideally using a fixed replacement; any removable design must have excellent retention and strength, usually with metal-backed teeth. Acrylic components must be considered likely to fracture and should be reinforced with carbon fibre or mesh to prevent fragments separating, and made radiopaque in case radiographic localisation in the lung is required (Fig. 38.2). Large posterior restorations are best dealt with by metal coverage to avoid cusp fracture, and porcelain is avoided because of the risk of fracture. Implants are not contraindicated but require careful planning to avoid overloading.

Management of the fit itself and its most dangerous complication, status epilepticus, are discussed in Chapter 43.

Dental treatment for epilepsy PMID: 12050884 and 18450188

Dentistry for patients with seizures PMID: 17000276

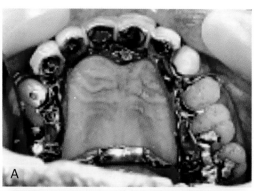
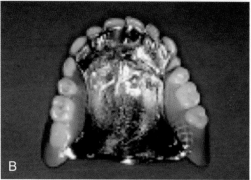

Fig. 38.2 Adapted denture designs for patient with epilepsy using metal reinforcement for all teeth. *(Reproduced from Fiske, J., Boyle, C., Epilepsy and oral care. Dental Update 29, 180–187.)*

Summary chart 38.1   Steps in the diagnosis of important causes of facial pain.

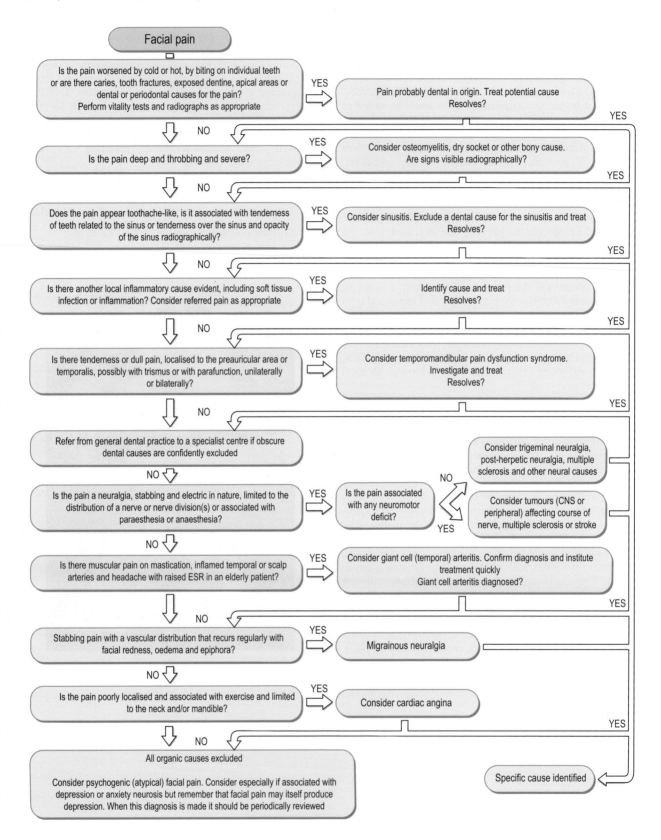

Physical and learning disability

39

The terminology for disability is sometimes confusing and constantly evolving. Healthcare professionals often demand clearcut definitions of degrees of disability that can be used to plan dental services or an individual's treatment. Unfortunately, this approach oversimplifies the problems.

People with disability see their needs in social terms rather than just the sum of their medical problems and, rightly, demand individualised care. The dentist must consider what each patient can do, and is prevented from doing, rather than concentrating on the physical or mental impairments themselves. This way of thinking focuses on the social and environmental aspects of disability and highlights ways in which the individual's environment can be adapted to limit, or even abolish, handicap. Current terminology for disability is shown in Table 39.1.

Nowhere is terminology more difficult than in the area of intellectual impairment. The terms mental retardation, deficiency or handicap are considered stigmatising and no longer acceptable in the UK but may be standard usage elsewhere. In practice, intellectual impairments cause a wide range of disability. Some patients are intelligent but cannot cooperate (e.g. cerebral palsy), others are intelligent but uncooperative (e.g. hyperactivity), yet others are intellectually impaired but may sometimes be easily treated (e.g. mild Down's syndrome). The specific diagnosis and its severity are much more helpful in planning treatment than non-specific labels such as 'moderate' learning difficulty.

The prevalence of inherited disability is estimated at 1.5 to 2 per 1000 live births. Intellectual impairments account for approximately 0.9 per 1000 and major physical impairments account for the remainder. The prevalence is rising as a result of better medical care for adults and improved survival for babies with congenital disorders. There are nearly one and a quarter million individuals in the UK with mild-to-moderate learning difficulty and another quarter of a million with severe difficulty. The management of their dental care is affected by both the disability and parents' motivation and attitudes. However, mental or physical disability does not necessarily mean that dental care has to be compromised, although this may sometimes be inevitable.

Children and adults with disability present a wide variety of challenges for dental management, but as many as 90% of them can probably be managed by good behaviour management, clinical technique and treatment planning. Sedation or general anaesthesia are essential for only a minority. Nevertheless, people with disability are a dentally neglected group, even though valiant attempts have been made to overcome this deficiency in recent years.

Preconceptions that 'the disabled' are difficult to work with are misplaced, and those who manage people with disability find the work highly rewarding.

There is a welcome concern about the dental care of children with disability, but it should be remembered that disability persists for life. The transition from special school to community care can worsen dental disease because dental care must be provided in a less controlled setting, and intensive prevention is more difficult to maintain. The elderly probably suffer more disabilities than children because of the additional problems of declining health.

Challenges in the provision of dental care for people with disability are summarised in Box 39.1. Unless the disability is severe, most of these difficulties can be overcome with patience, training, experience and suitable facilities. It should be remembered that when disability is viewed in its social context, many difficulties become the responsibility of the dentist rather than problems associated with the patient.

European curriculum special care dentistry PMID: 24423174

Web URL 39.1 British Society Disability and Oral Health: http://www.bsdh.org/

Mental illness (Ch. 40) often manifests itself as challenging behaviour, and patients suffer many problems in common with people with disability, particularly

Table 39.1	Current terminology for disability
Term	Definition
Impairment	Any loss or abnormality of physiological function or anatomical structure
Disability or limitation of activity	Restriction or lack of ability to perform a function considered normal
	Legally defined as having a physical or mental impairment that has a 'substantial' and 'long-term' negative effect on ability to do normal daily activities
Learning disability	A significant impairment of intelligence and social functioning acquired before adulthood
Handicap	The disadvantage for the individual, resulting from their disability, which prevents them from performing a normal role in society

Box 39.1 Typical challenges providing dental care for patients with disability

- Reduced cooperation with dental treatment
- Reduced ability to perform oral hygiene and manage diet
- Associated systemic disease
- Difficulties with transport and access to the surgery
- Possible need for sedation or general anaesthesia
- Medications or diets promoting caries
- Dysphagia, drooling, bruxism
- Oral effects of medications
- Competence to give consent
- Financial problems for patients
- Discrimination or prejudice in healthcare

Box 39.2   Common impairments affecting dental
            management

Learning disability

- Low intelligence
- Down's syndrome
- Microcephaly and hydrocephalus
- Metabolic disorders
- Hypoxia at birth
- Some syndromes

Behavioural disorders

- Autism
- Attention deficit hyperactivity disorder

Physical impairment

- Cerebral palsy
- Severe defects of the hands or arms
- Muscular dystrophies
- Spina bifida
- Epilepsy
- Some syndromes
- Communication problems: visual and hearing
  impairment
- Cleft palate (Ch. 3)

Box 39.3   Some factors to ameliorate disability in
            dental practice

Access	Level access, ramps, easy-grip door handles, doors hold open easily, wide corridors and aisles, obstructions clearly marked, if necessary provide off-site or domiciliary visits. Provide for guide dogs
Design and structure of buildings	Colour schemes, contrast floors and walls, well lit, alarms in toilets (visible and audible)
Signs and practice leaflets and paperwork	Large type, succinct, good colour contrast, easy to read, use symbols and words, use sans serif fonts, no justification of right hand margins, simple page layouts Consider Braille and audio versions
Websites	Should meet British Standard Specification for accessible websites
Staff and policies	Provide equality and diversity training for staff, record and survey needs of disabled users and consult local disability groups Each practice should have an equality policy

discrimination and poor access to dental care. Those with personality defects can sometimes be totally uncooperative, and their dental treatment may be severely compromised.

The importance of good prevention cannot be overemphasised. Many of the problems arising from treatment of people with disability would be solved by good preventive regimens.

Disabilities relevant to dentistry are summarised in Box 39.2.

Physical and learning disability are frequently combined, as in Down's syndrome and some cases of cerebral palsy. Learning disability (often associated with physical disability) affects by far the largest group of children with disability needing dental care. All patients with Down's syndrome, many with cerebral palsy and some with epilepsy also have learning disability. These four groups account for approximately 70%–75% of children with disability. Conversely, many patients with cerebral palsy have normal intelligence but may be misjudged because of communication difficulties.

The improved survival of preterm infants and better neonatal care mean that the number of children with disability is increasing.

UK DISCRIMINATION LEGISLATION

The United Nations Convention on Disability rights is enshrined in law in the Equality Act 2010. The entire Act does not apply to Northern Ireland, where the Disability Discrimination Act 2005 performs a similar role. The intention is to ensure all individuals are treated equally, and these Acts apply to all employers and service providers including dentists and cover race, gender, age and religion, as well as disability among the 'protected characteristics'.

The Act defines disability as physical or mental impairment that has a 'substantial' and 'long-term' (more than 1

year) negative effect on ability to perform normal daily activities. The definition is broad and applies equally to conditions such as colour blindness, visual or hearing impairment and fear of the dentist. It applies to all the policies and procedures of a dental provider, as well as to clinical care.

Under the Act, service providers must not use any reason related to patients' disability as an excuse to treat disabled people less favourably than others. Dentists must make 'reasonable adjustments' so that disabled people can access and use their services. This means more than providing wheelchair ramps. All aspects of the clinical practice and business of dentistry must comply. Some examples of the measures expected under the Act are shown in Box 39.3. Which are reasonable in any particular setting depends on guidance from the Disability Rights Commission and will change with time and with legal precedents.

Practices that are 'disability-friendly' will also be more suitable for the elderly and many other groups of non-disabled patients.

Web URL 39.2 UK disability definition: https://www.gov.uk/definition-of-disability-under-equality-act-2010

LEARNING DISABILITY

Learning disability is an all-inclusive term to describe those with intellectual impairment, whether caused by a specific disorder or an unknown cause. Down's syndrome, fragile X syndrome and hypoxia at birth are the more common causes, and the specific features of these conditions are dealt with later in this chapter. Learning difficulties may be unrelated to any physical disorder, or physical defects may be severe, as in some cases of cerebral palsy. A minority of patients with genetic syndromes have craniofacial anomalies associated with intellectual impairment.

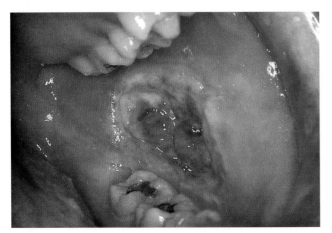

Fig. 39.1 Lip, tongue and cheek biting are frequent and distressing activities that are seen in learning difficulty and a range of neurological disorders. In this instance, biting followed local analgesic in a patient with insufficient understanding of its effects.

Intellectual impairment is classified according to the level of learning difficulty, and children are taught either in mainstream schools or special schools, according to the degree of impairment. Institutional care is avoided if possible. Unfortunately, the learning difficulty classification gives no more than a broad indication of probable problems with dental care because patients vary so widely and needs do not correlate simply with intelligence.

Learning disability has several facets. There is reduced intelligence, making learning new information and complex tasks difficult, together with impaired social functioning and ability to cope independently.

Children with mild learning difficulty can usually be coaxed into accepting regular treatment and (if the parents are supportive) to maintain acceptable standards of oral hygiene. However, oral hygiene is usually suboptimal or poor and depends on motivation and skill of parents or carers. At the other extreme, all that may be possible is first-aid dentistry under general anaesthesia. All intermediate grades exist, but the level of dental health that can be achieved depends greatly upon the level of the dentist's skill and devotion to the task and prevention by carers (Fig. 39.1).

Learning disability is rarely a solitary feature. Most individuals also have physical or sensory impairments, increased incidence of ill health, behavioural problems or mental illness and a high risk of dementia on ageing.

Lip biting in disability PMID: 11819955

Down's syndrome

Down's syndrome is the most common clinically recognisable syndrome with learning disability. It is caused by trisomy of chromosome 21 giving a total complement of 47 chromosomes instead of 46. This is usually caused by failure of the chromosomes to separate during meiosis in the ovum, a defect closely linked to maternal age. The risk rises to 1 in 25 in mothers aged 45 years or older. Because the defect arises in the ovum, both parents are healthy, and the condition is not inherited.

In contrast, approximately 4% of Down's patients have the additional chromosome 21 genetic material translocated to another chromosome. The translocation is transmitted in a familial pattern, but the parents are normal and the risk of an affected child is relatively low.

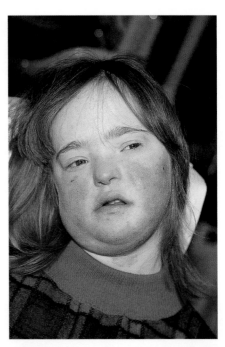

Fig. 39.2 **Down's syndrome.** This patient shows both the characteristic facial appearance and a cyanotic flush caused by associated congenital heart disease.

The rarest form is mosaic Down's syndrome in which the trisomy arises during early development, and the patients are a mosaic of cells with and without trisomy 21. In this type of Down's syndrome, the features are variable, and intelligence may be normal despite the typical appearance.

Ultrasound screening and cytogenetic diagnosis for mothers at highest risk allow two-thirds of affected embryos to be detected prenatally, and in the UK approximately 90% of affected pregnancies are terminated. This has more than halved the incidence to just more than 1 in 1000 live births.

General features

Down's children have a characteristic facial appearance (Fig. 39.2), abnormalities of the skull and frequently of the dentition, abnormal susceptibility to infection (particularly viral) due to multiple immune defects and congenital cardiovascular disease in as many as 50%.

The prominent medial epicanthic skin fold gives the eyes their readily recognisable appearance. There is hypoplasia of the midface, poorly developed paranasal sinuses and a malformed upper respiratory tract. Upper respiratory tract infections are common, and breathing is often partially obstructed. Underdevelopment of the maxillae is usually associated with a protrusive mandible and class III malocclusion, with anterior open bite (Fig. 39.3, Box 39.4). The ears are frequently malformed, and there is excess skin on the neck.

Upper lateral incisors are often absent, and the teeth have short roots. Despite a higher than normal incidence of enamel hypoplasia, caries risk is low. The low caries activity has been ascribed to the form and spacing of the teeth and to the high bicarbonate content and pH of the saliva. Any caries resistance is readily overcome by poor diet.

Plaque accumulation and poor oral hygiene, due to difficulty cleaning and made worse by mouth breathing, together with the systemic predisposition to infection, contribute to the early onset of periodontal disease and early tooth loss (Fig. 39.4). Acute ulcerative gingivitis is also common if oral hygiene is poor and often recurs.

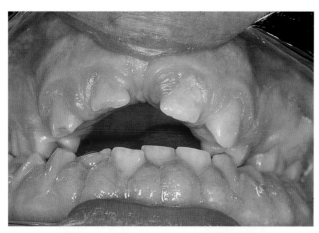

Fig. 39.3 Down's syndrome. Typical open bite and gingival hyperplasia from phenytoin for concomitant epilepsy.

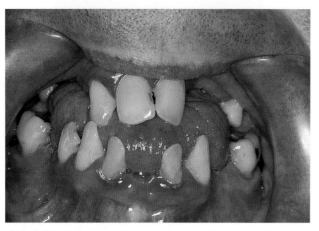

Fig. 39.4 Down's syndrome. Congenitally missing teeth with the hypotonic tongue protruding between them and gingivitis.

Box 39.4 Down's syndrome: features relevant to dentistry

- Class III malocclusion with hypoplastic maxilla
- Protrusive, fissured and apparently enlarged hypotonic tongue
- Lip hypotonia, mouth breathing and drooling
- Everted, thick, dry and crusted lips
- Oligodontia
- Delayed eruption of permanent teeth
- Hypoplastic dental defects and short roots
- Low caries activity
- Gross plaque accumulation
- Rapidly progressive periodontal disease
- Bruxism
- Short stature with short limbs
- Weak muscle tone
- Generalised susceptibility to infection
- Visual or hearing impairment in 50%
- Cardiac anomalies in 40%
- Weakness of atlantoaxial joint
- Susceptibility to leukaemia
- Alzheimer-like dementia in later life

Management

All Down's children have learning difficulties, some severe, but they continue to learn throughout life and may develop many skills if supported by good educational programmes and occupational therapy. Some can maintain an independent life.

Patients with Down's syndrome are often, but not invariably, good natured, cooperative within their ability and affectionate and receptive to dental care. However, this stereotype fails to recognise many who are frightened or more severely affected and completely uncooperative. The success of dental treatment depends mainly on the level of care provided. Those with milder learning disability can be treated normally in the dental chair, whereas the more severely affected may require general anaesthesia.

Control of periodontal disease is usually difficult, and success depends entirely on prevention by good oral hygiene. Teeth may be lost relatively early because of their short roots. Retention of teeth is important because dentures are usually poorly tolerated and retained because of the large protrusive tongue, poor muscle tone and poor comprehension. The apparently large tongue results from muscle hypotonia and forward posture, which also cause problems with mastication and swallowing.

Other features of the syndrome may affect dental treatment. The unstable atlanto-occipital joint is at risk of dislocation with severe consequences if the head is manipulated, particularly during general anaesthesia or sedation. All Down's syndrome patients should have been screened for this anomaly during early childhood. Deafness and visual problems are common. With improved medical care, life expectancy in Down's syndrome has lengthened and patients often live into their sixth decade. Unfortunately, almost half of older Down's patients suffer an Alzheimer-like dementia, which further compromises their independence.

Cardiac defects are present in 40%, and half of these are severe enough to warrant surgical intervention. Atrial and ventricular septal defects, mitral and tricuspid valve defects, Fallot's tetralogy and patent ductus are common. These are repaired in childhood but, in later life, valvular regurgitation and prolapse may develop. Despite many contributory factors, the incidence of infective endocarditis does not appear to be increased.

General and oral review PMID: 17899715

Dental treatment and oral features PMID: 11819976

Fragile X syndrome

Fragile X syndrome is the next most common chromosomal defect with learning disability after Down's syndrome; it affects at least 1 in 4000 males, being an X-linked dominant condition. Female carriers show variable partial features and only mild learning disability.

In this syndrome, the tip of the X chromosome appears as a thin thread of chromatin that is weakly attached and may break off.

Clinical features include moderate to severe learning disability, hyperactivity and behaviour similar to that of autism. Open bite and crossbite are frequent. After growth, males develop a large head with a long face, prominent forehead and chin, and large protruding ears.

Other chromosomal abnormalities

Edwards' syndrome (trisomy 18) affects 0.7 and Patau syndrome (trisomy 13) 0.3 per 1000 pregnancies, but spontaneous

Box 39.5   Features of Edwards' and Patau syndrome

Edwards' syndrome

- Heart defect in 85%
- Fixed flexed fingers
- Renal anomalies
- Oesophageal atresia
- Diaphragmatic hernia or abdominal wall defect
- Cleft lip or palate
- Neural tube defects

Patau syndrome

- Heart defect in 85%
- Failure of forebrain development
- Microphthalmia
- Cleft lip and palate
- Severe growth retardation
- Severe learning disability
- Polydactyly
- Kidney malformation

Box 39.6   Autism: typical features

- 'Aloneness'
- Lack of social interaction
- Lack of eye contact with others
- Communication problems
- Apparent unawareness of others
- Prefer constant daily routines
- Fixation on a single object or toy
- Persistent hand-slapping or other repetitive activity
- Rarely, extreme mathematical or artistic talents
- Learning difficulties in 70%

abortion reduces incidence in live births dramatically to approximately 1 in 8000–9000. Learning disability is severe in those that survive the medical complications, shown in Box 39.5.

BEHAVIOURAL DISORDERS

Behavioural problems and the more severe conduct disorders form a complex group of interlinked conditions with multiple causes. Autistic spectrum disorders have the best evidence of neurodevelopmental abnormality but all probably have both genetic and environmental components. Most autistic patients have learning disability

Autism

Autism is a neurodevelopmental defect causing lack of emotional development, disordered use of language, defective communication and extreme 'aloneness'. The condition is much more common in males, affects 1% of children and adolescents and has onset in the first 3 years of life. At one extreme, there is severe learning disorder and repetitive behaviour so that it may be impossible to communicate with, or manage, an autistic child without general anaesthesia. At the other, a clear understanding of the condition may allow management for effective prevention, though operative treatment will often require a general anaesthetic.

Conventional child and adult behaviour management techniques are ineffective in autism. Autistic patients are highly dependent on a regular routine and dislike noise and anything unexpected. Applied behavioural analysis is commonly used in education for autistic children and uses a series of rewards to change behaviour. The dentist must ensure that such rewards are not cariogenic (if they are food, often they are not) and can also use the established reward system to achieve changes in dental behaviour. Those with autism take everything literally. Idiomatic expressions will not be understood or be taken at face value, and clear simple speech is necessary.

Asperger's syndrome is the mildest form of autism, with normal intelligence and no delay in developing communication. Such individuals often lead normal lives.

Those in the autistic spectrum may possess, incomprehensible skills, often mathematical. Although very few of them match the widely known 'Rain Man' stereotype, as many as 10% of autistic individuals have some special skill or ability, and Asperger's syndrome patients often have a forceful interest in some well-ordered aspect of life, such as timetables.

Typical features of autism are summarised in Box 39.6.

Patient view dental treatment PMCID: PMC4228704 and PMID: 23943360

Planning treatment PMID: 25470557 and 24929596

Related issues in treatment PMID: 20675420

Attention deficit hyperactivity disorder

Attention deficit and hyperactivity are separate conditions but frequently occur together.

Attention deficit is characterised by daydreaming and limited ability to concentrate and perform complex tasks. Hyperactivity is characterised by constant movement, inability to concentrate on one task, being impulsive and, sometimes, making repetitive movements. The number of children diagnosed with these conditions has risen dramatically, and it is now considered that 3%–5% of children are affected, more commonly boys.

Drug treatment with methylphenidate (Ritalin) is safe and effective, but it is a potentially addictive drug. Atomoxetine (Strattera) is also used. Some cases seem to respond to dietary modification, but only if there is a behavioural association with a specific food.

There is no agreed dividing line between this disorder and normal child behaviour, so it has been suggested that some children labelled as affected are no more than mildly disruptive underachieving children. Conversely, severe hyperactivity is profoundly disturbing and may be associated with self-harm. Thus, mild cases can be expected to respond to appropriate behaviour management, whereas others may require sedation or anaesthesia.

Hyperactivity reduces with age, but poor concentration and impulsive behaviour usually persist, and many affected adults suffer from depression.

Review dental management PMID: 24011294 and 17403737

PHYSICAL IMPAIRMENTS

Cerebral palsy

Cerebral palsy is common, with an incidence of 1:1000, and can be one of the most severe disabilities with various types of neuromuscular dysfunction (Box 39.7). The cause is

Box 39.7   Types of cerebral palsy

- Spastic
  - Monoplegic
  - Paraplegic
  - Diplegic
  - Quadriplegic
- Athetotic
- Ataxic
- Hypotonic
- Mixed types

Box 39.8   Cerebral palsy: key dental features

- Usually class II malocclusion and anterior open bite
- Muscle hypotonia
- Frequently severe caries and periodontal disease
- Bruxism and masseteric hypertrophy
- Impaired swallowing reflex but exaggerated gag reflex
- Dental erosion and gastric reflux
- Enamel hypoplasia
- Mouth breathing
- Dental trauma
- Delayed eruption
- Drooling
- Epilepsy in 30%
- Frequently wheelchair users

cerebral damage from infection, trauma, hypoxia and other insults before, just after or at the time of birth. Many patients are born prematurely, and the risk rises with shorter gestation. Occasionally, childhood disease is the cause.

Neuromuscular dysfunction

Spasticity affects half of the patients and causes fixed contraction of affected muscles and general stiffness. This may be so great that it may not even be possible to move an affected limb passively.

Hemiplegia is the most common type: in such cases intelligence is usually normal but other neurological disorders, such as epilepsy, are frequent. Those with quadriplegia, by contrast, frequently have learning disability but are less often epileptic.

Athetosis refers to involuntary jerking movements, often of a wriggling character, sometimes accompanied by grimacing, and is seen in almost half the patients. Muscle spasm during growth distorts the skeleton.

Ataxia is least common and characterised by lack of balance, an unsteady gait and poor control over voluntary movements. In addition to variants of these three main types of disease, different parts of the body may be affected to a greater degree than others. Vision and hearing may be impaired.

Neuromuscular dysfunction can be so severe as to make speech unintelligible (dysarthria) and cause the person to appear intellectually impaired.

Dental aspects

Access to dental care may be difficult, whether the patient is wheelchair dependent or not. Patients using wheelchairs customised to support a distorted skeleton may prefer to be treated in it, using a wheelchair-tilting platform. Otherwise, many of these patients can be treated satisfactorily in the dental chair.

Without aggressive prevention, periodontal disease can be severe. Ability to maintain oral hygiene varies and may be adequate with adapted brushes or, when both arms are affected, completely dependent on a carer.

Communication is usually the main challenge but can often be possible if time is spent learning to comprehend the speech. Many cerebral palsy patients have visual speech aids or computerised devices to help them communicate.

Bruxism and masseteric hypertrophy are frequent, and drooling may result from the open mouth posture, head tilting and defective swallowing. Abnormal tongue posture and swallowing are associated with development of malocclusion. These latter complaints often most trouble these patients.

Restorative treatment can be difficult. The chief difficulty is with athetosis as unpredictable irregular movements may make it impossible to carry out good restorative work. It is also easy for the patient to be injured by sharp dental instruments. The mildest cases may respond well to relaxation with inhalation sedation or pre-operative benzodiazepines, but some will need full sedation or general anaesthesia.

It is always essential to use a mouth prop with conscious athetotic patients, as the jaws may suddenly clench.

Many cerebral palsy patients suffer epilepsy and drug-induced gingival overgrowth. Epilepsy, falls and sudden uncontrolled movements also render patients with cerebral palsy prone to dental injury.

Key features are summarised in Box 39.8.

Review dental management PMID: 19269401

Multiple sclerosis

Multiple sclerosis is a demyelinating disease causing both physical and mental illness. Onset is usually in the third or fourth decades; a late onset is often associated with progressive severe disease. The disease is most common in those of Northern European descent, and the UK has a very high incidence. It is the most common cause of neurodisability in young adults and affects more than 1 in 1000 UK adults, more than 2 or 3 per 1000 in Scotland.

The cause involves genetic and environmental elements, possibly viral infection, triggering a cell-mediated auto-immune reaction against oligodendrocytes. This causes focal demyelination of axons and inflammation in the white matter. Symptoms are varied depending on the part of the brain affected and increase in number and severity with progression.

Common initial features include optic neuritis with transient blindness of one eye, odd sensory symptoms, subacute loss of function of motor supply to an arm or, particularly, palsy of the VIth cranial nerve producing a convergent squint and diplopia. The outcome is highly variable; in the great majority there are short acute attacks of disability but, in approximately 10%, there is progressive deterioration culminating in widespread paralysis and sensory loss. Progression is more likely in males.

Disease progresses in periods of activity that can be modified but not prevented. Treatment of a relapse relies on high-dose corticosteroids. Long-term treatment to prevent relapse depends on a range of disease-modifying drugs including beta interferon, glatiramer acetate or natalizumab

> **Box 39.9 Multiple sclerosis: key features, these vary markedly between patients**
>
> - Onset usually in young adults
> - Neurological deficits in several sites
> - Many experience remittent episodes lasting 24 hours or have slow progression
> - Fatigue
> - Loss of mobility
> - Limb spasticity and tremor
> - Neuropathic pain
> - Cognitive problems
> - Incontinence
> - Poor swallowing and speech
> - Occasionally trigeminal neuralgia-like pain
> - Frequently wheelchair users, sometimes later bed bound

or mitoxantrone in severe disease. Gabapentin, baclofen or clonazepam are used for eye involvement and tizanidine and dantrolene for muscle spasm. Depression and neuropathic pain may require amitriptyline. The range of medications is as wide as the symptoms and signs. Many have significant side effects or significance for dentistry.

Dental aspects

The majority of minor cases can be treated normally, and in the remainder treatment altered to match the abilities of the patient. Treatment should be carried out in a phase of remission. For severely disabled patients, treatment under local anaesthesia is acceptable, but they should not be put in the supine position because of possible respiratory difficulties. Early-day appointments are favoured because of fatigue. As disease progresses, oral hygiene can deteriorate, and early intensive preventive care is necessary to avoid problems in late disease.

Glatiramer acetate and mitoxantrone cause oral ulceration and glatiramer acetate causes parotid enlargement and facial oedema, although very rarely. Many of the drugs used are mildly immunosuppressant. Dry mouth and candidosis are common. The concern that amalgam restorations can cause or worsen the disease is unjustified.

The key role for the dentist is in recognising unusual symptoms of pain or neuropathy that do not fit typical diagnoses, present in younger patients than expected, are recurrent or progressive and respond poorly to conventional drug treatments. Very occasionally, orofacial signs or symptoms are the first presentation, including numbness or paraesthesia or mouth or face, trigeminal neuralgia, facial palsy or unusual spasms of facial muscles.

Key features of multiple sclerosis are summarised in Box 39.9.

Multiple sclerosis oral health PMID: 23767394

Oral effects multiple sclerosis PMID: 19716502

Pain in multiple sclerosis general review PMID: 22909889

Cranial neuralgias in multiple sclerosis PMID: 22130044

Hydrocephalus

Hydrocephalus is caused by failure of drainage of cerebrospinal fluid causing increased intracranial pressure. It may be seen in isolation or associated with spina bifida or a variety of other conditions including intrauterine infection. Compression of the cerebral tissue during development can cause severe learning disability, epilepsy and muscle spasticity.

Treatment is to relieve the intracranial pressure by insertion of a catheter and, in the past, this released the cerebrospinal fluid directly into the right atrium (Spitz–Holzer valve). Younger patients are more likely to have a shunt into the peritoneal cavity. These catheters are prone to infection, more likely with the peritoneal type, but antibiotic prophylaxis for dental treatment is not recommended. Some types are associated with a risk of latex allergy.

Severe hydrocephalus in childhood can cause the skull to be so distended and heavy that the head has to be supported during treatment.

Dental treatment PMID: 20415804

Spina bifida

Spina bifida is failure of fusion of the vertebral arches and may be inherited or environmental in aetiology. Approximately 1:1000 children are affected. The mildest form (spina bifida occulta) is common but no more than a radiographic finding, sometimes with a tuft of hair overlying the defect. In the severe form there is a gross defect in the lower vertebral canal. The meninges and, often, nerve tissue protrude through it as a sac, which may be covered by skin. The consequences are paralysis and deformities of the lower limbs with loss of sensation and reflexes, incontinence and other complications. Meningitis is an obvious hazard, and epilepsy and learning disability are frequently associated because the brain is usually also structurally abnormal. Hydrocephalus is associated in almost all cases.

Since the upper part of the body is normal, the main difficulties in dentistry are management of access, wheelchair use, epilepsy, incontinence and these patients' high risk of latex allergy (Ch. 30).

Dental relevance and treatment PMID: 23270130 and 11460784

The muscular dystrophies

Muscular dystrophies, of which the Duchenne type is the most common (approximately 1 in 5000 male births), are the main crippling diseases of childhood. A range of genetic single gene defects cause different presentations with differing severity. Weakness of the muscles leads to progressively severe disability and is frequently associated with cardiomyopathy and respiratory impairment. Facial muscles are rarely affected (myotonic and facioscapulohumeral types of muscular dystrophy). A quarter of cases have learning disability.

There appear to be no specific dental problems. Most patients with Duchenne type are wheelchair-dependent by the age of 12 years and scoliosis develops, making treatment in a dental chair difficult. General anaesthesia is dangerous in the presence of cardiac disease or respiratory impairment.

Review dental relevance PMID: 19068065

Myasthenia gravis

Myasthenia gravis is a disabling autoimmune disease that causes weakness and rapid fatigue of voluntary muscles. Women between 20 and 30 years are mainly affected. Circulating autoantibodies to the nicotinic acetylcholinergic receptor of the neuromuscular end plates cause the disease by weakening the response to acetylcholine.

Clinically, there is rapidly developing, severe fatigue. Disability is worsened by cold, emotional stress and overexertion. Involvement of the respiratory muscles is potentially lethal and is most likely to affect the elderly. In many patients the initial signs involve twitching or weakness of the muscles around the eye.

Serum antibodies to acetylcholine receptors are detectable in approximately 85% of patients. Anticholinesterases, such as pyridostigmine, are the mainstay but cholinergic effects such as nausea, diarrhoea and bradycardia may be troublesome. Alternatives are corticosteroids in combination with azathioprine or ciclosporin.

Dental aspects

Weakness of the masticatory muscles causes the 'hanging jaw sign' for which patients characteristically support the jaw with a hand. Other effects include difficulties with speech, mastication and swallowing. Paresis or atrophy of the tongue, often with longitudinal grooves, are occasional complications. In the rare syndrome of thymoma, myasthenia gravis and depressed cell-mediated immunity, there is chronic mucocutaneous candidosis. Other rare autoimmune associations are pemphigus vulgaris and Sjögren's syndrome. Use of anticholinesterases can cause excessive salivation. Patients may also suffer gingival overgrowth from ciclosporin and candidosis from immunosuppressants.

Dental treatment should be undertaken shortly after medication and early in the day to avoid fatigue. Stress and anxiety worsen the severity of symptoms. A mouth prop may help patients reduce the muscular effort of mouth opening. The tongue may fall back, or feel as if it will, and patients may feel safer treated upright rather than supine. Denture control is often poor. Poor muscular control may compromise swallowing and clearance of pieces of dental debris, so rubber dam may be helpful. It is recommended that all local analgesics are used with caution, that is, with vasoconstrictor and reduced maximum doses, and penicillins are the preferred antibiotics.

Intravenous sedation is contraindicated because of the respiratory involvement. Many drugs used in anaesthesia, particularly muscle relaxants, can severely aggravate myasthenic manifestations. Severely affected patients or the very anxious are at risk of myasthenic crisis with respiratory failure and are best treated in a specialist centre.

Dental treatment considerations PMID: 9582706 and 22732850

Mental health disorders

Mental, or psychiatric, illness is common, affecting as much as one-third of the population at some time in their life, and as much as one-half of the population in some developed countries. When mild, it is frequently unrecognised. Classification and differentiation of mental illnesses are complex. The main disorders are summarised in Box 40.1.

The causes of mental illness are both genetic and environmental, poorly understood and linked to physical disease and external stresses, upbringing, drugs and social factors, as well as organic brain disease. Mental illness still carries a stigma, and dentists must be non-judgmental in discussing it.

Difficult behaviour is common in mental illness, so patients, like those with disability, suffer discrimination and poor access to dental care. General aspects of psychiatric disorders that can affect dental management are summarised in Box 40.2.

Dementia is covered in Chapter 41.

Oral disease in mental illness PMID: 21881097

Box 40.1   Types of mental illness

- Anxiety disorders
- Attention deficit hyperactivity disorder (see page 491)
- Disturbances of mood
  - Depression and manic-depressive psychosis
  - Chronic fatigue syndrome
- Personality disorders
- Obsessive-compulsive disorder
- Psychoses
  - Bipolar disorder
  - Schizophrenia

Box 40.2   Aspects of mental illness that may affect dental management

- Erratic attendance
- Oral neglect
- Inability to cooperate
- Difficult or aggressive behaviours
- Drug therapy
- Psychosomatic disorders
- Phobia of dental treatment
- Associated alcoholism
- Violence
- Munchausen's syndrome

PAIN WITHOUT MEDICAL CAUSE

Pain is not a simple sensation but has been described as the unpleasant experience felt 'when hurt in body or mind'. The psychological aspects of pain are often overwhelmingly important, and the patient's reaction is affected by such factors as mood, emotional characteristics, personality and cultural background. Some stoical patients tolerate constant pain well, but others complain bitterly and persistently about trivial lesions.

Pain without a cause is a very difficult problem, and dental surgeons cannot deal with unexplained pain without medical help. It is the dentist's role to exclude dental causes for any pain before making a differential diagnosis to allow an appropriate onward referral. This requires an understanding of both organic causes of orofacial pain and psychiatric illness. It is also important to avoid unnecessary dentistry or surgery when a psychiatric cause is likely. This is both damaging and causes delay in definitive diagnosis.

Now that atypical facial pain and burning mouth (Ch. 38) are considered either neuralgias or partially neurological, neuroimmunological and psychosomatic disorders, there are very few occasions when a dentist may need to consider a diagnosis of purely psychogenic pain.

Patients with atypical facial pain or burning mouth need to be seen in a specialist centre, and the role of the dentist in primary care is largely to be understanding, to reassure that dangerous disease and frightening possibilities such as cancer can be confidently excluded and to support patients after treatment is instituted. Such patients need to be referred to a specialist pain clinic, ideally one with dental expertise.

By definition, unexplained pain is a diagnosis of exclusion. It can be difficult to know how intensively to investigate possible causes, but the clinician cannot be complacent. A pain should not be labelled as psychogenic lightly. It is acutely embarrassing to diagnose a poorly localised severe and depressing facial pain as atypical odontalgia and then discover that it has been cured by restoration or extraction of a tooth with pulpitis, root perforation or undetected crack. Similarly, some conditions such as nerve invasion by adenoid cystic carcinoma produce unexplained unusual pain. Any diagnosis of psychogenic pain must be continually reviewed in case a physical or psychological cause becomes evident. Truly psychogenic pain is often associated with other bizarre symptoms, but even when these are present, it is not appropriate for the dentist to make a diagnosis of a purely psychosomatic pain.

All pain is affected by mental state, and all types of pain can become less bearable in depression. The mechanism of central pain, neuropathic pain and depression are inextricably linked, and depression may even be caused by alterations in some of the shared pathways. Because mental illness, even now, carries with it a stigma, patients frequently suppress the depression on presentation. The patient may also fear (often rightly) that doctors or dentists are intolerant of what is regarded as a weakness. Conversely, prolonged

Box 40.3 Anxiety states

- Phobias
  - Dental
  - Social
  - Others
- Panic disorder
- Anxiety with depression
- Generalised anxiety disorder
- Post-traumatic stress disorder

Box 40.4 Manifestations of anxiety

- Muscle tension
- Rapid breathing and heart beat
- Sweating, pallor
- Excessive talking
- Dry mouth
- Aggression or uncooperative

Box 40.5 Management of dental phobia

- Accurate history to identify anxiety level
- Identify triggers, smells, noise, needles, vibration
- Cognitive behavioural therapy
  - Relaxation techniques
  - Systematic desensitisation
  - Cognitive restructuring
- Avoid waiting time before appointment
- Conscious sedation
- Premedication with benzodiazepine
- General anaesthesia

Box 40.6 Typical manifestations of depression

- Feeling 'low' or miserable
- Uncontrollable pessimism
- Inability to sleep or early wakening
- Disturbance, usually loss, of appetite
- Loss of libido
- Tiredness
- Irritability
- Inability to look forward to any pleasurable activity
- Difficulty making decisions
- Resorting to alcohol, smoking or drugs
- Thoughts of suicide or death

severe pain can cause depression. It is usually impossible to decide which came first in a purely dental environment.

Chronic neuropathic pain PMID: 26685473

Idiopathic pain mechanisms PMID: 25483941

ANXIETY DISORDERS

Anxiety is a disproportionate fear of everyday events, an abnormal 'fight or flight' reaction mediated by catecholamines. Anxiety disorders include several distinct conditions summarised in Box 40.3.

Social phobia is the term given to uncontrollable anxiety in normal social situations. Persistent and chronic fear of being watched or judged by others, and fear of being humiliated by behaviour or appearance, are typical features.

The main significance to dentistry is fear of dentistry itself, together with the adverse effects of antidepressant medications.

Fear of dentistry

It is perfectly normal to feel anxiety at the prospect of dental treatment, but the healthy person can overcome these fears because there is desire for dental care.

Mild anxiety can be suppressed by the patient or missed by the dentist, who is used to dealing almost entirely with people exhibiting some degree of fear. Recognition is important as anxiety may manifest in different ways in different patients (Box 40.4). Anxiety is greater in children than adults.

In most cases, reassurance, simple behaviour management, distraction and sometimes a benzodiazepine or inhalational sedation are sufficient to manage anxiety.

Dental phobia is an extreme manifestation of anxiety and may sometimes result from painfully traumatic dental experiences as far back as in childhood. Truly phobic patients will not turn up for, or even request, appointments and suffer the consequences of repeated emergency dentistry. As much as 11% of the population fear dentistry sufficiently to accept pain and suffer detriment to their oral health. The majority are female. Specialist intervention is required using

the principles outlined in Box 40.5. Cognitive behavioural therapy is the most effective intervention, and sedation and general anaesthesia should be methods of last resort.

Characteristics of dental anxiety PMID: 26611310

Management dental anxiety PMID: 22996472 and 21838825

DEPRESSION

Depression is a serious illness, the impact of which on life is frequently underestimated. It is common and may sometimes underlie oral symptoms. Typical manifestations of depression are summarised in Box 40.6. Even severe depression is often undiagnosed.

A short period of depression following unpleasant experiences such as bereavement or financial difficulties is normal, but abnormal if symptoms are prolonged and quality of life is impaired. Unfortunately, depression is widely regarded as 'weakness', particularly in Britain, and suppression by alcohol is common. In other countries, the healthy outward expression of grief is thought to be therapeutic. Causes are complex, partly genetic, environmental and social. Serious, particularly life-threatening illnesses can also be triggering factors. Age of onset is approximately 30 years of age, and most patients are female. As much as 10% of the population have depression.

Dental aspects of depression

Depressed patients may sometimes be 'difficult' or even aggressive and need to be treated particularly tactfully and sympathetically. Dentists need to be alert for depression as it is common and often denied by patients in their medical history. Some patients will increase their carbohydrate

- Burning mouth syndrome
- Atypical facial pain and atypical odontalgia
- Temporomandibular joint pain dysfunction
- Factitious oral injury
- Neglect of oral health
- Adverse effects of medication

- Lack of correspondence with any recognisable disease
- Bizarre configuration with sharp outlines
- Usually in an otherwise healthy mouth
- Clinical features inconsistent with the history
- In areas accessible to the patient

intake in the belief that it boosts serotonin levels, risking caries.

Depression is found with many oral conditions, either as a cause, effect or simple association (Box 40.7).

The main problem with those under treatment is the oral effects of antidepressant drugs. Xerostomia is an almost universal effect of antidepressants and may lead to candidosis and ascending sialadenitis. Other effects appear rare, but include bruxism, dysgeusia, angioedema and, with tricyclic antidepressants, black tongue. The tricyclic antidepressants are now little used as first-line treatment because of adverse effects. Ibuprofen should be avoided with antidepressants, and paracetamol should be avoided with tricyclic antidepressants.

It should also be remembered that stress, anxiety and depression are commonly seen in dentists, although the frequently reported high suicide rate is not borne out by the evidence.

Dental management PMID: 8042134, 8486855

Obsessive-compulsive disorder

Obsessive-compulsive disorder is a manifestation of anxiety in which patients have uncontrollable ritualistic thoughts or behaviour that interfere with normal life. The condition is common, affecting approximately 1% of the population. Obsessive-compulsive states can lead to depression and are sometimes secondary to schizophrenia.

Treatment is with cognitive behavioural therapy or antidepressants, usually selective serotonin reuptake inhibitors.

Obsessions affecting dental management may include compulsive toothbrushing, possibly causing dental abrasion, excessive use of antiseptic mouthwashes, or fear of oral infections, of cancer or of halitosis, and refusal to be reassured.

Factitious ulceration

Factitious or self-inflicted traumatic ulcers in the mouth are very uncommon but important as indicators of self-harm in those with mental illness. Rarely, factitious oral ulceration has been a prelude to suicide.

Patients usually cause ulcers by repeated trauma to the lips or anterior visible parts of the mouth, in sites accessible to their dominant hand. Fingernails or instruments can be used, and repeated picking at the gingival margin or over bone can induce bone loss through chronic inflammation or, eventually, tooth exfoliation. Occasionally, a patient will extract their own teeth or cause mucosal ulceration and inflammation by rinsing with caustic fluids.

The diagnosis of self-inflicted injuries is difficult because the patient conceals the cause, but suspicious features are shown in Box 40.8. Frequently, the diagnosis can be con-firmed only by discreet observation after admission to hospital.

Case series PMID: 7776171 and case: 2887598

ANOREXIA NERVOSA AND BULIMIA NERVOSA

Anorexia nervosa is an eating disorder characterised by a desire to be slim associated with voluntary restriction of food intake and fear of weight gain, even to the point of emaciation and occasionally death. There is a distorted body image that prevents patients recognising their actual weight and shape. Bulimia nervosa is characterised by binge eating and vomiting to restrict food intake and is not necessarily associated with low body mass. Both are diseases of urban populations in developed countries.

Causes of both are complex, but there is a strong genetic predisposition on which psychological and social factors act. There are shared personality traits among anorexia, obsessive-compulsive disorder and autistic spectrum disorder.

Both conditions particularly affect females younger than 20 years but are increasingly recognised in males.

Oral and perioral effects of anorexia and bulimia are parotid swelling (sialadenosis, Fig. 22.23) and dental erosion and sensitivity due to vomiting (Ch. 6). Iron and vitamin deficiency may predispose to angular cheilitis or candidosis. Dentists may be able to identify such signs and make an early referral to medical care. Vacuum-formed splints can be used to protect teeth during vomiting. Low body weight must be taken into account when prescribing.

Oral manifestations eating disorders PMID: 18826377 and 11862200

PSYCHOSES

Schizophrenia

Schizophrenia is the most common form of severe mental illness. It can be chronic and severely disabling and affects 1% of the population, usually with onset between 20 and 30 years of age.

A great range of symptoms and abnormal behaviour is possible, probably reflecting different causes and subtypes. In the chronic phase, mood, thoughts and behaviour become abnormal and disorganised with inability to concentrate. Confusion, unpredictability and inappropriate behaviour and blunted or flattened mood are common. Patients may not follow or be able to construct a logical chain of thought. Intelligence is unimpaired, and insight may even be retained. Schizophrenic individuals do not necessarily behave abnormally all the time.

In the acute phase, there may be hallucinations and delusions with failure to distinguish reality from what is experienced. Patients may fear persecution, hear voices and, occasionally, perform violent acts. Signs of normal emotion are absent, and there is often withdrawal from social contact.

A wide range of drugs may be taken including phenothiazines and butyrophenones.

Dental aspects

Mild schizophrenia may appear merely to be stupidity or result in inappropriate behaviour. Responses to questions may indicate a failure to get through or elicit entirely inappropriate answers. Calm manner and avoidance of sudden stress are important. There is a risk that some patients will become violent, but only a small minority.

Provided that the patient is cooperative, there are no major restrictions on the form of dental treatment that can be provided. Any reaction between epinephrine in local anaesthetics and phenothiazines appears to be no more than theoretical.

Phenothiazines and some other neuroleptics can cause severe xerostomia, particularly in long-term use. Phenothiazines can also cause involuntary facial movements (dyskinesias) or parkinsonism. *Tardive dyskinesia* can develop in approximately 30% of patients treated long-term with phenothiazines. Involuntary movements particularly involve the face and are irreversible. Repeated grimacing and chewing movements may be violent and result in scarring and deformities of the tongue. Newer antipsychotics are almost free from this adverse effect, apart from aripiprazole, which seems prone to cause it.

Dental significance review PMID: 15119719 and 8258570

Dentistry and elderly patients

41

The ageing population of the UK and many countries is a well-recognised phenomenon, caused by increased lifespan and enhanced by falling birth rates. By 2040, it is estimated that 1 in 4 people will be aged older than 65 years (Fig. 41.1) and the overall UK population will have risen from its present 70 million to 90 million. Similar changes affect other countries, and in some the effect is even more marked.

Elderly individuals do not think of themselves as aged or in decline until very late in life and expect the same treatment as younger individuals as they are entitled to under the Equality Act 2010. However, increasing age is associated with a number of social, healthcare and dental challenges (Box 41.1).

These can become significant handicaps when an elderly patient experiences a significant oral disease, such as a carcinoma. Mobility, communication and illness are the key issues in the management of elderly patients. Neurological factors are particularly problematic (Box 41.2).

The edentulous elderly are more likely to suffer significant medical disease than the dentate elderly.

Edentulousness and medical disease PMID: 26371954

DEMENTIA

Mental deterioration is a common consequence of ageing and is something we all have to risk if we live long enough.

Dementia is a chronic progressive failure of mental processes affecting all aspects of mental activity, such as intelligence, memory, emotional state and personality. These different functions tend to be affected to a variable and unpredictable extent. Dementia is caused by Alzheimer's disease in two-thirds of cases, but also by vascular disease, Parkinson's disease or stroke. The incidence rises with age, from approximately 5% of those aged 70 years to half of those aged 85 years. Nevertheless, dementia and Alzheimer's disease are not obligatory elements of ageing. While HIV infection has become a chronic treatable infection and

---

Box 41.1 Challenges for elderly patients (older than 65 years)

- Age discrimination
- Disease: two-thirds have a chronic illness or disability
  - Osteoporosis
  - Depression, 40% of institutionalised individuals
  - Poor vision: cataracts or macular degeneration
  - Poor hearing and communication
  - Incontinence
  - Dementia
- Lack of carers, carers likely to be elderly too
- Reduced mobility
- Lack of social contact, loneliness and isolation
- Lack of financial resources
- Likely to be single or living alone
- One-third are at risk of malnutrition
- One-quarter are edentulous
- Only half are registered with a dentist

Percentage age distribution, United Kingdom, 1971–2085

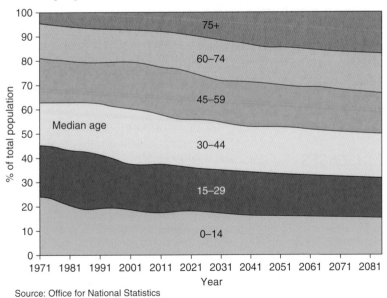

Fig. 41.1 UK population projections for different age groups. *(From Office for National Statistics. 2011. Results, 2010-based national population projections. [Online.] [Accessed 16 December 2016] Available from: http://www.ons.gov.uk/ons/dcp171776_237753.pdf)*

is now found in elderly patients, dementia from HIV infection may increase.

The features of dementia are shown in Box 41.3.

In the early stages the patient may seem bright enough but may immediately forget instructions, for example, about how to look after dentures. Other patients become confused, querulous, or even aggressive, behave in an irresponsible fashion, have delusions of persecution and can be generally 'difficult'. It is important to obtain as high a standard of oral health as possible in the early stages, ideally with a care plan, to prevent problems later. Dental pain can worsen the confusion in dementia. Caries may develop as a result of high-energy food supplements, and oral hygiene gradually worsens. Denture loss is a common problem, and duplicate sets of dentures and denture marking are helpful as adaptation to new dentures is likely to be impossible.

In late dementia, diagnosis of dental pain by conventional means may not be possible and should be suspected if there is failure to eat, restlessness and pulling or poking the face or mouth, drooling, ceasing denture wear, disturbed sleep or aggression.

Consent for treatment will eventually lie with another individual with Power of Attorney under the Mental Capacity Act 2005.

Selected patients with mild or moderate disease may be prescribed anticholinergic drugs to improve cognition, such as donepezil, rivastigmine or galantamine or the NMDA receptor blocker, memantine. The anticholinergics all cause dry mouth and potentially predispose to caries and make denture wearing more difficult.

Orofacial pain diagnosis in dementia PMID: 21359232

Creutzfeldt-Jakob disease in dentistry PMID: 18502958

Dental management PMID: 26556259 and 16158799

OTHER SYSTEMIC DISEASES

Systemic diseases which particularly affect the elderly are shown in Box 41.4.

A variety of drugs used for cardiovascular disease can also cause oral reactions (Ch. 42). Malnutrition is particularly likely to affect the elderly. Poverty, poor mobility (which interferes with both cooking and shopping) and mental deterioration are some of the contributory factors. Poorly functioning dentures and impairment of taste sensation may make matters worse.

However, deficiency states, particularly scurvy and vitamin B group deficiencies, are remarkably rare nowadays, even in

old age. It is important, nevertheless, that denture function should be the best possible in order not to worsen nutritional problems in older patients. Sore tongue or signs of atrophy of the mucosa should be investigated by haematological examination.

Parkinson's disease

This common idiopathic disease caused by loss of basal ganglia neurones is characterised by rigidity, slow movements and tremor with impaired coordination. It affects 1 in 1000 individuals older than 65 years.

Patients have a mask-like fixity of facial expression, with tremor sometimes affecting the lower jaw and often dribbling as a result of impaired neuromuscular function. Parkinson's disease is not usually a cause of intellectual deterioration but is a risk factor for dementia. Important features are summarised in Box 41.5.

Sympathetic management is essential. It is particularly important that the poverty of facial expression is not mistaken for incomprehension, and the defective speech be not thought to be due to impaired mental function.

Box 41.5   Parkinson's disease: key features

General

- Expressionless face
- Soft indistinct speech
- Stooping posture
- Slowness in starting or repeating movements
- Impaired fine movements especially of fingers
- Fatigue

Gait

- Slow to start
- Rapid small steps and tendency to run
- Impaired balance on turning

Tremor

- Usually first in fingers and thumb
- Can affect limbs, jaw and tongue
- Present at rest
- Diminished by activity

Rigidity

- 'Cogwheel' type particularly in the arms
- 'Lead-pipe' type particularly in the legs

Box 41.6   Some causes of limitation of mobility in the elderly

- Ataxia
- Strokes
- Arthritis
- Heart disease
- Late Alzheimer's disease
- Blindness
- Poor balance

Drooling may be particularly troublesome, but conveniently the antimuscarinic drugs sometimes given, such as benzhexol or orphenadrine, can cause dry mouth. Reduction in salivary flow can also be achieved using botulinum toxin in the parotid glands. Involuntary orofacial movements, due to levodopa or bromocriptine, may make use of rotating dental instruments hazardous. Parkinson's disease can cause difficulties with the management of dentures because of the loss of fine control of muscular movement. Oral hygiene is impaired. Postural hypotension is common, and patients must rise slowly from the dental chair.

The effects of Parkinson's disease can be diminished by giving a range of drugs including dopaminic agents such as levodopa, dopamine agonists, monoamine oxidase B inhibitors, anticholinergic drugs and catechol-O-methyl transferase (COMT) inhibitors such as entacapone. The last interacts with epinephrine, theoretically at least, so that epinephrine-free local anaesthetics or minimal doses may be preferable to avoid tachycardia and arrhythmias. L-Dopa causes taste disturbance and colours urine, sweat and saliva red.

However, complete success of treatment is rarely achieved, and virtually all the drugs have significant side effects, particularly in long-term use.

Access and neurological conditions PMID: 18953303

ORAL DISEASE IN THE ELDERLY

Illustrative of the dental problems of the elderly are the findings in a survey of care home managers, almost half of whom considered the oral and dental needs of their inhabitants were poorly met. Common problems are candidosis, difficulty eating, difficulty maintaining oral or denture hygiene and access to dental care.

Factors affecting dental care of the elderly

Many medical factors limit the mobility of elderly patients (Box 41.6), and they may simply be unable to afford the cost of dental care or transportation. Availability of domiciliary visits varies but is limited. Even when access to care is easy, elderly patients tend to become even more infrequent visitors to the dentist than they once were, especially when complete dentures have been provided. Oral hygiene is compromised by arthritis and the neurological disorders discussed previously.

Oral disease in elderly patients is likely to require time and special skills from the dentist. Even among the institutionalised elderly, complete dentures are no longer the norm, and the main dental need of most elderly patients is no longer effective and comfortable dentures. Those teeth that remain are less likely to suffer periodontitis but are prone to caries if sugar intake is not controlled and may be heavily restored, requiring long-term maintenance and repair. In the future, mouths with partial dentures and implants will pose significant challenges as teeth are progressively lost. The loss of adaptability with age requires good forward planning for prosthetics. It is also important to remember that good oral health is important in maintaining self-esteem.

The teeth

The teeth can undergo attrition, abrasion and, frequently, continued destruction by caries. Attrition increases with a reduced dental arch, and tooth wear may be accelerated by erosion. The roots gradually also become hypercalcified by progressive obliteration of the dentinal tubules by peritubular and circumpulpal dentine. The roots may as a consequence become completely calcified, impossible to root treat and brittle, so they are more likely to fracture during extraction. There is increased need for restorations with occlusal coverage to prevent fractures.

Caries is often on the root surface in the elderly. This is partly because caries-prone fissures or contacts have already become carious in earlier life and partly as a result of recession, dry mouth, poor oral hygiene and altered diet (Ch. 4). Dietary control of sugars is equally important at all ages. Fluoride varnish is a useful evidence-based intervention in institutions for the elderly.

Periodontitis is less of a problem. Patients who are prone are likely to have lost the most susceptible teeth before the age of 60 years, and only slow progression is expected. However, this depends on ability to maintain good oral hygiene.

The alveolar bone and dentures

In the edentulous elderly, progressive loss of denture-bearing bone reduces retention and stabilisation of dentures. Later, as excessive amounts of bone become resorbed, pain can be caused by the dentures pressing upon anatomical structures, such as the mylohyoid ridge or genial tubercles.

In general, the older the patient, the less adaptable they are likely to be. Although preservation of teeth for as long as possible may be desirable, it may create greater problems if extractions have to be postponed until very late in life. The wearing of full dentures demands a remarkable feat of adaptation at any age, and older patients face greater difficulties. Also, some older patients may no longer care about appearance, may have few social contacts and may prefer a soft diet. Motivation, which plays so large a part in adaptation to denture wearing, may also therefore be diminished. The importance of denture duplication and marking was noted earlier in the section on dementia.

Problems of edentulousness PMID: 24446979

The temporomandibular joints

Osteoarthritis of the temporomandibular joints is not a significant problem (Ch. 14).

Pain or other symptoms from the temporomandibular joints in the elderly are remarkably uncommon. However, pain on mastication may be due to temporal arteritis and, if so, requires urgent treatment because of the risk of loss of sight (Ch. 14).

Salivary function

Salivary secretion does not appear to be significantly reduced with age alone, but dry mouth is overall more common in the elderly as a result of diseases such as Sjögren's syndrome or the use of drugs with diuretic or antimuscarinic activity (Ch. 22). Elderly patients who have a dry mouth must therefore be investigated accordingly. Dehydration is common in institutionalised patients, particularly in those with urinary incontinence who avoid fluids.

Mucosal diseases in the elderly

Some changes in the oral mucosa are directly related to age. Examples include enlarged Fordyce's granules, lingual varicosities and foliate papillae (Ch. 1). These are often causes of anxiety in the elderly, who need to be reassured.

Mucosal diseases that may affect the elderly are summarised in Box 41.7 and discussed in more detail in previous chapters.

It must be emphasised that recurrent aphthae are uncommon in older persons but, when seen, it is important to look for some underlying cause such as pernicious anaemia or iron deficiency.

The mucosa also heals more slowly with age.

Box 41.7 Mucosal diseases more common in elderly patients

- Lichen planus
- Mucous membrane pemphigoid
- Pemphigus vulgaris
- Herpes zoster
- Glossitis
- Burning mouth syndrome
- Leukoplakia and erythroplakia
- Medication-related osteonecrosis
- Carcinoma

Malignant neoplasms and irradiation

In the institutionalised elderly population, 1 in 50 may have red or white oral lesions. Cancer of the mouth, which both becomes more common as age advances and is insidious in development, is particularly likely to be missed or ignored in its earlier stages, especially in institutions and in those with dementia.

Because of the rising frequency of carcinoma with advancing age, the elderly are more likely than the young to have had radiotherapy. They may therefore suffer from xerostomia or be at risk from osteoradionecrosis. Denture trauma can occasionally precipitate the latter complication, and wearing lower dentures after radiotherapy carries a risk that needs to be assessed patient by patient.

Elderly patients, who are more likely to have suffered metastatic carcinoma from breast, prostate or other carcinomas, may be at risk of medication-related osteonecrosis (Ch. 8).

Cardiovascular disease

Elderly patients are overall at the highest risk from infective endocarditis. A possible contribution to this is periodontal or dental sepsis. In addition, drugs given for cardiovascular disease can be a cause of oral lesions (Chs 32 and 42).

Access and neurological conditions PMID: 18953303

General review PMCID: PMC4334280

Epidemiology oral disease in elderly PMID: 26504122 (UK) and PMCID: PMC3487659 (US)

Complications of systemic drug treatment

42

The 2013 Health Survey in England revealed that 45% of adults were taking prescription drugs and 25% took three or more, the number rising with age. The most frequently used drugs are statins, antihypertensives and non-steroidal anti-inflammatory drugs. In some parts of the UK, one in five women use antidepressants. When non-prescription drugs and complementary medicines are added, and account is taken of the many new and highly potent targeted therapies, there is great potential for adverse reactions and drug interactions.

It has never been appropriate to try to remember more than the most significant interactions with drugs prescribed in dentistry. The British National Formulary and other national prescribing guidance in other countries must be consulted whenever the dentist is unfamiliar with a drug.

The patient's medical history must include a complete drug list, ideally with doses and frequency because these often determine actions taken in response. Patients may misconstrue the word 'drugs' and should be asked whether they are taking 'medicines, tablets, injections, or any sort of medical treatment for *any* purpose' or have received any medications recently, or whether they have been given any sort of hospital card. If unsure, their medical practitioner's practice computer should be able to produce a list of current and past prescriptions quickly and easily.

Unfortunately, of the 2.7 million items prescribed each day at a cost to the taxpayer of some £9 billion each year, much is either not taken or taken incorrectly. When prescribing, always give clear concise advice on how to take the medication, remind patients of the importance of completing antibiotic courses and of not sharing medications with others.

Drugs may complicate dental treatment itself, react with drugs given for dental purposes or have adverse effects in the head and neck. A selection of key interactions are given in Table 42.1, and some specific examples and types of reaction are summarised in Box 42.1 and shown in Figs 42.1 and 42.2.

Review oral adverse effects drugs PMID: 24929593 and 24697823

Interactions with complementary agents PMID: 23813259

Adverse effects novel biological agents PMID: 22420757

Box 42.1 Important types of oral drug reactions

I. **Local reactions to drugs**
- Chemical irritation
- Interference with the oral flora

II. **Systematically mediated reactions**
- Depression of marrow function
- Depression of cell-mediated immunity
- Lichenoid reactions
- Erythema multiforme (Stevens-Johnson syndrome)
- Fixed drug eruptions
- Toxic epidermal necrolysis

III. **Other effects**
- Gingival hyperplasia
- Pigmentation
- Dry mouth

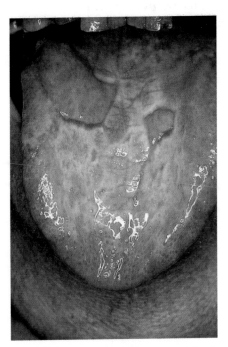

Fig. 42.2 Lichenoid reaction to gold treatment for rheumatoid arthritis. There is extensive ulceration of the dorsal tongue, atrophy and keratosis. Biopsy showed changes very similar to lichen planus.

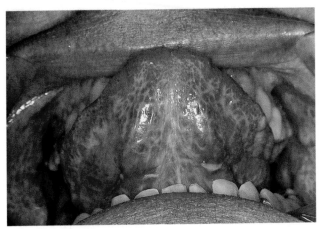

Fig. 42.1 Lichenoid reaction to captopril. In this milder reaction, there are several small ulcers, but the main effect is the production of striae covering the whole ventral surface of the tongue.

Table 42.1 Examples of prescribed drugs having dentally relevant adverse effects

Type of drug / drug	Dentally relevant adverse effects
Allopurinol	Oral lichenoid reactions Taste disturbance
Angiotensin-converting enzyme inhibitors, Captopril	Angio-oedema Burning mouth Oral lichenoid reactions
Antibiotics	Superinfection (usually candidosis), Allergy (mainly penicillin). Tetracyclines are prone to cause candidosis, sometimes within 48 hours. Several classes of antibiotics potentially interfere with contraceptive pill effects, but the effect seems largely theoretical. It is only significant with rifampicin and drugs not used in dentistry. Ampicillin causes rashes during glandular fever Erythromycin and tetracycline potentiate digoxin Erythromycin potentiates benzodiazepines (theoretical risk only for sedation, possible risk with long-term benzodiazepines) Erythromycin potentiates warfarin Tetracyclines stain forming teeth, minocycline causes tooth discolouration, even sometimes in adult teeth Erythromycin, metronidazole and cephalosporins potentiate warfarin Co-trimoxazole, chloramphenicol may cause marrow suppression leading to opportunistic oral infection and ulceration or purpura and bleeding
Anticoagulants	Risk of post-operative haemorrhage
Antihistamines	Dry mouth, drowsiness, potentiate sedatives
Antimalarials	Oral lichenoid reactions (including those available over the counter without prescription) Mucosal pigmentation
Aspirin	Potentiation of any haemorrhagic tendencies and anticoagulants Avoid in children because of risk of Reye's syndrome Causes mucosal burn if applied to mucosa
Bisphosphonates	Necrosis of mandible and maxilla (see Ch. 8)
Calcium channel blockers (e.g. nifedipine, verapamil)	Gingival overgrowth
Captopril	Oral lichenoid reactions Taste disturbance
Carbamazepine	Facial muscle spasms Taste disturbance
Catechol-O-methyltransferase inhibitors	Potentiate epinephrine in local anaesthetics, but not at low doses
Chlorhexidine	Mucosal discolouration, especially the tongue
Ciclosporin	Gingival overgrowth
Corticosteroids	Opportunistic infections Risk of circulatory collapse (see also Ch. 36) Cushing's syndrome, hypertension and diabetes Depression of inflammatory and immune responses Impaired wound healing Mood changes Moon face Depressed protein metabolism Raised blood sugar Sodium and water retention Feeling of wellbeing may mask significant disease
Cytotoxic drugs	Oral ulceration (especially methotrexate), opportunistic infections Cisplatin can cause grey gingival line ('lead line'), vincristine can cause jaw pain and weakness of the facial muscles
Diltiazem	Gingival overgrowth
L-DOPA	Colours saliva dark red or brown at high dose
Fluconazole and miconazole antifungals	Potentiate warfarin, even topical use in large amounts can have this effect Adverse interaction with statin drugs
Gold injections	Potent cause of oral lichenoid reactions and toxic epidermal necrolysis
Hypnotics and sedatives	Potentiation of general anaesthetics and other sedating drugs

Table 42.1 Examples of prescribed drugs having dentally relevant adverse effects (Continued)

Type of drug / drug	Dentally relevant adverse effects*

Immunosuppressive drugs
    Ciclosporin
    Methotrexate
    Steroids
    Azathioprine
	Oral ulceration (especially methotrexate), opportunistic infections particularly viral and fungal, recurrence of zoster, measles, herpes virus infections
	Taste disturbance

Insulin	Risk of hypoglycaemic coma
Iron supplements	Mucosal discolouration
Isotretinoin	Exfoliative cheilitis
Metformin	Oral lichenoid reactions Metallic taste Vitamin B12 deficiency
Metronidazole	Disulfiram reaction with alcohol Taste Do not prescribe to patients taking lithium Potentiates warfarin
Metoclopramide	Clenching of jaw muscles
Monoamine oxidase inhibitors	Dry mouth, dangerous interactions with opioids, particularly pethidine
Nicorandil	Oral ulceration (Ch. 16)
Non-steroidal anti-inflammatory analgesics	Oral lichenoid reactions rarely Longer doses reduce effectiveness of many anti-hypertensives Angio-oedema rarely
Opioid drugs of all types, sedatives and analgesics	Potentiate benzodiazepines and cause markedly increased risk of respiratory depression
Phenothiazine antipsychotics ('major tranquillisers')	Dry mouth Tardive dyskinesia (uncontrollable facial movements) Parkinsonian tremor Oral mucosal pigmentation
Phenytoin	Gingival overgrowth Lymphadenopathy occasionally Folate deficiency occasionally leading to exacerbation of aphthous stomatitis Salivary gland swelling
Rifampicin	Colours saliva red
Tricyclic antidepressants (e.g. amitriptyline)	Dry mouth *Do not* cause significant interactions with epinephrine in local anaesthetics

*Allergy to any drug is possible and so excluded.

Local analgesics with vasoconstrictors

In the past many drugs, notably tricyclic antidepressants and monoamine oxidase inhibitors, have been thought to cause significant interactions with vasoconstrictors in local analgesics. The passage of time and national audit of adverse reactions have shown that the fears were unfounded.

Current evidence indicates that despite theoretical possibilities, there are no significant interactions between dental analgesics and any other drugs, provided both the analgesic and medication are used at normal doses. In 1995, a dentist was convicted of manslaughter after causing the death of a patient on beta-blockers by giving her 16 cartridges of lidocaine with epinephrine. However, it appears overdose of lidocaine rather than hypertension, the theoretical risk, was the cause.

The only significant possible interactions with epinephrine (adrenaline) are a drug user who has recently taken cocaine, at risk of hypertensive crisis, and patients taking catechol-O-methyl transferase inhibitors for Parkinson's disease. Caution appears pragmatic with these latter relatively new classes of drugs, but even with these, normal maximal doses of epinephrine appear safe. It might only be suggested that extra care be taken to avoid intravascular injection until further evidence accumulates.

It is not logical to avoid lidocaine with adrenaline on theoretical grounds when it is the safest and most effective analgesic. Choosing a less effective analgesic is unfair on the patient and failure of analgesia may compromise treatment.

Allergic reactions are discussed in Chapter 30.

Local analgesics review PMID: 23660127 and 22822998

Adverse reactions to local analgesics PMID: 22959146

Prolonged analgesia PMID: 21623806

CHEMICAL DEPENDENCE

The British Drugs Survey suggests that one in five adults are recreational drug users to some degree, most using drugs relatively infrequently. Leaving alcohol and tobacco aside, the commonest drugs used are marijuana, amphetamines, cocaine and ecstasy (MDMA). The majority of users do not become dependent, but alcohol, cocaine, tobacco and benzodiazepines have, perhaps surprisingly, a somewhat similar risk of inducing physical and mental dependence. There is no risk of dependence from use of benzodiazepines for dental conscious sedation.

There are few direct oral effects of drug dependence.

Alcohol is associated with many maxillofacial injuries, and erosion results from acidic drinks such as wines and carbonated mixers. Aspirin and non-steroidal anti-inflammatory drugs carry a risk of severe gastric or oesophageal bleeding and will potentiate a haemorrhagic tendency caused by cirrhosis. Metronidazole must be avoided if a patient cannot reduce their alcohol intake or cease it during treatment.

Cocaine applied topically to be absorbed through oral mucosa causes vasoconstriction. This can result in ischaemic ulcers and necrosis if applied repeatedly to the same site. Cocaine inhaled to the nose causes avascular necrosis of the septum and necrosis may extend to perforate the hard palate.

Methamphetamine ('speed'), in particular, is likely to cause considerable oral damage in long-term use. It is acidic and also causes dry mouth. Great thirst, which tends to be relieved by almost continuous consumption of carbonated drinks, some of which have a high sugar content, is a common response. This drug is the most closely associated with gross oral disease

All those with a serious dependency are likely to suffer personality change and ignore their health and nutrition, including their mouth. Gross caries and periodontal neglect are common, compounded if the drug(s) induce dry mouth.

Difficulties in management are common (Box 42.2). Addicts may manipulate dentists into prescribing drugs, particularly opioids, by complaining of pain. Multiple drug abuse is also common, and attempts may be made to obtain any drugs, such as benzodiazepines or antihistamines, that are mood altering or sedative. Because of the risk of dependence, benzodiazepines should only be prescribed for short periods.

Liver function damaged by alcoholism or hepatitis impairs drug metabolism. This makes general anaesthesia, in particular, hazardous, as does respiratory disease or covert use of drugs of abuse pre-operatively. Benzodiazepines have an

---

Box 42.2 Implications of drug dependence for dental management

- Stealing prescription pads
- Attempts to manipulate dentists into prescribing drugs
- Carriage of hepatitis viruses or HIV by intravenous addicts
- Maxillofacial injuries, particularly among alcoholics
- Impaired liver function secondary to alcoholism or hepatitis
- Lymphadenopathy secondary to drug injection in unusual sites
- Infective endocarditis secondary to dirty injections
- Severe infections such as osteomyelitis among alcoholics
- Increased risks from general anaesthesia
- Gross oral neglect and sometimes enhanced sensitivity to pain
- Rarely, ulceration of the palate secondary to cocaine-induced ischaemia of the nasal cavity
- Occasionally, parotid swelling in alcoholics
- Interactions with other drugs

---

extended beta half-life (metabolism phase) leading to prolonged elimination but full eventual recovery.

Injecting drug users are at high risk of infective endocarditis from reusing needles. The damaged heart is then vulnerable to further episodes of endocarditis of dental origin (Ch. 32).

Oral manifestations marijuana use PMID: 23420976

Methamphetamine oral effects PMID: 18992021 and 25952435

Cocaine use oral significance PMID: 18408681

Alcohol abuse role dentist PMID: 16262033

Management methadone users PMID: 16262036

MDMA ecstasy oral significance PMID: 26268009 and 18268544

Medical emergencies

43

Dentists must know how to recognise and manage medical emergencies, rare though they may be. Their professional skills and equipment should enable them occasionally to save patients' lives. City traffic and the load on ambulance services are so heavy that hospital transfer can be delayed. Under such circumstances, measures taken by the dental team may be critical.

Dentists are required to ensure that all members of their staff are able to provide practical assistance in these circumstances. This involves training, keeping up to date and regular practice.

Many types of emergencies may have to be faced (Box 43.1). Many can be prevented by good history-taking and appropriate precautions.

References for the emergency procedures discussed here may be found in the following guidelines and databases. The BNF website provides drug information.

Risk assessment and prevention PMID: 23470404

Incidence of emergencies in US PMID: 20388811

Incidence in UK PMID: 10488938 and 10800238

Web URL 43.1 Standards for training and clinical practice UK: https://www.resus.org.uk/ and enter 'standards primary dental care' into search box

Web URL 43.2 Drugs for medical emergencies BNF: http://www.evidence.nhs.uk/ and enter 'emergencies dental practice' into search box

SUDDEN LOSS OF CONSCIOUSNESS

Common themes

The ABCDE approach to emergencies (assess **A**irway, **B**reathing, **C**irculation, **D**isability, **E**xposure) has become almost universally used, although in dental practice situations it is the first three and an assessment of consciousness that are immediately useful. It is also important to remember that patients in an emergency situation may still be in danger from the environment or their position.

Calling for help is also key. Additional personnel not only provide more pairs of hands but also emotional and intellectual support and, if they are members of the dental team, help trigger practiced automatic responses. When calling for an ambulance, it is important to have information about the patient ready. In cities, the response may be an ambulance, car, motorcycle or bicycle, and the equipment and skills of the paramedic need to be tailored to the emergency based on the information given.

It is also suggested that practices with an automatic defibrillator register it with their local ambulance service so that it can be of use to others in the neighbourhood.

Web URL 43.3 ABCDE approach: https://www.resus.org.uk/resuscitation-guidelines/abcde-approach/

Fainting

Fainting, caused by transient hypotension and cerebral ischaemia, is the most common cause of sudden loss of consciousness in primary dental care (in hospitals, fits are of similar incidence). There are several predisposing factors (Box 43.2), but some patients are particularly prone to faint and frequently do so. The cause is peripheral vasodilatation, usually combined with an element of bradycardia.

Signs and symptoms are usually readily recognisable (Box 43.3). Sometimes consciousness is lost almost instantaneously. Minor convulsions or incontinence are occasionally

---

Box 43.1   Emergencies that may arise during dental procedures

Sudden loss of consciousness (collapse)

- Fainting
- Anaphylactic shock
- Acute hypoglycaemia
- Myocardial infarction
- Cardiac arrest
- Strokes
- Circulatory collapse secondary to corticosteroid therapy

Acute chest pain

- Angina
- Myocardial infarction

Difficulty in breathing

- Asthma
- Anaphylactic shock
- Left ventricular failure
- Convulsions
- Epilepsy
- Any other cause of loss of consciousness, including fainting

Other emergencies

- Haemorrhage
- Drug reactions and interactions
- Major maxillofacial injuries

Box 43.2   Factors predisposing to fainting

- Upright posture
- Anxiety
- Pain
- Injections
- Fatigue
- Hunger

Box 43.3   Fainting: signs and symptoms
• Premonitory dizziness, weakness or nausea
• Pale, cold moist skin
• Initially slow and weak pulse becoming full and bounding
• Loss of consciousness

Box 43.4   Management of a fainting attack
• Lower the head, preferably by laying the patient flat*
• Loosen any tight clothing round the neck
• If no rapid improvement,
    • the legs can be raised or pressure applied to the abdomen to increase venous return
    • apply pulse oximeter if available
    • administer oxygen
• Give a sweetened drink when consciousness has been recovered
• If no recovery within a few minutes, consider other causes of loss of consciousness

*To keep the patient upright worsens cerebral hypoxia and is harmful.

Box 43.5   Signs and symptoms of acute hypoglycaemia
• Premonitory signs are similar to those of a faint, but little response to laying the patient flat
    may include aggressiveness or excitation
    may include period of worsening drowsiness
• Unconsciousness that steadily deepens

Box 43.6   Management of hypoglycaemia
• Patients often aware of what is happening and able to warn the dentist
• Before consciousness is lost, give glucose tablets or powder, or sugar (at least four lumps) as a sweetened drink, repeated if symptoms not completely relieved
• If consciousness is lost, give subcutaneous glucagon (1 mg) then give sugar by mouth during the brief recovery period. Intravenous glucose (as much as 50 mL of a 50% solution) is an alternative but difficult to use in an emergency situation. Glucagon may be repeated once, but after that has no effect as all glycogen stores have been mobilised.
• Hypostop, a gel containing glucose, may provide sufficient glucose absorbed through the oral mucosa to combat declining consciousness
• If consciousness is lost, call ambulance, provide oxygen, apply pulse oximeter if available and move to recovery position

Box 43.7   Typical features of acute anaphylaxis
• Initial facial flushing, itching, paresthesiae or cold extremities
• Facial oedema or urticaria
• Bronchospasm (wheezing), hoarseness, stridor
• Loss of consciousness
• Pallor going on to cyanosis
• Cold clammy skin
• Rapid weak or impalpable pulse
• Deep fall in blood pressure
• Death if treatment is delayed or inappropriate, from cardiac or respiratory arrest

associated. Principles of management are summarised in Box 43.4.

Prevention

Loss of consciousness in a faint is impossible when supine. Performing injections and all treatment with the patient flat is helpful, but the physiological mechanisms still act: the patient may feel unwell, ask to sit up and then faint.

Regular fainters are frequently helped by an appropriate dose of a minor anxiolytic on the night before and again an hour before treatment, but they must then be accompanied by a responsible adult and follow the usual precautions about their use.

Acute hypoglycaemia

Hypoglycaemia affects patients with diabetes whose insulin dose is too high, either after an overdose of insulin or if prevented from eating at the expected time (Box 43.5). If there is any doubt about the cause of loss of consciousness, in an emergency situation always assume hypoglycaemia in a patient with diabetes. *Hyper*glycaemic coma is much less frequent and tends to affect patients with type 2 diabetes who are dehydrated and is a more chronic process. Insulin must never be given as it can be fatal to a patient with hypoglycaemia.

If there is sufficient time and hypoglycaemia is suspected, the patient may be able to check their own blood glucose using their own portable monitor.

Management of hypoglycaemia is shown in (Box 43.6).

Web URL 43.4 Hypoglycaemia: http://emedicine.medscape .com/article/767359

Anaphylactic reactions

Penicillin is the most common cause of these type I hypersensitivity reactions. Anaphylactic reactions can also be precipitated by insect stings, foods (nuts or shellfish particularly) and, exceptionally rarely, by aspirin.

In general, the quicker the onset, the more severe the reaction. A severe reaction to penicillin may start within a minute of an injection, but immediate loss of consciousness is more likely to be due to fainting. A reaction starting 30 minutes after an injection is unlikely to be dangerous. Acute reactions to oral penicillins are rare but can develop after half an hour or more because of slower absorption from the gut.

Collapse is due to widespread vasodilatation and increased capillary permeability causing potentially fatal hypotension.

Signs and symptoms

The clinical picture is variable (Box 43.7).

Management

Epinephrine is the mainstay of treatment (Box 43.8) and the lifesaving element. It raises cardiac output, combats excessive capillary permeability and bronchospasm, and also inhibits release of mediators from mast cells.

Circulatory collapse is probably largely due to histamine release, which is inhibited by parenteral chlorphenamine. Hydrocortisone is slow to take effect but maintains the blood pressure for some hours and combats the continued effect of the antigen–antibody reaction.

Rapid transfer to hospital is necessary to provide circulatory support by intravenous fluids and other measures. The patient must also be given a card and educated against the use of the causative drug.

Minor anaphylactic reactions, with slow onset and no respiratory signs, can be managed by laying the patient flat, raising the legs and providing oxygen. Urticarial rashes and other mild signs benefit from oral or intramuscular chlorphenamine and bronchospasm from salbutamol inhaler. Many patients with severe allergies carry an 'EpiPen' or similar emergency epinephrine autoinjector. These are useful in an emergency but deliver a slightly lower dose than is normally administered in an emergency and may need to be repeated more rapidly than conventional doses.

Web URL 43.5 Anaphylaxis UK: https://www.resus.org.uk/anaphylaxis/

Web URL 43.6 NICE clinical pathway postevent: http://pathways.nice.org.uk/pathways/anaphylaxis

Web URL 43.7 Anaphylaxis US: http://www.aaaai.org/ and enter 'practice parameter anaphylaxis' into search box

Web URL 43.8 International guideline: http://www.bsaci.org/ and enter 'anaphylaxis guideline' into search box

Myocardial infarction

A patient typically has severe chest pain, but may suddenly lose consciousness as a result of a myocardial infarct. Treatment is therefore either as angina or cardiac arrest.

Cardiac arrest

Cardiac arrest can follow myocardial infarction, any cause of severe hypotension such as an anaphylactic reaction or adrenal crisis, or hypoxia. Dentists should be aware of and alert to the possibility of cardiac arrest and be able to recognise it (Box 43.9) and manage it (Box 43.10) when it happens. Detail cannot be given here; practice in a simulated emergency setting is essential.

Speed of response is critical and there is a legal obligation that the dental team should be trained in cardiopulmonary resuscitation (CPR) and be able to carry it out immediately. Resuscitation must be started within a few minutes.

Guidelines were recently simplified (2015) and adapted to recognise the wide availability of automatic electronic defibrillators (AEDs). These are now kept in many public places and should available to the dental surgery. Defibrillation within 5 minutes of infarction is associated with a recovery rate of 70%, much higher than with cardiopulmonary resuscitation alone. Each minute of delay to defibrillation reduces survival by 10%, so this has become a critical procedure; CPR alone rarely restarts the heart.

In a clinical dental setting the dentist and team should be prepared to provide basic life support (BLS; defined as life support without equipment) and use their airway skills to provide oxygen by bag or mask and use an AED.

Basic life support should be started immediately the patient becomes unresponsive and is not breathing normally. This last point must be carefully assessed. In the first minutes after arrest there may be 'agonal' gasps, slow deep breaths with a snoring sound. These, as well as lack of breathing, indicate a need to start cardiopulmonary resuscitation. It is now considered that giving CPR to a patient who is not in arrest causes no significant risks; do not allow uncertainty about diagnosis to cause delay. Cyanosis, pupil dilatation and loss of reaction to light, and absence of measurable blood pressure are late signs that should not be sought. Mild seizures or fits may follow cerebral anoxia and should not be confused with epilepsy and trigger the wrong emergency response.

CPR requires a firm surface, ideally the floor. If the patient is too heavy to lift out of a dental chair but can be laid supine there, resuscitation can be carried out by the operator and assistant standing beside the chair. An operator's stool can be placed under the headrest to stabilise the chair. The optimal pressure for chest compression is about 40 or 50 kg (the weight of the upper part of the body applied through stiffly extended arms). Ensure the chest recoils fully between compressions. External cardiac massage is tiring, and another person should preferably alternate with the first operator at intervals of 2 minutes. CPR starts with compressions rather than breaths because the lungs already contain oxygenated blood that must be pumped to the brain as soon as possible. Continued effective compressions with minimal interruption is the key element.

'Rescue' breaths should be given over a period of approximately 1 second, ensuring that the chest rises. As soon as possible, mouth-to-mouth breaths should be switched to positive pressure inflation with 100% oxygen and a self-inflating bag and mask.

Signs of restoration of blood pressure are disappearance of facial pallor and a good spontaneous pulse, contraction of the pupils, return of reflex activity such as the blink reflex and reaction of the pupils to light, lightening of unconsciousness and purposeful spontaneous movements, not twitching or convulsions.

Resuscitation of children is an unlikely requirement in a dental setting. Specialised techniques are not critical. If in doubt, use the adult procedures rather than delay. Children have a greater requirement for oxygenation, so ideally 5 rescue breaths or ventilations should be given first. Chest compressions should be 4 cm for a young, and 5 cm for an older, child.

Causes of failure are summarised in Box 43.11.

The chances of having to provide CPR in a dental surgery are low, and members of the dental team need to be prepared to use their skills outside the surgery.

Commentary on guidelines PMID: 22240694

Web URL 43.9 Resuscitation Council guidelines: https://www.resus.org.uk/information-for-professionals/

Case report PMID: 26866410

Box 43.11   Causes of failure of cardiopulmonary resuscitation

- Interrupting cardiac compression for ventilation
- Failing to clear the airway or to keep it open by failing to hyperextend the head adequately
- Failing to close the nose during mouth-to-mouth ventilation
- Failing to fit the mask closely onto the patient's face when using an inflating bag
- Failing to make sure that ventilation is adequate, as shown by movement of the chest
- Timidity in applying external cardiac compression, and using insufficient force to compress the heart. The risk of cracking a rib should be disregarded
- Failing to release pressure on the chest completely between compressions and thus preventing cardiac filling
- Compressing the chest too rapidly to allow the heart to fill between compressions
- Putting the hands in incorrect positions
- Failing to act sufficiently quickly and fretting about details rather than getting on with it
- Lack of practice. The response should be near automatic

Box 43.12   Signs and management of a stroke

Signs

- Loss of consciousness
- Weakness of an arm and leg on one side
- Drooping of the side of the face
- Often stertorous breathing

Management

- Maintain the airway, administer oxygen
- Call an ambulance for transfer to hospital

Web URL 43.10 Guidance US: http://cpr.heart.org/ and enter 'healthcare professional BLS' into search box

Strokes

Patients are usually hypertensive and middle aged or elderly. The clinical picture varies with the size and site of brain damage (Box 43.12). Typical features are unilateral paralysis, often of the face, or sensory disturbance, disorientation, difficulty with speech or unilateral loss of vision. Transient ischaemic attacks, mild minor strokes, should be recognised and treated by referral to hospital. Rapid transfer is important as thrombolytic treatment must be given rapidly to be effective.

Subarachnoid haemorrhage from a ruptured berry aneurysm on the circle of Willis is the main cause of stroke in a younger person. It typically causes intense headache followed by coma.

Circulatory collapse in patients on corticosteroid treatment

Steroids given therapeutically are sensed by the pituitary in the same way as natural steroids and the high levels suppress corticotrophin-releasing hormone and adrenocorticotropic hormone (ACTH) secretion through the physiological feedback mechanism. With time, the lack of ACTH suppresses the adrenal and the gland atrophies, so that stressful situations that would normally cause a rapid adrenal response no longer do so. Adrenocortical function may take as long as 2 years to recover after ceasing steroids, although in most patients 2 months is sufficient.

The response of patients on long-term corticosteroid treatment to surgery is unpredictable. It has generally been considered that all patients who are taking or have been taking systemic corticosteroids are at risk, even those using high-potency topical steroids on a large area of skin. However, adverse effects do not appear to arise unless the dose of prednisolone exceeds 10 mg per day.

Although near-fatal circulatory collapse has been reported to follow dental extractions in a patient taking as little as 5 mg of prednisone per day, few cases are well documented. In the past, a large additional dose of steroid 'cover' (usually 100 mg prednisolone) was given before surgery, but this is now considered an overprotective and unnecessary precaution.

It is currently considered that only surgery under general anaesthesia carries significant risk of adrenal crisis. Even surgical removal of lower third molars is not stressful enough to cause a significant release of cortisol physiologically, and a doubling of the normal daily dose preoperatively and for 24 hours is sufficient precaution for surgery under local analgesia. High-dose cover is reserved for general anaesthesia. The risk of adrenal crisis is almost negligible in dentistry.

Although steroid cover is no longer routine, there remains a significant risk of collapse in patients who have recently had their steroid dose reduced or stopped. During the recovery period, they are at risk of adrenal crisis and a lower threshold for steroid cover is required.

Thus, patients with primary Addison's disease, those on the highest doses or with recently reduced doses of steroid remain at risk, and ability to prevent and manage a steroid-related collapse remains important (Box 43.13).

Steroid cover PMID: 15592544

CHEST PAIN

Angina pectoris

Acute chest pain due to myocardial ischaemia is the only symptom. Pain is centred on the chest, often described as tightness, squeezing or pressure or indigestion. It may radiate to the inner left arm or jaw. Additional signs such as nausea, vomiting and shock may occur in a severe attack, but suggest a myocardial infarct. A first anginal attack may come as a consequence of an emotional response to dental treatment. Stop treatment and give glyceryl trinitrate sublingually (Box 43.14).

Many patients have already had attacks and carry medication. Unless treatment is immediately effective, the patient should be transferred to hospital.

Patients whose angina is induced by anxiety may benefit from premedication with a benzodiazepine for dental treatment. Those with unstable or recent hospital admission for angina should not be treated in dental practice until stable.

Myocardial infarction

Myocardial infarction is a common cause of death and must be recognised quickly (Box 43.15), as the patient's fate may be decided by the first few minutes' treatment. Several aspects of dentistry, particularly apprehension, pain or the effect of drugs, might contribute to make this accident more likely in a susceptible patient.

Most patients will have a history of angina or be a known risk patient, but this is not absolute. The symptoms range from those of severe angina to loss of consciousness depending on the area of the heart involved. Pain can radiate to the left shoulder or down the left arm but, very occasionally, is felt only in the left jaw. The pain does not respond to trinitrate. Vomiting is common, and there is sometimes shock or loss of consciousness. Principles of management are summarised in Box 43.16. Some patients die within a few minutes after the start of the attack, and it is rash to try over-ambitious treatment. Prompt ambulance attendance will be the most useful response, as they can administer fibrinolytic and other drugs and monitor the cardiac condition. There should be no concern about giving aspirin as the beneficial effects far outweigh any potential disadvantages.

Box 43.13   Signs and management of corticosteroid-related collapse

Signs

- Pallor
- Rapid, weak or impalpable pulse
- Loss of consciousness
- Rapidly falling blood pressure

Management

- Lay the patient flat and raise the legs
- Give at least 200 mg hydrocortisone sodium succinate intravenously*
- Call an ambulance for immediate transfer to hospital
- Give oxygen and, if necessary, artificial ventilation
- Consider other possible reasons for loss of consciousness

*The intramuscular route can be used if a vein cannot be found but absorption is slower.

Box 43.14   Management of angina

- Give the patient their anti-anginal drug (usually 0.5 mg of glyceryl trinitrate sublingually) *or*
- Glyceryl trinitrate spray* (400 mg) gives rapid relief
- Administer oxygen
- If there is no relief within 3 minutes the patient has probably had a myocardial infarct

*Glyceryl trinitrate spray has a better shelf-life for the emergency kit.

Box 43.15   Typical signs and symptoms of myocardial infarction

- Severe crushing retrosternal pain
- Shallow strained breathing
- Vomiting
- Weak or irregular pulse
- Pale clammy skin

Box 43.16   Management of myocardial infarction

- If there is loss of consciousness, proceed as for cardiac arrest (mentioned previously)
- Otherwise, put the patient in a comfortable position that allows easy breathing. Do not lay flat if there is left ventricular failure and pulmonary oedema
- Send an assistant to telephone for an ambulance
- Constantly reassure the patient
- Use glyceryl trinitrate spray or the patient's own anginal medication
- Give 50/50 nitrous oxide and oxygen from a relative analgesia machine, to relieve pain and anxiety, or, if unavailable, oxygen alone
- Unless allergic, give aspirin 300 mg by mouth as soon as more urgent measures have been carried out
- Monitor for possible cardiac arrest

Box 43.17   Signs and management of status asthmaticus

Signs

- Breathlessness
- Inability to talk
- Expiratory wheezing (may be disguised as rapid shallow breathing)
- Rapid pulse (usually over 110 per minute). Progress to bradycardia is a danger sign
- Accessory muscles of respiration come into action
- Cyanosis

Management

- Reassure the patient
- Do *not* lay the patient flat
- Give normally used anti-asthmatic drugs (such as salbutamol) by inhaler (2 puffs, repeated as necessary). If the patient cannot inhale effectively, use a spacer device. Better, administer salbutamol by nebuliser
- If no response or tachycardia develops, call an ambulance for transfer to hospital
- Give oxygen and continue salbutamol
- In emergency, if patient continues to deteriorate or has other signs suggesting an allergic reaction as a cause, give epinephrine (adrenaline) as for anaphylaxis.

RESPIRATORY DIFFICULTY

Severe asthma and status asthmaticus

Causes

Loss of, or forgetting to bring, a salbutamol inhaler, anxiety, infection or exposure to a specific allergen are possible causes. Inability to complete sentences in one breath indicates severe dyspnoea; if the patient becomes cyanosed, exhausted or confused, or their pulse falls to 50/min or less, the condition is life threatening.

Giving hydrocortisone in dental practice is no longer recommended.

Features and management are shown in Box 43.17.

Box 43.18   Signs and management of a tonic-clonic epileptic attack

Signs

- Sometimes a brief warning cry as the chest muscles contract and air is forced through a closed larynx
- Consciousness lost immediately
- The body becomes rigid (tonic phase) and cyanosis appears, usually about 30 seconds
- Widespread jerking movements start (clonic phase), for a few minutes
- Sometimes incontinence or frothing of the mouth
- Flaccidity sometimes follows after a few minutes
- Consciousness regained slowly after a variable period
- Confusion or drowsiness may persist

Management

- Put the patient prone in the coma ('recovery') position as soon as possible, usually after the clonic phase
- Prevent patients from injuring themselves
- Do not try to put anything in the mouth in the attempt to prevent the patient biting the tongue
- Make sure the airway is clear after convulsions have subsided
- Do not give any medication but await recovery
- Reassure patients as soon as consciousness returns
- For any first attack, the patient should be sent to hospital
- Only allow patients to return home when fully recovered and accompanied by a responsible adult

Left ventricular failure

Extreme breathlessness with increased respiratory rate is the main sign. It may be associated with chest pain if secondary to myocardial infarction. Apart from measures for an infarction, sitting the patient upright and giving oxygen, little can be done in the dental surgery apart from immediately calling an ambulance.

CONVULSIONS

Epilepsy

Hunger, menstruation and some drugs such as tricyclic antidepressants, alcohol or frequently flashing lights (not merely turning the operating lamp on and off) may sometimes precipitate a seizure (Box 43.18). Recognition, types and avoidance of an epileptic seizure are covered in Chapter 38.

Status epilepticus

If convulsions do not stop within 15 minutes or are rapidly repeated, the patient can die from anoxia (Box 43.19). Any individual's seizures normally last a consistent length of time and stop by themselves. This time is useful information to record in the medical history. Continuous or repeated seizures without recovery between them for 30 minutes or more constitutes status epilepticus. Any seizure type may develop into status epilepticus. Status in a tonic-clonic seizure is potentially life threatening, and an ambulance should be called if the clonic phase lasts more than 5 minutes; do not wait for the 30-minute defining time as urgent medical help is needed.

Box 43.19 Management of status epilepticus

- Treat initially as any fit (earlier)
- If continuous or repeated more than 5 minutes, call for an ambulance
- Continue to administer oxygen
- Give 10 mg, buccal midazolam ('midazolam oromucosal solution') to an adult patient or child older than 10 years (1–5 years, 5 mg; 5–10 years, 7.5 mg) from a prefilled emergency oral syringe. Some patients or carers may carry an emergency supply of oral or rectal midazolam
- Other preparations of midazolam or diazepam should NOT be used
- Repeat midazolam if no recovery within 5 minutes
- Maintain the airway and give oxygen

Web URL 43.11 Actions for seizures: https://www.epilepsysociety.org.uk/ follow menu about epilepsy>first aid

OTHER EMERGENCIES

Haemorrhage

Prolonged bleeding is usually due to traumatic extractions. A major vessel is unlikely to be opened during dental surgery, and patients are unlikely to lose any dangerous amount of blood if promptly managed (Box 43.20). Post-extraction bleeding is usually only an emergency in the sense that the dentist may be woken up at 3 o'clock in the morning by a frightened patient.

Occasionally, bleeding is due to unsuspected haemophilia or other haemorrhagic disorders.

Post-extraction bleeding PMID: 24930250

Violence

Violence toward healthcare workers is steadily growing. Aggressive behaviour can be the result of mental illness, particularly schizophrenia, drug abuse (particularly of alcohol) or brain damage. The risk to dental clinical staff can be significant, especially because of the ready availability of sharp instruments. All practices should have a policy for dealing with violent patients, although the risk is much higher in secondary care.

The ambulance service is not equipped to deal with such cases so that the police must be called. Patients who abuse National Health Service staff may have their access to healthcare limited after investigation.

General principles of managing potential violence are given in Box 43.21. These are designed for patients with mental illness but are equally applicable to all aggressive patients.

Box 43.20 Management of prolonged dental haemorrhage

- Reassure the patient
- Clean the mouth with swabs and locate the source of bleeding
- If there is point bleeding from bone, crush the vessel with a small instrument. Soft tissue bleeding will usually respond to pressure alone
- Give epinephrine (adrenaline)-containing local anaesthetic, remove ragged tissue, squeeze up the socket edges and suture it. A small piece of oxidised cellulose (Surgicel) may be placed loosely in the socket below the suture to aid haemostasis, but is usually unnecessary
- When bleeding has been controlled, ask about the history and especially any family history of prolonged bleeding
- Check for anticoagulant or antiplatelet drugs
- If bleeding continues despite suturing or if the patient is obviously anaemic or debilitated, transfer to hospital for investigation and management of any haemorrhagic defect
- Meanwhile, limit bleeding as much as possible with a pressure pad over the socket and by supporting the patient's jaw with a firm barrel bandage
- Tranexamic acid mouthwash may stabilise what clot forms while awaiting transfer to hospital

Box 43.21 Management of potential violence

- Reassure the patient that everyone is working in their best interests
- Be sensitive to changes in mood or composure that may lead to aggression or violence
- Seek help, but devolve dealing with the patient to one person
- Separate agitated patients from others and staff, do not allow staff to become isolated and at risk
- Train in verbal and non-verbal skills to avoid or manage adverse situations without provoking aggression
- Communicate respect for and empathy with the patient at all times
- Ensure staff control their own anxiety or frustration when dealing with the patient and do not escalate the situation inadvertently

Learning guide

44

Textbooks such as this grow in size from edition to edition, adding much that can only be described as reference material. Undergraduate students will never see most of the conditions in it, before or after graduation. Despite this, on qualification they are expected to not only diagnose them, but also institute appropriate referral or treatment.

It is unsurprising that students often ask despairingly what they need to know. The breadth of oral medicine, pathology, surgery, radiology and the medical aspects of dentistry is immense, and students need to prioritise their limited time to make sure that they know details only when required. Teachers of these subjects would much prefer students to enjoy these interesting subjects, be led by interest and curiosity and not learn facts obsessively.

In the past, national regulatory bodies would prescribe the topics to be taught in undergraduate courses. More recently, there has been an almost complete shift to practical learning outcomes and competencies expected of the graduating dental surgeon. This produces a welcome emphasis on higher-level learning and the synthesis and application of knowledge to clinical problems. Unfortunately, the competencies are often somewhat generic. Both teachers and students no longer have a defined syllabus of knowledge to form the essential factual foundation required for these higher-level skills.

In the UK there has been a change in both undergraduate and specialist education to focus on the expected future roles of dental surgeons and curriculum space has had to be made for many new topics. This has led to a concentration on 'what the general dental practitioner really needs to know'. Knowledge-based topics such as those in this book are thus at risk of being downgraded in the mind of the student. However, it is important to remember that before reaching dental practice, many dentists will work in secondary care in specialist departments where a lack of knowledge could be severely detrimental to patients. Many dentists go on to become specialists.

The average-sized UK dental practice will have 20 or so patients with lichen planus, one or two with mucous membrane pemphigoid or severe desquamative gingivitis, more than 100 red or white patches, numerous cysts and inflammatory conditions, and every once in a while a patient with a malignant tumour that must not be missed. Those in primary care fulfil an important screening role and act as gatekeepers in national health systems. They need breadth of knowledge rather than detail.

This chapter attempts to provide a syllabus of topics for students of dentistry to concentrate on. It is based on published curricula from the UK specialist societies of Oral and Maxillofacial Pathology and of Oral Surgery, the Scandinavian Fellowship for Oral Pathology and Oral Medicine, the Profile and Competencies for the Graduating European Dentist of the Association of Dental Education in Europe, US and North American publications and competencies defined by the Dental Council of India and other accrediting bodies. Some of these are referenced at the end. It is impossible to define a syllabus that would be appropriate for all countries or dental schools. Some teach these subjects independently, others in integrated courses and yet others in problem-based learning format. Those practising in tropical areas may well omit Paget's disease and orofacial granulomatosis and other diseases that affect Northern populations and replace them with deep mycoses and other diseases of local importance. This is a guide for students based on the author's views and experience.

In using this table it must be accepted that there are conflicts. For instance in giving a differential diagnosis of a mixed radiolucent lesion in the jaws it will be necessary at a basic level to include lesions that are listed in the third or fourth columns. This table is to be used as a guide to the importance of *detailed* knowledge. Rarer lesions will often merit more attention because of the importance of the diagnosis to the patient.

How much needs to be known about each topic? Students should focus on information that allows understanding of the clinical presentation, differential diagnosis and would equip them to discuss the significance and implications of the condition with a patient and other professionals. Those topics in the core curriculum need to be thoroughly understood and are very much a minimum expectation. They are listed from the perspective of pathology and medicine. It is quite possible that a topic such as cleft palate would be a core topic in paediatric dentistry or orthodontics where the emphasis would be on clinical aspects.

Students often ask whether they need to know histopathology. Certainly, undergraduate courses should not attempt to teach students to become diagnostic pathologists. Diagnostic histopathology is a postgraduate speciality. Nevertheless, there are good reasons why knowledge of disease at the tissue level is important. It aids understanding of disease processes and enables students to see the biology of a disease in progress. There is no better illustration of how the patient is affected and a picture provides considerably more understanding than could be transmitted by words alone. Knowing how diseases affect tissues informs the decision whether or not to perform a biopsy, what type of biopsy is appropriate and how the disease can be investigated and managed. It has been interesting to see how virtual microscopy systems have made histopathology more accessible to students, who often felt isolated and stressed looking down a microscope on their own. Histopathological knowledge is required in many areas, to a variable degree as indicated in this book, but not in the detail required of a diagnostic pathologist.

From the patients' perspective, dentists, whether in primary or secondary care, are expected to be the experts on oral and dental conditions. Medical practitioners receive only very limited, if any, training in oral disease. An incorrect differential diagnosis and referral by a dentist may well start the patient along the wrong, and possibly a harmful, care pathway.

Table 44.1

Minimum core topics, detailed knowledge expected	Core+ key topics for dentistry required for differential diagnosis but less extensive knowledge acceptable	Otherwise important concepts requiring overview knowledge but not detail	Supplementary and reference topics, primarily for postgraduates and those in secondary care
The processes of differential diagnosis, principles of history taking, examination, selection and interpretation of investigations for oral and head and neck disease			
Medical history taking, relevance of disease to dentistry and follow-up questions for history taking			
Detailed knowledge of biopsy procedures for the mouth and selection of conditions for which biopsy is a useful investigation	Fine needle aspiration	Principles of other biopsy techniques	
Relative value of imaging techniques and selection for specific purposes			
Biopsy specimen handling and interpretation of histology reports and other investigation results	Immunofluorescence	Molecular tests	
An appreciation of the relative incidence of lesions and conditions			
Correct definition, use and spelling of medical and pathological terms			
Missing and supernumerary teeth Normal teething and dental development chronology Cleft lip and palate	Minor tooth anomalies Ankyloglossia	Dental effects of common syndromes Submucous cleft	Clefts in syndromes Craniofacial syndromes
Amelogenesis imperfecta, molar incisor hypomineralisation, hereditary opalescent teeth and dentinogenesis imperfecta	Regional odontodysplasia Hypophosphatasia	Segmental odontomaxillary dysplasia Congenital syphilis Vitamin D–resistant rickets	Dentinal dysplasia Ehlers-Danlos syndromes
Chronological hypoplasia and fluorosis. Tetracycline pigmentation			
Resorption and hypercementosis			
Delayed eruption and accelerated tooth loss			
Normal enamel, dentine and pulp structure. Pathology of caries as it relates to prevention and operative treatment, epidemiology and risk management	Pathogenesis and structural changes in enamel, dentine and cementum *Streptococcus mutans*	Microbiology of caries, ecological plaque theory	
Pulpitis and pulpal reactions to damage, relationship to treatment, pulp stones			
Apical periodontitis and the sequelae of pulp necrosis or pulp removal, periapical granuloma, radicular cyst, dentoalveolar abscess and spread of infection			
Tooth wear and the processes of attrition, abrasion and erosion Bruxism		Abfraction	
Osseointegration	Causes of failure		

Table 44.1 (Continued)

Minimum core topics, detailed knowledge expected	Core+ key topics for dentistry required for differential diagnosis but less extensive knowledge acceptable	Otherwise important concepts requiring overview knowledge but not detail	Supplementary and reference topics, primarily for postgraduates and those in secondary care
Normal periodontium structure Plaque-related gingivitis, periodontitis and their variants, classification, aetiology, pathogenesis and tissue changes. Diseases mimicking gingivitis and periodontitis and their differential diagnosis Effects of systemic disease			
Aggressive periodontitis			Papillon–Lefèvre syndrome
Acute ulcerative gingivitis, periodontal abscess, pericoronitis	Noma and HIV periodontitis		Localised spongiotic gingivitis
Localised and generalised gingival enlargement Drug-induced overgrowth	Hereditary types		
Common mucosal lesions, fibrous epulis, fibroepithelial hyperplasia., pyogenic granuloma, pregnancy epulis, peripheral giant cell granuloma, squamous papilloma, papillary hyperplasia of palate		Multiple endocrine neoplasia type 2b Condylomas Multifocal epithelial hyperplasia Calibre-persistent artery	Verruciform xanthoma
Haemangioma and the range of vascular anomalies			
Traumatic injuries to soft tissue and teeth, Amalgam tattoo		Eosinophilic ulcer	
Infection of dental origin, abscess, cellulitis, oedema, fascial space infections, their anatomy and treatment, role of antibiotics and antibiotic stewardship	Antibiotic abscess Cavernous sinus thrombosis		
Other infections, tuberculosis, actinomycosis		Mucormycosis	Systemic mycoses
Viral infections, primary and recurrent herpes simplex infection, herpes zoster infection. Epstein–Barr virus infection and its sequelae	Herpangina and hand foot and mouth disease	Herpetic whitlow	Ramsay Hunt syndrome Measles Chicken pox Cytomegalovirus ulcers
Syphilis, primary and secondary			Tertiary syphilis
Candidosis, all oral presentations			Chronic mucocutaneous and endocrine syndromes
Recurrent oral ulceration and aphthous stomatitis, minor, major and herpetiform	Behçet's disease	HIV-associated ulcers Nicorandil ulcers	
Lichen planus and lichenoid reactions, topical and systemic	Lupus erythematosus	Malignant change in lichen planus Graft versus host disease	Vulvovaginal-gingival syndrome Plasma cell gingivitis Chronic ulcerative stomatitis
Immunobullous diseases, pemphigus, mucous membrane pemphigoid	Angina bullosa haemorrhagica	Linear immunoglobulin (Ig)A disease	Paraneoplastic pemphigus
Erythema multiforme		Stevens-Johnson syndrome	
Erythema migrans, anaemic glossitis, oral hairy leukoplakia	(Black) hairy tongue Amyloidosis of tongue	Lingual papillitis	Patterson-Kelly syndrome Keratosis of renal failure

Table 44.1 (Continued)

Minimum core topics, detailed knowledge expected	Core+ key topics for dentistry required for differential diagnosis but less extensive knowledge acceptable	Otherwise important concepts requiring overview knowledge but not detail	Supplementary and reference topics, primarily for postgraduates and those in secondary care
Granulomatous disease, Crohn's disease and orofacial granulomatosis, foreign body reactions	Sarcoidosis		Reactions to injected cosmetic agents
Frictional and reactive keratoses Idiopathic lesions, White sponge naevus, leukoedema Fordyce granules Cheek and tongue chewing		Stomatitis nicotina	
Physiological pigmentation, melanotic macules, melanocytic naevi. Melanoma	Peutz–Jegher disease Inflammatory pigmentation	Addison's disease Melanoacanthoma Heavy metal poisoning	Other syndromes with pigmented lesions
Oral potentially malignant disorders, concept, all diseases other than those listed to the right, epithelial dysplasia, factors potentiating malignant change, differential diagnosis and management. Oral submucous fibrosis Prevention from a public health perspective		Genetic concepts of field change, clonal selection and transformation Human papillomavirus (HPV)–associated dysplasia	Dyskeratosis congenita Syphilitic leukoplakia
Oral squamous cell carcinoma, epidemiology, aetiology, spread, prognosis and principles of management. Early and late signs. Staging and grading. Radiation exposure and the effects of radiation and adverse effects of treatment for head and neck cancer. Role of dental practitioner. Prevention from a public health perspective	Oral cancer screening and prevention Outline and concepts of patient cancer pathway including referral pathways Verrucous carcinoma	Lip carcinoma	Fanconi anaemia
HPV oropharyngeal carcinoma	Basal cell carcinoma of skin	Nasopharyngeal carcinoma	
Tori and exostoses	Osteomas Osteosarcoma	Gardner's syndrome Cleidocranial dysplasia Hyperparathyroidism	Osteochondroma Chondrosarcoma Ewing's sarcoma Osteogenesis imperfecta Osteopetrosis
Normal healing of tooth socket, dry socket			
Acute and chronic forms of osteomyelitis of the jaws and osteoradionecrosis, healing fracture and tooth socket, Prevention of infection in bone Correct use of antibiotics	Proliferative periostitis Dense bone islands and osteoporotic bone marrow defects	Chronic focal low grade osteomyelitis Diffuse sclerosing forms Traumatic sequestrum	SAPHO and CRMO syndromes
Medication-related osteonecrosis, causes, prevention and treatment			
Principles of classification of jaw cysts. Odontogenic cysts, radicular, residual, collateral, dentigerous cysts and odontogenic keratocyst. Differential diagnosis, role of biopsy, treatment	Basal cell naevus syndrome Lateral periodontal and calcifying odontogenic cysts	Botryoid cyst Glandular odontogenic cyst	Orthokeratinised odontogenic cyst Gingival cysts

Self-assessment questions

These self-assessment questions are based on the material of the previous section but may also link to material covered elsewhere. They are not intended to be comprehensive, but give an indication of the understanding and problem solving abilities expected at an undergraduate level. You will not find all the information you require to answer these questions in this textbook of essential facts. Use these questions to guide your additional reading and learning.

CHAPTER 1

- How might poor history taking inhibit a patient from providing the information you seek?
- Can you draw a family tree from a patient's family history and interpret inheritance patterns from it?
- Which features in a pain history might suggest pain of odontogenic, neurological or vascular origin?
- What is the difference between a medical history and a medical history questionnaire?
- Could you justify all the questions asked in a medical history to a patient?
- What features of the extraoral head and neck examination might suggest systemic disease?
- What are the advantages and disadvantages of the various methods for testing the vitality of teeth? How is it possible to be certain about the vitality of a specific tooth?
- What features in the examination of the hands suggest systemic disease?
- How would you decide whether or not a lesion was appropriate for a biopsy in primary care?
- When is a punch biopsy appropriate in the mouth?
- Could you undertake a mucosal biopsy and submit the specimen for diagnosis correctly?
- What features in the history and examination would prompt you to send a biopsy for immunofluorescence testing?
- What is the difference between a screening and diagnostic test?
- What are the advantages of tests based on molecular biology (DNA and RNA sequence)?
- When would a plain radiograph be a better imaging technique than a cone beam or medical CT scan?
- Which blood investigations might be useful to investigate a patient with oral ulceration?
- How should a sample of pus for culture and antibiotic sensitivity be collected?
- When constructing a differential diagnosis, how would you decide the appropriate order for the various possible diagnoses?
- Which oral conditions may be diagnosed on the basis of the history alone?
- Which normal oral structures may be mistaken for lesions?

- What is the difference between a lesion, a disease and pathology?

SECTION 1

CHAPTER 2

- What are the causes of failure of eruption of teeth?
- What are the causes of early loss of deciduous teeth?
- How would you differentiate developmental defects of the teeth from those with other causes?
- Why are only females affected by vertical ridging of the teeth in some types of amelogenesis imperfecta?
- The challenges of restoring dentitions affected by amelogenesis imperfecta and dentinogenesis imperfecta are different. Explain why in terms of the tooth structure.
- How is molar-incisor hypomineralisation different from other presentations of defective enamel formation?
- What are the differences between dentinal dysplasia and dentinogenesis imperfecta?
- How might radiographic features of the jaws predict colon carcinoma?
- How would you distinguish tetracycline staining and fluorosis?
- How would you explain the risk of fluoride mottling to a patient?
- What might cause loss of tooth vitality shortly after eruption?

CHAPTER 3

- Why might a cleft palate indicate a cardiac defect? What are the underlying mechanisms that link these conditions?
- Why is the timing of cleft lip and palate surgery critical?
- What features in the medical history and examination might make you suspect a submucous cleft?
- What features of a Stafne bone cavity should allow confident radiological diagnosis?

CHAPTER 4

- How may caries be prevented by reference to the four major aetiological factors?
- Can caries activity be predicted by investigating the oral or plaque flora?
- How is the ecological plaque theory different from the specific pathogen theory of dental caries?
- If *Strep. mutans* did not exist, would caries develop?
- Can you explain how different sugars and differing bacterial flora affect the Stephan curve?

- Is frequency or amount of sugar intake more important in dental caries?
- What are the effects of dietary fluoride on dental caries?
- How does an intact layer of plaque over a carious lesion affect its structure?
- What is the importance of cavitation to the treatment of dental caries?
- How does enamel etching for restorative procedures differ from dental caries?
- How does the viability of the dentine and pulp protect against the sequelae of dental caries?
- How can the activity of an individual carious lesion be estimated clinically?
- How does knowledge of enamel caries influence treatment decisions?
- How does knowledge of dentine caries influence treatment decisions?
- How is the concept of minimally-invasive dentistry supported by the pathology of caries?
- How is infected and affected dentine identified clinically?
- Is a tax on sugary drinks justified?

CHAPTER 5

- How is pulpitis diagnosed and how may it be differentiated from periapical periodontitis?
- What conditions may mimic the symptoms of pulpitis?
- What operative procedures foster resolution of reversible pulpitis?
- Can you trace the possible pathways from pulpitis to life-threatening infection?
- Why, even when dental caries is untreated, are these life-threatening complications so rare?
- What is the aetiology of tooth-wear and how may it be associated with general health?
- Are there bacteria in a periapical granuloma
- What is the role of antibiotics in treatment of periapical periodontitis and periapical abscess?
- Are pulp stones of any significance?

CHAPTER 6

- Why do patients with erosion caused by dietary acid intake not usually have problems with excessive dental caries?
- Is there benefit in distinguishing attrition, abrasion and erosion?
- Does bruxism cause temporomandibular joint pain or myofascial pain?
- How does differentiating internal from external resorption aid treatment?
- What is the clinical significance of excess cementum?
- How long can an implant remain in situ?
- How does the absence of a periodontal ligament around an implant affect restoration and complications of implant placement?

CHAPTER 7

- How do the plaque flora and host immunological responses to plaque mature through life?

- Does the classification of periodontal diseases in current use aid treatment?
- What is the significance of the histological stages of gingivitis and periodontitis?
- How does the ecological plaque theory differ from the specific pathogen theory ?
- What is the rate of progression of chronic adult periodontitis?
- What conditions predispose to periodontitis in children and in adults?
- Which is the key host defence mechanism against periodontitis?
- What are the pathological differences between acute necrotising ulcerative gingivitis and chronic adult periodontitis?
- How does HIV infection predispose to periodontal destruction?
- What clinical features of gingivitis or periodontitis might suggest underlying HIV infection?
- Which systemic medical conditions may present with gingival signs and symptoms?
- A middle-aged adult presents with advancing periodontal destruction in a previously healthy mouth. How would you investigate this patient?
- What diseases have similar presentations to plaque-induced gingivitis and periodontitis?
- What gingival manifestations might lead to diagnosis of important systemic disease?

CHAPTER 8

- When and how might healing of an extraction socket lead you to suspect important underlying disease?
- Osteomyelitis of the jaws often has local or systemic predisposing causes. How would you identify these?
- How do the radiographic changes in osteomyelitis develop with time?
- What are the differences between chronic osteomyelitis and florid cemento-osseous dysplasia?
- Why is dry socket not considered a form of osteomyelitis?
- Why is chronic osteomyelitis difficult to treat?
- What is the role of antibiotics in osteomyelitis?
- Is proliferative periostitis an osteomyelitis?
- What medications cause osteonecrosis and how to they do this?

CHAPTER 9

- Which microbial species are associated with facial infections of odontogenic origin?
- Which of the various odontogenic soft tissue infections of the face may be life-threatening and why?
- What investigations are required when a patient presents with a soft tissue infection of suspected odontogenic origin?
- What determines whether a periapical granuloma progresses to a facial abscess?
- How do you determine when and which antibiotic to prescribe for a soft tissue swelling suspected of being an abscess?

- Can poor dental prescribing increase the risk of serious odontogenic infections?
- How is cavernous sinus thrombosis recognised and what are its dental causes?
- How does the presentation of deep fungal infections differ from bacterial infections?
- What systemic mycoses are important to dentistry in the part of the world where you practise?

CHAPTER 10

- What is cortication radiologically and what does it mean if a lesion is corticated?
- What features of the history and examination would lead you to suspect a cyst rather than any other localised radiolucency in the jaws?
- How may hyaline or Rushton bodies aid cyst diagnosis?
- When should you undertake an incisional biopsy of a cyst?
- When is a biopsy of a suspected cyst not indicated?
- Which cysts have diagnostic histological features?
- How does the growth pattern of a cyst aid diagnosis?
- What are the arguments for and against considering the odontogenic keratocyst to be an odontogenic tumour?
- How does the orthokeratinising odontogenic cyst differ from the odontogenic keratocyst?
- A young adult presents with bilateral odontogenic keratocysts. How would you investigate and manage this patient?
- Which types of cyst may recur following treatment?
- How would you differentiate an inflammatory collateral cyst from a dentigerous cyst?
- How is marsupialisation different from decompression?
- Is endodontic treatment effective for radicular cysts?
- How would you differentiate a sublingual dermoid cyst from a ranula?
- How may ranulas be treated conservatively?
- Why is the age of the patient critical in diagnosis of cystic neck swellings?

CHAPTER 11

- When presented with a lesion in the jaws, what features would suggest an odontogenic tumour rather than a cyst, primary bone tumour or other cause?
- How is a unicystic ameloblastoma defined and how may one be diagnosed?
- There is a recent tendency to try to treat ameloblastoma conservatively. How is this achieved and what are the advantages and disadvantages of this approach?
- Which odontogenic tumours would be expected to recur following removal by enucleation and curettage?
- Which odontogenic tumour might present as localised periodontitis?
- The odontogenic myxoma is benign but requires excision with a margin for effective treatment. Why?
- Which odontogenic tumours contain radiopacities?
- You notice a radiopaque lesion attached to the root of a tooth; how would you investigate and manage the patient?

- How would you investigate and treat a patient with a radiolucency in the posterior body of the mandible?
- Does the finding of Braf mutations in ameloblastoma have any significance?
- Does cemento-osseous dysplasia matter to a patient? How would you advise them?
- Why are only some ossifying fibromas considered odontogenic?

CHAPTER 12

- A lesion in a child is found to be a giant cell lesion on biopsy. How does the site affect treatment?
- How would you further investigate a patient whose intra-osseous lesion proved to be a giant cell lesion on biopsy?
- How can surgery for giant cell granuloma be avoided? How would you advise a patient making a decision on treatment?
- What radiological features might suggest an intra-osseous haemangioma?
- How does the clinical course of osteosarcoma of the jaws differ from that of osteosarcoma of the long bones?
- How does the position of a radiolucency either above or below the inferior dental canal aid differential diagnosis?
- It is often said that a sharply demarcated radiopaque lesion in bone is almost certainly benign. Is this correct?
- What clinical features help differentiate benign from malignant neoplasms of the jaws?

CHAPTER 13

- How is osteogenesis imperfecta linked to dentinogenesis imperfecta and why are the teeth not affected in some types of osteogenesis imperfecta?
- What are the causes of failure of eruption of teeth?
- What abnormalities are seen in the bones and teeth in the different forms of rickets?
- What investigations would aid the differentiation of a central giant cell granuloma from a brown tumour of hyperparathyroidism?
- What conditions may be confused with Paget's disease radiographically and how may they be differentiated?
- What is the cause of fibrous dysplasia and how may it be differentiated from cemento-ossifying fibroma?

CHAPTER 14

- How would you investigate a patient with trismus?
- How would you investigate a patient complaining of limited jaw opening?
- How would you investigate a patient complaining of locking of the temporomandibular joint?
- What radiographs and other imaging techniques are appropriate for assessment of the temporomandibular joints?
- Does a normal temporomandibular joint radiograph exclude joint disease?
- How would you investigate and treat a case of temporomandibular pain dysfunction syndrome with particular emphasis on excluding organic disease?

SECTION 2

CHAPTER 15

- How do you distinguish an ulcer from a white patch or other mucosal alteration?
- What features of oral ulcers would suggest viral infection as the cause?
- What tests are available to identify the presence of viral infection? For which orofacial infections might they be diagnostic?
- What treatment and advice would be appropriate for the parent of a child with primary *Herpes simplex* infection?
- What are the significant complications of *Herpes zoster* infection of the head and neck?
- A child has small ulcers on the palate suggestive of viral infection. How would you investigate them? Should they be advised to take time off school?
- Are universal infection control procedures sufficient for a patient with oral primary syphilis?
- Why do candidal infections tend to recur?
- A patient presents with angular stomatitis. How should they be investigated and treated and what would you do if treatment failed?
- Is dental prescribing of antifungal agents as important as antimicrobial stewardship for antibacterial prescribing?

CHAPTER 16

- How may a traumatic ulcer be differentiated from squamous cell carcinoma?
- How would you investigate a patient with recurrent aphthous stomatitis to exclude underlying predisposing causes?
- What treatments are available for recurrent aphthous stomatitis? What are their advantages and disadvantages?
- What drugs can lead to oral ulcers?
- What questions would you ask a patient to pursue the possible diagnosis of Behçet's disease?
- Which chronic mucosal diseases cause persistent ulcers?
- How may lichen planus and lichenoid reactions be differentiated?
- What is the value of biopsy in the diagnosis of lichen planus?
- How would you investigate a patient with desquamative gingivitis to differentiate the possible causes?
- What are the similarities and differences between the lesions of lupus erythematosus and lichen planus?
- How may the chronic ulcers of vesiculobullous diseases be differentiated from those in lichen planus?
- What special precautions are required when taking a biopsy for the diagnosis of pemphigus or pemphigoid?
- Primary herpetic gingivostomatitis and severe erythema multiforme may present with similar lesions. How would you differentiate these two conditions?

CHAPTER 17

- Which laboratory investigations may aid diagnosis for a patient with a sore but apparently normal tongue?
- What conditions would you consider as possible causes of a sore red tongue?

- How many distinctive oral presentations of candidosis can you identify?
- Why is a smear for microscopy a better diagnostic test than microbiological culture in candidal infection?

CHAPTER 18

- List the white patches that affect the oral mucosa. How may they be differentiated?
- Would any special precautions be necessary to undertake a biopsy of suspected oral hairy leukoplakia?

CHAPTER 19

- Which white lesions of the oral mucosa carry a risk of malignant transformation?
- Which white lesions of the oral mucosa carry no significant risk of malignant transformation?
- What diseases cause red patches of the oral mucosa?
- Which conditions presenting as red patches carry a risk of malignant transformation?
- What investigations would be appropriate for a patient presenting with an oral white lesion?
- Why is a biopsy considered mandatory for all oral white lesions?
- How does biopsy aid the diagnosis and management of risk of malignant transformation?
- What are the earliest signs of oral squamous carcinoma and how do they differ from those in the later stages of the disease?
- What interventions would be appropriate for a patient with a dysplastic oral lesion?
- How would you select the appropriate area of a red or white patch for biopsy?
- How would you decide whether a red or white lesion was suitable for biopsy in a general practice setting?
- What information about a red or white lesion should be provided to the histopathologist after biopsy?
- Is human papilloma virus a cause of oral potentially malignant lesions?
- How is smoking cessation made effective in dental practice?

CHAPTER 20

- What public health measures might reduce the incidence of oral carcinoma? Why are they so difficult to implement?
- What is the difference between staging and grading of carcinomas?
- How is oral squamous carcinoma staged and what is the importance of the stage for treatment and survival?
- How can the general dental practitioner contribute to the management of a patient with oral squamous carcinoma?
- Are any young patients at particular risk of oral squamous carcinoma?
- How may the dental practitioner contribute to the prevention of oral carcinoma?
- Why does oral squamous carcinoma have such a high mortality?
- How does the growth and spread of oral carcinoma determine treatment?

- How does the growth and spread of oral carcinoma cause death?
- Is it ethical to promote a low risk tobacco habit as preferable to a high risk habit?
- Which benign oral lesions may be mistaken for carcinoma, either clinically or histologically?

CHAPTER 21

- What advice and guidance should a dentist provide to prevent lip carcinomas?
- Do human papillomavirus (HPV) carcinomas arise in any identifiable potentially malignant conditions in the oropharynx or mouth?
- Why might an HPV-associated carcinoma have a better prognosis than a tobacco induced carcinoma?
- Why might virally induced carcinomas be so much more common in Eastern countries?

CHAPTER 22

- What are the causes of 'meal-time syndrome'?
- What investigations aid the differentiation of salivary calculi from salivary duct strictures?
- What other lesions may resemble a mucous extravasation in the lower lip?
- What investigations aid the diagnosis of mumps? For how long is the condition infectious?
- How would you identify possible causes of dehydration in a patient with dry mouth?
- Does the clinical presentation of dry mouth aid the differential diagnosis of its possible causes?
- What combination of laboratory investigations would be required to make a diagnosis of Sjögren's syndrome?
- What is the role of the general dental practitioner in management of dry mouth?
- What is the role of the hospital dental specialties in the management of Sjögren's syndrome?
- What is the importance of sudden salivary swelling in a patient with Sjögren's syndrome? How would you investigate a patient with this complaint?
- A young adult presents with bilateral salivary gland swelling. What features in the history, examination and special investigations aid your differential diagnosis?

CHAPTER 23

- What are the potential complications of an incisional biopsy of the parotid gland?
- A young adult presents with a unilateral salivary gland swelling. What features in the history, examination and special investigations aid your differential diagnosis?
- Which salivary gland swellings should be subjected to incisional biopsy and which should not? Explain why.
- What alternative investigations might you consider when a biopsy of a mass in a salivary gland is contraindicated?
- What features of a salivary neoplasm would suggest that it is malignant?
- A 35-year-old male presents with an ulcerated mass on the palate. Discuss the differential diagnosis and appropriate investigations.

- How is a sialogram performed? What information can a sialogram provide?
- How may ultrasound aid the diagnosis of swellings of the head and neck?
- There are so many salivary neoplasms. Does it really matter which one a patient has, provided it is clear whether it is benign or malignant?

CHAPTER 24

- What are the common causes of nodular lesions of the attached gingiva?
- What happens to fibrous hyperplastic lesions if left untreated?
- How would you differentiate a pyogenic granuloma from a Kaposi's sarcoma?

CHAPTER 25

- Why is it important to know about the pathology of the granular cell tumour?
- Does a lymphangioma differ from a cystic hygroma?
- How might you check a lesion for potentially dangerous vascularity before biopsy?
- Many lesions are called haemangiomas. Why is their terminology so confusing and which lesions, if any, are benign neoplasms as suggested by the name?

CHAPTER 26

- Which features in the history, examination and investigations would allow the differential diagnosis of oral pigmented lesions?
- Which oral pigmented lesions should be subjected to biopsy and why?
- What features of an oral pigmented lesion suggest melanoma?
- How are syndromic pigmented lesions recognised?

SECTION 3
CHAPTER 27

- How would you investigate a patient presenting with a sore uniformly depapillated tongue?
- How would you differentiate the various causes of anaemia using investigations?
- Which malignant neoplasms may present as gingival swellings or gingival enlargement?
- How might a dentist notice the first signs of lymphoma or leukaemia?
- What are the oral complications of chemotherapy for lymphoma and leukaemia?

CHAPTER 28

- How would you manage a patient presenting with post-extraction haemorrhage?
- How may post-extraction haemorrhage be prevented?
- How does the management of patients on newer anticoagulants differ from that for those taking warfarin?

CHAPTER 29

- Is an HIV-infected dentist safe to practice?
- What systemic complications of HIV infections may impact the provision of routine dental care?
- Which oral lesions might raise suspicion of immunodeficiency?
- How do the presentations of gingivitis and periodontitis in patients with immunodeficiency differ from those in normal patients?

CHAPTER 30

- How would you investigate and manage a patient with an enlarged upper lip?
- Discuss non-infectious occupational risks of the practice of dentistry. How may they be prevented?
- If lupus erythematosus was suspected, what questions might reveal evidence of systemic disease?

CHAPTER 31

- Which features of an enlarged cervical lymph node would suggest malignancy?
- Which features of an enlarged cervical lymph node would suggest a reactive cause?
- How may tuberculosis present in the head and neck?
- What investigations should be performed to aid diagnosis for a patient with a chronically enlarged cervical lymph node? What is the value of each test?
- Which causes of lymph node swelling are more important in children and young adults as opposed to the elderly?
- Does a history of bacille Calmette-Guérin (BCG) vaccination exclude tuberculosis as a cause of an enlarged lymph node?
- How does the neck level and site of an enlarged lymph node provide information about possible causes?

CHAPTER 32

- Why has the recommended antibiotic prophylaxis for infective endocarditis in dental patients changed over the last few years?
- What other measures should be taken instead of antibiotic prophylaxis in the prevention of infective endocarditis in dentistry?
- How and why has the prevalence of the different risk factors for infective endocarditis changed over the last decades?
- How will you explain to a patient why they may no longer be offered antibiotic prophylaxis for dental treatment?

CHAPTER 33

- When should antibiotics be prescribed for acute or chronic sinusitis?
- How would you diagnose and treat an oroantral communication?
- What are granulomas and why do they form?
- Are there connections among granulomas, granulation tissue and pyogenic granuloma?
- Which diseases of the head and neck, excluding the oral mucosa, show granulomatous inflammation histologically?
- Discuss the differential diagnosis for a patient with diffuse enlargement of the gingiva.
- How might a carcinoma in the maxillary antrum present to a dentist?

CHAPTER 34

- How may a patient with hepatitis B or C be identified and their infectivity assessed?
- Is a hepatitis B vaccination sufficient protection for the dentist against hepatitis?
- What are the causes of lip swelling?
- What are the causes of granulomatous inflammation in the oral mucosa?
- What is the difference between oral Crohn's disease and orofacial granulomatosis?

CHAPTERS 35, 36 AND 37

- Are any nutritional supplements of benefit to the oral health of the normal population?
- How does diabetes mellitus affect the provision of dental treatment?
- What are the causative connections between endocrine disease and gingival enlargement?
- How might a dentist aid diagnosis of thyroid diseases, including neoplasms?
- How would you recognise a patient with multiple endocrine neoplasia syndrome?
- How does renal dialysis affect the mouth and dental treatment?

CHAPTER 38

- How easy is it to completely exclude dental causes for pain?
- Now that burning mouth is considered a neuralgia, should primary and secondary forms be identified?
- Is occlusal adjustment effective in migraine?
- How may dental causes for facial pain be identified?
- What are the features of pain of vascular origin and how do they differ from those of pain of neural origin?
- How can the dentist help a patient with loss of taste or smell?
- What information would you record in the medical history of an epileptic patient and why?
- How would you decide whether or not to refer a patient with intractable pain to their medical practitioner?
- For which types of facial pain might a computerised tomogram or magnetic resonance scan be indicated?
- How may atypical facial pain be identified and how should it be treated?
- What analgesics might be prescribed by a dentist to treat orofacial pain?

CHAPTER 39

- What features of Down's syndrome might affect provision of dental treatment?

- Explain handicap, disability and impairment using examples in dentistry.
- Why do normal behaviour management techniques not work in children with autism?
- How must dental treatment be adapted for a patient with each disorder in this chapter?
- In which conditions is there an increased risk of trauma to teeth and oral tissues? How may this be managed?

CHAPTER 40

- How may anxiety about dental treatment be managed?
- How is depression linked to central pain and what are mechanisms?
- How do drugs for mental illness impact on dental treatment?
- How may depression present in a dental setting?

CHAPTER 41

- How might a dentist aid the diagnosis of diseases common in the elderly?
- How may preventive regimens be adapted to suit patients with the conditions in this chapter?
- How may consent for dental treatment be obtained in patients with learning difficulties or mental illness?

- Why are patients with renal disease prone to latex allergy?
- How does Parkinson's disease impact on oral health?

CHAPTER 42

- Which drugs can cause lichen planus–like reactions?
- Which drugs can cause symptoms of burning mouth?
- Which drugs can cause oral or facial pigmentation?

CHAPTER 43

- How would you differentiate the causes of loss of consciousness?
- How would you treat each of the medical emergencies listed in this chapter?
- In each case, which of the actions are most critical to a successful outcome?
- What adverse effects might ensue if you inadvertently administered the wrong treatment for a medical emergency?
- Where could you check the current Resuscitation Council UK guidelines for basic life support?
- Are you able to use an automatic defibrillator?

Index

Page numbers followed by "*f*" indicate figures, "*t*" indicate tables, and "*b*" indicate boxes.

A

ABCDE approach, to emergencies, *507*
Abfraction, *87*
Abrasion, *85–86, 85f–86f*
Abscess
  antibiotic, *133, 516t–520t*
  apical, acute, *79–81, 80f*
  dentoalveolar, *79–81, 80f*
  periapical, *129*
    acute, *82*
    chronic, *82f*
  periodontal, *107b, 110, 110f–111f, 474*
  submasseteric, *223*
Absence (petit mal) seizure, *484*
Acanthomatous ameloblastoma, *167, 167f*
Acesulfame K, *59t*
Achondroplasia, *207–208, 208b*
Aciclovir, *237–238*
Acid
  bacterial, *53*
  production in plaque, *56–57*
Acinar cells, *355*
Acinic cell carcinoma, *362, 362f*
Acquired clotting defects, *403–404, 403b*
Acquired immunodeficiency syndrome (AIDS), *408–411, 408f, 433*
  clinical course of, *410*
  diagnosis of, *410*
  key features of, *412b*
  purpura associated with, *401*
  tuberculosis and, *242*
Acquired melanocytic naevi, *384*
Acromegaly, *211, 463–464, 463f–464f*
Actinomyces species, in gingivitis, *98*
Actinomycosis, *135–136, 135f, 136b*
Acute angina, *437*
Acute disseminated Langerhans cell histiocytosis, *190–192, 190t*
Acute myelomonocytic leukaemia, gingival swellings in, *115–116, 115f–116f*
Acute osteomyelitis, of jaws, *120–122, 121b*
  clinical features of, *120–121, 121f*
  complications and resolution for, *122, 122b*
  management of, *121–122, 122b*
  pathology of, *121, 121f–122f*
Acute pericoronitis, *110–112, 111b, 111f*
Acute sinusitis, *443, 443f*

Addison's disease, *383, 466–467, 466b, 467f*
Additional teeth, *24–25*
  effects and treatment of, *25*
Adenocarcinoma
  basal cell, *367t–368t*
  polymorphous, *362–363, 362f*
Adenoid cystic carcinoma, *361, 361f*
Adenolymphoma, *359*
Adenoma
  basal cell, *359*
  canalicular, *359*
  pleomorphic, *357–358, 357f–358f, 358b*
Adenomatoid odontogenic tumours, *172, 172b, 172f, 516t–520t*
Adjunctive treatment, for acute osteomyelitis, *122*
Adrenaline, *438*
Adrenocortical hypofunction, *466–467*
Adults
  caries in, *69*
  gingival cyst of, *158, 158f*
Agranulocytosis, *109, 398, 408*
Albright's syndrome, *216, 218*
Alcian blue, *14*
Alcohol
  abuse, *506*
  in oral cancer, *320, 320f*
Alkaline phosphatase, hypophosphatasia, *209–210*
Allergic angio-oedema, *423*
Allergic fungal sinusitis, *444–445*
Allergic reactions, *419–422*
Allergy, *419–427*
  latex, *420–421, 421b*
  to local anaesthetic, *421–422*
  mercury, *422–423, 423f*
  metals, *422–423*
  nickel, *422*
Allopurinol, adverse effects of, *504t–505t*
Alpha-thalassaemias, *393*
Alternaria sp., *444*
Alveolar bone
  destruction of, *102, 104f*
  in elderly, *501–502*
  resorption, *100b*
Alveolar mucosa, *96*
Alveolar osteitis, *117–120*
  aetiology of, *117–119, 119b*
  clinical features of, *119, 119f*
  pathology of, *119*
  prevention of, *119–120, 120b*
  treatment of, *120, 120b*
Alveolar rhabdomyosarcomas, *380*

Alveolar ridge, carcinomas in, *326*
Amalgam restorations, *423*
Amalgam tattoo, *386–387, 387f*
Amelanotic melanomas, *389*
Ameloblastic carcinoma, *183, 183f*
Ameloblastic fibro-odontome, *173*
Ameloblastic fibrodentinoma, *173*
Ameloblastic fibroma, *172, 173b, 173f, 516t–520t*
Ameloblastic fibrosarcoma, *183, 185f*
Ameloblastomas, *165–168, 165b, 166f*
  acanthomatous, *167, 167f*
  behaviour and treatment of, *168*
  desmoplastic, *168–169, 169f*
  follicular, *166–167, 167f*
  granular, *167, 168f*
  islands of, *167, 168f*
  key features of, *168b*
  maxillary, *168*
  metastasising, *169*
  pathology of, *166–168*
  plexiform, *166–167, 167f*
  solid/multicystic, *165–166, 166f*
  unicystic, *169–170, 169f–170f*
Amelogenesis imperfecta, *25–28, 29f*
Amyloid deposition, *200*
Amyloidosis, *200, 287–288, 287f–288f, 287t*
  of tongue, *516t–520t*
Anaemia, *391–392*
  aplastic, *398*
  clinical features of, *391, 391b*
  pernicious, *391*
  in recurrent aphthae, *392*
  resistance to infection and, *392*
  sickle cell, *391–393*
  types of, *391t*
Anaerobes, suppurative parotitis, *344*
Anaesthesia
  general, dangers of, *392*
  of lower lip, *479–480, 480b*
Analgesia, local, *437–438, 437f*
Anaphylactic reactions, *508–509, 508b–509b*
Aneurysmal bone cyst, *188b, 220–221, 220b, 220f*
Angina
  acute, *437*
  Ludwig's, *131–132, 132f*
Angina bullosa haemorrhagica, *400, 400f, 516t–520t*
Angina pectoris, *511, 511b*
Angio-oedema, *421t, 423*
Angiofollicular lymph node hyperplasia, *434*
Angiomatosis, bacillary, *413*

Angiotensin-converting enzyme inhibitors, adverse effects of, 504t–505t
Angular stomatitis, 246, 246f
anaemia in, 392
Anhidrotic (hereditary) ectodermal dysplasia, 23–24, 24b, 24f
Ankyloglossia, 49–50, 50f, 516t–520t
Ankylosing spondylitis, 228
Ankylosis
temporomandibular joint and, 223, 226
and tooth resorption, 88
treatment of, 226
Anodontia, 23
isolated, 23
with systemic defects, 23–24
Anorexia nervosa, 497
Antibiotic stomatitis, 246–247, 247f
Antibiotics
abscess, 516t–520t
adverse effects of, 504t–505t
prophylaxis see Prophylaxis
Antibodies, periodontitis and, 103
Anticoagulants, adverse effects of, 504t–505t
Antifungals, adverse effects of, 504t–505t
Antihistamines, adverse effects of, 504t–505t
Antimalarials, adverse effects of, 504t–505t
Antimicrobial treatment, of acute osteomyelitis, 122
Antineutrophil cytoplasmic antibodies (ANCA), 447
Antiretroviral drugs, 411b
see also Highly active anti-retroviral treatment (HAART)
Antral carcinoma, 449f
Antral polyp, 446, 446f
Antrum, maxillary see Maxillary antrum
Anxiety disorders, 496, 496b
Apatite crystals, 61
Aphthous stomatitis, 256–259, 256t, 258f
aetiology of, 257–258, 258b
clinical features of, 256–257
diagnosis of, 258, 259t
features of, 256b
herpetiform, 257, 257f
major form, 257, 257f
treatment for, 259
management of, 258–259
minor form, 256–257, 256f
pathology of, 258
types of, 257b
Aphthous ulcers, in AIDS/HIV, 416f
Apical periodontitis, 53
acute, 78–79, 78f
clinical features of, 78
pathology of, 78–79
possible complications of, 79b
sequelae, 78–79, 79f
chronic, 81–83
clinical features of, 81, 81f

outcomes for, 83b
pathology of, 81, 81f–82f
treatment and sequelae of, 81–83, 82f
Apixaban, 404
Aplastic anaemia, 398
Appliances, for bruxism, 87
Artefactual polyp, 12f
Arteritis, temporal, 476
Arthralgia, 224
Arthritis, 226
oral signs in, reactive, 277–278, 277f
osteoarthritis, 227–228, 228b, 228f, 502
other types of, 228
psoriatic, 228
rheumatoid, 226–227, 424, 424b
suppurative, 223
Aspartame, 59t
Asperger's syndrome, 491
Aspergillus spp., 444
Aspirin, adverse effects of, 504t–505t
Asthma, 422, 447, 447b
severe, 512
Ataxia, 492
Atherosclerosis, 107b
Athetosis, 492
Atopic dermatitis (eczema), 419
Atopic disease, 419
effects of drugs used for, 419b
Atopy, 419
Atrophic candidosis, 246
Attached gingiva, 95–96, 95b
Attention deficit hyperactivity disorder, 491
Attrition, 85, 85f
Atypical facial pain, 479, 479b
Atypical odontalgia, 479
Autism, 491, 491b
Autoantibodies, 424
in Sjögren's syndrome, 348t
Autoimmune disease, 414, 419–427
Autoimmune polyendocrine syndrome I, 250–251, 250b
Autoimmune polyendocrine syndromes, 467
Autoinflammatory disease, 423–425
types and examples of, 424b
typical features of, 424b

B

B-cell lymphoma, immunostaining techniques for, 17t
B lymphocytes, 407
Bacillary angiomatosis, 413
Bacteraemias, 438
Bacteria, associated with chronic periodontitis, 100b
Bacterial infections, in AIDS/HIV, 413
Bacterial parotitis, 344–345, 344f
Bacterial plaque see Plaque
Bacterial polysaccharides, 55–56

Bacteriological diagnosis, of acute osteomyelitis, 122
Bacteroides, 121
Bartonella henselae, 432
Basal cell adenocarcinoma, 367t–368t
Basal cell adenoma, 359
Basal cell carcinoma, of skin, 516t–520t
Basal cell naevus syndrome, 153–154, 154b, 154f, 516t–520t
Basic life support (BLS), 509b, 510
Behavioural disorders, 491
Behçet's disease, 259–261, 516t–520t
erythema nodosum in, 260f
International Criteria for, 260t
Bell's palsy, 478, 480–481, 481f
Bence-Jones proteinuria, 199
Benign chronic white mucosal lesions, 291–297
Benign epithelial tumours, 165–176
Benign mesenchymal tumours, 177–179
Benign nerve sheath tumours, 377
Benign tumours, 377–380
Beta-thalassaemias, 393
Betel quid, 319t
in oral cancer, 320
Biofilm, 53
Biopsy, 11
brush, 13–14, 14b
essential principles of, 13b
fine needle aspiration, 13, 13b
frozen section technique, 13, 13b
site, selecting, 11
types of, 11b
Biopsy punch, 12
Bipolaris sp., 444
Bisphosphonate-induced osteonecrosis, 125, 126b, 127f
Bisphosphonates
adverse effects of, 504t–505t
Paget's disease, 213
Black tongue, 285
Bleeding disorders, combined, 404
Bleeding, prolonged, 513
Blood blisters, 273
Blood investigations see Haematology
Blood vessel abnormalities, 399–401
Bloodstream metastasis, in oral cancer, 325, 325b
Blue naevus, 384
Bohn's nodules, 157–158, 158f
Bone
cysts, 218–221
aneurysmal, 220–221, 220b, 220f
solitary, 218–220, 219b, 219f
dead, 121
destruction, 212f
genetic diseases of, 205–221, 205b
haemangioma of, 194–195, 195f
malignant neoplasms of, 196–202
non-odontogenic tumours of, 187, 187b
resorbing factors, 101, 101t
radicular cyst and, 143
resorption, 99, 213–214

Bone islands, sclerotic, *128, 128f*
Bone marrow
    osteoporotic defect, *221, 221f*
    transplantation, *408, 408b*
Borrelia burgdorferi, 432
Botryoid odontogenic cysts, *155–156, 155b, 155f–156f*
Botulinum toxin, for bruxism, *88*
Branchial clefts, *161–162*
Branchial cyst, *161–162, 162f*
Brittle bone disease, *205*
Bronchogenic carcinoma, *449–450*
Brown spot lesion, inactive, *69*
Brush biopsy, *13–14, 14b*
    in oral cancer, *333*
Bruxism, *87–88*
    daytime, *87*
    effects of, *87b*
    features of, *87b*
    management of, *87–88*
    nocturnal, *87*
Buccal mucosa, carcinomas in, *326*
Bulimia nervosa, *497*
Bullous pemphigoid, *275*
Burkitt's lymphoma, *395–396, 396f, 414*
Burning mouth 'syndrome,' , *478, 478b–479b*
Burns, chemical, *279f*

C

Calcific barriers, in pulpitis, *74, 76f*
Calcifications, pulp, *77*
Calcifying epithelial odontogenic tumours, *170–171, 171b, 171f*
Calcifying odontogenic cysts, *156–157, 156f–158f, 157b, 176, 176b*
Calcium
    hyperparathyroidism and, *211*
    as plaque minerals, *57*
Calcium channel blockers, adverse effects of, *504t–505t*
Calculus
    salivary, *341–342, 341f, 342b*
    subgingival
        in gingivitis, *98, 98f*
        in periodontitis, *99*
Caldwell-Luc approach, *445*
Calibre-persistent artery, *375, 375f–376f*
Canalicular adenoma, *359*
Cancellous osteoma, *192*
    of mandible, *192f*
Cancer, oral, *317–334*
    aetiology of, *318–321, 318b*
    age and gender incidence of, *317, 317f*
    alcohol in, *320, 320f*
    causes of death in, *331*
    clinicopathological features and behaviour of, *325b*
    dentist in, role of, *331–332, 332b, 332t*
    diagnostic catches in, *334*

diet in, *320–321*
distribution of, *322, 323f*
'early' and 'late,' , *321–322, 321f–322f, 322t*
epidemiology of, *317, 317f*
genetic predisposition in, *321*
histopathology in, *322–323, 323f–324f*
immunosuppression in, *320*
infections in, *320*
key features of, *318b*
local spread of, *323–324, 324f*
malnutrition in, *320–321*
management of, *326–331, 326b*
    novel treatments for, *331*
    outcome of, *329–330, 330b, 330f*
    palliative care for, *331*
    preoperative assessment for, *326, 328t*
    survivorship in, *331*
    treatment failure in, *331*
    treatment for, *326–329, 328b, 328f*
metastasis in, *324–325*
other habits in, *321*
pathology of, *322–326*
patients without risk factors in, *321*
poor oral health in, *321*
potentially malignant disorders in, *321*
screening of, *332–333*
site variation in, *325–326*
tobacco use in, *318–320*
UK patient 'pathway' for, *327t*
see also Carcinoma
Cancrum oris, *134, 134f–135f*
Candida sp., 244
Candidosis, *244–251, 244b*
    acute antibiotic stomatitis, *246–247, 247f*
    in AIDS/HIV, *412–413, 412f*
    anaemia in, *392*
    angular stomatitis, *246, 246f*
    chronic, *299t*
    chronic hyperplastic, *249–250, 249f, 296*
    chronic mucocutaneous, *296*
    denture-induced stomatitis, *248–249, 248b, 248f*
    erythematous, *246, 246b, 246f*
    management of types of, *252f*
    thrush, *244–245, 245b, 245f, 296*
    tongue, *285*
Capillary haemangioma, *379, 379f*
Captopril, *504t–505t*
    lichenoid reaction to, *503, 503f*
Carbamazepine
    adverse effects of, *504t–505t*
    for trigeminal neuralgia, *477*
Carbonated drinks, and erosion, *86*
Carcinoma
    acinic cell, *362, 362f*
    adenoid cystic, *361, 361f*
    ameloblastic, *183, 183f*
    clear cell, *367t–368t*

epithelial-myoepithelial, *363*
ex pleomorphic adenoma, *363, 363f*
human papillomavirus-associated oropharyngeal, *335–339, 336f–338f*
lip, *335, 335f–336f*
lymph node, *429*
lymphoepithelial, *367t–368t*
maxillary antrum, *448–449*
metastatic
    bronchogenic, *201f*
    of mandible, *201f*
mucoepidermoid, *360–361*
myoepithelial, *367t–368t*
nasopharyngeal, *339*
oncocytic, *367t–368t*
remote, *383*
salivary duct, *363*
second primary, *330*
secretory, *362*
squamous, *321f–324f, 322t, 323, 327t*
squamous cell, *367t–368t*
of tonsil, *337f–338f*
undifferentiated, *363*
verrucous, *333–334, 333f*
Carcinoma in situ, *309–310*
Cardiac arrest, *509–510, 509b*
Cardiopulmonary resuscitation, *510, 510b*
Cardiovascular disease, *437–441*
    dental implications/side-effects of drugs used for, *437t*
    in elderly, *502*
    general aspects of management, *437–438*
Caries
    in elderly, *501*
    prevalence and mottling of, *40f*
Cartilage-capped osteoma, *187–188*
Castleman's disease, *434–435, 435f*
Cat-scratch disease, *432, 432b, 432f*
Cathepsin C gene, *110*
Cavernous haemangioma, *379, 379f*
Cavernous sinus thrombosis, *133, 516t–520t*
Cavitation, *64, 64f–65f*
    radicular cyst and, *143*
CD4 cells, *409*
Cellulitis, *223*
    facial, *130–132, 131f–132f, 133b*
Cemento-osseous dysplasias, *181–183, 218*
Cemento-ossifying fibroma, *180–181, 180f–181f, 193, 193t*
    juvenile, *181*
    management of, *180*
    microscopy of, *180*
    multiple, *181*
    syndromic, *181, 181t*
Cementoblastoma, *178–179, 179b, 179f*
Cementomas, *179, 179b*
Cementum, *91*
    cellular, *91*
    cervical, *70*

Central giant cell granuloma, *188b*

Cerebral palsy, *491–492, 492b*

Cerebrovascular accidents, *482*

Cervical lymphadenopathy, *429–436, 429b, 429f*
  investigation of, *429–430, 430b*
  tuberculous, *430–431, 430b*

C1esterase inhibitor deficiency, *408*

Cetuximab, for oral cancer, *329*

Challacombe scale, for assessing dry mouth, *346t*

Cheek, biting, *293, 293f*

Chemical burns, *279f*

Chemical dependence, *505–506, 506b*

Chemicals, corrosive, and erosion, *86*

Chemistry, clinical, *18*

Chemoradiotherapy, for human papillomavirus-associated oropharyngeal carcinomas, *338*

Chemotherapy, for oral cancer, *329*

Cherubism, *188b, 208–209, 209f–210f, 210b*

Chest pain, *511*

Chewing tobacco, *319t*

Chicken pox, *241–242*

Chicken tongue, *224–225*

Children, resuscitation of, *510*

Chimarrão, in oral cancer, *321*

Chlorhexidine, *259*
  adverse effects of, *504t–505t*

Cholesterol clefts, in radicular cyst, *143, 144f*

Cholesterol crystals, in radicular cyst, *145f*

Chondromatosis, synovial, *229, 229f*

Chondrosarcoma, *197–198, 198f*

Chorioretinitis, *433*

Christmas disease, *403*

Chromium allergy, *422*

Chronic candidosis, *299t*
  in oral cancer, *320*

Chronic gingivitis, *96–99*
  clinical features of, *97, 97b, 97f*
  management of, *98, 99f*
  microbiology of, *97–98*
  pathology of, *97, 97b, 97f*
  pregnancy and, *99*
  systemic predisposing factors of, *99*

Chronic hyperplastic candidosis, *304*

Chronic hyperplastic gingivitis, *97*

Chronic mucocutaneous candidosis syndromes, *250–251, 250f*

Chronic multifocal Langerhans cell histiocytosis, *190, 190t*

Chronic obstructive airways disease (COAD), *447*

Chronic osteomyelitis, *122–123, 123b, 123f*

Chronic renal failure, *471, 471b*

Chronic sialadenitis, *345, 345f*

Chronic sinusitis, *443–445, 444f*

Chronic unifocal Langerhans cell histiocytosis, *190t*

Chronological hypoplasia, *29–30, 30f–31f*

Chvostek's sign, *466*

Cicatricial pemphigoid, *273*

Ciclosporin, adverse effects of, *504t–505t*

Cigarette smoking, in oral cancer, *318–319*

Cinnamon stomatitis, in lichenoid reactions, *269*

Circulatory collapse, *510–511, 511b*

Circumvallate papillae, *7t*

Claudication, jaw, *231*

Clavicles, absence of, *208f*

Clear cell carcinoma, *367t–368t*

Clear cell odontogenic carcinoma, *183, 184f*

Cleft lip, *45–48*
  dental defects, *48*
  management of, *47–48, 47b*

Cleft palate, *45–48, 47f*
  dental defects, *48*
  management of, *47–48, 47b, 48f*

Clefts of lip or palate, *45–48, 45b*
  development of, *45, 46f*
  sites of, *45, 47f*
  types of, *45, 46f*

Cleidocranial dysplasia, *208, 208b, 208f–209f*

Clinical chemistry, *18*

Clinical differential diagnosis, *8–9*

Closed questions, *1t*

Clostridium difficile, *454*

Clot, formation of, *117*

Clotting disorders, *402–403, 402b*
  acquired, *403–404, 403b*

Cluster headache, *482–483*

Cocaine, abuse, *506*

Codman's triangles, *196*

Coeliac disease, *451*

Cold sores, *238*

Colitis
  pseudomembranous, *454*
  ulcerative, *453–454*

Collateral oedema, *129, 129f*

Combined bleeding disorders, *404*

Compact osteoma, *192f*

Complex odontoma, *174, 174f–175f*

Compound odontoma, *174, 174f–175f*

Computerised tomography (CT), *10t*
  with contrast medium, *10t*

Concrescence, *91, 92f*

Condylar hyperplasia, *228–229, 229f, 516t–520t*

Condylar neck fracture, *223*

Condyles, rheumatoid arthritis and, *227*

Cone beam CT, *10t*

Congenital epulis, *378, 379f*

Congenital naevi, *384*

Congenital syphilis, *36–37, 37f*

Connective tissue diseases, *424*

Consciousness, sudden loss of, *507–511*

Consent, *5–6, 6t*

Consumption coagulopathy, *404*

Contact dermatitis, *419–420, 420b, 420f*

Conventional radiography, *10t*

Convulsions, *512–513*

Core or needle biopsy, *11–12, 12b*

Corticosteroids, *470*
  adverse effects of, *504t–505t*
  circulatory collapse, *510–511, 511b*
  recurrent aphthae, *259*

Corundum, *387*

Cosmetic implants, *376, 376f*

Coumarin anticoagulants, *403–404, 403b*

Cowden's syndrome, *50, 50f*

Cracked teeth, *474*
  as cause of pulpitis, *73, 73f*

Craniofacial malformations, *50, 51t*

CREST syndrome, *225*

Cretinism, *464*

Crohn's disease, *451, 452f, 453b, 459f*

Cryptococcosis, *136*

Curettage, of cysts, *142*

Cushing's disease, *467, 467b*

CUSP, *270*

Cyclamate, *59t*

Cyclic neutropenia, *398*

Cystadenocarcinoma, *367t–368t*

Cystic fibrosis, *449*

Cysts
  bone *see* Bone, cysts
  definition of, *139b*
  infected, *142*
  in jaws *see* Jaw(s), cysts in
  salivary, *342–344*

Cytology, exfoliative, *13–14*

Cytomegalovirus
  in AIDS/HIV, *414*
  associated with ulcers, *240*

Cytotoxic chemotherapy, *38*

Cytotoxic drugs, adverse effects of, *504t–505t*

D

Dabigatran, *404*

Dane particle, *455*

Darier's disease, *279t*

Dark zone, *62*

Dead bone, *121*

Dead tracts, *67t, 69f*

Debridement, of acute osteomyelitis, *122*

Decalcified sections, *14*

Deciduous teeth
  caries in, *69*
  defects of, *25*
  resorption of, *88*

Decortication, for osteomyelitis, *122*

Deep tongue tie, *50*

Delayed eruption, of teeth, *43, 43f, 44b*

Delphian node, *436*

Delta agent, *457*

Dementia, *499–500, 500b*

Dens evaginatus, *41, 42f*

Dens in dente, *41f*

Dens invaginatus, *41, 41f*

Dental bleeding, prolonged, 399
Dental care, of elderly, 501
Dental caries, 53–70
    actions of fluoride on, 60b
    in adults, 69
    aetiology of, 53, 53f
    arrested, 68–69, 69f
    in deciduous teeth, 69
    development of
        essential requirements for,
            53b
        and Westernisation, 58
    and experimental studies on
        humans, 58–59, 59f
    hidden, 70
    microbiological aspects of, 56b
    microbiology of, 54–57, 55b, 55f
    pathology of
        clinical aspects of, 68–70
        dentine, 65–68, 65f–67f, 67b
        enamel caries, 61–64, 61f, 65b
        relevance of, to progression
            and treatment of, 71t–72t
    prevalence of, 57
    reactions to
        clinical aspects of, 70
        protective, of dentine and pulp
            under, 67–68, 67t, 68f–69f
    remineralisation and, 68–69
    root surface, 70
    and saliva, 60
    sucrose and, 57–59
        epidemiological studies on,
            57–58
    susceptibility of teeth to, 59–60
Dental disturbance, localised, 25f
Dental follicle, normal, in
    odontogenic myxoma, 178
Dental phobia, 496, 496b
Dentigerous cysts, 146–148, 146f–
    147f, 208
    clinical features of, 147, 149b
    definition of, 147b
    differential diagnosis of, 148
    histopathology of, 147–148, 148f
    pathogenesis of, 147, 147f–148f
    radiography of, 147, 147f
    treatment of, 148
Dentinal dysplasia, 32–33, 33f
    type 1, 33, 34f
Dentinal hypersensitivity, 86
Dentine
    caries, 65–68, 65f–66f
        advanced, 66f
        arrested, 69
        development of, key events in,
            67b
        zones of, 66–67, 67f
    decalcified, 66
    defects of, 33–35
    infection of, 65–66, 66f
    protective reactions of, under
        caries, 67–68, 67t, 68f–69f
Dentinogenesis imperfecta, 31–32,
    32f–33f, 206–207
    tooth structure in, 32, 33f
    type I, 30

Dentinogenic ghost cell tumour, 176,
    176f
Dentist, role in oral cancer, 331–332,
    332b, 332t
Dentoalveolar abscess, 79–81, 80f
Denture-induced granuloma, 369–
    370, 369f
Denture-induced stomatitis, 248–249,
    248b, 248f
Dentures, in elderly, 501–502
Depression, 496–497, 496b
    dental aspects of, 496–497, 497b
Dermatitis, contact, 419–420, 420b,
    420f
Desmoplastic ameloblastoma,
    168–169, 169f
Desquamative gingivitis, 262, 262f,
    273
    result of mucous membrane
        pemphigoid, 274f
Development, disorders of tooth,
    45–50, 45b
Diabetes mellitus, 468–469, 469b
    gingivitis and, 97b
Diagnosis
    differential, 8–9
    plan, 20
    principles of, 1–20, 1b
Diagnostic tests, 9
Dialysis, 471, 471b
Diet, for oral cancer, 320–321
Diffuse calcification, pulp, 77
Diffuse mucosal pigmentation,
    383
Diffuse sclerosing osteomyelitis,
    123–124
Dilaceration, 40, 40f
Diltiazem, adverse effects of,
    504t–505t
Disability, 487b–488b, 487t
    in elderly patients, 500b
    learning, 488–491, 489f
    physical, 487–494
Disability Discrimination Act 2005,
    488
Discoid lupus erythematosus, 299t
Dislocation, of temporomandibular
    joint, 232–233, 233f
Disseminated intravascular
    coagulation, 404
Dissolvable tobacco, 319t
DNA ploidy analysis, in dysplastic
    lesions, 311
Dorsal tongue fur, 7t
Down's syndrome, 489–490, 489f–
    490f, 490b
    gingivitis and, 97b
    in prepubertal periodontitis,
        109–110
    syndromic cleft lip and palate
        and, 48
Drug(s)
    adverse effects of, 504t–505t
    causing taste disturbances, 483t
    in diffuse mucosal pigmentation,
        383
    effect on teeth, 37–38

impaired metabolism, 454–455,
    455b
lichenoid reactions, 268, 268b
oral reactions to, 279
side-effects of heart disease, 437t
temporomandibular joint trismus,
    224
used for atopic disease, 419
Drug-associated lymphadenopathy,
    435, 435b
Drug-associated purpura, 401, 402b
Drug-induced gingival hyperplasia,
    437f
Drug-induced melanin pigmentation,
    383f
Dry mouth, 345, 483
Dry (nasal) snuff, 319t
'Dry' socket, 117
Dyskeratoma, warty, 279t
Dyskeratosis congenita, 299t, 306,
    306f, 321
Dyskinesia, tardive, 224
Dyspepsia, 451
Dysplasias, 300
    cemento-osseous, 218
    cleidocranial, 208, 208b,
        208f–209f
    epithelial, 309, 309t
    fibrous, 203f
        monostotic, 216–218, 218b
        polyostotic, 218
    gnathodiaphyseal, 207
    koilocytic, 306
    lichenoid, 305–306
    mild, 309, 309f
    moderate, 309, 310f
    severe, 309–310, 310f
Dysplastic lesions, 307–312
    grading of, 309–311, 309f–311f,
        309t–310t
    other investigations for, 311, 312f
    principles of, 308b
    risk assessment of, 308–312
        biopsy, 308–309
        clinical, 308, 308b
    treatment of, 311–312, 311b
Dysplastic leukoplakia, 299t
Dyspnoea, 512
Dysrhythmias, 438

E

'Early' oral carcinoma, 321–322,
    321f–322f, 322t
Ecological plaque hypothesis, 55
Edentulous patients, pain in, 474–
    475, 474b
Edwards' syndrome, 490–491, 491b
Ehlers-Danlos syndromes, 36, 36f
    pulp calcifications and, 77
    temporomandibular joint
        dislocation, 233, 234t
Eikenella corrodens, 100b
Elderly patients, dentistry and,
    499–502, 499b, 499f
    cardiovascular disease in, 502

Elderly patients, dentistry and *(Continued)*
disability in, *500b*
limitation of mobility in, *501b*
oral disease in, *501–502*
systemic diseases in, *500–501, 500b*
Electric pulp testing, *7–8, 7b, 8t, 11b*
Electrocautery, *12*
Electronic cigarettes, for smokeless tobacco-induced keratoses, *303*
Embryonal rhabdomyosarcomas, *380*
Enamel, *61*
caries
early lesion, *61–63, 62f–64f*
pathology of, *61–64, 61b, 61f*
process of, *65b*
defective, formation of, *25–30*
defects of, *33–35*
demineralised, *63f*
maturation of, and saliva, *60*
mottled, *38, 39b*
organic matrix of, *64f*
raised fluoride levels, effects on, *39t*
zones, *61, 62t*
Enamel pearls, *41–42, 42f*
Endocarditis, infective, *138, 438–439, 438b, 438f*
Endocrine disorders, *463–470*
Endotoxin, *101, 101t*
Enucleation, of cysts, *141, 141b*
Enzymes, *101t*
Eosin *see* Haematoxylin and eosin (H&E)
Eosinophilic granuloma, *255*
solitary or multifocal, *190*
Eosinophilic ulcer, *255, 340t*
Epidermoid cyst *see* Sublingual dermoid cyst
Epidermolysis bullosa, *36–37, 279t*
Epidermolysis bullosa acquisita, *275*
Epilepsy, *484–485, 484b, 485f, 492, 512–513, 512b*
Epinephrine, *438, 509*
Epithelial attachment, *95, 95f, 102, 104f*
Epithelial dysplasia, *309, 309t*
Epithelial-myoepithelial carcinoma, *363, 367t–368t*
Epithelial proliferation, radicular cyst and, *143*
Epstein Barr ulcers, *340t*
Epstein-Barr virus (EBV), *294, 432*
AIDS/HIV and, *413*
in nasopharyngeal carcinoma, *339*
Epstein's pearls, *158*
Epulis, *369–370, 369f–370f*
congenital, *378, 379f*
differential diagnosis of, *372f*
giant-cell, *371–373*
pregnancy, *371*
Erosion, *86, 87f*
Eruption cysts, *148–149, 149f*
Erythema migrans, *283–284, 284f*

Erythema multiforme, *275–277, 275b, 276f*
clinical features of, *276b*
Erythema nodosum, in Behçet's disease, *260f*
Erythematous candidosis, *246, 246b, 246f*
Erythroleukoplakia, *300*
Erythroplakia, *299t, 300*
malignant change in, clinical risk factors for, *308b*
in oral submucous fibrosis, *304, 305f*
Erythroplasia, *300, 300f*
Ewing's sarcoma, *198–199, 198f–199f*
Examination
clinical, *6–8*
extraoral, *6*
medical, *8*
oral, *6–8*
Excisional biopsy, *12*
Exfoliative cytology, *13–14*
Exophthalmos, *464b*
Exostoses, *187, 188f*
Extraction socket, normal healing of, *117, 118f*
Extraoral disease, pain from, *476b*
Extraoral examination, *6*
Exudate, gingival, *96*

F

Face, major infections of, *129–138*
Facial cellulitis, *130–132, 131f–132f, 133b*
Facial clefts, *48–49, 49f*
Facial pain, *486f*
Facial palsy, *480–482, 480b*
Factitious ulceration, *255–256, 256b, 497, 497b*
Fainting, *507–508, 507b–508b*
Familial adenomatous polyposis, *36*
Familial gigantiform cementoma, *182–183*
Familial hypophosphataemia, *37*
Fanconi anaemia, *321*
Fascial space infections, *129–130, 130b, 130t, 131f*
Fear, of dentistry, *496, 496b*
Ferritin, *285*
Fetal alcohol syndrome, *40*
Fibrinolytic drugs, for purpura, *401*
Fibro-osseous lesions, *215–218, 216b*
Fibroepithelial polyp, *369–370, 369b, 369f–370f*
Fibrolipoma, *377*
Fibroma
cemento-ossifying, *193, 193t*
giant cell, *370*
leaf, *370f*
ossifying, *193*
psammomatoid ossifying, *193, 194f*
Fibromatosis, hereditary gingival, *113–114, 114f*

Fibroosseous odontogenic lesions, *179–183*
Fibrosarcomas, *380*
Fibrosis, oral submucous, *224*
Fibrous ankylosis, *227*
Fibrous dysplasia, *203f, 216, 216f–218f, 516t–520t*
monostotic, *216–218, 218b*
polyostotic, *218*
Fine needle aspiration, *516t–520t*
Fine needle aspiration (FNA) biopsy, *13, 13b, 434*
First-bite syndrome, *476*
Fish mouth, *224–225*
Fissure caries, *63*
Fistula, oroantral, *446, 446f*
Fixation, *14, 14b*
Flap operations, for periodontitis, *105–106*
Floor of mouth, carcinoma of, *325–326*
Flora, microbial, *70*
Florid cemento-osseous dysplasia, *182, 182f*
Fluid accumulation, radicular cyst and, *143*
Fluorescent in situ hybridisation (FISH), *17–18*
Fluoride
actions of, on dental caries, *60b*
effects of, *60*
as plaque mineral, *57*
raised, *39t*
Fluoride mottling, *39f*
Fluorosis, *38–40, 38b, 39f–40f*
Focal cemento-osseous dysplasia, *182, 183f*
Focal epithelial hyperplasia, *374f*
Focal sclerosing osteomyelitis, *124, 124b*
Folate
deficiency, *258, 391*
serum, *286*
Foliate papillae, *283*
Folic acid deficiency, *461*
Follicular ameloblastoma, *166–167, 167f*
Fordyce's spots, *7t, 291, 291f–292f*
Foregut cyst, *162*
Fragile X syndrome, *490*
Free gingiva, *95b*
Frictional keratosis, *292, 292f–293f*
Frozen section technique, *13, 13b*
Fructans, *55*
Fructose, *59t*
Fungal sinusitis, *444, 444f–445f*
Furred tongue, *283*
Fusobacterium nucleatum, *100b*

G

Gardner's syndrome, *36, 36f, 192–193, 193f, 454*
Garrè's osteomyelitis, *126b*
Gastric regurgitation, *451, 451f*